Cross-Sectional

ECHOCARDIOGRAPHY

Cross-Sectional
ECHOCARDIOGRAPHY

ARTHUR E. WEYMAN, M.D.
Director, Cardiac Ultrasound Laboratory,
Massachusetts General Hospital
Associate Professor of Medicine,
Harvard Medical School

Lea & Febiger • *Philadelphia* • *1982*

Lea & Febiger
600 Washington Square
Philadelphia, PA 19106 U.S.A.

Library of Congress Cataloging in Publication Data

Weyman, Arthur.
  Cross-sectional echocardiography.

  Bibliography: p.
  Includes index.
  1. Ultrasonic cardiography. I. Title.
[DNLM: 1. Echocardiography. WG 141.5.E2 W549c]
RC683.5.U5W49 1981   616.1′207543   81-8440
ISBN 0-8121-0794-2   AACR2

PRINTED IN THE UNITED STATES OF AMERICA

Print Number   3   2   1

This book is dedicated to the memory of Dr. William J. Grace

Preface

This book is the end product of 7 years of almost full-time commitment to the development of cross-sectional echocardiography. It is the sum of numerous individual and collaborative research efforts, the experience gained in attempting to teach both the technical and interpretive aspects of this imaging modality, extensive discussion and contemplation, and the often painful wisdom that results from paths taken in error and mistakes made. The text itself was begun nearly 3 years ago. It was originally intended as a simple guide to others starting out in cross-sectional echocardiography to facilitate their efforts and to help them to avoid many of the technical and interpretive pitfalls we encountered in the early years of this work. It was decided, at that point, to limit the discussion to cross-sectional echocardiography because there were a number of excellent books available on the M-mode method. Writing such a book did not appear to be a major undertaking because the clinical applications of cross-sectional echocardiography, at that time, were limited, and the scope of the text was, likewise, expected to be narrow. Unfortunately, a series of personal and professional transitions interrupted this undertaking almost at its start and delayed its completion for several years. During the intervening period, there has been enormous growth in both the technical and clinical applications of cross-sectional echocardiography, and as a result, this volume is far larger than originally conceived.

Also during these years, the relative role of cross-sectional and M-mode echocardiography has shifted, and the cross-sectional technique, which was only a small component of the echocardiographic examination when this book was begun, has now become the primary imaging modality. As the role of the cross-sectional method expanded, that of the M-mode component of the echocardiographic examination became more restricted, and at this point, it would be much less of a task to include pertinent M-mode applications. This might seem even more appropriate because many of these applications, although not illustrated, are alluded to. Further, this omission might be taken to indicate that the M-mode examination is no longer considered important. This is clearly not the case. A discussion of M-mode echocardiography is omitted simply because it is almost impossible to change the philosophy of a book in mid-writing and attempting to do so would have delayed this project even further. The book, therefore, remains as it was initially conceived—a text almost exclusively confined to cross-sectional echocardiography. Anytime the term, echocardiography, is used in this context, it refers to the cross-sectional format.

One exception can be found in Chapter 12 in the section on interventricular septal motion. It was impossible in writing this section to describe septal motion using the cross-sectional format alone, and it was necessary, in this one area, to include several M-mode records.

The text is conceptually divided into three sections. The first two chapters deal with the physical principles of ultrasound and its application in cross-sectional imaging. Similar information can be found at the beginning of most textbooks on echocardiography and is included here because of its critical importance in determining the nature and quality of the data that are available for clinical evaluation. These chapters are written at a relatively basic level, which is consistent both with my level of understanding and with the needs of the average clinician.

The second section, which includes Chapters 3 and 4, deals with the general principles of the cross-sectional examination and describes the standard imaging planes. I feel that this is the most important section in the book. Almost anyone can be taught to interpret a high-quality cross-sectional echogram. There are few skilled operators, however, who can consistently record high-quality cross-sectional images in the heterogeneous patient population encountered in the routine laboratory. Obviously, it is impossible to convey or teach a technical skill in a book. This section, therefore, approaches the examination from a conceptual viewpoint and, hopefully, will allow the reader to appreciate, at least in theory, the steps that are necessary to produce consistent images of optimal quality.

When reading Chapter 3, several of our fellows felt that this section was overly long and repetitious. At one time, I considered shortening this chapter; however, after subsequently observing that the recording errors made by these same individuals could have been overcome by closer attention to the principles set forth in this chapter, I decided that possibly even more repetition would be helpful. I strongly feel that if the concepts set forth in this chapter can be firmly grasped and incorporated into the routine examination, the attainment of high-quality cross-sectional images will be far easier than if one were to follow the natural tendency to rely on pattern recognition.

Chapter 4, which describes the standard imaging planes, is a tedious chapter that was difficult to write and I am sure will be difficult to read. It is based on the presumption that, in recording these standard planes, the observer actually looks at only a few points within the image and seeks to optimize the recording of these structures. This can be compared to photographing a ship on the horizon. If the ship is appropriately framed, then the sky and sea will be in their proper proportions. It is hoped that, by focusing on these primary structures, the orientation of the individual planes can be more easily envisioned and the effects of slight changes in angulation or rotation likewise understood. Much time is spent on describing the optimal method for recording these planes. This is again done because of a strong conviction that it is only through rigid standardization that useful quantitation is possible.

The third section of this book deals with the clinical applications of cross-sectional echocardiography. This section is organized and written from the perspective that cross-sectional echocardiography displays "functional anatomy." The individual chapters generally follow the path of blood flow through the left and right sides of the heart. The order in which individual structures are considered in each chapter is further influenced by their relative echocardiographic importance. I have attempted in these chapters to describe both the functional and pathologic anatomy of different structures and lesions in sufficient detail that the examiner can anticipate the principal anatomic variations that may be encountered. This, again, is done in the hope that the greater the level of understanding, the less the reliance on pattern recognition.

The chapters that deal with ventricular structure and function are written at a time when methods for evaluating both the right and left ventricles are in rapid evolution. Because there are no generally accepted approaches to many of these questions, it was necessary to discuss a number of different alternatives and suggest those that, in my opinion, might be the most useful. In some areas, the approaches presented are recognized as less than optimal; however, there is no general agreement on a better method. An example is the segmental evaluation of left ventricular wall motion. The method presented in the text will probably not become the accepted standard. This particular system, however, has been used in a number of clinical studies and forms the basis for most of the correlations contained later in the chapter. It is included, therefore, as an example of how such a system might be employed and because the data derived using the nine-segment format are representative and should be clinically useful. Another example can be found in the truncated-cone method for defining endocardial surface area also contained in the chapter on the left ventricle. Again, it is not my intention that this method be viewed as the appropriate or only method to derive this type of data. The model and formulas are presented only as examples of one approach with the recognition that other figures or other models might, in time, prove more appropriate.

The discussion of the right ventricle is, likewise, highly theoretical. Little echocardiographic data are available concerning methods of deriving right ventricular volume or function. In the absence of this type of information, it seemed useful to review some of the figures and approaches that have been used in other imaging modalities because these have formed the basis for the echocardiographic evaluation of the left ventricle and, it can be assumed,

will likewise be used in approaching right ventricular volume and function.

The approach to congenital heart disease is significantly different from that found elsewhere. Isolated congenital lesions, such as the bicuspid aortic valve or Ebstein's anomaly, are included in the discussion of the aortic or tricuspid valves, respectively. Chapter 13, which presents a diagnostic approach to the patient with congenital heart disease, deals solely with those patients in whom there are multiple congenital anomalies. This chapter takes the approach that the echocardiographer is not presented with a patient with double-outlet right ventricle or tetralogy of Fallot, but rather with an unknown patient with suspected complex, congenital heart disease. It is only during the course of the examination that the various components that lead to an appropriate overall diagnosis become apparent. As a result, this chapter presents an organized and orderly method for assembling the various pieces of the puzzle rather than a description of how the puzzle looks when it is completed. This presumes that the observer can recognize the whole from the sum of its parts. Although unorthodox, this is an approach that I have found helpful in teaching residents and fellows and that, hopefully, will help the reader when faced with an unknown patient with complex, congenital disease.

As with all things, it is only in doing something that one learns how to do it. So it was with this first edition, which was a learning process in many ways. As one learns how to assemble material and organize thoughts, there is a great temptation to go back and rewrite earlier sections. This is particularly true of areas that are rapidly evolving and in which important new information is appearing almost daily. At some point, however, a project such as this must come to an end.

This book, although written primarily by a single author, obviously could not have been accomplished without support and input from a number of other sources. So many people have aided by gathering the data on which this work is based, by proofreading, by commenting, and by just being generally supportive that it is impossible to acknowledge all of these contributions. There are a number of people, however, who have played a particular role in the completion of this endeavor and whose contributions must be acknowledged. First of all, I would like to thank my family, Jean, Jenny, Shannon, and Robert, for their patience and continued encouragement throughout the writing of this book. Much of the time spent in preparing this text was, of necessity, taken away from family activities, and despite this, they were always fully supportive of this effort. Likewise, Mrs. Willie Mae Tate, without whose help neither this family nor this text could have been completed.

I should also like to thank Dr. Charles Fisch, who provided the environment, support, and, most importantly, the time to pursue these endeavors. Dr. Harvey Feigenbaum, in whose laboratory the vast majority of this work was undertaken and without whose enormous knowledge and historical perspective in M-mode echocardiography these efforts could not have been accomplished. Mrs. Sonya Chang, who initially taught me echocardiography, instilled in me a great respect for the technical demands of this technique, and helped me to understand that the technician is at the heart of all quality echocardiographic studies.

Over the course of these 7 years, I have had the good fortune to work with a number of highly skilled technical specialists who performed many of the studies on which this book is based. These persons include Janie Stewart, Jane Marshall, Debbie Green, Kevin McInerney, M.C. Clark, and Licia Mueller. It is because of the personal and professional quality of such people that this is such an enjoyable profession to be a part of.

Many of my colleagues throughout the years have, to a large part, been responsible for the clinical and research efforts on which this text is based. Their names can be found scattered repeatedly throughout the bibliography to the various chapters. There are others, however, who were of particular help in the actual preparation of this manuscript. These persons include Reg Engleton, Frank Fry, Tom Franklin, Ken Johnston, and Paul Goldberg, who provided much of the basic science input for the earlier chapters and aided in the critical review of these sections; Drs. Tom Gibson, Bob Godley, Larry Rink, Dan Doty, John Butterly, Pres. Wiske, and Mary Etta King, who aided in proofreading many of these chapters and provided invaluable editorial critique; and Phil Wilson, who was responsible for much of the art work found in the first four chapters and without whose enormous talent and creativity the preparation of this text would not have been possible. Also, Nancy Kriebel, Cheryl Childress, and Brent Bauer who helped with many of the diagrams and charts found throughout the clinical section. The typing of this manuscript was, likewise, an enormous task, and for this, I thank Linda Williams and Kathleen Cavanaugh. And last, but not least, I must acknowledge the early efforts of my good friend Dr. Dennis Greenbaum, who "first translated Weyman into English."

Boston, Mass.   Arthur E. Weyman

Contents

Section 1

Physical Principles of Ultrasound
and Its Application in
Cross-Sectional Imaging

Chapter 1

Physical Principles of Ultrasound

Sound is a mechanical vibration in a physical medium, such as air or water, that, when it stimulates the auditory apparatus, produces the sensation of hearing.[1] Ultrasound is sound with a frequency higher than the audible range for man or greater than 20,000 cycles per second. The acoustic laws that govern the behavior of low-frequency sound (audible sound) also apply to ultrasound. Ultrasound, however, can capitalize on properties that are not so apparent at lower frequencies (because of the relatively large wavelength to object size relationship). These properties make ultrasound particularly useful in clinical medicine. Most significantly, ultrasound can be beamed in a particular direction and is reflected by relatively small objects (in the millimeter and submillimeter range).[2] The use of pulsed reflected ultrasound to visualize intracardiac structures noninvasively is termed echocardiography.[3]

Historically, echocardiography can be traced to the demonstration by the Curie brothers in 1880 that a suitably cut plate of quartz, when subjected to a mechanical stress, develops electrical charges on its surface (Fig. 1–1).[4] This production of electrical energy or voltage by the application of a mechanical stress to a crystal is known as the piezoelectric or pressure-electric effect.

The following year (1881), the same observers noted the converse of this principle; specifically, when a piezoelectric crystal is appropriately placed in an alternating electric field, it rapidly changes shape or is thrown into vibration in a characteristic fashion (Fig. 1–1). These basic principles of piezoelectricity—the transformation of electrical energy into mechanical energy and the subsequent transformation of mechanical energy into electrical energy—form the basis for all ultrasonic cardiac visualization.

Figure 1–2 illustrates, in simplified form, the application of these principles in clinical echocardiography. Initially, a piezoelectric crystal or transducer is briefly subjected to a rapidly alternating electrical voltage. This alternating pulse shock excites the crystal, thereby causing it to change shape rapidly or to vibrate (Fig. 1–2, A). As the crystal vibrates, it produces alternating areas of rarefaction and con-

3

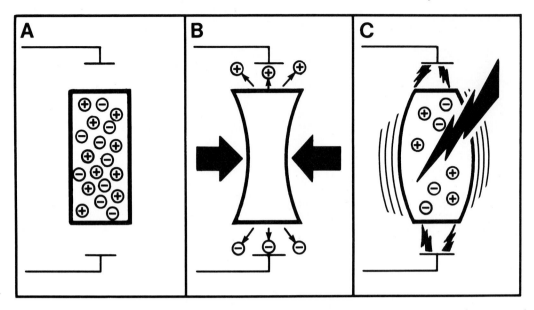

Fig. 1–1.   Diagram illustrates the principles of piezoelectricity. *A,* A quiescent rectangular polar crystal is positioned between two electrodes. *B,* An external stress is applied, thereby deforming the crystal. This mechanical stress causes electrical charges bound within the crystal to shift to the surface, where they can be measured as a voltage. *C,* An electrical current is applied to the crystal. The interaction of this external electrical field with the charges in the ionic lattice of the crystal alters the crystal's shape. When the electric field is rapidly alternated, the crystal is thrown into a correspondingly rapid vibration, which produces a sound wave of like frequency.

densation of the molecules in the surrounding medium, which are, in effect, sound waves.[5] Once produced, these vibrations or sound waves are propagated into the surrounding medium, at a rate proportional to the speed of sound in that particular medium (Fig. 1–2, *B*), until a reflecting interface is encountered (Fig. 1–2, *C*). At this point, a portion of the sound energy is reflected back toward the transducer.[5] When the returning sound energy or echo strikes the now quiescent transducer element, the sound energy produces stresses within the crystal that cause electrical charges to form on its surface (Fig. 1–2, *D*). By measuring the strength of the electrical charge reflected as a voltage, one can determine the amount of stress applied to the crystal and, hence, the amount of returning acoustic energy or echo strength. In addition, if one knows the speed of sound in that particular medium, by measuring the time taken for the sound pulse to travel from the transducer to the structure in question and return, one

can calculate the total distance traveled by the pulse using the simple relationship $d = v \times t$ (distance equals velocity $\times$ time). Because the distance from the transducer to the reflecting interface is only one-half the total distance traversed by the sound wave (which must travel from the transducer to the reflecting target and back), one can divide the distance by two or utilize half the speed of sound in the equation (as is done in most commercial echographs), thereby making possible the direct determination and appropriate display of the distance of the reflector or target from the transducer.[5]

Multiple factors may contribute to the character of the transmitted and returning ultrasonic pulse and, as a result, to the echocardiographic image. These factors include: (1) the properties of sound itself that govern its formation and transmission, (2) the specific characteristics of ultrasound that distinguish it from low-frequency sound and facilitate its use in cardiac diagnosis, (3) the spatial configu-

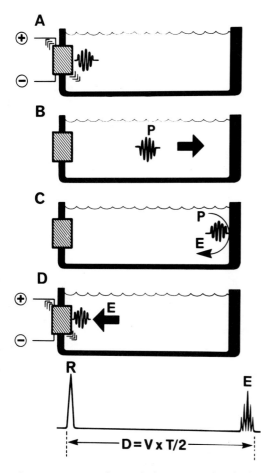

Fig. 1–2. Diagram depicts the basic principles of echo-cardiographic imaging. R = reference spike indicating transducer position; P = transmitted pulse; E = echo; D = distance from transducer to reflector; V = velocity or speed of sound in that particular medium; T = time from pulse transmission to echo return. Because the distance of the target from the transducer is only one half of the total distance that the sound pulse must travel, the equation is divided by two. (See text for details.)

ration of the ultrasonic beam, which defines the area of the heart through which the ultrasonic energy passes and, hence, the area that can be illuminated and visualized, (4) the piezoelectric element or transducer, which determines the character of the generated ultrasonic pulse as well as the shape of the ultrasonic beam, (5) the properties of the medium through which the sound passes and the interfaces or targets encountered that affect the intensity of the sound energy and the am-

plitude of the returning echoes, and finally, (6) the types of echo amplification and display that govern the properties of the final recording. Each of these elements contributes to the final ultrasonic image and, hence, is worthy of consideration.[6]

PROPERTIES OF SOUND

Sound energy travels through a medium in the form of a wave. During the passage of sound, the particles of the medium are thrown into vibrations that are either parallel to the line of propagation (longitudinal waves) or perpendicular to the line of propagation (transverse waves). Although both types of waves occur in solids, only longitudinal waves can be supported in fluids and air. A typical sound wave consists of areas in which the particles of the medium are tightly packed or compressed alternating with areas in which the particles are spaced relatively farther apart (areas of rarefaction). Although the passage of a sound wave throws the particles of a medium into oscillation, no net particle motion occurs.[5] Figure 1–3, A, is an example of a simple sound wave.

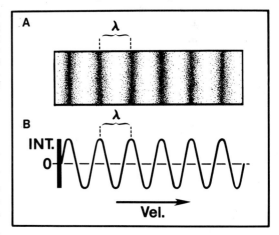

Fig. 1–3. Diagram illustrates the characteristics of a sound wave. A, The alternating compression and dispersion of the particles in any medium that occur during the passage of a sound wave. B, The amplitude and frequency of particle displacement are expressed graphically as a sine wave. INT. = the intensity that is related to the degree of particle displacement. Vel. = velocity of sound in a particular medium. λ = wavelength.

The characteristics of a sound wave can be expressed graphically as a sine wave (Fig. 1–3, B). When depicted in this manner, the height of the sine wave above and below the baseline represents the degree of particle compression and rarefaction, respectively. The degree of particle displacement is a reflection of the sound energy or the intensity of the wave. The distance between two similar areas along the wave path (e.g., two areas of maximum compression) is termed a wavelength (λ). The number of wavelengths per unit time is the frequency of the sound wave. Wavelength and frequency are, therefore, inversely related. Frequency may be expressed either in cycles per second (cps) or in hertz (Hz) (after the German physicist, Heinrich Hertz). 1 cps = 1 hertz; 1000 cps = 1 kilo-hertz (kHz); and 1,000,000 cps = 1 mega-hertz (MHz). The number of wavelengths passing a given point in space per unit time multiplied by the wavelength equals the velocity of sound in that medium.

A consideration of our auditory environment provides further understanding of the chief properties of sound waves that are important in echocardiography (i.e., intensity, frequency, and velocity). All sounds have intensity or loudness. A bell or piano key struck lightly produces a soft or low-intensity sound. The same sound source struck more forcefully produces a higher-intensity or stronger sound. Similarly, in echocardiography, the force or voltage applied to the piezoelectric element determines the amplitude of vibration of the crystal which, in turn, governs the sound pressure and, hence, the intensity of the transmitted pulse.

The intensity of the transmitted pulse is important for two reasons. First, the amount of reflected energy or echo strength produced at any interface is a percentage of the strength of the ultrasonic wave striking that surface. Thus, if all other elements of a system are constant, the intensity of the transmitted pulse determines the strength of the returning echo. Second, high-intensity sound may damage or destroy biologic systems.[7] Although the energy levels utilized in clinical echocardiography have not, to date, been associated with any recognized toxicity, the effect of sound on biologic tissues is an important consideration and is one of the factors limiting the intensities that may be utilized clinically.[7] The biologic effects of ultrasound are discussed in more detail later in this chapter.

Again, a consideration of our environment suggests several important characteristics of sound frequency. First, sounds of different frequencies travel at the same speed in the same medium. If one listens to an orchestra, the sounds produced by the high-frequency instruments arrive at the ear simultaneously with those produced by the low-frequency instruments. If sounds of varying frequencies traveled at different rates, harmony would be impossible. Second, high-frequency sounds have a much lower penetration than do low-frequency sounds. If one stands close to a jet engine, one hears a high-frequency, ear-piercing whine. Conversely, at a distance from the same engine, only a low roar is audible. The high-frequency components in this example are more intense and predominant when one is close to the source of sound, whereas at a greater distance, only the low-frequency components are transmitted. In addition, as is considered later in the discussion of resolution, the higher the frequency of the sound wave, the smaller the structures that reflect it without entering the range in which scattering is apparent. Because small, closely spaced structures are examined in echocardiography, this characteristic of frequency is of paramount importance.

Finally, echocardiographic determination of interface location requires knowledge of the velocity or speed of sound. The velocity of sound in any medium depends on the density and elasticity of that medium.[5] The elastic constants of a medium are temperature dependent, and as a result, velocity varies with temperature.[5] Because the temperature of the body is maintained within well-defined limits, the effects of temperature on velocity are generally disregarded in clinical echocardiography. In some media, velocity partially depends on the frequency of the sound wave, a phenomenon known as velocity dispersion. Velocity dispersion, when it does occur, is usually small and, hence, is likewise disregarded.

In general, as the density of a medium increases, the velocity of sound through the medium also increases. Thus, sound travels faster through such solids as bone than through either liquids or air. The velocity of sound in fluids is generally between 1000 and 1600 meters per second. In human tissue, the mean value for the velocity of sound is 1540 meters per second or 1.54 millimeters per microsecond.[6] For simplicity, 1.5 millimeters per microsecond is used for the speed of sound in the examples throughout this book.

PROPERTIES OF ULTRASOUND

All the properties of low-frequency sound apply also to ultrasound. Ultrasound, however, has specific characteristics that are particularly useful in cardiac diagnosis. Ultrasound can be beamed in a particular direction; obeys the laws of geometric optics regarding reflection, transmission and refraction; and can be reflected by relatively small, closely spaced objects.

The Ultrasonic Beam

The sound energy produced by an ultrasonic generator (transducer) is propagated into an adjacent medium in the form of a beam. In the immediate vicinity of a typical disc-shaped transducer, the beam is cylindric with a diameter comparable to that of the disc. Farther from the transducer, the margins of the beam diverge, and the beam widens into a cone.[8] The well-columnated portion of the beam in close proximity to the transducer is called the near field or Fresnel zone, whereas the diverging conical portion of the beam is referred to as the far field or Fraunhofer zone. The junction of the near and far fields is the transition zone (Fig. 1–4).

The length of the near field can be calculated from the formula $L = r^2/\lambda$, where r is the radius of the sound-generating surface and λ is the wavelength of the transmitted pulse. This formula shows that the length of the near zone increases when either the surface area of the transducer increases or the wavelength decreases. Because wavelength and frequency are inversely related, a decrease in wavelength is the same as an increase in frequency.

In the far zone, the angle of the divergence of the beam (α) can be derived from the formula, $\alpha = 0.61 \lambda/r$. Here again, an increase of either frequency or transducer size decreases the spread of sound energy, thereby producing a narrower, more intense beam. Larger high-frequency transducers, therefore, produce beams with longer near fields and less divergence in the far field, whereas smaller lower-frequency transducers have shorter near fields and greater beam divergence. The beam configurations for a series of transducer elements of various sizes and frequencies are illustrated in Figure 1–5.

The shape of the ultrasonic beam is important because it determines the areas of the heart from which echoes may be recorded, affects the intensity of the ultrasonic energy at any point along the beam path, and governs the lateral resolution of the system. In general, narrower beams are preferable to broad beams because they (1) produce echoes from a more limited area of the heart, thereby reducing ambiguity of echo origin, (2) are more intense and thus generate stronger echoes, and (3) have superior lateral resolution.

In addition to varying transducer size and frequency, one can also change the shape of the beam by focusing. Conven-

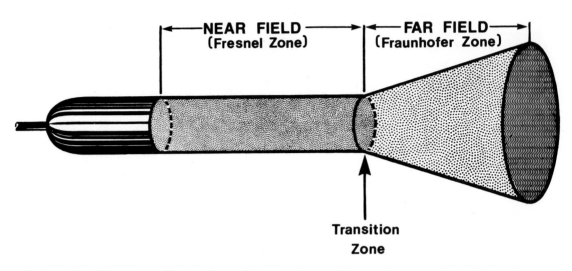

Fig. 1–4. Simplified diagram illustrates the configuration of a sound beam as it progresses from the transducer. The near field is the region closest to the transducer face. The beam is relatively well columnated in this zone. In the transition zone, the beam begins to diverge. The far field is the conical diverging portion of the beam. The sound energy in an actual sound beam is not as uniformly distributed and the beam margins are not as sharply demarcated as indicated in this diagram.

tional focusing is achieved by placing a concave acoustic lens in front of the transducer.[8] By varying the concavity of the lens, one can bring the beam to a narrowed or focal zone at a predetermined distance from the transducer. Decreasing the cross-sectional area of the beam within the focal zone increases its intensity, assuming constant transducer power output. Because the strength of the returning echoes is related to beam intensity, focusing increases the intensity of the echoes from all structures within the focal zone, both absolutely and in relation to targets elsewhere in the beam path. Beyond the focal zone, the beam again diverges. Because focusing decreases the radius (r) of the beam in the focal zone, the angle of divergence in the far field is greater for a focused beam than for an unfocused beam. Because beam divergence begins from a smaller cross-sectional area, however, the overall beam area within the working range of the transducer is generally smaller for a focused than for a nonfocused beam. The effects of focusing on beam pattern are illustrated in Figure 1–6.

Reflection, Refraction, and Transmission

When an ultrasonic beam meets the boundary between two different media, part of the acoustic energy is reflected and part continues into the second medium. When the linear dimensions of the boundary are large with respect to the wavelength, the amount of energy reflected is proportional to the difference in acoustic impedance, or the acoustic mismatch, of the two media.[9] The acoustic impedance of a medium is the product of the density of the medium and the speed of sound in that particular medium. Reflectors that are large relative to the wavelength of the ultrasonic pulse and have a smooth surface (i.e., are mirror-like) are called specular reflectors.

When reflection occurs, the reflected wave is returned in a negative direction through the incident medium at the same velocity with which it approached the boundary. As in optics, the angle of re-

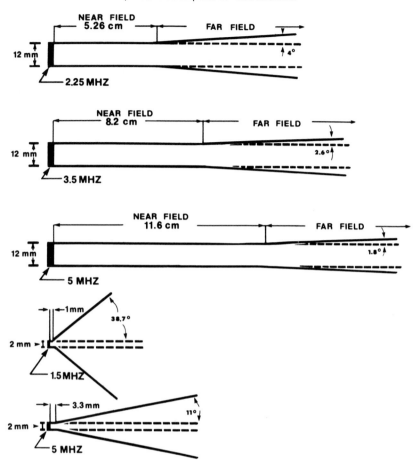

Fig. 1–5. Diagram illustrates the effects of transducer size and frequency on ultrasonic-beam configuration. For transducers of similar size, an increase in frequency results in a longer near field and less beam dispersion in the far field. A decrease in transducer size, however, decreases near-field length and increases beam dispersion, even at higher frequencies.

flection equals the angle of incidence in the same plane (Figure 1–7, A).[5]

The energy returning to the transducer from any reflective interface is related not only to the acoustic mismatch at the interface but also to the angle of the incident beam relative to the plane of the reflector. As indicated in Figure 1–8, when the transducer is perpendicular to the plane of the reflector, a large percentage of the reflected energy returns directly to the transducer. As the angle between the transducer and the reflecting interface increases, however, the amount of reflected energy returning to the transducer rapidly diminishes. The strength of the recorded

echo, therefore, is a function of both the acoustic mismatch at an individual interface and the angle of the transducer relative to the plane of that interface.

The portion of the ultrasonic energy that is transmitted beyond the interface is propagated into the second medium at a speed proportional to the speed of sound in that medium. When sound travels through both media at the same speed, the angle of incidence equals the angle of transmission (see Fig. 1–7). When the speed of sound in the two media differs, the sound wave is refracted. The difference between the angle of incidence and the angle of transmission is proportional

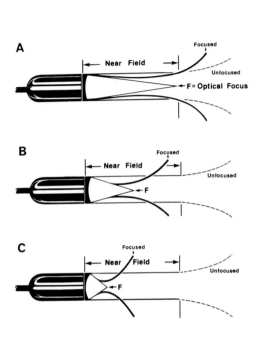

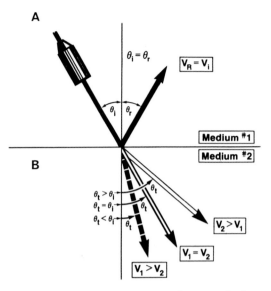

Fig. 1–6. Diagram illustrates the effects of focusing on beam patterns for a series of acoustic lenses with increasing radii of curvature. In each of the three examples, the beam pattern for an unfocused transducer of comparable size and frequency is indicated by the outer interrupted lines. The inner solid lines illustrate the beam pattern produced by the acoustic lens, and the innermost conical area is the focal pattern for a corresponding optical lens. Point F is the optical focus. A, The radius of curvature of the lens is such that the optical focus occurs at the transition zone for the unfocused beam. At this optical focus, the point of maximal acoustic focusing occurs slightly beyond the midpoint of the near field. Beyond the region of the acoustic focus, the beam diverges to a width that corresponds to the width of the unfocused transducer at the transition point. Beyond the transition point, the focused beam diverges more rapidly than the unfocused beam. B and C, As the radius of the curvature of the acoustic lens increases, the optical focus is brought closer to the transducer face, and the acoustic focus more closely approximates the optical focus. The degree of beam narrowing at the acoustic focus increases; however, the beam width at the transition point is greater than that for an unfocused transducer and increases as focusing is increased. As indicated by this figure, focusing always occurs in the near field of the corresponding unfocused transducer, and the acoustic focus always occurs closer to the transducer face than does the optical focus. As the focal point is brought closer to the transducer face, the acoustic focus more closely approximates the optical focus. When focusing is desired at a specific point in space, therefore, one must select a transducer with a sufficiently long near field so that the point of desired focusing lies within this range.

Fig. 1–7. Diagram illustrates the reflective and refractive characteristics of ultrasound. A, When a sound beam strikes an interface between two media of differing acoustical impedance, a portion of the sound energy is reflected into the incident medium. Because the velocity of the reflected wave (V_r) equals the velocity of the incident wave (V_i), the angle of reflection (θ_r) equals angle of incidence (θ_i) in the same plane. B, The portion of the sound energy that continues into the second medium is propagated at an angle relative to the incident beam (θ_t), which is determined by the relative speed of sound in the two media. When the speed of sound in the second medium (V_2) is greater than that in the first (V_1), the sound energy in the left-hand portion of the incident beam begins to accelerate before the sound energy in the right-hand portion of the beam reaches the interface. This situation causes the sound wave to bend to the right and to be propagated at an angle that is greater than the angle of incidence. Conversely, when the speed of sound in the second medium (V_2) is slower than that in the first medium (V_1), the left-hand margin of the beam, which reaches the interface first, begins to decelerate as it enters the second medium. The right-hand margin of the beam continues at its original speed. This situation deflects the beam to the left, and the angle of transmission (θ_t) is less than the angle of incidence (θ_i). When the speed of sound in both media is the same, ($V_1 = V_2$) there is no refraction, and the angle of transmission (θ_t) equals the angle of incidence (θ_i).

to the difference between the sound velocities in the two media. Because the velocity of sound in human tissue is fairly constant, little refraction occurs, and the beam path is considered to remain straight.

In addition to specular reflectors, sound waves may encounter structures that are smaller than the wavelength of the ultra-

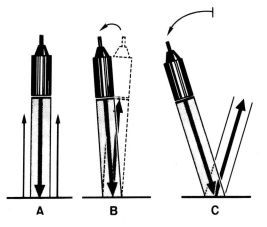

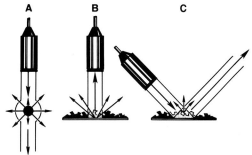

Fig. 1–9. *A,* Interaction of a sound wave with a target that is smaller than the wavelength of the ultrasonic pulse. *B,* Interaction of a sound wave with a rough or irregular but perpendicular surface. *C,* Interaction of a sound wave with a rough surface, which it strikes obliquely. The irregularity of the interface causes a portion of the sound energy to reflect back to the transducer. This reflective pattern can be contrasted to that depicted in Figure 1–8, *C,* where no sound energy was reflected toward the transducer when the beam intersected a smooth surface at a similar angle.

Fig. 1–8. Diagram illustrates the effects of transducer angle on the amount of reflected acoustic energy that returns to the transducer and, hence, is recorded as an echo. *A,* The transducer is perpendicular to the reflective interface. In this situation, the majority of the returning energy is transmitted directly toward the transducer and, hence, can be recorded. *B,* The transducer is at a slight angle to the reflecting interface. In this orientation, only a portion of the reflected energy strikes the transducer face and is recorded. *C,* The transducer lies at a relatively acute angle to the reflective interface and most, if not all, of the reflected energy is directed away from the transducer face. In this case, although the amount of energy reflected into the incident medium may be great, little if any of the reflected energy strikes the transducer face and, hence, is recorded.

sonic pulse as well as structures that are large with rough or uneven surfaces. When the sound waves strike an obstacle that is comparable to or smaller than wavelength, diffraction occurs, and a portion of the sound energy changes direction and bends around the obstacle. The remainder is scattered in all directions (Fig. 1–9, *A*). A sound wave that strikes a relatively large but rough surface produces a specular reflection with an additional scattered field (Fig. 1–9, *B*). The presence of scattering is of clinical importance because, although the amount of energy returned to the transducer from a scatterer is significantly less than that from a specular reflector, scattered energy is propagated in all directions and, hence, is less angle dependent (Fig. 1–9, *C*). The echoes from the normal mitral

valve, although relatively stronger when the transducer is directly perpendicular to the valve, diminish rapidly as the angle between the transducer and the reflecting surface decreases.[10] In contrast, although the peak amplitude of echo production from a deformed thickened mitral valve may be less, the echo strength remains fairly constant through a wide range of incident angles reflecting the omnidirectional nature of the scattered field.

Resolution

When examining the heart, the examiner is attempting to separate and record small, rapidly moving structures that may be only 1 or 2 millimeters apart. The smallest distance between two points at which the points can be distinguished as separate by an imaging system is referred to as the resolution of the system. Echocardiography deals with two types of resolution, axial resolution and lateral resolution. Axial resolution is the ability to differentiate between points lying along the path or axis of the beam, whereas lateral resolution refers to the ability to differentiate points lying side by side relative to the beam path.

Axial Resolution

The axial resolution of an ultrasonic beam is related to its wavelength or frequency and to the duration of the transmitted pulse. To illustrate the effects of wavelength and pulse duration on resolution, let us first calculate the wavelengths of two pulses of ultrasound: one of 300 kHz and a second of 3 MHz. Both of these sound frequencies are within the ultrasonic range; however, the difference in resolving power is significant. The wavelength of an ultrasonic pulse is calculated by using the formula, wavelength equals velocity divided by frequency $(\lambda = \dfrac{V}{F})$.

$$(1) \quad F = 300{,}000 \text{ Hz}$$
$$\lambda = \frac{1.5 \text{ mm/sec or } 1500 \text{ m/sec}}{300{,}000 \text{ cps}}$$
$$\lambda = .005 \text{ m or } 5 \text{ mm}$$

$$(2) \quad F = 3{,}000{,}000 \text{ Hz}$$
$$\lambda = \frac{1.5 \text{ m/sec or } 1500 \text{ m/sec}}{3{,}000{,}000 \text{ cps}}$$
$$\lambda = .0005 \text{ m or } 0.5 \text{ mm}$$

The wavelength of the 300-kHz pulse, therefore, is 5 mm, whereas that of the 3-MHz pulse is 0.5 mm.

Assume that a sound pulse of 4 cycles is transmitted into a test medium (such as that illustrated in Fig. 1–10) in which 2 targets (T_1 and T_2) are located at 10 and 11 cm from the transducer. At the lower frequency (300 kHz), the total length of the sound pulse is 20 mm (λ = 5 mm × 4 cycles = 20 mm). With a pulse train of this length, the echo from the closer of the two targets (T_1) is still striking the transducer when the echo from the second target (T_2) returns. The echocardiograph, therefore, senses and displays one long echo rather than two discrete echoes representing each of the reflecting surfaces. If a third reflector were placed between T_1

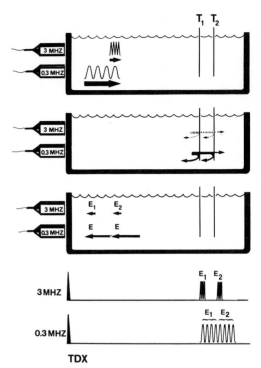

Fig. 1–10. Illustration of the effects of frequency on axial resolution. In the upper panel, 2 pulses of 4 cycles each, one from a 3 MHz transducer and one from a 0.3 MHz transducer, are emitted into a test medium. Because of the higher frequency, the pulse from the 3 MHz transducer is much shorter than the corresponding pulse from the lower-frequency transducer. When these pulses strike two targets, T_1 and T_2, echoes are reflected at both interfaces. Because of the shorter pulse duration at the higher frequency (3 MHz), separate reflections (E_1 and E_2) arise from each target and are recorded as distinct. At the lower frequency (0.3 MHz), the pulse length is such that the echoes from T_1 and T_2 are continuous, and hence, these targets cannot be "resolved" as separate.

and T_2, it would be undetected. In contrast, when a frequency of 3 MHz is utilized, the wavelength is only 0.5 mm. With the same 4-cycle pulse train, the total pulse length is only 2 mm. At this pulse duration, there is a relatively long interval between the return of the echo from the first target and that from the second target. Thus, two separate echoes are displayed by the echocardiograph, and the presence of two distinct reflecting interfaces is "resolved." In addition, at 3 MHz, a third structure placed between T_1 and T_2 could still be resolved. This example, shows that the higher the frequency of the transmitted pulse, the better the resolution along the path or axis of the beam. It also shows that resolution is a function not only of the wavelength or frequency but also of pulse duration. Because the shortest pulse duration is a single half cycle, the wavelength sets the limit of resolution of the system. The determinants of frequency and pulse duration will be discussed in the section on transducers.

Lateral Resolution

Although the ability to differentiate between points along the axis of the beam depends on frequency and pulse duration, the differentiation of points laterally oriented relative to the beam path is a function of beam width. Beam width, as indicated in Figures 1–5 and 1–6, is a function of transducer size, frequency, and focusing.

To understand lateral resolution, one must first realize that the echocardiograph displays all structures within the beam path along a single line representing the axis of the beam. Figure 1–11 illustrates the types of distortion this display characteristic can produce. In A, three pairs of reflectors, separated by 1 centimeter, are placed along the path of an ultrasonic beam. Reflectors A1 and A2 are oriented parallel to the path of the beam, and hence, their degree of separation is appropriately displayed. Reflectors B1 and B2 are separated by the same distance, but lie at an angle to the beam axis. In this example, their true lateral separation is not evident, and hence, only their axial distance is displayed. In the final example, reflectors C1 and C2 are beside each other in the ultrasonic beam. In this example, not only is the true distance between the two reflectors not apparent, but the echoes from each source are superimposed on one another. The presence of two distinct reflecting sources cannot be detected. For this reason, parallel structures must be separated by more than the width of the ultrasonic

beam to be "resolved" as laterally distinct.

Because of its effect on beam width, the overall gain or sensitivity of the system may also affect the apparent lateral resolution. This situation occurs because sound energy is not evenly distributed across the beam and tends to be most intense in the center and to decrease toward the margins. Thus, similar reflectors in the center of the beam produce stronger echoes than do those at the beam margin. When the sensitivity of the system is low, the weaker echoes from the beam margins are not recorded, and the beam appears narrower (Figure 1–11, B). When the gain is high, the echoes at the beam margins are recorded, and the effective beam width appears greater.

Finally, as Figure 1–11, C, illustrates, the limitations encountered in displaying laterally positioned objects also apply to lateral motion. Thus, when the beam is held stationary, only the components of motion oriented parallel to the axis of the beam are appropriately displayed. Because both frequency and beam shape are determined by transducer design, transducer selection sets the theoretic limitations of resolution for any system.

THE TRANSDUCER

Transducers are devices capable of converting one form of energy into another. The piezoelectric materials, which convert electrical energy into sound energy, fall within this larger group of devices known as transducers and are commonly referred to as such. All piezoelectric materials lack a center of symmetry or are anisotropic.[11] The electric charges bound within the ionic lattice of the crystals, therefore, can interact with an applied electrical field, thereby changing the shape of the crystal and producing a mechanical effect. This alteration in the shape of the crystal following the application of an electric charge is known as the direct piezoelectric effect. The amount of deformity

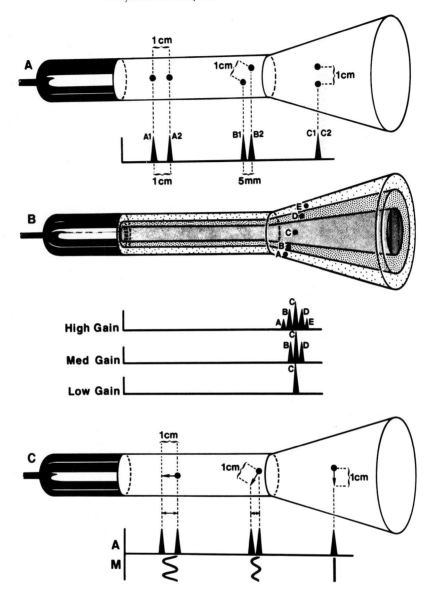

Fig. 1–11. Diagram illustrates the effects of beam width and gain on lateral resolution and the recording of off-axis motion. (See text for further details.)

is directly proportional to the applied voltage within the elastic limits of the crystal. Similarly, the voltage that appears across a piezoelectric material following a mechanical stress (the inverse piezoelectric effect) is directly proportional to the applied stress. A number of naturally occurring crystals, such as quartz, lithium sulfate, and potassium sodium tartrate (Rochelle salts), exhibit this piezoelectric property. At present, however, a group of artificial ceramic materials, known as ferroelectrics (e.g., barium titanate and lead zirconate titanate), which show strong piezoelectric properties, are utilized as the active element in most transducers.

Figure 1–12 is a diagram of a conventional echocardiographic transducer. The complete "transducer" consists of the piezoelectric element, which both generates

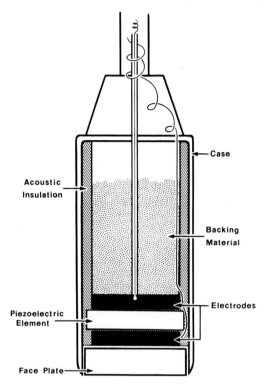

Fig. 1–12. Diagram of a conventional echocardiographic transducer with the principal components labelled. (See text for further details.)

and receives the acoustic impulse; the electrodes, which transmit the current required to shock-excite the crystal and record the voltage produced by the returning echoes; backing material, which helps to control the length of time the transducer vibrates following an electrical excitation; acoustic insulation, which prevents transmission of the ultrasonic energy to the housing of the transducer, thereby causing interference with the returning signal; the transducer case, which provides a means of holding and directing the piezoelectric element; and finally, the face plate, which permits contact of the piezoelectric element with the chest wall and focusing of the transducer when a lens is placed in this position.

As already noted, the most important features of the transducer are its characteristic frequency, the length of time it oscillates after shock-excitation, and its overall size. The characteristic frequency of a transducer is determined by the thickness of the piezoelectric element. This occurs because shock-excitation of a piezoelectric crystal results in the transmission of sound energy from both the front and the back faces of the crystal. Unless the acoustic impedance of the surrounding medium is identical to that of the crystal, a portion of the sound energy is reflected at each interface back into the crystal. The sound energy then traverses the crystal at a speed proportional to the speed of sound in that material. The time taken to reach the opposite face is proportional to the width of the crystal. When the thickness of the element is exactly one-half the wavelength, the reflected and transmitted stresses at each surface reinforce each other, and the transducer resonates with a maximum displacement amplitude. The frequency that corresponds to a half-wavelength thickness is called the fundamental resonant frequency of the transducer. When the element is of wavelength thickness, the stresses at each surface are opposite, and the displacement amplitude is at a minimum. Because the thickness of a half-wavelength transducer at any frequency depends on the propagation velocity of sound in the particular material utilized in making the transducer, the half-wavelength thickness must be calculated specifically for each piezoelectric material. A representative thickness for a standard, commercial, 1-MHz transducer is approximately 2 mm. Because wavelength is inversely related to frequency, the thickness of the piezoelectric element is inversely proportional to the frequency generated.

Because the resolution of an ultrasonic system depends on the total pulse duration (not just on the individual wavelength) and because the shortest pulse duration theoretically achievable is one half cycle, the theoretic limit of resolution can be set at any frequency. Piezoelectric materials used in ultrasonic transducers, however, have a relatively long response to excitation. These ringing responses produce a long ultrasonic pulse, which, if undamped, results in poor range resolution. The placement of a specially composed backing material behind the piezoelectric element shortens this ringing response by decreasing the length of time the crystal "rings," thus shortening the pulse length. In addition, this damping material absorbs sound energy emitted from the back face of the transducer. Such energy would otherwise reflect within the housing of the transducer and would interfere with echoes returning from the examined medium. A high degree of transducer damping decreases pulse duration, but also decreases transducer sensitivity, whereas poorly damped crystals have better sensitivity but degraded range resolution. Figure 1–13 illustrates the effect of varying degrees of damping on pulse configuration.

Finally, transducer size must be considered because it contributes to the shape of the ultrasonic field. In general, large transducers yield better circumscribed beams (longer near fields) and are easier to focus. When the area through which the ultrasonic beam can be directed to deeper structures (the acoustic window) is limited, use of a smaller transducer may be necessary.

ATTENUATION AND ABSORPTION

As a sound wave passes through the body, there is progressive loss of the sound energy or attenuation. In homogeneous tissue, attenuation occurs as a result of both absorption and scatter. Absorption implies that the amplitude of sound is weakened primarily by inner friction or viscosity, which transforms sound energy into other forms of energy (heat).[5] Scattering occurs at the many small interfaces or elastic discontinuities encountered as the beam passes through even the most homogeneous medium.[5] The scattering of the sound energy at each of these interfaces decreases the amount of energy available to penetrate more deeply into the body. Attenuation may also be produced by deviation from a parallel beam. Any increase in beam diameter increases the cross-sectional area over which the sound energy is spread and, hence, decreases intensity per unit area.

In nonhomogeneous media, a portion of the sound energy is reflected at each interface encountered by the beam, thereby further attenuating beam strength. Figure 1–14 illustrates the effects of reflection, scattering, and beam dispersion on the intensity of the sound beam and the resulting display characteristic of sequentially encountered targets. Because higher-frequency sound is reflected by smaller interfaces, the attenuation of the sound beam increases as its frequency increases. The term, "half-value layer," is frequently used to compare the attenuation of sound in different media. The half-value layer is the distance a sound wave travels in a given tissue before its energy is attenuated to half its original value. Some representative half-value layers include plasma—100 cm; whole blood—35 cm; and muscle—3.6 cm. As a rule of thumb, the attenuation of sound in tissue is said to be approximately 1 db/cm/MHz.

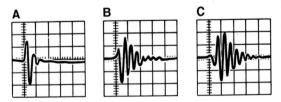

Fig. 1–13. The effects of damping on pulse configuration. *A,* A highly damped transducer with a short "ringing" response, which emits a pulse composed of a small number of cycles. *B,* and *C,* The "ringing" response is increased by decreasing the damping of the transducer, and the pulse duration is correspondingly longer.

CHOICE OF APPROPRIATE TRANSDUCER FREQUENCY

From the foregoing discussion, it should be evident that increasing transducer fre-

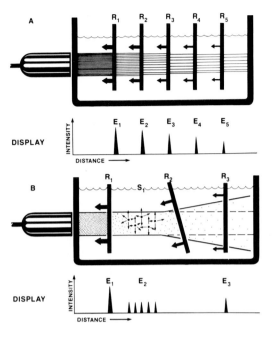

Fig. 1–14. Illustration of the factors contributing to the attenuation of an ultrasonic pulse. *A,* The sound beam is transmitted into a homogeneous medium containing a series of equally spaced reflectors (R1–R5). As the sound beam propagates into the medium, its intensity gradually decreases because of absorption and scattering. In addition, a portion of the sound energy at each interface is reflected toward the transducer as an echo (E). This further attenuates the sound beam, thereby decreasing the energy available to propagate beyond that reflector. When both the medium and reflector spacings are constant, the echo strength on the resultant display gradually and predictably decreases (E1–E5). *B,* A more complex situation that is more comparable to that encountered in cardiac imaging. In this example, the beam is initially transmitted into a relatively homogeneous medium, resulting in some sound energy loss due to absorption and scattering. At reflector R1, a larger amount of energy is directed toward the transducer as an echo (E1). This action weakens the beam. The beam then encounters a series of larger scatterers (S1), each of which further decreases the intensity of the beam. Beyond the scattering field, the beam begins to diverge, which further decreases its intensity. The beam then encounters a reflector at an angle to the transducer face that produces echoes. These echoes are reflected into the incident medium but are propagated at an angle that prevents them from being recorded. The weakened beam then continues in a diverging pattern until reflector R3 is encountered. The reflectivity of target R3 is similar to that of R1; however, the recorded echo (E3) is much less due to the loss in beam intensity that occurred because of the attenuation prior to this point. Because the in vivo system is complex and because many reflectors and scatterers significantly attenuate the ultrasonic beam without being detected, direct correction for this energy loss is virtually impossible.

quency improves axial resolution as well as improving beam characteristics by both elongating the near field and diminishing beam divergence in the far field. Unfortunately, an increase in frequency also increases attenuation, thereby diminishing the ability of the beam to penetrate to deeper cardiac structures. In this trade-off between penetration and resolution, penetration is of primary importance because resolution becomes irrelevant when the echo beam cannot reach the structures of interest. As a general rule, therefore, one seeks to use the highest frequency that can still penetrate to the structures one wishes to examine. In adults, a 2.25-MHz transducer ordinarily provides sufficient penetration to reach the back wall of the heart while still providing satisfactory resolution. In younger children, a 3.5-MHz transducer can frequently be utilized, whereas in infants and neonates, a 5-MHz transducer provides excellent resolution and still has sufficient penetrating power to examine the entire cardiac area in these smaller subjects. In unusual circumstances, lower-frequency transducers in the range of 1 MHz may be required to provide adequate penetration in thick-chested subjects or in older patients with emphysema or pulmonary obstructive changes.

THE ECHOGRAPH

In the preceding section, the factors that determine the source, characteristics, and intensity of the echoes returning to the transducer from within the heart were examined. This section considers the methods of acoustic pulse generation and the different formats by which the returning echoes can be recorded and displayed.

The circuitry necessary to transmit, receive, amplify, and display the acoustic pulse is contained in the basic echograph.[6] Figure 1–15 is a simplified block diagram of such an instrument. The main control component of the echograph is the master clock or oscillator (Fig. 1–15-1). The mas-

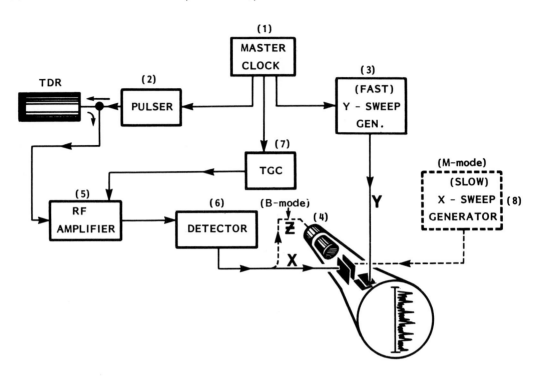

Fig. 1–15. Block diagram of a basic echograph. The primary components are labelled. (See text for further details.)

ter clock is preset to transmit pulses at a designated frequency. Initially, the master clock signals the pulser to discharge stored electrical current into the transducer (TDR) (Fig. 1–15-2). This shock excites the transducer, thus generating the acoustic pulse. Simultaneously, the master clock activates the vertical or Y-sweep generator (Fig. 1–15-3), initiating the fast or downward deflection of the electron beam of the cathode ray tube (CRT) (Fig. 1–15-4). The cathode ray tube consists of an electron gun that produces a focused beam of high-velocity electrons, a set of vertical and horizontal deflection plates that position the electron beam, and a display surface coated with a phosphor that glows where the electrons impinge on its surface. The CRT is ideally suited to display echocardiographic data because the electron beam has a low mass and, hence, can be deflected rapidly. In addition, the position of this beam can be determined accurately by the voltage applied to the deflection plates.

Once activated, the Y-sweep generator rapidly displaces the electron beam vertically at a rate equal to half the speed of sound in tissue. Sweeping the beam at this fixed rate makes possible the conversion of time to distance and, hence, the display of echoes on the CRT at a distance from a reference point that is proportional to the physical distance of the echo-producing structures from the transducer face. Using half the speed of sound corrects for the "round-trip" passage of the acoustic pulse thereby permitting the display of echoes from axially related structures at an appropriate depth and correct spatial relationship to each other.

METHODS OF AMPLIFICATION

As the transmitted pulse passes through tissue, echoes from successively deeper interfaces are received by the transducer. Each packet of ultrasonic energy or echo that strikes the transducer produces a transient vibrational stress within the crystal. This stress is converted by the piezoelectric element to oscillatory electrical signals. The intensity of the electrical energy produced by these echoes is generally weak (in the low microvolt range). Because much higher voltages are needed to drive the display apparatus, some form of amplification is required. In addition, enormous variation (many thousandfold) in intensity may exist between the weakest and strongest echoes. Because of the difficulty in displaying variations in signal strength of this magnitude on a linear scale, some form of nonlinear amplification or dynamic compression must also be introduced during the amplification process.

In its raw state, the oscillatory electrical signal is called an RF or radio frequency signal. This RF signal is initially received and amplified by the RF amplifier (Fig. 1–15-5). The basic RF signal contains both amplitude and phase information. The amplified RF signals may be further processed to improve the resolving characteristics of the echo system. Commonly, the RF signal is first transformed to a video signal by displaying only the envelope of its positive components (Fig. 1–16). This signal processing occurs in the second component of the amplifier train, the detector (Fig. 1–15-6).

In the video format, the signal reflects both the amplitude and the duration of the pulse train. Because the entire pulse train is displayed, a relatively long signal is produced. This prolonged signal makes differentiation of closely spaced structures difficult. In addition, because the leading edge of the pulse most appropriately reflects the position of the echo-producing interface, it is desirable to shorten the duration of the displayed echo while emphasizing the leading edge of the signal. This combination of features can be achieved by differentiating the signal and displaying only its positive components (see Fig. 1–16). Differentiation has the added advantage of making the width of

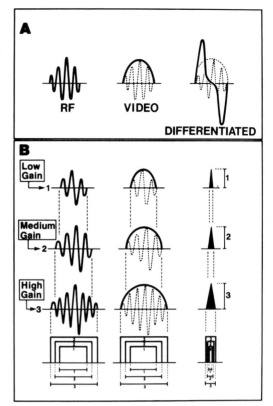

Fig. 1–16. *A,* Diagram illustrates the effects of amplification on the radio frequency (RF), video, and differentiated signal. The RF signal is the oscillatory electrical output of the transducer. In the video format only, the envelope of the positive components of this signal is displayed. Differentiating the signal accentuates the leading edge and effectively shortens the signal duration. *B,* The effects of increasing gain on these signals. When the gain is increased, both the amplitude and duration of the RF signal are increased because the lower intensity components of the RF signal are displayed at higher gains. This characteristic is also true of the video signal. With a differentiated signal, in contrast, signal width increases minimally with increasing amplitude.

the echo less gain sensitive. In the RF or video format, an increase in system gain causes amplification of all signals. As a result, more of the lower-intensity echoes at the onset and the termination of the pulse are displayed. Both signal amplitude and duration increase as gain increases. The differentiated signal also increases in amplitude with increasing gain; however, as illustrated in Figure 1–16, *B,* the duration or width of the displayed echoes does not change significantly. This characteristic is important because if one is attempting to measure the distance between two echoes that are constantly changing in width as gain is varied, the measurements will also vary and, hence, will be unreliable. With a differentiated signal, the echo intensity may be increased without significantly changing the distance between echoes, thereby making measurements more reproducible.

Another component of the amplifier chain is the time-gain compensation (TGC) or gain as a function of depth (Fig. 1–15-7). The TGC compensates for the relative decrease in the amplitude of echoes from more distant structures. This decrease occurs as a result of the attenuation of the sound beam as it progresses deeper into the body. When this attenuation is constant, it can be corrected for directly. Because, clinically, attenuation varies from patient to patient, this correction must be individualized, and hence, the depth-dependent increase in gain must be adjustable. Amplification circuitry in the TGC selectively increases the strength of far-field echoes to achieve this adjustability. In addition, it permits individual control of the rate at which this amplification is brought into play. In this manner, one can compensate for some of the normal depth-related decrease in echo intensity, and the relative intensities of both near- and far-field echoes can be displayed more appropriately (Fig. 1–17). After passing through the amplifier train, the amplified processed echo is transmitted to the CRT for final display.

DISPLAY FORMATS

There are two basic formats for displaying echocardiographic data: the A-mode and the B-mode. In each of these formats, individual echoes are displayed along a line that represents the beam axis. The difference between the two formats lies in the method of depicting echo amplitude.[6] In both the A- and the B-mode, the horizontal deflection plates of the CRT are attached to the fast or Y-sweep generator. When signalled by the time-base circuit (the master clock or oscillator), the Y-sweep generator sweeps the electron beam vertically at a rate corresponding to the speed of penetration into the heart of the interrogating sound beam. In the A-mode system, amplification circuitry is connected to the vertical deflection plates of the CRT, thereby producing horizontal deflections of the vertically sweeping electron beam each time a change in voltage is recorded (see Fig. 1–15, solid lines).

The amplitude of these horizontal deflections is proportional to the voltage transmitted to the CRT from the amplifier chain and, hence, reflects the relative strength of the recorded echoes. The A-mode format, therefore, displays individual echoes as spikes along a vertical line that represents the beam axis. The distance of these echoes from the start of the sweep is proportional to the distance of the echo-producing structure from the transducer. The amplitude of these spikes is proportional to the strength of the returning echo (Fig. 1–18, A). When moving structures are recorded, these spikes also move along the vertical axis in a pattern corresponding to the motion pattern of the structure from which they are reflected. The A-mode technique makes possible the detection of highly reflective structures that produce dominant spikes and of structures with characteristic motion patterns, such as the mitral valve or aortic root. Unfortunately, less highly reflective structures or those spaced closely together with similar motion patterns are difficult to differentiate and thus restrict the diagnostic value of A-mode echocardiography. Because of these inherent limitations, the A-mode method is not currently used as a primary clinical display format.

The second major display format, the B-mode or brightness-modulated mode, differs from the A-mode in that the amplified echoes are transmitted to the electron gun

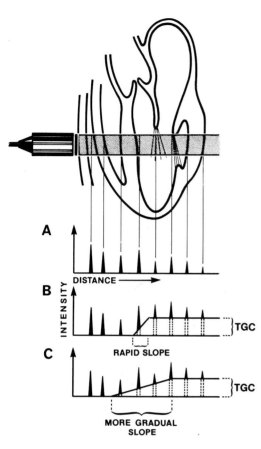

A

DISTANCE →

B

INTENSITY

}TGC

RAPID SLOPE

C

}TGC

MORE GRADUAL
SLOPE

Fig. 1–17. Illustration of the effect of the time-dependent gain (TGC) on the echoes from more distant structures. *A*, The normal loss in echo strength due to the decreasing intensity of the beam as it propagates through the heart. *B*, The effect of the TGC in boosting the intensity of far-field signals. Intensity is selectively increased to display far-field signals at an appropriate height relative to the near-field echoes. *C*, The position of this gain function and its rate of employment can be individualized to suit the needs of the operator.

of the CRT as the Z-axis input rather than to the vertical deflection plates (see Fig. 1–15, interrupted line). Variations in the voltage from the amplifier train through the Z-axis input intermittently intensify the electron beam during its vertical sweep, producing points of increased brightness. The distance of these points along the vertical axis represents the depth of sequentially encountered, echo-producing structures, whereas the brightness of the points indicates the intensity of these reflectors (Fig. 1–18, *B*). In this basic for-

mat, the B-mode line contains little useful information. Conversion to the B-mode format, however, frees the vertical deflection plates, which can then be used to vary the pattern in which the B-mode lines are assembled and displayed. The individual B-mode lines form the basic building blocks for all subsequent echocardiographic imaging formats. The manner of display is varied to achieve particular clinical goals.

The first modification of the B-mode format, the M-mode or time-motion display,[12] utilizes a slow-sweep or X-axis generator to sweep sequential B-mode lines across the face of a CRT (see Fig. 1–15, interrupted line). With an appropriate amount of persistence in the phosphor of the CRT, the B-mode lines leave a trail of echoes as they move. Sweeping the lines at a fixed rate permits the recording of the position and motion pattern of the echoes from intercardiac structures relative to time (see Fig. 1–18). The high resolution, rapid sampling rate, and convenient graphic format of M-mode echocardiography are ideal for imaging localized areas of the heart and analyzing time-related events. As a result, M-mode echocardiography, until recently, was the primary clinical method for displaying echocardiographic data.

Unfortunately, the M-mode format provides only axial information concerning structure, motion, and depth. It is therefore limited because it fails to convey any appreciation of the true lateral distances between structures or to accurately reflect off-axis motion. Initial attempts to provide more spatial information led to the development of M-mode scanning (Fig. 1–19). An M-mode scan is obtained by manually sweeping the transducer from one area of the heart to another while continuously recording the resultant echocardiographic data on a strip-chart recorder.[13] This technical development provided some qualitative information concerning lateral structure relationships. Unfortunately, these scans vary with the speed and path

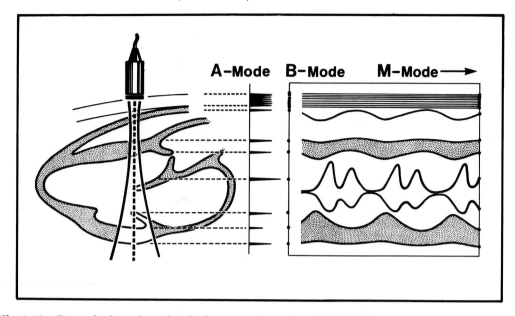

Fig. 1–18. Types of echocardiographic displays currently used. To the left of the figure, an ultrasonic beam is directed through the heart at the level of the mitral valve. In the A-mode format, the distance of the echo-producing interfaces from the transducer is depicted by a series of spikes along the vertical axis of the display. The strength of the echoes from each interface is indicated by the length of the horizontal spikes. In the B-mode format, distance is again depicted along the vertical axis by a series of dots. The intensity or brightness of the dots corresponds to the strength of the reflected echoes. In the M-mode format, the B-mode line sweeps across the face of a cathode-ray tube. Because of the persistence of the phosphor of the tube, the B-mode dots leave a trail as they move. This trail depicts the motion of intracardiac structures relative to time.

of transducer movement, and because each of these variables changes from sweep to sweep and from examination to examination, the reproducibility of these data is limited.

The desire to add quantitative spatial information to the echocardiographic examination led to the development of the second modification of the B-mode format which, in the clinical context, is termed two-dimensional or cross-sectional echocardiography. Cross-sectional echocardiography is an imaging format in which the ultrasonic reflections from a predetermined cross-sectional or tomographic plane through the heart are recorded and displayed. To assemble a cross-sectional image, one moves the sound beam from one area of the heart to another through a fixed plane while continuously transmitting sound pulses and recording the resulting echoes. To display the acquired data in a coherent fashion, one continu-

ously senses and transmits to the CRT the transducer position so that the resultant B-mode lines can be displayed in a position that corresponds to the spatial position of the ultrasonic beam at the time the data are recorded. Figure 1–20 illustrates how these B-mode lines can be assembled into a cross-sectional image of a fixed area of the heart.

The simplest example of this type of cross-sectional imaging is a static manual B-mode scanning system. Figure 1–21 is a block diagram of such a system. In this format, methods of pulse generation and echo amplification are similar to those previously described for the basic echograph. The chief differences in the scanning format are (1) the transducer is attached to an articulated arm, which limits the transducer's motion to a single plane, and (2) position sensing devices in the arm continuously relay the transducer coordinates via the summing circuitry to the

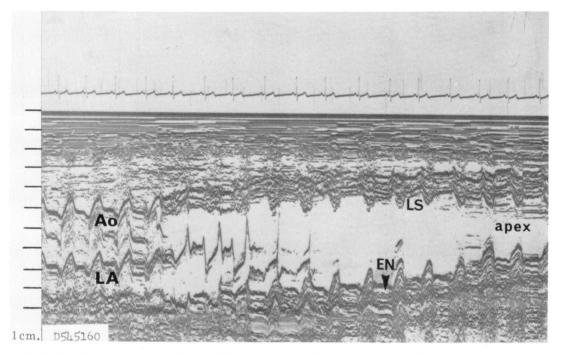

Fig. 1–19. Representative M-mode scan. This scan is obtained by sweeping the transducer from the aorta (AO) and left atrium (LA) on the left through the left ventricle to the cardiac apex to the right. The overall configuration of the left ventricle, as well as the motion patterns of specific areas, can be appreciated. The distance from the aortic root to the apex, however, is a function of the speed with which the transducer is angled and does not represent a true anatomic distance.

vertical and horizontal deflection plates of the CRT; the CRT then positions the path of the fast or Y-sweep on the oscilloscope to conform to the relative position of the ultrasonic beam in space. Because each B-mode line is recorded and can be stored in its appropriate spatial position, one can gradually assemble an image that depicts a two-dimensional or tomographic plane of the heart by manually moving the transducer across the precordium while continuously sampling.

Because cardiac structures are in constant motion, if data are randomly recorded at a slow rate during unselected portions of the cardiac cycle, the interfaces from which the data arise constantly vary in position, resulting in a blurred image. To overcome the effects of cardiac motion, slow manual or mechanical scanners are commonly modified, using a gating circuit triggered by the R wave of the electrocar-

diogram. The gating circuit allows the recording oscilloscope to accept pulses only during specific portions of the cardiac cycle and, thus, effectively stops cardiac motion. Delay and duration controls within the gating circuitry vary the elapsed time between the R wave and the onset-duration of the unblanking signal of the gate. Echoes received when the unblanking signal is active are recorded, whereas those received during the remainder of the cardiac cycle are eliminated. Multiple independent gates can be incorporated to permit the assembly of multiple images from varying points in the cardiac cycle.

During actual performance of a manual cross-sectional study, the transducer is slowly moved along the chest wall by the operator. With each cardiac cycle, a line representing the path of the sound beam during that cycle is written on a storage oscilloscope. Between the writing of in-

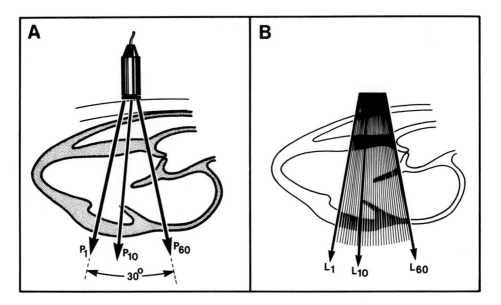

Fig. 1–20. Diagram of the method of pulse transmission and image recording and display in the cross-sectional format. *A,* Pulses are continuously transmitted as the transducer is moved in a fixed plane through a 30-degree arc from the papillary muscles to the left atrium. *B,* B-mode lines, which correspond to each of these pulses, are recorded and are assembled and displayed in a pattern that corresponds to the pattern of pulse transmission. The first data line (L₁), therefore, corresponds to the position of the first pulse (P₁), the tenth data line (L₁₀) to the tenth pulse (P₁₀), and so on.

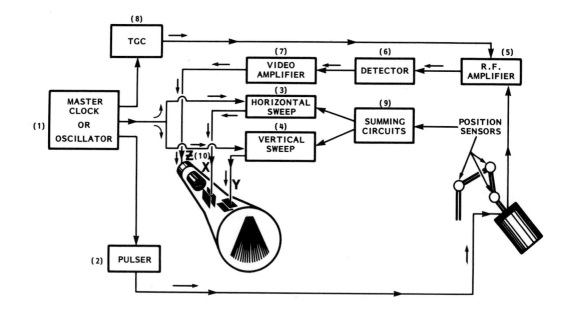

Fig. 1–21.   Block diagram of a simple B-mode scanning system.

dividual lines, the direction of the sound beam is adjusted slightly to record additional anatomic information, and in this fashion, an image is gradually accumulated. Figure 1–22 is an example of such a scan. In this figure, the path of the transducer motion is parallel to the long axis of the left ventricle in a plane extending from the left ventricular apex to the aortic root. This type of image displays the spatial geometry of the heart, the interrelationship of various structures, and the lateral as well as axial distance between areas of interest.

If the B-mode scanning system is further modified to permit more rapid electronic or mechanical beam scanning, images can be accumulated at a sufficiently high rate

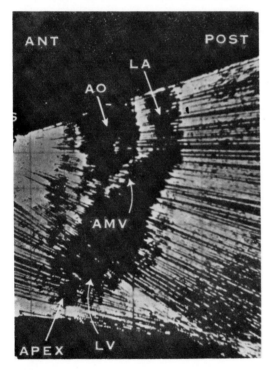

Fig. 1–22. Cross-sectional scan of the heart. This scan is assembled by recording sequential gated B-mode lines. These lines are displayed in a spatially oriented fashion to gradually build a two-dimensional image of the heart at a selected point in the cardiac cycle. LA = left atrium; AO = aorta; AMV = anterior mitral valve; LV = left ventricle. (From King, DL: Cardiac ultrasonography: cross-sectional ultrasonic imaging of the heart. Circulation, 47:843, 1972. Reproduced by permission of the American Heart Association.)

to display dynamic cardiac motion in "real time." These "real-time" or dynamic B-mode instruments are discussed in detail in Chapter 2. The data derived from them form the basis for the clinical section of this book.

SYSTEM CONTROLS

The types of signal processing and variations in display that occur in an echograph are characteristic of the individual instrument and are not under operator control. Certain features of the display, however, can be controlled by the operator; these variable controls will be discussed in the next section.

All echocardiographs provide certain operator controls that, regardless of the kind of display, permit (1) the absolute amplitude of all echoes within the field of examination to be varied, (2) the selective amplification of echoes within specific portions of the field, or (3) echoes of only specified amplitudes to be included in the final display. The primary system controls that perform these functions and are common to most echocardiographic instruments include the system gain or coarse gain, the time-gain compensation (TGC) or gain as a function of time or depth, the near-field gain, the damping circuit, and the reject circuit.

System Gain or Coarse Gain

The system gain uniformly increases the amplitude of all echoes within the display. Depending on the degree of differentiation of the displayed signal, an increase in the overall gain may increase not only the amplitude of the displayed echo, but also its duration or width. In addition, as previously noted, an increase in the overall gain permits display of weaker echoes and effectively increases beam width. Higher coarse gain settings, therefore, increase the ability to display weak or less distinct echoes; however, this ability always occurs at the expense of lateral resolution and, depending on display configuration, may also decrease axial resolution.

Time-Gain Compensation (TGC) or Gain as a Function of Depth

The TGC is an amplifier circuit that compensates for the natural loss in echo intensity or strength that occurs as the beam penetrates more deeply into the chest. To achieve these ends, the TGC consists of an amplification circuit, which selectively increases the strength of far-field echoes, as well as a ramp function, which permits individual control of the level and of the rate at which this depth-dependent amplification is brought into play. By varying the slope of this ramp, one can rapidly employ full amplification at a particular level or can gradually increase amplification as a function of time or depth (Fig. 1–17). In both M-mode and cross-sectional echocardiography, delineation of the interventricular septum is a difficult problem. Conventional practice, therefore, places the leading edge of the ramp at the right-ventricular border of the septum, thereby abruptly boosting the level of all echoes in the septal region and onward to the posterior wall of the heart. This placement separates the septum from the less intensely amplified right ventricular cavity and highlights this region of the heart.[14]

Near-Field Gain

Because the strength of the echocardiographic beam is greatest in the near field, the echoes from structures most closely opposed to the transducer are the strongest and, if kept in their raw form, tend to dominate the display. To permit more detailed analysis of structure, configuration, and motion in the near field, one must frequently decrease the strength of the near-field echoes to a greater degree than that of those returning from more distal structures. This situation is, in effect, the reverse of the TGC function. For this reason, a selective near-field gain control is conventionally supplied to control the amplitude of these strong near-field echoes. This control determines the amplitude of all echoes in the portion of the display from the transducer to the ramp of the TGC. This near-field gain control, therefore, affects a variable portion of the display, depending on the position of the ramp, and must be distinguished from the near field of the ultrasonic beam, which depends on transducer properties and not on gain.

Damping Circuit

The damping circuit controls both the amplitude and the time constant of the transmitted pulse. This effectively decreases the power output of the transducer and shortens the pulse duration. The damping circuit decreases effective beam width and improves resolution. It does so, however, at the expense of signal strength. Although the coarse gain and the damping controls affect different portions of the signal, their net effects on the overall image are similar.

Reject Circuit

The echoes returning from within the heart vary widely in amplitude. Numerically, the low-intensity signals from weak or off-axis reflectors and from scattering sources exceed the higher amplitude echoes from the more prominent structures of primary interest. When displayed in an unaltered state, these weak echoes dominate the display and obscure the higher amplitude signals. A reject circuit is incorporated into most echographs to eliminate the weak echoes. This circuit filters out all signals below a fixed amplitude, thereby removing weaker echoes and background noise from the final display and permitting the higher amplitude signals to be displayed in greater contrast.

BIOLOGIC EFFECTS OF ULTRASOUND

Ultrasound at relatively low intensities has been used for many years without reported ill effect as a noninvasive imaging tool in clinical medicine. One must recognize, however, that sound waves that contain sufficient mechanical energy to damage or to destroy biologic tissue can be produced.[15,16] The original Langevin underwater detection apparatus could generate intensities in the sound field sufficient to kill small fish or to induce severe pain in the human hand.[17] Subsequent reports have noted a variety of functional and structural changes in a wide range of biologic systems, including human beings, following ultrasonic radiation. These effects appear primarily related to the local heating properties of ultrasound, mechanical stresses induced during passage of the sound wave, and cavitation. Because the goal of any medical diagnostic technique is to obtain as much information as possible concerning the state of the human organism without adversely affecting that organism, the properties of ultrasound that determine its safe application must be understood.

The biologic effects of ultrasound depend on the total energy flux across a particular area, the spatial distribution of energy within the sound beam, the time duration and pattern over which a biologic system is exposed to the sound energy, the frequencies contained within the sound wave, and the sensitivity of the exposed tissue system. In addition to the ultrasonic field parameters to which the tissue is exposed, the quantity of ultrasonic energy absorbed by the tissue elements as a consequence of this exposure (the "dose") is also an important consideration.

The amount of acoustic energy per unit time produced by a sound-emitting device determines its ability to do work or to create a biologic effect. This amount is termed the acoustic power of that device. Such power is measured in watts; 1 watt equals 1 joule per second. A joule is equal to 0.239 calories (the calorie is the amount of heat energy required to raise the temperature of 1 g of water by 1° C). When actually transmitted into a tissue system, the acoustic power is concentrated within the margins of the sound beam. The concentration of power within a specific area is the *intensity*. Intensity is commonly expressed as either watts per meter squared or milliwatts per centimeter squared. Measurement of the intensity of a sound beam is not simple because the intensity at any given time is not constant throughout the beam. Because the intensity can vary, depending on the point within the sound beam at which it is measured, intensity is often referred to in terms of (1) the average intensity over the cross-sectional area of the sound beam or relative to some other representative area, (2) the peak intensity within the sound beam, or (3) the recorded intensity at a particular point in space. The average intensity of the sound beam, or the so-called spatial average (SA), can be calculated by dividing the total power output of the device by a representative area, such as the area of the transducer face. Thus, for an ultrasonic device that employs a disc-shaped transducer that has a radiating area of 2 cm² and emits a power of 2 milliwatts, the spatial average intensity would be 1 milliwatt per cm².

Although relatively easy to determine, the spatial average intensity has the disadvantage of depending somewhat arbitrarily on the area selected to calculate this average and generally does not reflect the actual energy levels to which local tissue areas within the sound beam are exposed. For many purposes, therefore, intensity levels are referred to in terms of the peak intensity encountered by any tissue area within the path of the sound beam. When examining a typical sound beam, the highest intensity, the *spatial peak intensity*, generally occurs a few centimeters in front of the transducer face and on its axis. For a nonfocused transducer, the spatial peak intensity typically exceeds the spatial average value by a factor of 2 to 3. If the transducer is focused, the factor may be larger.

In addition to the total amount of acoustic energy produced by a sound-emitting device and the spatial distribution of that energy as it passes through a tissue system, the biologic effects on that system also depend on the time of exposure. The exposure time depends on whether the sound-emitting device transmits a continuous or an intermittent sound wave. A sound-emitting device that produces a constant sound wave is said to operate in a continuous or CW (constant wave) mode, whereas a device that transmits a series of identical pulses, each consisting of only a few cycles, is said to operate in a *pulsed mode*. Most imaging systems operate in a pulsed mode; therefore, the tissue system imaged is subjected to sound energy intermittently. In a pulsed system, the exposure time is a function of both the length of each pulse, or the *pulse duration*, and the number of pulses transmitted per unit time, the *pulse repetition frequency*. The time between the onset or other corresponding points of successive pulses is the *pulse repetition period*. The pulse repetition period, therefore, equals the reciprocal of a pulse repetition frequency. Thus, if pulses are transmitted at a frequency of 1000 per second, the pulse repetition period is 1/1000 of a second or 1 millisecond. The fraction of the total time the instrument is operating (the time the sound is actually "on") is termed the *duty factor* and is expressed by the ratio of the pulse duration to the pulse repetition period. Therefore, if the pulse duration is 1 microsecond and the pulse repetition period is 1000 microseconds or 1 millisecond, the duty factor is 1/1000 or 0.001 (0.10%). Duty factors for diagnostic ultrasonic instruments are typically in the range of 0.0005 to 0.002.

The power output of an ultrasonic device operating in the pulsed mode is the same when the device is "on" as that of a CW device operating at the same frequency. Likewise, the spatial distribution of intensities is similar. Because tissue is subjected to these energy levels only intermittently in the pulsed mode, such energy levels can be described either in terms of the intensities to which tissue is subjected when the instrument is "on," the *temporal peak intensity*, or in terms of the average intensity received by the tissue over the entire time period the instrument is in operation, the *temporal average intensity*. The temporal average is then the power transmitted during the time the instrument is "on" averaged over the entire pulse repetition period. Because intensity in the pulse mode varies relative to both space and time, intensity can be expressed in four ways:

1. The *spatial average, temporal average* (SATA). This value is obtained by measuring the average power output of the device over time and dividing it by an appropriate area, usually that of the transducer face. This measurement of intensity is the most quickly determined and most frequently quoted by manufacturers. It also yields the lowest values of the four commonly utilized measures of intensity.

2. The *spatial average, temporal peak* (SATP). The spatial average, temporal peak intensity gives the average intensity over an appropriate area, such as the transducer face, that occurs when the ultrasonic emitting device is "on." This value is obtained by dividing the SATA value by the duty factor.

3. The *spatial peak, temporal average* (SPTA). This intensity measurement represents the intensity occurring at the spatial peak or the point of maximum intensity within the sound beam averaged over time. It is calculated by multiplying the SATA value by the ratio of the spatial peak to the spatial average, or the SP/SA factor.

4. The *spatial peak, temporal peak* (SPTP) is the intensity at the spatial peak during the time the ultrasonic emitting device is "on." It is the highest of the four intensities. This intensity is calculated by

dividing the SATA value by the duty factor and then multiplying by the SP/SA factor.

The spatial peak, temporal average is apparently the most meaningful of these measurements because it describes the peak energy level to which any of the tissue areas lying within the sound beam are exposed (averaged over the total time of exposure). The total time of exposure reflects not only the actual exposure time, but also the period available for potential recovery between pulses. In general terms, SPTA intensity levels in the low milliwatt per cm^2 range are employed in medical imaging, whereas higher intensities in the low watts per cm^2 range are used in therapeutic techniques, which rely on tissue heating and intensities of greater than 10 watts per cm^2 in lesioning devices. The frequency of a sound wave also influences its biologic effects. Higher frequency tends to favor heat production due to the increased absorption of sound energy at increasing frequencies, whereas lower frequency (in the low kHz range) favors cavitation.

Relating these ultrasonic field parameters to patient safety, the committee on bioeffects of the American Institute of Ultrasound in Medicine has stated that, as of October 1978, no independently confirmed significant biologic effects had been observed in mammalian tissues exposed to intensities (SPTA as measured in a free field of water) below 100 milliwatts per cm^2. Furthermore, such effects had not been demonstrated for ultrasonic exposure times (total time, which includes "off" time as well as "on" time for repeated pulse regimen) of less then 500 seconds and more than 1 second, even at higher intensities, when product of intensity and exposure time is less than 50 joules per cm^2.[18]

Despite this optimistic clinical experience, large gaps exist in the knowledge base concerning the effects of ultrasound in human beings. A threshold level below which sound can be used for an unlimited period without any ill effect has not been defined. Likewise, the cumulative effects of multiple, repeated ultrasonic pulses are poorly characterized. One must also remember that effects that occur on a gross scale are easily identified and, hence, appreciated. More subtle effects, which are not readily evident, may be retained within the system and may accumulate or be passed to subsequent generations. Thus, despite the apparent safety of the low-intensity sound levels used in diagnostic imaging, these instruments should be employed judiciously and with sufficient medical justification.

In cross-sectional cardiac imaging, the actual exposure at any point within the heart is further affected by the variation in the pattern in which pulses are transmitted and by the attenuating properties of the tissues through which the sound energies must pass to reach the heart. In the cross-sectional format, pulses are directed in a variable scan pattern. Consequently, a particular tissue area may actually receive sound energy from only a small fraction of the total number of transmitted pulses. Likewise, in the sector format, the amount of energy concentrated near the apex of the sector (where pulses tend to overlap) is greater than that encountered in the far field (where the individual waves are more widely separated). In addition, the sound energy emitted by the transducer face is attenuated as it passes through the superficial skin and muscle layers that overlie the heart. As a result, the sound intensity levels experienced by specific areas within the heart vary not only with the temporal and spatial field characteristics of the sound beam, but also with the frequency at which a particular region is interrogated by the sound energy and with the characteristics of the tissue layers lying between the transducer and that area. Actual cardiac exposure, therefore, may represent a small fraction of the total energy level produced by the ultrasonic instrument.

REFERENCES

1. Lord Rayleigh: Theory of Sound. New York, Dover Publications, 1945.
2. Rschevkin, SN: The Theory of Sound. Translated by OM Blunn, and PE Doak. New York, Pergamon Press, 1963.
3. Feigenbaum, H: Echocardiography. 1st Ed. Philadelphia, Lea & Febiger, 1974.
4. Curie, J, and Curie P: Comptes rendus, page 204, July (1880).
5. Kinsler, LE, and Frey, AR: Fundamentals of Acoustics. New York, John Wiley & Sons, 1962.
6. Wells, PNT: Biomedical Ultrasonics. New York, Academic Press, 1977.
7. Fry, FJ: Intense focused ultrasound. *In* Ultrasound: Its Applications in Medicine and Biology. Edited by FJ Fry. Amsterdam, Elsevier Scientific Publishing, 1978.
8. Kikuchi, Y: Transducers for ultrasonic systems. *In* Ultrasound: Its Applications in Medicine and Biology. Edited by FJ Fry. Amsterdam, Elsevier Scientific Publishing, 1978.
9. Fry, WJ, and Dunn, F: Ultrasound: analysis and experimental methods in biologic research. *In* Physical Techniques in Biological Research. Vol. 4. Edited by WL Nastuk. New York, Academic Press, 1962.
10. Reid, J: A review of some basic limitations in ultrasonic diagnosis. *In* Diagnostic Ultrasound. Edited by CC Grossman, JH Holms, C Joyner, and EW Purnell. New York, Plenum Press, 1966.
11. Meitzel, AH: Piezoelectric transducer materials and techniques for ultrasonic devices operating above 100 MHz. *In* Ultrasonic Transducer Materials. Edited by OE Mattist. New York, Plenum Press, 1971.
12. Edler, I: Diagnostic use of ultrasound in heart disease. Acta Med Scand, *308*:32, 1955.
13. Feigenbaum, H: Use of echocardiography in evaluating left ventricular function. Second World Congress on Ultrasonics in Medicine. Excerpta Medica, June, 1973.
14. Chang, S: M-Mode Echocardiographic Techniques and Pattern Recognition. Philadelphia, Lea & Febiger, 1976.
15. Langevin, P: French Patent. 505, 703, 1918.
16. Fry, FJ: Biological Effects of Ultrasound. A Review. Proc IEEE, 67:604, 1979.
17. O'Brien, WD, Jr: Safety of ultrasound. *In* Handbook of Clinical Ultrasound. Edited by M DeVleiger et al. New York, John Wiley & Sons, 1978.
18. Report of the American Institute of Ultrasound in Medicine's Bioeffects Committee. J Clin Ultrasound, 5:2, 1977 (updated August 1978).

Chapter 2

Cross-Sectional Scanning: Technical Principles and Instrumentation

History of Cross-Sectional Imaging

The first two-dimensional ultrasonic imaging system was developed by Wild and Reid in 1952.[1] This "two-dimensional echoscope" consisted of a single, pivot-mounted crystal enclosed in a water-filled chamber (Fig. 2–1). The crystal was arced synchronously through a 45-degree sector by an oscillating cam. The cam was also mechanically attached to an electronic position-sensing unit, which synchronized the position of the sweep on a cathode ray tube with the path of the sound beam in space. (Fig. 2–2).

The same year, Howry and Bliss developed a conceptually similar instrument called a "sonoscope" which utilized a large, mechanically driven transducer submerged in a water tank to generate cross-sectional images of the extremities (Fig. 2–3).[2] Not until 1957, however, did Wild, et al., using a mechanically driven, linear scanning instrument, first examine the freshly excised human heart and produce cross-sectional images of the poste-

rior wall, aorta, and a segment of the left coronary system.[3]

For the greater part of the next decade, advances in two-dimensional imaging were largely limited to studies of the abdomen and other areas that provided ready access to the exploring ultrasonic beam. Although preliminary attempts were made to generate two-dimensional cardiac images, the failure to appropriately display dynamic cardiac motion and the difficulties in gaining access to the heart limited progress.

In 1967, a group of Japanese investigators, led by Ebina, obtained the first large clinical series of static cross-sectional images of the cardiac chambers and great vessels using a compound, mechanically driven, water-path scanner (Fig. 2–4). In addition, by synchronizing their ultrasonic sampling with the R wave of an electrocardiogram, they were able to generate cardiac "ultrasonotomograms" during both systole and diastole (Fig. 2–5).[4]

During the same period, Ashberg, using a scanning transducer and parabolic mir-

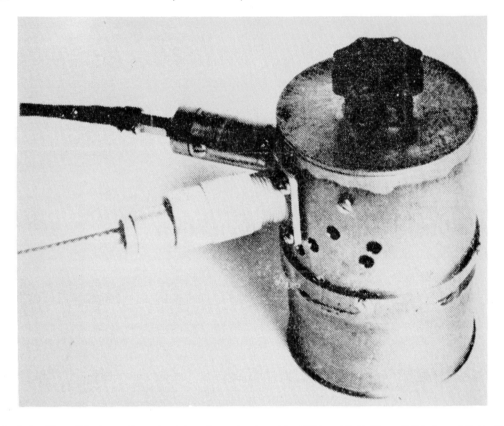

Fig. 2–1.   The original two-dimensional transducer developed by Wild and Reid. (From Wild, JJ, and Reid, JM: Application of echo ranging techniques to the determination of structure of biologic tissue. Science, *115*:226, 1952.)

ror system, introduced dynamic motion to the cross-sectional format.[5] This technique, which he called "ultrasonic cinematography," produced cardiac images at a rate of seven frames per second. Although all the early scanning systems involved either mechanical or manual scanning of the transducer, Somer demonstrated in 1968 that, using existing electronic scanning techniques, a medical instrument could be developed in which beam scanning and position sensing could be achieved electronically.[6]

Despite steady improvement in cross-sectional instrumentation and increasing interest in cross-sectional cardiac scanning, these techniques were not applied clinically in a routine fashion until the appearance of the "real-time" imaging systems in the early 1970s.

The development by Bom, et al., of an electronically activated linear array system was the first practical method for deriving spatially correct, dynamic images of the moving heart.[7,8] This linear array consisted of a series of small transducers, aligned in a row, that could be activated in rapid sequence either individually or in groups (Fig. 2–6). The linear arrangement permitted the transmitted pulse to shift rapidly down the line of transducers, thereby achieving the same type of beam movement that had previously been attained by manual or mechanical motion of an individual transducer. Figure 2–7 is an example of how the resulting parallel data lines were recorded and assembled into a composite image.

Rapid electronic switching between transducers permitted image assembly at

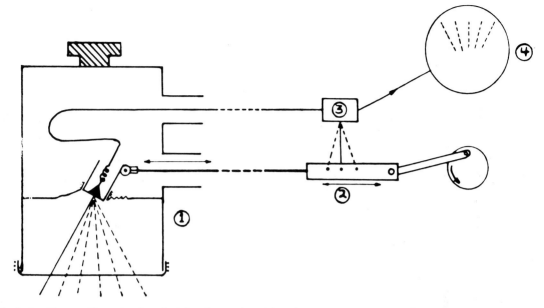

Fig. 2–2.   Diagram illustrating the principles of operation of the echoscope. A pivot-mounted crystal (1) was driven by an oscillating ram (2), which was mechanically connected to an electronic position sensing device (3). This device, in turn, synchronized the position of the transducer with the orientation of the displayed data lines on the oscilloscope (4). (From Wild, JJ, and Reid, JM: Application of echo ranging techniques to the determination of structure of biologic tissue. Science, *115*:226, 1952.)

a sufficiently high frame rate to record dynamic cardiac motion. In addition, individual transducers could be used to generate M-mode recordings from preselected areas of the heart, thus adding spatial orientation to the derived M-mode data and improving understanding of the M-mode record. The linear array format, however, failed to achieve general acceptance because of (1) the almost compulsory use of small crystals, which had poor inherent beam characteristics and limited lateral resolution;[9] (2) the large composite transducer size, which was poorly suited to the available echocardiographic windows; and (3) the limited line density of the final image. This concept, however, represented a major advance because it proved that dynamic cardiac imaging not only was possible, but could be applied to large groups of patients and could provide useful clinical information.[10,11]

The demonstration of the feasibility of dynamic cardiac imaging was followed by rapid advances in cross-sectional echocardiography from both the engineering and clinical standpoint. In 1973 and 1974, Griffith and Henry at the National Institutes of Health,[12] Eggleton and Johnston at Indiana University,[13–15] and McDicken in Scotland[16] developed prototype instruments for rapid mechanical sector scanning. These instruments provided both the high frame rate and line density required for high-resolution cardiac imaging in a relatively simple and flexible format. During the same period, Thurstone and VonRamm, at Duke University,[17–19] utilizing the principles suggested by Somer, developed a phased array system, which permitted electronic steering of the ultrasonic beam in a sector format. This sophisticated system, in addition to providing dynamic two-dimensional images of the heart, also incorporated transmit and receive focusing of the ultrasonic pulse. Subsequently, a number of other phased array systems have been developed with proven clinical

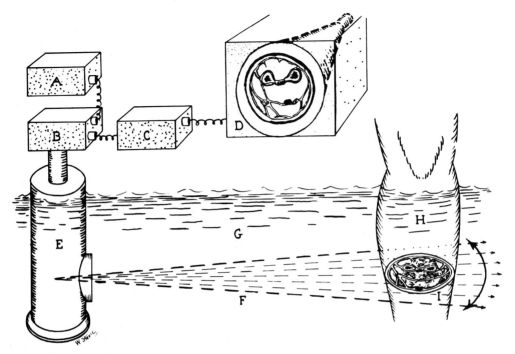

Fig. 2–3. Diagram of the components and principles of operation of the sonoscope developed by Howry and Bliss. The pulser (A) activated the ultrasonic crystal, which was contained in a large submerged housing. The horizontal beam scanning and synchronization system (B) moved the transducer and recorded its position. The large submersible transducer and housing (E) directed sequential ultrasonic pulses in a controlled scan through a submerged extremity, such as that indicated to the right (H). The received echoes were then amplified in the amplifier chain (C) and displayed in a spatially correct format on the oscilloscope (D). (From Howry, D, and Bliss, W: Ultrasonic visualization of soft tissue structure of the body. J Lab Clin Med, *40*:579, 1952.)

application and reliability. In the intervening years, these basic systems have undergone extensive clinical trials in a number of centers throughout the United States and elsewhere. The results of these and subsequent studies form the basis for this book.

SCAN FORMATS

In all cross-sectional scanning systems, the sound beam is moved or scanned in a fixed plane across the precordium. As the beam moves, the echoes returning from structures along its path are continuously recorded. Each time a pulse is transmitted, the beam coordinates are simultaneously sensed and relayed to the cathode ray tube so that each new line of echocardiographic data can be oriented and displayed in a pattern that corresponds to the relative

path of the sound beam in space. If the beam is swept rapidly enough, images can be assembled at a sufficiently high frame rate to depict dynamic cardiac motion.

Three predominant scan formats have been employed, either alone or in combination, to generate and record these images. These formats include the linear scan, the sector scan, and the arc scan (Fig. 2–8, A through E). In the linear format, the point of origin of the ultrasonic pulse is moved in a straight line across the precordium so that the resulting sound waves propagate parallel to one another. This type of scan can be accomplished by (1) manually or mechanically moving a single transducer from one point to another (Fig. 2–8, A), (2) aligning a number of transducers next to one another and activating them in sequence (Fig. 2–8, B) or (3) utilizing a rotating transducer(s) to reflect sequential

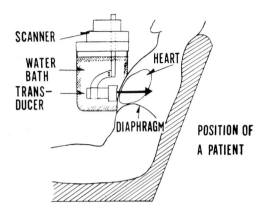

SCANNER

WATER
BATH

TRANS-
DUCER

HEART

DIAPHRAGM

POSITION OF
A PATIENT

Fig. 2–4. Diagram of the mechanically driven water path scanner developed by Ebina, et al. During the examination, the patient was seated, and the scanning instrument was applied directly to the anterior chest wall. (From Ebina, T, et al.: The ultrasono-tomography of the heart and great vessels in living human subjects by means of the ultrasonic reflection technique. Jpn Heart J, 8:331, 1967.)

pulses off the face of a parabolic mirror so that the pulses enter the chest in a parallel fashion (Fig. 2–8, C). In the linear format, the scan area is of equal width in both the near and far field. The line density or the number of individual B-mode lines contained in each image depends on the method of scanning. When a single transducer is moved across the precordium (Fig. 2–8, A), beam movement can be as slow as desired, and the resultant line density, therefore, may be high. Unless the scan rate is uniform, however, the image may be degraded by uneven line density. When a number of transducers are combined in a linear array (Fig. 2–8, B), each transducer generates a single data line. The number of lines in the image, therefore, equals the number of transducers in the array and is, of necessity, limited. The regular spacing of the transducers in this format results in an even line distribution and a more visually acceptable image.

In the sector format (Fig. 2–8, D), the transducer is held in a stationary position on the precordium, and from this fixed point, the sound beam is swept through a predetermined arc. A sector scan, therefore, is narrow in the region close to the transducer face and becomes wider as the imaging plane progresses farther from the transducer.

In the arc scan (Fig. 2–8, E), the transducer is moved in an arcuate fashion while the ultrasonic beam is directed at a constant point in space. The arc scan permits examination of an individual point from multiple directions, thereby optimizing target description. A compound scan consists of a combination of two or more of the previously described scanning formats.

From the display standpoint, the linear scan has obvious advantages because it encompasses a large cross-sectional area that is the same in both the near and the far field. From a visualization standpoint, the compound scan, which permits individual points to be examined from multiple aspects, optimizes the chances for recording a given target. In clinical practice, however, the sector format, which is most readily adapted to the limited echocardiographic window and thus permits the greatest amount of information to be obtained in the largest number of patients, has become the scan pattern of choice. Instruments employing this format have gained the widest acceptance.

INSTRUMENTATION

The various types of instruments that have been employed to obtain cross-sectional cardiac images are summarized in Table 2–1. These cross-sectional systems can be broadly classified as either static or dynamic, based on the rate at which individual frames are assembled. The static systems include both manual and mechanical scanning devices, which generate single composite images. When applied to the heart, these instruments are usually time gated so that data are acquired only during specific points in the cardiac cycle. Each static image is assembled, therefore,

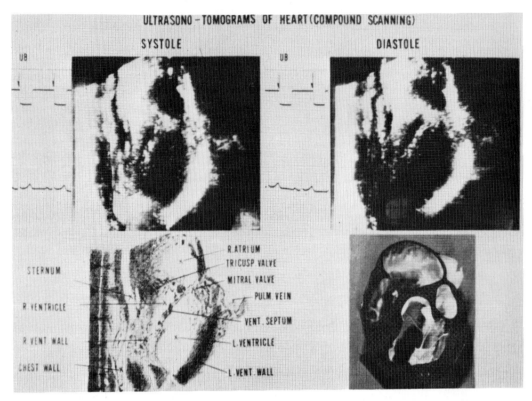

Fig. 2–5. Ultrasono-tomograms of the human heart recorded during diastole and systole. The path of the scan transects the right atrium, the left ventricle, and a portion of the interventricular septum. Changes in left ventricular and right atrial cavity sizes from systole to diastole are apparent. An anatomic section corresponding to the path of the imaging plane used to record these sections appears in the lower right of the figure. (From Ebina, T, et al.: The ultrasono-tomography of the heart and great vessels in living human subjects by means of the ultrasonic reflection technique. Jpn Heart J, 8:331, 1967.)

from data derived from a number of cardiac cycles.

TABLE 2–1
CROSS-SECTIONAL INSTRUMENTATION

1. Static
   —Manual
   —Mechanical
2. Dynamic
   —Mechanical sector scanners
     a) Oscillatory
     b) Rotary
   —Transducer arrays
     a) Linear arrays
     b) Phased arrays

Dynamic systems involve fast movement of the ultrasonic beam across a predetermined area of the precordium at sufficiently high-data acquisition rates to permit image assembly at a rapid frame rate. These instruments can also be conveniently subclassified, based on the method of the beam movement, into mechanical scanning systems and transducer arrays.

From a diagnostic standpoint, the dynamic nature of the heart makes assessment of cardiac motion at least as important as visualization of cardiac structure. Imaging systems that display dynamic cardiac motion in real time are therefore essential to an adequate assessment of cardiac performance. For this reason, only

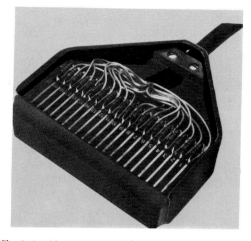

Fig. 2–6. Linear array transducer similar to that developed by Bom, et al. (From Bom, N, et al.: Multiscan echocardiography 1: a technical description. Circulation, *48*:1066, 1973. Reproduced by permission of the American Heart Association.)

dynamic systems are currently in use and will be discussed further.

At present, two types of two-dimensional real-time echocardiographic imaging systems combine the sector format with a real-time display. They are the mechanical sector scanning and the phased array scanning systems. Both perform the functions previously described; however, they accomplish the desired goal in two different ways. Linear arrays, although poorly suited to adult cardiac imaging, are important from a historical viewpoint and are still utilized in many areas as research instruments and in pediatrics.

DYNAMIC CROSS-SECTIONAL IMAGING SYSTEMS

Mechanical Sector Scanning

In the mechanical sector scanning format, the ultrasonic beam is swept through a fixed plane by rapid mechanical oscillation of a single transducer or by rotation of multiple transducers. The transducer(s) is housed in a small hand-held scanning probe that permits flexible angulation and rotation of the scan plane. In addition to the transducer(s), the probe normally con-

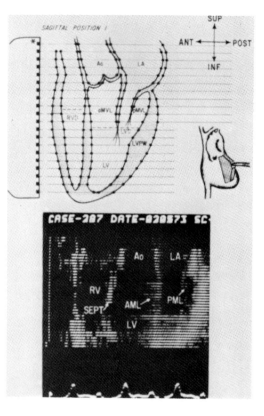

Fig. 2–7. Diagram illustrating a linear array transducer oriented parallel to the long axis of the left ventricle (LV) and aortic root (AO). The path along which the sound pulses generated by the individual transducers transect the heart in this orientation is indicated. Also shown is the type of image obtained by assembling the resultant echoes. (From Sahn, DJ, et al.: Multiple crystal cross sectional echocardiography in the diagnosis of cyanotic congenital heart disease. Circulation, *50*:230, 1974. Reproduced by permission of the American Heart Association.)

tains a position-sensing device and a small motor to drive the crystal(s). The transducer(s) is similar to those used in conventional one-dimensional imaging systems. In oscillating systems, the transducer is generally constrained with a pivot bearing about which it is driven through a selected arc at a predetermined rate. The transducer drive is also connected to a position-sensing apparatus so that the position of the ultrasonic beam is continuously recorded as it sweeps through its arc. Various methods for position sensing have been employed, including variable differ-

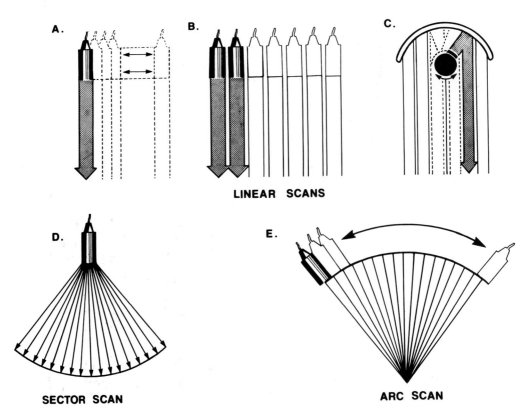

Fig. 2–8. Series of diagrams illustrates the different scan formats that have been used to produce cross-sectional images. Panels *A, B,* and *C* indicate the various methods used to generate linear scans. *A,* A single transducer is rapidly moved from one point to another while maintaining a constant orientation relative to the heart. *B,* A series of transducers is aligned in a row and activated in sequence to produce a series of parallel pulses. *C,* A rotating transducer is used to reflect pulses off a parabolic mirror such that they enter the tissue in a parallel orientation. *D,* A sector scan. In this format, the transducer is held in a fixed location while the sound beam is gradually swept through an arc of varying width. *E,* An arc scan in which the transducer is moved along an arcuate path while the beam is directed at a fixed point in space.

ential transformers, resistance pads, potentiometers, and photo-optical sensing devices. Figure 2–9 is an example of one of the early mechanical scanners that was developed at Indiana University.[14,15]

The mechanical sector scanning concept proved advantageous when compared to the earlier dynamic systems (i.e., the linear array or parabolic mirror and rotary transducer) for a number of reasons. First, the mechanical scanners utilized single, relatively large, focused transducers that had comparatively well-columnated beam patterns. This construction improved lateral resolution as well as system sensitivity. Second, the smaller, more

flexible probe could be placed in a variety of interspaces or echocardiographic windows, thereby permitting the examiner to adapt freely to the configuration of the patient's chest. In addition, the high pulse repetition frequency and relatively small scan angle of the mechanical scanners provided a high line density and resulted in a more pleasing and recognizable cross-sectional picture. The mechanical scanning concept was also relatively simple, and the amount of hardware required to drive the transducer and sense its position was limited. Figure 2–10 illustrates the original prototype mechanical scanner developed by Eggleton and Johnston. This

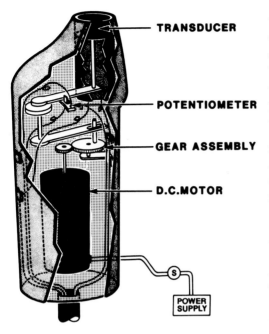

TRANSDUCER

POTENTIOMETER

GEAR ASSEMBLY

D.C.MOTOR

POWER SUPPLY

Fig. 2–9. Diagram illustrates the components of one of the early probes used for mechanical sector scanning. In this model, a small D.C. motor was attached to a gear assembly, which drove an oscillating transducer through a 30-degree arc. The probe position was sensed by a low-noise potentiometer, which recorded changes in the position of the drive shaft and, hence, of the transducer. The actual area of transducer contact with the skin was small, and the probe could be easily maneuvered to fit into any intercostal space.

scanner was assembled largely from existing components and was designed so that the scan module could be inexpensively retrofitted in an available M-mode system.

Limitations of the mechanical scanning format included the small scan area of early instruments, limited width at the apex of the sector, uneven line distribution with oscillating probes, and mechanical vibration, which could be felt by the patient. Figure 2–11 compares the scan areas encompassed by a linear array with those encompassed by the 30- and 90-degree sector formats. The diagram shows that the sector format causes significant loss of near-field information at the apex of the sector. In the trade-off between the rectangular display and the ability to utilize a small echocardiographic window, the lat-

ter has proved more important in adult clinical practice. In the far field, the scan area depends on the size of the sector. In the mechanical systems, sector size is, to some extent, limited by the type of probe and method of transducer motion. Oscillating probes with scan angles as high as 60 degrees have been developed; however, rocking the transducer through such a large angle tends to cause excessive vibration on the patient's chest and becomes annoying. In general, most successful oscillating scanners have employed the 30-degree format with occasional widening of the sector to 45 degrees.

More recently, rotary transducer systems that provide a wider scan angle have become increasingly popular. Figure 2–12 is an example of a commercially available rotary transducer system. In this system, 4 single transducers are oriented at 90 degrees to one another. Each transducer is then rotated through a full 360-degree arc. The individual transducers are activated only as they pass through an ultrasonic window in the probe head. The result in this example is an 82-degree sector. Transducer rotation occurs within a fixed plastic case. The wide scan area therefore can be achieved without discomfort to the patient because no moving parts come in contact with the chest. In addition to the wider scan angle, the rotary system produces a line distribution that is more even than that achieved with the early oscillatory transducers. Uneven line distribution is frequently encountered in oscillating systems because the transducer is required to slow down, stop, reverse direction, and accelerate again at each border of the sector. When the activation rate of the transducer is constant, the line density at the margins of the sector (where the transducer is moving more slowly) is greater than the line density in the midportion of the sweep (where the transducer is moving at its most rapid rate). This uneven line density can be overcome by making the pulse frequency a function of scan speed.

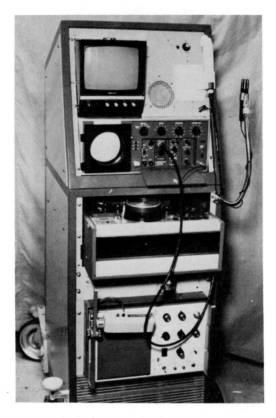

Fig. 2–10. The original prototype mechanical scanner developed by Eggleton and Johnston. This instrument, known as "the blue goose," provided much of the early cross-sectional data on which this book is based.

In the rotary format, the speed at which the transducer passes through the aperture in the transducer head is always constant, and hence, the line density throughout the 90-degree sector is uniform. No variation in pulse frequency is required.

Transducer Arrays

Transducer arrays are composed of a group of individual transducers or transducer elements. Transducers have dimensions of several wavelengths and, thus, can transmit a highly directional beam. Transducer elements, in contrast, are small in comparison to the wavelength and are practically nondirectional. Transducers function independently, whereas transducer elements are effective only in groups.[20] A group of transducers or transducer elements, which are aligned next to one another in a straight row, is referred to as a linear array.

Linear Arrays

Linear arrays may be composed of a group of transducers or transducer elements. A linear array that is composed of a row of equidistant transducers that are activated individually by switching the activation pulse from one transducer to another is termed a "simple switched array." An array that is composed of a large series of transducer elements that are activated in groups such that each group forms a composite transducer is referred to as a "grouped switched array."

The original linear array system developed by Bom, et al., was a simple switched array.[7,8] In this system, 20 individual transducers, each 4 × 10 mm, were aligned

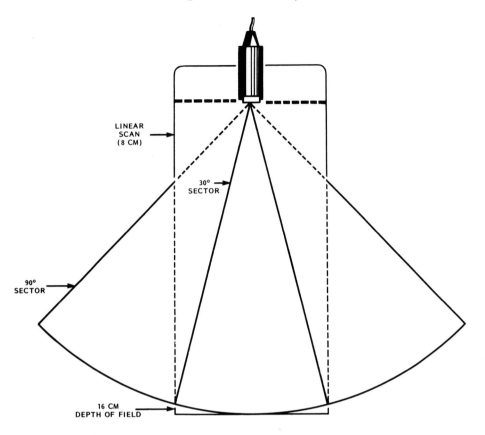

Fig. 2–11. Diagram illustrating the relative areas encompassed by a linear array with an 8-cm transducer face, a 16-cm depth of field, and 30- and 90-degree sector scans with comparable depths of field.

to yield a composite array with a transmitting surface of 1 × 8 cm. By briefly pulsing each transducer and leaving it on as a receiver for approximately 200 msec, one could record 20 individual B-mode data lines from a scan area (disregarding beam dispersion) of 1 × 8 × 16 cm with a line density of 1 line per 4 mm. By pulsing each transducer twice and displaying the second line at half the distance between two adjacent transducers or by electronically doubling each line, one could increase the line density to 1 line per 2 mm at a frame rate of either 80 or 160 per second. This line density still failed to produce a visually pleasing image. Increasing line density by decreasing transducer size would result in unacceptable lateral resolution. To overcome the problem of low line density in a linear array, grouped

switched arrays were developed. Figure 2–13 compares a simple switched linear array with a "grouped switched array." In the grouped format, multiple small transducer elements are arranged in a linear array. Groups of elements are then activated together and collectively form a large effective transducer face. This grouping results in an improved beam profile and, at the same time, increases the image line density. The large composite transducer, however, still lacks flexibility and requires a large "window" to obtain access to the heart. Such characteristics limit its value in adult cardiac imaging.

Phased Arrays

Phased arrays are multiple element transducers that sweep the sound beam

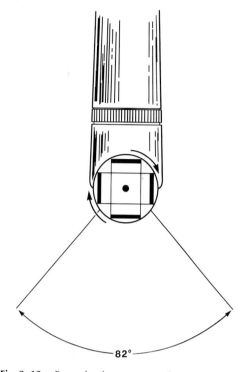

Fig. 2–12. Example of a rotary transducer system used in cross-sectional imaging.

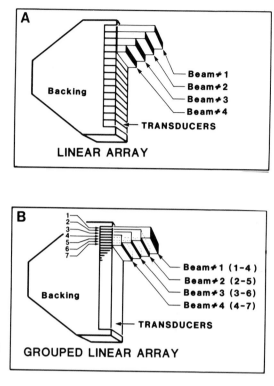

Fig. 2–13. Diagram comparing a simple switched linear array (A) with a grouped switched linear array (B). In the simple switched array, each transducer produces a separate ultrasonic beam. In the grouped array, groups of transducer elements are simultaneously activated, thereby producing a larger effective transducer face and increasing the image line density. In Figure 2–13, B, beam #1 is produced by a composite waveform resulting from the activation of transducer elements 1 through 4. Beam #2 is produced by the simultaneous activation of elements 2 through 5, beam #3 is produced by the activation of elements 3 through 6, etc.

through a predetermined arc electronically rather than manually or mechanically. Each element in the array is narrow so that the divergence angle of the beam is wide and the element can be considered to emit a spheric wave front. Electronic beam steering is achieved using the principle of summation of time-sequenced wavelets first described by Huygens in the seventeenth century. Simply stated, when each of a series of linear oriented transducers in an array is excited simultaneously, the resulting wavelets emanating from the individual transducers summate to form a single wave that propagates in a direction normal to or directly away from the transducer face. Conversely, when the transducers are excited in rapid sequence rather than simultaneously, the wavelets emanating from each transducer are propagated at an angle to the transducer face. This resultant angle is proportional to the time interval or delay between activation of the transducers. By rapidly varying the time sequence in which the transducers are excited, one can electronically direct or steer the wave front at correspondingly variable angles from the transducer face. Because the position of the array is fixed and the beam is swept from side to side, the resultant image is in a sector format. The first clinically useful phased array system was designed by Thurstone and VonRamm and can serve as an example of this type of imaging.[17,18]

When describing the physical principles of any phased array system, the transmit and receive operations are customarily considered separately. In the transmit mode, ultrasonic energy is formed into a beam and propagates along a predetermined path by the constructive and destructive interference of sequentially created acoustic wave fronts. In the receive mode, ultrasonic energy is sensed from a predetermined direction by the addition and subtraction of incoming ultrasonic energy of varying phase.

The method by which the ultrasonic beam is generated and steered in a phased array system is illustrated graphically in Figures 2–14, *A* and *B*. In these examples, 19 elements are depicted in each array; however, for simplicity, only the wavelets

A

B

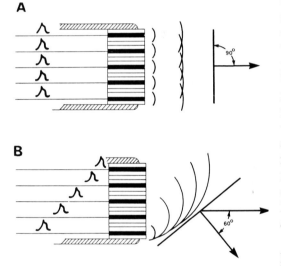

Fig. 2–14. Diagram illustrating the method of beam transmission and steering in the phased array format. *A,* A series of electrical pulses is depicted moving from left to right toward the transducer elements in the array. The pulses activate the elements, simultaneously producing a series of small wavelets. As these wavelets move from the transducer face, they summate to form a beam that propagates away from the transducer. *B,* The transducer elements are activated slightly out-of-phase. In this example, the upper transducer is activated first, producing an acoustic wavelet that propagates to the right and away from the array. Rapidly thereafter, the second element is excited, producing a second wavelet slightly behind the first. The sequence continues until the bottom element in the array is activated. In tissue, these five individual wavefronts summate to produce an acoustic beam that approximates in shape and direction the beam that would be produced by a transducer aimed in that direction.

produced by 5 of these transducer elements are indicated.

During beam transmission a cylindric gaussian focus can be produced at a specified range by imposing a spherical timing relationship on the excitation pulses (Fig. 2–15). The focusing produced by such a spherical wave front, however, allows the focusing of each sound transmission in only a single area along the beam axis. As with fixed focusing, a single transmit focus improves the resolution of the system in the focal region; however, outside this region, the resolution may be degraded because of increased beam dispersion. In addition, although some beam focusing can be produced by this manner, theoretic considerations and beam-pattern photographs indicate that the amount of sound energy along the axis of the beam outside the focal range is variable. Because each pulse must write one entire image line, blanks in the beam pattern result in gaps in the data line, thereby seriously degrading the resulting image. To produce a more uniform depth of focus throughout the scan area, the prototype system used five different focal points. Combining adjacent image lines recorded at different focal depths in an interlaced fashion was believed to improve the effective focal characteristics of the entire system.

In the receive mode, the array must appropriately record echoes from targets lying along the path of the transmit pulse.

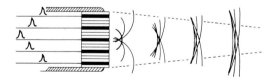

Fig. 2–15. Diagram illustrates the method of transmit focusing in the phased array format. In this diagram, the electrical pulses that activated the transducer elements have a spherical timing relationship. This relationship causes the elements at the margins of the array to activate slightly before those in the center. This activation sequence causes the consolidation of the sound energy in the central portion of the beam and effectively focuses the array at a fixed point within the near field of the transducer.

The width of the array, however, prohibits the echoes returning from an angle (with respect to the plane of the transducer face) from simultaneously striking each element on the array's surface. For the effective orientation of the array during reception to correspond to its orientation during transmission, delays in the processing of the echoes received by each element must be introduced. These delays are varied as necessary so that the echoes returning from a particular direction will be in phase and, hence, will summate (Fig. 2–16). Echoes received from all other directions will not be in phase and, therefore, will partially cancel out.

In the prototype system, accurate phasing was accomplished using delay lines, which passed the acoustic information with different delay times from each element. In this fashion, echoes from a desired azimuthal orientation tend to be favored at the summing preamplifier. In addition to maintaining the effective orientation of the array during reception, the delay circuitry also permits the focusing of the receiver at any desired range and allows tracking of this focus in synchrony with the range of the returning echoes.

Figure 2–17 illustrates the method for obtaining this type of receive focusing. As illustrated in this figure, echoes arising from a specific source at the center of the sound wave (reflector B) arrive at the individual transducer elements in the array at different times. This variation in timing is also indicated by the electrical pulses to the left of the array. Echoes from other reflectors at the same depth (A and C) strike the transducers in timing sequences that are slightly different from one another as well as from reflector B. The controlling computer delays all the signals by the amount of time required to appropriately

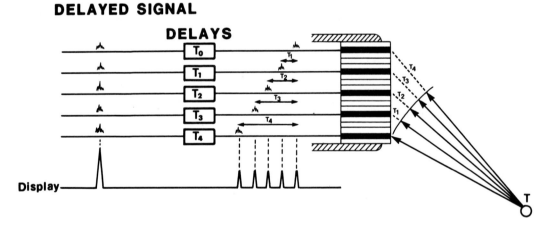

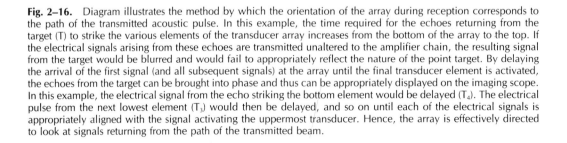

Fig. 2–16. Diagram illustrates the method by which the orientation of the array during reception corresponds to the path of the transmitted acoustic pulse. In this example, the time required for the echoes returning from the target (T) to strike the various elements of the transducer array increases from the bottom of the array to the top. If the electrical signals arising from these echoes are transmitted unaltered to the amplifier chain, the resulting signal from the target would be blurred and would fail to appropriately reflect the nature of the point target. By delaying the arrival of the first signal (and all subsequent signals) at the array until the final transducer element is activated, the echoes from the target can be brought into phase and thus can be appropriately displayed on the imaging scope. In this example, the electrical signal from the echo striking the bottom element would be delayed (T_4). The electrical pulse from the next lowest element (T_3) would then be delayed, and so on until each of the electrical signals is appropriately aligned with the signal activating the uppermost transducer. Hence, the array is effectively directed to look at signals returning from the path of the transmitted beam.

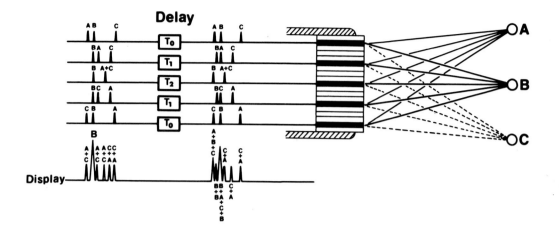

Fig. 2–17. Diagram illustrates the method by which the array can be focused to preferentially receive echoes from a particular point along the path of the transmitted beam. The echoes arising from a specific point target (B) arrive at the individual transducer elements in the array at different times. This variation in timing is reflected by the relationship of the electrical pulses to the left of the array. Echoes from other reflectors at the same depth (A and C) strike the transducer elements in timing sequences that are slightly different from one another as well as from those arising from reflector B. If all the pulses are delayed by the time required to appropriately summate and display echoes from target B, the echoes from this point will be in phase and, hence, will summate. Those from targets A and C will be further out of phase and, with appropriate filtering, can be eliminated.

summate and display echoes from the particular area of interest (reflector B). This effectively places echoes from reflectors A and C out-of-phase in relation to those from reflector B, thereby producing a type of focusing. Because the returning echo information results from a known interrogating pulse, the time of the returning echoes is directly related to the depth of the echo-producing source. In practice, therefore, as illustrated in Figure 2–18, the receive system is focused initially in the near field (target F_1) for the period immediately after interrogation. The system is then refocused at successively deeper levels (targets F_2 and F_3) as the pulse continues to propagate to the maximum focal distance allowed by the near-field characteristics of the transducer array.

The near field of the array, which is determined by the size of the composite transducer and by the ultrasonic frequency of operation, is the distance from the array in which the ultrasonic energy is mainly confined within the dimensions of the transducer face. As discussed in Chapter 1, when the transducer is a single element disc, the beam near the transducer is cylindric, propagating away from the transducer's face at a radius that approximates the radius of the disc (Fig. 2–19, A). In a phased array, this zone is rectangular (Fig. 2–19, B and C). Note that the near field for the lateral or Y dimension is greater than the near field for the elevation or X dimension because the height of the array elements is smaller than the total array width. Because the phased array has separate transducer elements only in the lateral dimension, the ability to create an electronically positioned moving focus on receive is confined to the lateral dimension of the beam.

Two types of focusing can be used to improve the elevation characteristics of the array's beam. First, an acoustic lens can be employed to focus the beam in the X dimension. Second, the technique of

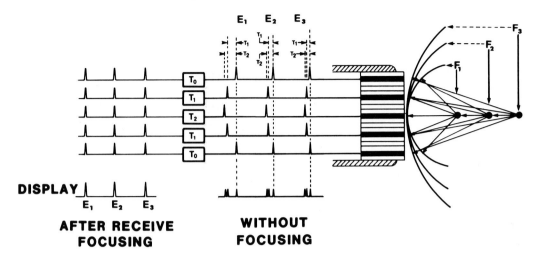

Fig. 2–18. Diagram illustrates the method by which the receive focus can be shifted to follow the progress of the transmitted pulse. The array is initially focused in the near field at F_1 by assigning the appropriate spherical timing relationship to the delays to place echoes from this point in phase. Then, by changing the spherical arrangement of the delays, the array can be sequentially refocused at increasingly deeper tissue depths, F_2 and F_3, thereby tracking the path of the transmitted pulse through the tissue.

"shading" can be used. This technique involves widening the array by adding additional lines of transducers or varying the power output at the margins of the transducer elements when compared to the center of the element. Each of these techniques decreases the power output at the edges, thereby minimizing the abrupt discontinuity found with a single element and reducing the side-lobe amplitudes (Fig. 2–20). These techniques for focusing the beam in the X or thickness dimension can be combined with the moving receive focus in the Y or lateral dimension to optimize beam configuration.

In operation, the controlling computer of the phased array first provides the X-Y deflection information to the CRT in the form of the sine and cosine of the deflection angle to be examined. The computer then sets the transmit timing circuits to produce a focused beam at the desired azimuthal direction. The transmit and deflection operations are then initiated, and the individual transmit pulses are triggered at appropriate times to produce the desired beam direction and focal point.

The returning echo data, which are received by the individual elements, are first amplified by a low-noise preamplifier and are then amplified with logarithmic compression before beam delay. The echo data are then delayed for an appropriate length of time to permit the synchronization of the signals from the individual transducers. Appropriately delayed acoustic information from all receiving channels is then summed, and the resulting signal after detection is used to modulate the brightness of the CRT (Z-axis input). Immediately after the initiation of the transmit pulse, the computer sets the receiver delay lines to focus in the immediate proximity of the transducer. As the pulse progresses and as echoes are received from sources deeper in the tissue, the controller changes the receiver delays to maintain the focus of the receiving system at the appropriate point along the beam path. In this fashion, an electronically steered beam, which is focused in both its transmit and receive modes, is produced.

As with mechanical sector scanning, the phased array approach has inherent advantages and limitations. Advantages of

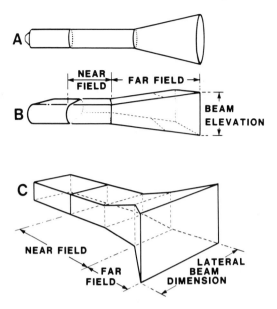

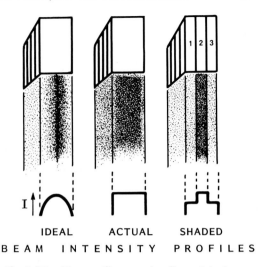

BEAM   INTENSITY   PROFILES

Fig. 2–19. Diagram comparing the configuration of the sound beam arising from a simple disc-shaped transducer with that generated by a rectangular transducer array. *A,* In the former instance, the beam is cylindric in the near field, paralleling the margins of the transducer face. In the far field, beyond the transition zone, the beam gradually diverges, thereby assuming a conical shape. The beam configuration of a rectangular array is more complicated. *B,* In the X or thickness dimension, the transducer width is relatively small, and hence, the near field is short and beam divergence begins relatively close to the transducer face. *C,* In the lateral or Y dimension, the near field is longer and beam divergence begins farther from the transducer because of the relatively greater length of the array.

Fig. 2–20. Diagram illustrates the effects of shading on a series of representative beam intensity profiles. In the ideal beam, peak energy is concentrated in the center of the beam and gradually decays as the beam margins are approached. In practice, the drop in intensity at the beam margins is relatively abrupt. This change in intensity contributes to side lobe formation. This abrupt discontinuity at the beam margins can be decreased by placing one or more transducers beside the center transducer and by activating them less intensely.

these systems include (1) flexibility of beam angulation, depth of field examined, and line density; (2) ability to record M-mode data from any azimuthal direction; (3) ability to focus in both the transmit and the receive mode. Limitations include the large size and the complexity of the required hardware, which limit portability and increases cost; limited transducer frequency; and increased side-lobe intensity. Finally, as described earlier, although transmit and receive focusing refine the lateral dimension of the beam, the beam pattern in the thickness or elevation dimension is poor despite acoustic focusing and shading. This characteristic is in direct contrast to the single element transducer used by the mechanical systems,

which simultaneously produces an acoustic focus in both dimensions.

PRINCIPLES OF DYNAMIC CARDIAC IMAGING COMMON TO ALL SYSTEMS

In dynamic or "real time," two-dimensional cardiac imaging, ultrasonic data are displayed in a spatially oriented format relative to time. The introduction of time into the two-dimensional image creates a number of obligatory constraints. Instead of leisurely assembling a single picture of the heart, images must now be created at a rapid predetermined or fixed rate. Because one begins with a limitation in the amount of ultrasonic data that can be collected in a given time period (limited by the speed of sound in tissue), the number of image frames to be assembled determines the amount of data that can be included in each frame. If the image frames are assembled at a fixed rate, the size of the scan area then determines how thinly the data must be spread over the final ultrasonic image. As a result, several additional terms are required to describe dynamic imaging. These include pulse or line repetition frequency, frame rate, line density, depth of field, scan angle, and dead time. Each of these variables is interdependent. An alteration in one of necessity alters the others. Although different methods have been designed for generating ultrasonic images, the same basic physical constraints apply to all systems.

The Pulse or Line Repetition Frequency

The rate at which individual sound pulses are transmitted, resulting in lines of returning ultrasonic data, is referred to as the pulse or line repetition frequency. The maximum line repetition frequency that can be employed is governed by the speed of sound in tissue and by the depth of tissue one wishes to examine.

Figure 2–21 illustrates these relationships. In this example, we have assumed that the distance from the anterior chest wall to the posterior wall of the heart is 15 cm. Assuming that sound travels through the heart at 1.5 mm per microsecond, 100 microseconds is required for a sound pulse to travel from the anterior chest wall to the posterior wall of the heart. Because the returning echoes must traverse the same distance back to the transducer, the entire transit time for the burst of ultrasonic energy from the transducer to the posterior wall of the heart and back is 200 microseconds. Each burst or pulse of acoustic energy results in the reception of a line of ultrasonic data. The maximum number of pulses that can be transmitted each second and consequently the resultant line repetition frequency at a 15-cm tissue depth therefore is 1 pulse/0.0002 sec or 5000 pulses per second.

If one were examining an infant or small child and thus needed to penetrate only 7.5 cm of tissue, the total transmit time of the pulse would be only 100 microseconds, and 10,000 pulses could be trans-

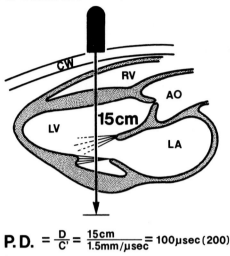

$$\textbf{P. D.} = \frac{D}{C'} = \frac{15\,cm}{1.5\,mm/\mu sec} = 100\,\mu sec\,(200)$$

$$\textbf{PRF} = \underline{.0002\ sec}/pulse\ \text{or}\ 5000\,pulses/sec$$

Fig. 2–21. Diagram illustrates the effects of the examined tissue depth on the pulse duration (P.D.) and, hence, on the number of pulses that can be transmitted in a given time period (the pulse repetition frequency, PRF). In this example, the tissue depth is 15 cm. If the speed of sound in tissue is 1.5 mm per μsec, the sound wave will require 100 μsec to reach this depth and an additional 100 μsec to return to the transducer. Because each pulse requires 200 μsec, a maximum of 5000 pulses can be transmitted per second.

mitted per second. In the alternative case, if one were examining a large subject or were examining the heart from a relatively long distance, such as from the subxiphoid region, a depth of field greater than 15 cm might be necessary. At a field depth of 21.5 cm, the transit time of the pulse increases to 300 microseconds, and the maximum pulse repetition frequency is 3333 pulses per second. The depth of field one must examine, therefore, determines the pulse repetition frequency and, hence, the number of ultrasonic data lines available per second.

The optimum depth of field required in cardiac imaging depends on the size of the patient and on the position from which the examination is attempted. In the standard adult population, a field depth of between 16.5 and 17 cm normally allows the recording of the posterior surface of the heart from the anterior chest wall. Examination from the apex and subxiphoid region requires a longer field depth in the range of 20 to 21.5 cm.

In addition to the time the pulse has to travel, additional time is lost between pulses because the echograph cannot be converted from a transmitter to a receiver instantaneously. This retrace time or dead time further limits the number of pulses that can be transmitted and the amount of data that can be collected and displayed per unit time.

Frame Rate

After the line repetition frequency of the system is established, the frame rate should next be determined. Frame rate is important when one is attempting to resolve the motion of rapidly moving structures. For example, if we assume that the aortic valve opens at a speed of 300 mm per second and that each leaflet moves approximately 1 cm from the open to the closed position, full excursion of the leaflet will occur in one thirtieth of a second. If the imaging system has a frame rate of 30 frames per second, the valve will be closed in one frame and open in the next. When one is attempting to analyze the pattern of valvular motion, a frame rate of more than 30 frames per second is required to examine intermediate positions along the leaflet's path. Increasing frame rate again allows more detailed motion analysis, although at a significant price. Because one begins with a fixed number of lines of information, an increase in frame rate decreases the lines available for each individual frame. When we assume a pulse repetition frequency of 4,500 pulses per second at a frame rate of 10 frames per second, we have 450 lines per frame. At 30 frames per second, we have only 150 lines per frame, whereas at 100 frames per second, we will have only 45 lines per frame. As the available ultrasonic data per frame are reduced, high-quality images become increasingly difficult to produce. Higher frame rates, therefore, result in a trade-off between frame rate and image quality.

Scan Angle

The next important consideration is the size of the scan or the scan angle. Remember, the depth of field determines the line repetition rate, the line repetition rate determines the number of lines of information available, the frame rate determines the number of lines per individual frame, and the scan angle or picture size determines the density of these lines over the image field (Fig. 2–22). Line density, to a large degree, determines the quality of the image. When the lines are widely spread, reconstruction of the image is difficult because of a deficiency of information. As a general rule, a line density of about 2 lines per degree with a range of approximately 1.5 to 2.2 lines per degree provides sufficient data to create a clinically acceptable image.

Field Versus Frame

In addition to the general operating characteristics of two-dimensional systems, a number of other concepts in cross-sectional imaging must be defined and understood. The first is the difference between a field and a frame. A field is comprised of the data recorded during one complete passage of the beam of ultrasound across the surface of an object. A frame is the sum of all data recorded until the beam returns to its original starting point and new information becomes superimposed in an identical pattern on previously recorded data. Thus, when the received ultrasonic data lines are recorded in the same position, direction, and pattern each time the ultrasound beam sweeps across the patient, each field is equal to a frame. However, when data lines are accumulated from different directions or in a different pattern during each of multiple sweeps, a number of fields are required to comprise a single frame.

To illustrate this more fully, consider two different types of mechanical scanning systems. In an oscillating sector scan-

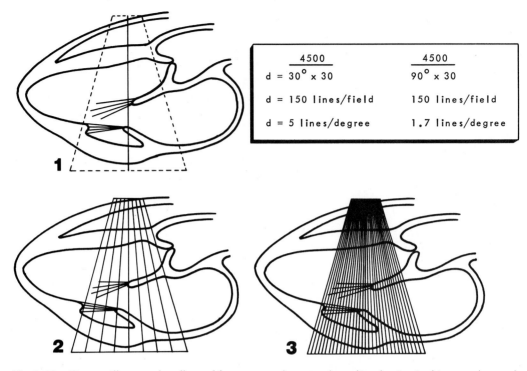

Fig. 2–22. Diagram illustrates the effects of frame rate and scan angle on line density. In this example, a pulse repetition frequency of 4500 per second is assumed. In example 1, the frame rate is also 4500, thereby resulting in only 1 line per frame and no cross-sectional image. When the frame rate is reduced, as illustrated in example 2, the line density improves; however, a poor-quality image is still present. By further reducing the frame rate, as shown in example 3, the line density increases sufficiently to produce a visually acceptable image. Numerically, if one divides the 4500 lines into a 30-degree sector at 30 frames per second, there will be 150 lines per field or 5 lines per degree. This line density is relatively high and results in a visually pleasing image. If the sector is widened to 90 degrees and the frame rate is held constant, the line density drops to 1.7 lines per degree. At this line density, the image is barely acceptable; below this density, the image quality becomes unacceptable to the average viewer.

ning system, the transducer and beam of ultrasound are initially swept from left to right across the surface of the chest. After reaching the opposite margin of its sector, the beam then returns from right to left before beginning the cycle again. Because each sweep and corresponding data display occur in opposite directions, they each constitute individual fields. The combination of the two fields, which are displayed before the transducer begins in its original direction, constitutes a single frame.

In a rotary transducer system, the motion of the transducers is always in the same direction. As illustrated in Figure 2–23, A, when the data lines that are recorded during each transducer sweep are displayed in the same position or on top of the lines from the preceding sweep, each field equals a frame. If, in contrast, lines from two or more consecutive transducer sweeps are displayed in the interspaces between the lines from preceding sweeps (interlacing), the number of fields required to complete a single frame depends on the number of lines that are interlaced (Fig. 2–23, C).

Side Lobes

Another important concept in cross-sectional imaging is the side lobe. Although side lobes occur in all systems, they are most prominent in the phased arrays and may be a source of significant image arti-

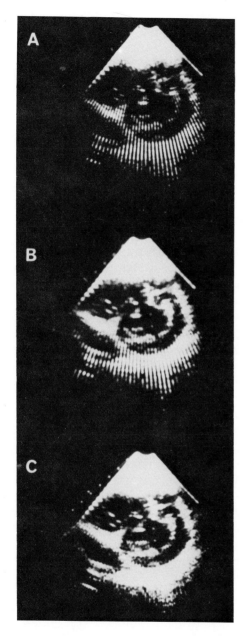

Fig. 2–23. Diagram illustrates two methods of increasing the apparent line density. *A,* A Single field of data is displayed. At the line density of this image there is a clear separation between the individual data lines producing a "spoking" effect. *B,* The system gain has been increased, causing the individual data points to bloom. The data lines widen, and the separation between lines decreases. *C,* The technique of interlacing has been used. In this example, a second field has been laid down such that the data lines are placed between the lines of the field illustrated in *A.* Interlacing further smooths the image; however, some blurring results because the data in the second field are recorded slightly later.

fact. The side lobe concept can again be explained on the basis of Huygens' principles of wave motion. According to these principles, each point along a wave front can be considered an independent sound source that generates a spherical wave front. In the midportion of the wave, these tiny wavelets summate to form a common wave front. At the lateral margins of the sound source, however, a portion of the sound energy is transmitted radially away from the main beam axis. Radial transmission of sound energy is referred to as the edge effect. When analyzing the intensity of the ultrasonic field in a 180-degree arc about the transducer face, the peak intensity of the sound energy occurs within the confines of the main sound beam. As one moves radially away from this main beam axis, a series of gradually decreasing sound intensity peaks are encountered. These peaks alternate with areas of diminished intensity. The areas of increased sound intensity, or side lobes, represent the energy originating from the transducer edges and transmitted radially into the surrounding medium. The variation in sound intensity occurs because the net energy arising from opposite "edges" arrives at varying points in space, either in phase or out of phase. When the sound energy from two opposite edges arrives in phase, the energy summates, and a region of high intensity occurs. Conversely, when the sound energy arrives out of phase, phase cancellation occurs, and a low-intensity sound field results. Figure 2–24 illustrates the effects of the distance from the individual edges of the sound source on the phase of the sound beam and the variable intensities encountered at any point along a 180-degree arc from the sound-generating source.

Because the distance from any two points or edges of the transducer face varies depending on the point along the 180-degree arc at which the sound intensity is sampled, the sound energy alternatively is in and out of phase, and is illustrated in

A

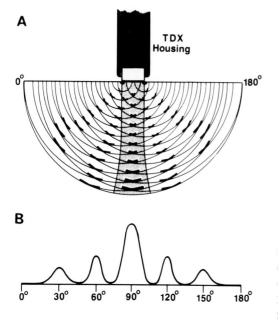

B

Fig. 2–24. Diagram illustrates the method of side lobe generation and the variations in sound intensity encountered at sequential sampling points through a 180-degree arc around the transducer face. In the upper panel, laterally directed echoes arise from the edges of the transducer. These echoes are alternately in and out of phase as they propagate radially away from the transducer face. Areas of increasing sound intensity can be detected at points where the echoes are in phase, whereas the sound intensity is relatively low in regions where the echoes are out of phase. In the lower panel, the relative sound intensities measured at various points in a 180-degree arc around the transducer are illustrated. The area of peak intensity represents the main beam. On either side of the main beam, regions of increasing intensity (corresponding to points where the radially directed sound energy is in phase) alternate with areas of lower intensity (where this energy arrives out of phase).

Figure 2–24, *B*, the intensity of the sound field varies accordingly.

The number of side lobes generated by any transducer is a function of the length of the transducer in relationship to the wavelength of the transmitted pulse. The smaller the transducer, the greater the side lobe generation. Conversely, an infinite transducer does not generate side lobes. In a single transducer system, such as a mechanical sector scanner, the side lobes, although present, are of relatively low intensity because there are only two transducer edges. In addition, the side lobes do not vary in intensity despite al-

teration in transducer position or direction.

Side lobes are a greater problem in a phased array system because one must utilize a number of small transducers, resulting in multiple edges. Each edge is capable of generating radially directed sound energy. The intensity of the side lobes also increases as the beam angle becomes more oblique relative to the transducer face. This situation results in increased side lobe intensity as the main beam approaches the margins of the sector.

Side lobes are significant from the standpoint of artifact production because all sound energy returning to the transducer is displayed as though it had originated along a line corresponding to the main beam axis. Although the intensity of the side lobes is usually considerably less than the intensity of the main beam, variability in reflector strength may cause an echo from a target within the side lobe to display as strongly as or stronger than a corresponding weaker source along the beam path. This side lobe can cause the image to become cluttered with meaningless echoes that reduce its interpretability.

For example, target B in Figure 2–25 lies in the path of a side lobe that has only 25% of the intensity of the main beam. Target B, however, has a reflectivity 10 times greater than that of target A, which lies along the path of the main beam. The resultant echo from target B is therefore $2\frac{1}{2}$ times that of the corresponding weaker target. If both targets lie at the same distance from the transducer, the echo from target A may be completely obscured. These side lobe artifacts permit the display of structures that are outside the path of the main beam as though they are lying along the beam axis and, hence, may produce gross distortions in image presentation. This problem is greater when logarithmic amplifiers are employed because they tend to increase the intensity of these weakened off-axis signals.

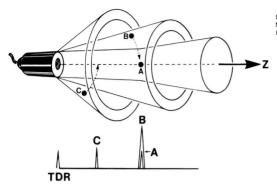

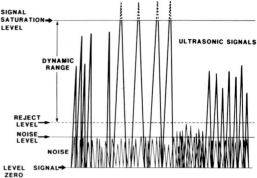

Fig. 2–25. Diagram illustrates the effects of side lobes on the displayed data. In this example, a disc-shaped transducer with a main beam and two side lobes is illustrated. Target A, a weak reflector, is located along the main axis of the sound beam. Target B, which is more highly reflective than target A, lies in the path of the inner side lobe. Target B is the same distance from the transducer as is target A. On the display, target A produces a much weaker echo than does target B and, hence, is completely overshadowed by the stronger reflection arising from the side lobe. Target C is encountered by the outer side lobe. This target is also displayed as though positioned along the central axis of the beam, and hence, its position on the display does not correspond to its true position in space.

Fig. 2–26. Diagram depicts the dynamic range of a representative echocardiographic display system. As indicated, all ultrasonic signals begin at a zero signal level and can increase in amplitude until they reach the system "signal saturation" level. Many of the low-intensity signals fall within the range of the background noise and are therefore obscured. All systems have a built-in system reject, which eliminates both the system noise and the low-intensity echoes that lie just above the noise level. The dynamic range of the system, therefore, is between the system reject level and the signal saturation level and represents the echoes that actually appear on the display scope.

Dynamic Range—Gray Scale

The acoustic transducers used in diagnostic echocardiography can record echoes over a range of pressures in excess of 100,000 to 1 (100 db). Display devices, such as television monitors, oscilloscopes, and black-and white video strip-chart recorders, used for the presentation of the ultrasonic information display an intensity range of only approximately 32 to 1 (30 db). To insure that the image presented to the diagnostician contains all the information present in the original echocardiographic signal, one must electronically manipulate the incoming ultrasonic data so that they can be faithfully displayed on the limited-range output device. To fully understand this important area, one must first define what is meant by the term, "dynamic range."

Figure 2–26 schematically depicts the "dynamic range" of a representative system. This illustration, in the form of A-mode display, indicates that all processed ultrasonic signals start at a "zero signal level" and can increase in amplitude until they reach the system's "signal saturation level." A portion of the ultrasonic information falls in the same amplitude range as that of background noise and, therefore, is obscured. Noise, which is present in all electronic systems, is a combination ·of acoustic signals that reach the transducer from structures that do not lie on the central axis of the ultrasonic beam and random electronic fluctuations that are produced in the amplifiers of the system. When amplified signals are converted from ultrasonic energy to voltage by the transducer and are processed by a linear system, the dynamic range is defined as the ratio of the largest signal that can be faithfully depicted before signal saturation to the smallest signal amplitude that can be detected above the system noise. For a 100-db range (100,000 to 1) this situation can include signal amplitudes ranging from 20 mv to 2 volts. This range is too broad for any linear system to handle.

Because all systems have a "built-in reject function" (i.e., they disallow the display of some small signal amplitudes), dynamic range is defined as the ratio of the largest signal amplitude that can be faithfully depicted before signal saturation to the smallest signal amplitude that can just be perceived above the reject level. This latter interpretation applies equally well to the display devices used in echocardiographic image acquisition and processing systems because they all possess "built-in reject functions" and signal saturation levels.

Because an imaging system cannot display simultaneously the entire range of echo amplitudes despite the use of the entire dynamic range of its acquisition, processing, and display subsystems, most echographs use some form of dynamic range compression. The resulting image depicts varying echo amplitudes as varying shades of gray.

The first dynamic-range compression method employed by commercially available echocardiographs is schematically depicted in Figure 2–27. This approach, called "clipping," simply clipped off all echoes above the amplitude at which the input signal exceeded the linear range of the amplifiers. Clipping thus restricted the range of output signals to one that the display devices could accept. This method produced an image that appeared to possess little gray scale (bistable). This loss of gray scale occurred because the gain controls were normally set to receive weak signals; consequently, the majority of signals exceeded the linear range of the amplifiers and were displayed only as maximum signals (white). These bright dots then tended to overpower the small, gray scale, presenting echoes from the weaker reflectors that were adjacent to them. This resulted in a black-and-white image with no intermediate shades of gray.

A variety of more recent devices has been developed that permits the selection of variable relationships between the input and output signals. In some instances, the operator can select the specific type of signal processing that is most appropriate to the study being performed. Figure 2–28 is an example of one type of signal processing that has been utilized to highlight higher-intensity echoes when looking for increases in reflectivity arising from diseased vascular walls. This format is only

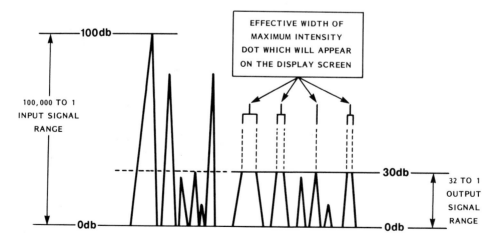

Fig. 2–27. Diagram illustrates the use of "clipping" to produce dynamic range compression. In this format, all echoes above the output capacity of the amplification and display apparatus are simply clipped when they reach a threshold level. Such action effectively restricts the range of the output signal to a level that the display devices can accept. The relative intensity of the signals above the clipping level is indicated by the width of the base of the remaining echo and, hence, by the intensity of the display dot on the imaging scope.

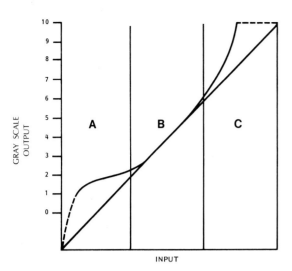

Fig. 2–28. Diagram illustrates one method of varying the relationship between the input and the output signals. In this format, the low-intensity signals (A) are logarithmically amplified and displayed over the lower two shades of gray on the output grade scale. The midrange signals (B) are then displayed in a linear fashion over the next four shades of gray. The high-intensity input signals (C) are exponentially amplified and displayed over the final four shades of the gray scale. This format compresses the lower-intensity signals into a relatively homogeneous field of gray while amplifying the higher-intensity signals, causing them to stand out in contrast to the homogeneous background.

one of an almost limitless series of relationships that can be established between the input and output signals.

The usefulness of various forms of gray-scale imaging is well established in obstetric and abdominal ultrasonic imaging. In cardiac imaging, where structure location and motion have received more attention than has echo quality, this methodology has been less completely studied. It is anticipated, however, that gray scale, as well as other forms of signal processing, will become increasingly more important as more and more echocardiographic imaging systems with the ability to display the full range of diagnostic information in levels of gray become available.

Persistence

When the electron beam of a cathode ray tube strikes the front surface of the tube,

the phosphor coating surface is illuminated and begins to glow. The length of time the phosphor glows after initial illumination is an inherent property of the phosphor and is termed persistence. Persistence is the basis of all image formation because, without some degree of persistence, the data would disappear immediately from the screen, and no image would result. The use of the persistence of the eye alone would require a high frame rate. Thus, an aircraft propeller appears to the eye as a disc; however, the revolutions per minute (rpm's) of the propeller are of a different order of magnitude than are those of standard imaging frame rates.

Persistence is seen and utilized daily in cardiology. The tracing on the standard bedside electrocardiographic monitor represents the persistent trail of the electron beam as it sweeps across the surface of the monitor, displaying voltage change relative to time. Similarly, the standard M-mode echocardiographic sweep represents information that is left behind or persists as the ultrasonic data line that displays echo amplitude and depth is swept across the face of the oscilloscope.

The same oscilloscopes (CRT) are utilized for repeated data visualization in most of these display formats; thus, the afterglow of the phosphor should gradually fade away so that the scope is available for the next image. If further images are not displayed, the time required for the initial images to fade can be appreciated. If, however, a second image is written before the first image has completely disappeared, one must rely on the increased intensity of the new information to dominate the display while the decaying data from the previous sweep become relatively less dominant. Because cross-sectional images are written rapidly, one on top of the other, four or more fields may be displayed before the recorded data from the first field totally fade.

The choice of phosphor determines the amount of "history" to be dealt with by the examiner. As a rule, the variation in intensity permits the eye to exclude data that are less intense or persistent and to concentrate on newly written or current information. In certain circumstances, however, the persistence may create significant artifacts. Thus, if a particularly strong echo source is displayed, the echo data from the first frame may be sufficiently bright to appear in the third or fourth frame. These dominant, persistent echoes may then be confused with more recently written, but less intense, echo information, creating a "persistence artifact" (Fig. 2–29). In addition, the position of an interface may change from frame to frame during real-time dynamic imaging, and as a result, persistent data may lie next to, rather than beneath, previously recorded data. Such positioning blurs the display.

The effect of writing one image on top of another is particularly apparent in oscillating transducer systems. As the oscillating transducer sweeps in one direction (left to right), it continuously writes information on the oscilloscope. When it reaches the full extent of its arc and reverses its course (right to left), it initially writes new data on top of the information from the end of the last sweep, which still persists brightly. Conversely, the data at the far end of the sweep have now been on the scope for a longer period of time and are beginning to fade. In this situation, on one half of the sector recent data are inscribed twice, whereas on the other half, nothing has been written for a relatively long time. As a result, half of the screen is bright, and the other half is relatively less intense.

While the inherent persistence in a single display tube may produce artifacts, many echocardiographic systems contain multiple cathode ray tubes in series leading to the final display. Each of these tubes has its individual persistence. The sum of the persistent artifacts from each tube may be considerable. In the standard display format utilized in many commercial in-

struments, the inital image is recorded directly on a cathode ray tube, which introduces persistence. The image on this cathode ray tube is then recorded using a television camera, which introduces a second persistence. The video information is then redisplayed on a television monitor, which introduces a third persistence. In addition to the variation in persistences of the individual instruments, the persistence of each tube may change over time as the phosphor ages. When one looks at an individual field, therefore, the resultant data represent the sum total of current data plus persistent data. The amount and complexity of the persistent data are determined by the relative persistences of the multiple components in the display chain.

Several display modifications have been attempted to eliminate, or at least to highlight, some of the persistence artifact. The first modification uses a phosphor that is initially illuminated in one color but persists in a second color. An example is the P7 phosphor utilized in at least one commercial instrument. The P7 phosphor is illuminated in blue and persists in yellow. In this format, "persistent" data can readily be distinguished from more recently acquired data. Another method for eliminating or controlling some of the persistence artifact is direct recording, which will be discussed in the section on types of display. Unfortunately, no universally acceptable approach to this problem has to date been identified.

Complex Signal Processing

Because of the difficulties in appropriately displaying the raw echo data, new approaches to signal processing are being explored. Many of the more sophisticated approaches to signal processing involve digitizing the returning echoes. Once in this form, the acoustic data can be mathematically manipulated with ease.

Digital signal processing can be used to simulate different amplifier transfer func-

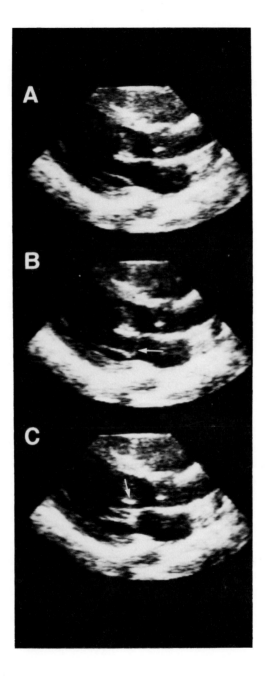

Fig. 2–29.   Series of parasternal long-axis recordings of the mitral valve during valve closure illustrates the effects of persistence of the resulting image. A, Recorded just prior to initial leaflet closure. The anterior mitral leaflet is in an open position and lies perpendicular to the path of scan plane. In this position, it is highly reflective and produces a bright echo. B, The anterior leaflet has closed, as indicated by the horizontal arrow. The bright echo from the open leaflet recorded in the previous frame still persists and is more obvious than the true echo from the closed leaflet, which now lies parallel to the path of the scan plane. C, A still later frame. The closed leaflets are now more prominent, but the echo from the previously open leaflet still persists (oblique arrow). If the effects of persistence were not recognized, the abnormal echo in Figure 2–29, B, might have been interpreted as an abnormality of the mitral leaflet itself.

tions. As a result, log, linear, exponential, and various other transfer functions can be obtained. Another signal processing approach is similar to the picture enhancement done for the space program. Echoes are selectively printed or deleted based on amplitude and density information of the surrounding echoes. These schemes can improve lateral and longitudinal resolution within their design limits. Fast Fourier transformation, auto correlation, and convolution are some of the many other techniques available to process acoustic data. Usually the signal is returned to analog form for display after processing is completed.

Image Recording Techniques

For maximum clinical utility, cross-sectional images must be displayed and recorded simultaneously. In addition, they should be available for instant playback and analysis. Detailed analysis further requires their availability for viewing in real-time, slow-motion, and stop-frame formats. In addition, the volume of data acquired in a single study makes a rapid scanning capability in both forward and reverse modes desirable. This flexibility is generally found only in a video recording format; consequently, cross-sectional images are primarily recorded on magnetic videotape.

Initially, movie film was tried because it is generally less expensive and more flexible than videotape, is easily spliced, and can be shown almost anywhere. The lack of an instant playback capability, however, makes this format impractical for routine studies.

Acoustic data can be transferred to videotape by two methods. The first and, by far, the most commonly utilized is to simply focus a television camera on the screen of the X-Y monitor. The "vidicon" then converts the ultrasonic image to a television image using an electron beam that scans a photoconductive target, which is placed in the focal plane of the camera lens. The resultant electronic signals from the television camera can then be displayed on a television monitor and/or recorded by a videotape recorder. Because the format in which the television image is formed on the television monitor is different from the scanning format associated with the ultrasonic image, this process is called "scan conversion."

Television recording is easy to implement and uses devices that are inexpensive and readily available. Several limitations of the method have been noted, however. These limitations relate to the persistence artifacts discussed earlier and the difference in scan rate of the ultrasonic and video images.

To overcome these problems, systems for direct ultrasonic recording have been developed. The electronic signals associated with the echocardiographic image are displayed and recorded without use of a scan converter.[21] As a result, the visualized image is a direct reproduction of the original cardiac imaging signals. This image is achieved by recording each ultrasonic data line and its spatial coordinates directly on videotape and, at the same time, precisely synchronizing the ultrasonic field rate with the corresponding video field rate. This procedure eliminates the persistence artifacts associated with scan conversion. It also allows the stored data to be processed and its display characteristic to be varied at a later point in time because all the original ultrasonic data are recorded. The complexity of this system, however, and the necessity for reassembling and displaying all data through the original recording system, thereby making replay on other television systems impossible, have limited its general acceptance.

FACTORS AFFECTING THE CROSS-SECTIONAL DISPLAY CHARACTERISTICS OF A POINT TARGET

A number of factors affect the manner in which a point target, swept by a cross-sectional beam, appears on the final display. These factors are summarized in Figure 2–30. *A*, illustrates a single circular point target. In panel *B*, an ultrasonic beam is swept across the point target from left to right. As the right-hand margin of the beam encounters the target, an echo is produced by the target. This echo, however, is displayed as though the point target were lying along the beam axis. When the beam has a width of 1 centimeter at the level of the point target, the target is displaced 5 millimeters to the left on the display. As the beam continues across the point target for an additional 5 millimeters, the target is then intersected by the true beam axis and, hence, is appropriately displayed. Further motion of the beam aligns the target at the left-hand margin. In this position the target again is displayed as though it were positioned along the beam axis and,

hence, is displaced 5 millimeters to the right.

Panel *C* illustrates the final display configuration of this single point target. Because an echo is continuously produced by this target while it lies within the sound beam, the point is effectively spread in a lateral dimension equal to the diameter of the beam. This "point-spread function," therefore, corresponds to the beam diameter. Targets positioned in the far field of the beam, where the lateral extent is greater, tend to undergo more spreading, whereas those in the narrower portion of the beam tend to be displayed more appropriately.

Panel *D* illustrates the effect of increasing gain on the displayed target. As the gain of the system is increased, the effective beam width also tends to increase, resulting in a greater point-spread function

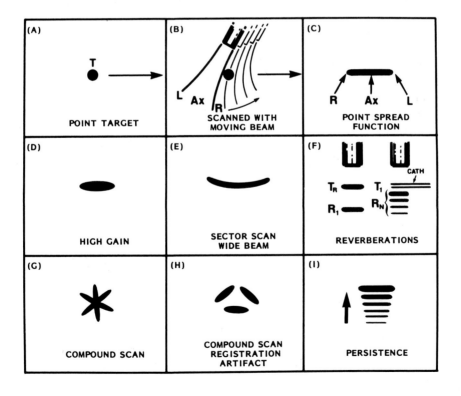

Fig. 2–30. Summary of factors influencing the cross-sectional display characteristics of a point target.

and image width. In the axial dimension, an increase in gain tends to increase the width of the echo, particularly in the video format as indicated in Chapter 1. Therefore, the point target is displayed as an elongated oval.

Panel E illustrates the effect of excessive beam width in a sector scanning format on the target echo. Because the beam sweeps in an arc, a target that is a constant distance from the transducer face is displayed in an arcuate fashion when scanned by a relatively wide beam. This phenomenon also affects targets that are scanned by narrower beams; however, when the beam width is limited, this effect is not as apparent and is generally undetected.

Panel F depicts two of the more characteristic patterns that can be seen as a result of internal reverberations of echoes. In the left-hand illustration, a single image (TR), produced by the actual target, is followed by a second image, R_1, which represents a reverberation. This phenomenon occurs because the sound energy is reflected back to the transducer from the target and strikes the transducer face. It can then be reflected back to the target and then to the transducer a second time. This motion produces a second echo that is twice the distance of the first echo from the transducer.

The right-hand panel illustrates the type of reverberation frequently seen when a pulse strikes a target composed of several highly reflected interfaces. In this example, an angiographic catheter has been used. The sound energy that strikes the catheter can be reflected back and forth a number of times by the interfaces that comprise the catheter walls before returning to the transducer. When this occurs, a series of echoes is produced behind the catheter, whose distance from the transducers is a reflection of the number of internal reflections that occur prior to the echo's exit from the catheter. This type of reverberation is frequently seen in patients with Swan-Ganz or other hemodynamic catheters in place during the echocardiographic study.

Panel G illustrates the appearance of a target that is scanned from several different directions. The point-spread function, which occurs perpendicular to the axis of beams originating from a variety of directions, results in a rosette-like display of the point target. Thus, although compound scanning enhances the operator's chances of recording an individual target, it may also distort the final display characteristics of that target.

The combined effects of compound scanning and registration artifacts are indicated in panel H. Registration artifacts arise because of variations in the speed of the sound wave as it approaches a target from different directions. The echograph assumes the speed of sound to be constant and, hence, displays all targets at a distance calculated from this assumed speed. The speed of sound through muscle, blood, and other tissues, however, varies slightly. As a result, a sound beam approaching a target along a number of different paths encounters each of these media in differing proportions. The actual time taken by the sound beam to reach the target, therefore, may vary slightly depending on the path taken. When this time variance occurs, the target appears on the display as a series of linear echoes that do not intersect at a common point (panel H).

The final artifact is produced by the persistence of the image frames themselves. Panel I illustrates the appearance of the persistence artifact when imaging a point target that is moving anteriorly toward the transducer. The upper linear echo is the reflection from the linear target. Each of the linear echoes beneath the dominant echo has a sequentially diminished intensity and represents the echoes from that target recorded in earlier frames. These earlier echoes are gradually fading with time. Because the echo is rapidly moving, any residual data from earlier frames are exposed and become evident. When the point target is a strong reflector, the residual data may persist for many frames and, hence, may blur the image.

REFERENCES

1. Wild, JJ, and Reid, JM: Application of echoranging techniques to the determination of structure of biological tissues. Science, 115:226, 1952.
2. Howry, D, and Bliss, W: Ultrasonic visualization of soft tissue structure of the body. J Lab Clin Med, 40:579, 1952.
3. Wild, JJ, Crawford, HD, and Reid, JM: Visualization of the excised human heart by means of reflected ultrasound or echocardiography. Am Heart J, 54:903, 1957.
4. Ebina, T, et al.: The ultrasono-tomography of the heart and great vessels in living human subjects by means of the ultrasonic reflection technique. Jpn Heart J, 8:331, 1967.
5. Ashberg, A: Cinematography of the living heart. Ultrasonics, 5:143, 1967.
6. Somer, FC: Electronic sector-scanning for ultrasonic diagnosis. Ultrasonics, 6:153, 1968.
7. Bom, N, Lancee, CT, and HonKoop, J: Ultrasonic viewer for cross-sectional analysis of moving cardiac structures. Bio-Med Engineering, 6:500, 1971.
8. Bom, N, et al.: Multiscan echocardiography I. Circulation, 48:1066, 1973.
9. Roelandt, J, et al.: Resolution problems in echocardiology: a source of interpretation errors. Am J Cardiol, 37(2):256, 1976.
10. Kloster, FE, et al.: Multiscan echocardiography II. Technique and initial clinical results. Circulation, 48:1075, 1973.
11. Bom, N, et al.: Evaluation of structure recognition with the multiscan echograph: a cooperative study in 580 patients. Ultrasound Med Biol, 1:243, 1974.
12. Griffith, JM, and Henry, WL: A sector scanner for real time two-dimensional echocardiography. Circulation, 49:1147, 1974.
13. Eggleton, RC, et al.: Visualization of cardiac dynamics with real time B-mode ultrasonic scanner (abstr). Circulation, (Suppl III), 49 and 50:26, 1974.
14. Eggleton, RC, and Johnston, KW: Real time mechanical scanning system compared with array techniques. Institute of Electrical and Electronic Engineers, Proceedings in Sonics and Ultrasonics, November 1974.
15. Eggleton RC, et al.: Visualization of cardiac dynamics with real time B-mode ultrasonic scanners. In Ultrasound in Medicine. Edited by D White. New York, Plenum Press, 1975.
16. McDicken, WM, Bruff, K, and Paton, J: An ultrasonic instrument for rapid B-scanning of the heart. Ultrasonics, 13:269, 1974.
17. Von Ramm, OT, and Thurstone, FL: Cardiac imaging using a phased array ultrasound system. I. System design. Circulation, 53(2):258, 1976.
18. Kisslo, J, Von Ramm, OT, and Thurstone, FL: Cardiac imaging using a phased array ultrasound system. II. Clinical technique and application. Circulation, 53(2):262, 1976.
19. Kisslo, JA, Von Ramm, OT, and Thurstone, FL: Dynamic cardiac imaging using a focused, phased-array ultrasound system. Am J Med, 63(1):61, 1977.
20. Somer, JC: Transducer arrays. In Handbook of Clinical Ultrasound. Edited by M deVlieger, et al. New York, John Wiley & Sons, 1978.
21. Goldberg, PR: Principles of two dimensional real time echocardiographic imaging. Acta Med Scand, Suppl, 627:7, 1978.

Section 2

The Cross-Sectional Examination—General Principles and Standard Imaging Planes

Chapter 3

Cross-Sectional Echocardiographic Examination

The goal of the cross-sectional examination is to optimally record the anatomic and functional characteristics of a particular area or areas of the heart in a number of tomographic imaging planes. If this goal can be achieved, the size, shape, relative position, and both absolute and relative motion patterns of multiple cardiac structures can be assessed.[1–5]

To achieve this goal, all cross-sectional echocardiographic instruments provide a small, flexible, hand-held probe, which can be easily manipulated by the examiner.[6–10] Figure 3–1 illustrates a typical probe and the fan-shaped imaging plane it generates. Three dimensions or axes characterize this imaging plane: (1) the depth of field or distance from the transducer face (the Z axis), (2) the width from one margin of the plane to the other (the Y axis), and (3) the thickness (the X axis). Although represented as a plane, the scan area is actually composed of a series of individual sound pulses or beams. The beam that propagates directly away from the transducer face and, as such, is an extension of the long axis of the probe is referred to as the central ray.

The flexibility of the probe permits almost limitless variation in the direction in which the imaging plane can be oriented to transect the heart. Despite this flexibility, aligning the probe and, hence, the examining plane to optimally record a particular structure may prove to be a formidable task for a number of reasons.

First, the examiner is attempting to visualize a specific area within an organ (the heart) which itself cannot be seen. External reference points on the chest wall may help to locate the heart; however, the position and orientation of individual cardiac structures within the chest are so variable that final plane orientation must be related to, and determined by, the particular area one wishes to visualize. This, in turn, requires that the examiner be able to (1) identify intracardiac structures from the images they produce, (2) define the plane in which they are visualized, (3) understand how to realign the imaging plane to achieve optimal visualization, and (4)

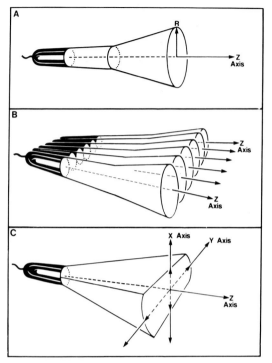

Fig. 3–1. Diagram illustrates the formation of a cross-sectional imaging plane from a series of individual ultrasonic beams or pulses. *A,* A single ultrasonic beam. The Z axis corresponds to a long axis down the center of the beam. It propagates away from the transducer face and can be considered an extension of the long axis of the transducer. R = the radius of the sound beam at any point along the Z axis for a disc-shaped transducer. *B,* An illustration of how the series of sound beams can be aligned next to one another to form a scan plane. *C,* An illustration of the resultant imaging plane. This plane can be described by three axes. The Z axis, which corresponds to the path of the scan plane as it propagates away from the transducer, is an extension of the long axis of the transducer. The Y axis is perpendicular to the Z axis and extends from one lateral margin of the scan plane to the other. The X axis is orthogonal to both the Y and Z axes and represents the thickness of the scan plane. These axes obviously vary in length, depending on where in the scan plane they are measured. Therefore, these axes have no absolute values.

recognize when such visualization is achieved. All these functions must occur almost simultaneously as the examination progresses to obtain the best final image.

Second, the flexibility of the transducer allows the imaging plane to be directed toward the heart from a number of different vantage points. From any of these transducer positions, the imaging plane

can be rotated 360 degrees, and at any degree of rotation, the plane can be angled through a wide arc. This enormous degree of flexibility presents the examiner with an equally enormous variety of potential image formats that must be recognized and interpreted.

Finally, the broad imaging plane encompasses a large area of the heart. Although the imaging plane configuration is fixed, the relationships of cardiac structures that fall within the plane are variable. Consequently, the plane may be appropriately aligned to optimally record a particular aspect of one structure while other areas within the same scan plane are poorly visualized. These nongeometric relationships of anatomic structures relative to the fixed planar area create further imaging artifacts, which must be recognized and their cause appreciated.

Despite these difficulties, one can perform a cross-sectional study that records high quality images that appropriately depict the structural configuration and motion of numerous areas of the heart. Appropriate performance of the cross-sectional examination, however, requires that the examiner have: (1) an appreciation of the three-dimensional anatomy of the heart, (2) the ability to conceptualize how the same structure might appear when viewed in a number of different projections, (3) an understanding of the patterns produced when a plane transects a variety of geometric figures along a number of paths, (4) a knowledge and understanding of a number of standardized imaging planes and an ability to recognize when these images are optimally recorded, and (5) an ability to recognize and make allowances for the effects of pathologic conditions on the appearance and orientation of a structure. The flexibility of the cross-sectional technique and the large variety of data that can be recorded therefore require a high degree of technical expertise to produce consistently useful clinical information.

The purpose of this and the following chapter is: (1) to describe the steps necessary to record optimal cross-sectional images, (2) to review the most commonly utilized imaging planes and the method for standardizing image orientation, and (3) to explore methods by which other ultrasonic imaging formats, particularly the M-mode echocardiogram, can be utilized to augment the data generated in a cross-sectional study.

THE CROSS-SECTIONAL EXAMINATION

The cross-sectional echocardiographic examination proceeds in a series of steps. These steps can be divided into those that are preliminary to the actual performance of the examination and those encompassed in the examination itself. Preliminary steps include: (1) the initial approach to the patient, (2) considerations in dealing with uncooperative patients, (3) transducer selection, and (4) initial instrument control setting. The examination itself proceeds in a stepwise, albeit more integrated, fashion. The sequence of the examination is: (1) location of the heart, (2) initial structure identification, (3) initial determination of plane orientation, and (4) fine plane positioning.

Preliminary Steps

Initial Approach to the Patient

The cross-sectional examination is appropriately performed on cardiac patients of all ages, from the premature infant to the elderly person.[11-14] The basic approach is similar for all patients regardless of age or sex. In preparation for the examination, the patient should be placed in the supine position on a comfortable examining surface. The room should be darkened slightly to permit maximal visualization of the display scope and also to provide a relaxed environment. The patient should be undressed to the waist. Exposure of a large area of the chest is necessary to make ad-

equate use of all the probe positions from which the examining plane can be directed toward the heart. For female patients, this exposure occasionally results in some embarrassment. Such embarrassment should be overcome before beginning the study so that it does not become a recurrent problem as increasingly larger areas of the chest must be explored to record an adequate examination. An examining gown, open in the front, allows the patient to be covered and yet permits broad access to the chest wall.

Some form of timing information should be recorded so that the events occurring during the echocardiographic examination can be temporally related. For this purpose, an electrocardiogram is customarily recorded with the cross-sectional study.[11-14] The electrocardiographic data then can be redisplayed with the individual image frames to help to establish the timing of each frame within the cardiac cycle. When recording the electrocardiogram, only the limb leads are utilized because the exploring chest electrode would interfere with transducer placement. Additional timing information can be obtained from other graphic recording devices, such as the phonocardiogram and arterial and venous pulse tracings. Unfortunately, the cross-sectional images are recorded at a relatively slow frame rate, which limits the timing value of many of these graphic recordings. When an M-mode study is recorded in conjunction with the cross-sectional examination, these recordings retain their inherent usefulness. When a number of studies are recorded simultaneously, all recording electrodes, microphones, or other sensing devices must be attached prior to initiating the echocardiographic examination.

Before beginning the examination, both the patient and the examiner must be as comfortable as possible. If the patient is in an uncomfortable position, he will move about, thereby necessitating continual readjustment of the examining plane. If the examiner is uncomfortable, he will rapidly become fatigued, thereby shortening the time that can be devoted to the examination and limiting the quality of the data that are finally collected.

The examiner should be seated at the patient's side at the same level as the patient and should be able to reposition the patient (e.g., by using an electric bed) or to adjust the controls on the echocardiographic equipment without moving. This environment is most aptly achieved in a well-designed echocardiographic laboratory. Whenever possible, the echocardiographic examination should be performed in such a controlled setting (Fig. 3–2). However, when dealing with critically ill patients, one must frequently perform studies on a portable basis. The examiner is rarely as comfortable and the patient is rarely as cooperative in such a setting. This is frequently reflected in the quality of the data.

The operator generally approaches the patient from the right side. The probe is then held in the right hand, and the instrument controls are adjusted with the left. The right-sided approach is preferable because: (1) the majority of examiners are right handed; therefore, the fine probe positioning, rotation, and angulation that are required during the examination can be performed more readily with the probe in the right hand rather than the left; (2) the right hand is generally stronger and does not fatigue as quickly as does the left; (3) many cross-sectional studies must be recorded with the patient on the left side and/or with the probe positioned at the cardiac apex. With the examiner on the patient's right side, the right arm naturally falls across the chest to the cardiac apex, thereby allowing easy probe manipulation in this area. Conversely, from the left side, the probe must be held in an awkward, backhanded fashion when attempting to

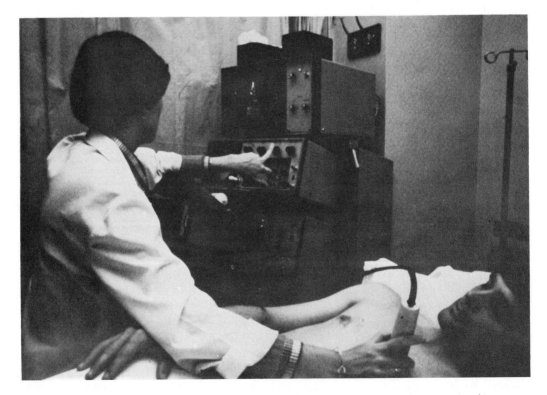

Fig. 3–2. Proper position of the echocardiographic technician relative to the patient and cross-sectional instrument.

examine a patient in the left lateral position or to record apical images. Such positioning limits probe control and flexibility.

Difficult or Uncooperative Patients

On occasion, the echocardiographic examination may be more difficult because of lack of patient cooperation, limited patient mobility, or restricted access to the precordium. In these circumstances, the approach to the patient may need modification.

Lack of patient cooperation is most frequently encountered in the pediatric age group. Lack of cooperation is most commonly due to fright on initial exposure to a strange procedure or to fatigue in the latter stages of the examination.

As a rule, once a child's cooperation has been lost, the examination is effectively over. Attempts to re-establish rapport using distractions, such as cookies, rattles or lollipops, may occasionally regain cooperation, but the cooperation is usually short lived. Although useful data are occasionally obtained from a "moving target," such a situation is less than optimal. The examiner is then faced with the option of accepting an incomplete study, repeating the examination at a later date, or sedating the child. It is best, therefore, to make every effort to establish good rapport at the onset and to be assured that the child is comfortable during the study.

Several steps may help to allay initial fear of the examination. If the child is old enough to understand, he should be introduced to the instrumentation and told how he will be able to "see his heart on television." He should be given a chance to hold the examining probe and to assure himself that the probe will not hurt. Such assurances are particularly helpful when using an oscillating probe because its noise and vibration sometimes cause even adults to expect that the examination will be painful. The probe should be initially applied to the hand or to the forearm as often as necessary to make the child comfortable. When actually applied to the chest, the probe can be supported by the examiner's little finger, thereby limiting actual skin contact. If the child still indicates discomfort, a sufficient amount of coupling gel can be used so that the probe never actually touches the chest during the examination. If parents are present, the examiner may inform them about the nature of the examination and may explain in general terms what is being recorded during the examination. This information puts them at ease, and their sense of calm is transmitted to the child. Once the examination has begun, the child should remain involved in the process and should be kept comfortable.

Another frightening aspect of the examination, particularly for small children, is the attachment of the EKG electrodes. Experience suggests that this procedure may be more frightening than the examination itself. When examining patients with congenital heart disease, structure orientation and identification are far more important than timing motion. If the electrocardiographic leads, therefore, prove disquieting, they can be easily omitted. Adequate timing information to establish the sequence of cardiac events generally can be derived from the cross-sectional echogram itself. But, if all else fails, sedation may be required. The decision to sedate a child is determined after considering the importance of the information to be derived from the study and after consulting with the responsible physician.

Adult patients may also be uncooperative and even openly combative. This reaction is usually a reflection of their underlying disease process. Again, a decision must be made in conjunction with the responsible physician as to whether the clinical question to be answered by the echogram warrants sedating or restraining the patient.

Other situations related to the patient's clinical condition may prevent the positioning required to obtain an optimal study. Such difficulties arise most commonly in patients on ventilators, with arterial or venous pressure-monitoring catheters in place, or in traction. In these situations, the operators should attempt to record as much information as possible, recognizing that the quality of the examination may not be optimal. These studies should be interpreted in this light, and if circumstances permit, the patient may need to be restudied at a later date in the more controlled environment of the echocardiographic laboratory.

Finally, there are a number of situations in which access to the chest may be limited. This occurs following cardiac surgery when the midportion of the patient's chest is commonly covered with bandages, in patients with acute myocardial infarction when monitoring electrodes may cover the principal echocardiographic windows, and in patients with chest wounds, burns, or extensive abrasions. Frequently, examinations in these situations are requested by physicians who are unfamiliar with the technical requirements of the echocardiographic study. When such requests are made, the primary physician should be contacted, and the requirements of the examination should be explained. Bandages or electrodes should never be removed by the operator independently, and the transducer should never be placed in an area of the chest in which the skin surface is not intact.

Selection of a Transducer

Transducers vary in size, frequency, and focal characteristics. Selection of the appropriate transducer for a particular clinical study is determined by the physical characteristics of the patient and by the requirements of the examination. The transducers used in M-mode echocardiography are relatively simple and inexpensive. As a result, many laboratories have a variety of M-mode transducers, and the examiner can select the transducer most appropriate to a particular situation. The probes used in cross-sectional imaging are far more complex and expensive. Probe design and operating characteristics may also be an integral part of the overall cross-sectional imaging system. As a result, the examiner frequently has little if any choice regarding the cross-sectional probe to be used for a given study.

Despite this current lack of flexibility in cross-sectional transducer selection, a discussion of the transducer is important for two reasons: (1) it can be anticipated that, with continued improvement in instrument design, more flexibility will be available in the future, and (2) the transducer is probably the most important component in any cross-sectional system. When transducers cannot be interchanged, the type of system initially chosen for a laboratory may be influenced by the characteristics of the transducer used by the system.

Transducer size refers to the area or diameter of the transducer face. The area of the transducer face in a single element system is a function of the size of the individual transducer. In an array of transducers, the area of the transducer face is the sum of the areas of all the transducers in the array. Both the size and shape of the transducer face are important from an imaging standpoint because they determine the area encompassed by the sound beam, the length of the near field in each dimension, the angle of divergence in the far field, and the depth at which the beam can be acoustically focused. As a rule, larger transducers have better beam characteristics and can be brought to a sharper, more intense focus at a deeper tissue depth (see Chap. 1).[15,16]

Transducer size also determines the size of the acoustic window required to transmit the examining plane into the chest. Because the window size for any patient is relatively fixed, transducer size must be appropriate to the clinical environment. The size of the transducer should correspond as closely as possible to the size of the echocardiographic window through which the imaging plane is directed. This relationship in size is important because the area of the raster* of the display corresponds to the physical area of the imaging plane. When transducer size is larger than window size, the portion of the imaging plane arising from the segment of the transducer face that lies outside the window is not transmitted, and the margins of the display raster are blank. When an interruption in the window lies beneath the transducer, information is missing in a more central portion of the raster, thereby producing an "acoustic shadow." Transducers that are small enough to fit cleanly within the clinical echocardiographic window provide uninterrupted images, whereas those that are too large for a single window or that overlie a number of separate windows produce truncated or interrupted images.

The second factor to be considered in transducer selection is frequency. When determining the appropriate transducer frequency, one must consider the relationship of resolution and penetration. Resolution is the ability to distinguish structures that are closely related in space as separate. Penetration is the ability of the sound beam to penetrate the heart and to reach the individual structures the examiner seeks to record. Resolution is directly related to frequency. As frequency increases, resolution also increases. Table 3–1 illustrates the wavelengths and, therefore, the relative resolving powers of a series of transducers of increasing frequencies. Increasing frequency, however, also increases attenuation. An increase in attenuation restricts the ability of the sound waves to penetrate the heart; consequently, frequency and penetration are inversely related. Without penetration, res-

*The raster is the area in the CRT in which the image is reproduced.

TABLE 3–1

RELATIONSHIP OF TRANSDUCER FREQUENCY TO WAVELENGTH

Frequency (MHz)	Wavelength (mm)	Wavelength (micron)
1	1.500	1,500
2.5	0.600	600
5	0.300	300
7.5	0.200	200
10	0.150	150
100	0.015	15

olution is meaningless. Penetration, therefore, is of primary importance when considering these two variables.

In adults, the sound beam must often penetrate to tissue depths of 20 cm or more. This requirement is particularly true when using the apical or subcostal windows. When an intensity loss of 1 db per cm per MHz is assumed, a pulse transmitted from a 2-MHz transducer loses 40 db in reaching this 20-cm depth. Because another 40 db are lost during the return trip to the transducer when using the pulsed echo method, a total of 80 db or a 10,000-fold loss in signal strength is encountered at this transducer frequency. At the same tissue depth, a comparable pulse from a 4-MHz transducer undergoes a 160-db intensity loss. By way of comparison, the dynamic range of the amplifiers of most echographs is only 80 to 100 db. Therefore, although the intensity of any echo is a function of the intensity of the input pulse, a signal loss of 80 db at conventional input intensities still permits the returning echoes to be recorded and amplified. A loss of 160 db places the returning echo beyond the recording and amplification capabilities of most commercial instruments. An increase in the intensity of the input signal can compensate for the loss in signal strength encountered during tissue passage; however, at high input intensities, attenuation becomes nonlinear and increases as input power increases.

In the adult population, therefore, transducers with a frequency range of 2 to 2.5 MHz provide the penetration necessary to record the back wall of the heart and to still maintain an axial resolution in the range of 1 millimeter. Several recently developed instruments utilize 3.5-MHz transducers. Surprisingly good penetration has been achieved with these instruments in some patients while providing the increased resolution inherent in a higher frequency element. When evaluating such an instrument for routine use, however, one must examine typical rather than optimal patients to be sure that the penetration of the transducer is adequate for the routine clinical population of the laboratory.

Penetration may prove to be a particular problem in certain circumstances—most commonly in the barrel-chested or obese patient. Theoretically, a lower-frequency transducer (in the 1-MHz range) would be most useful. In practice, however, the number of times this situation actually occurs rarely justifies the additional expense of such a low-frequency probe. In addition, the increased field of vision and spatial orientation provided by the cross-sectional technique permit the examiner to approach the heart from a number of different vantage points, thereby increasing the opportunity to obtain useful data in all types of patients.

In infants and small children, the back wall of the heart is closer to the exploring probe, and penetration is less of a problem. For these situations, higher-frequency transducers can more easily be used. Thus, when the back wall of the heart is 10 cm from the transducer, a 2-MHz probe encounters only a 40-db loss in signal strength, whereas at 5 cm, this loss is only 20 db. Thus, in a small infant, one can theoretically use a frequency as high as 10 MHz and still generate echoes with intensities within the recording and amplification capabilities of the instrument.

The choice of transducer frequency may also be limited by the operating characteristics of a particular system. In mechanical scanning systems, transducer frequency is not limited by instrument design, and hence, almost any frequency can be selected. In the phased array format, the choice of frequency is limited by the system itself. To date, the highest frequency obtained by using a phased array system has been 3.5 MHz.

In addition to defining the limits of frequency (as discussed in Chap. 2), the depth of field also determines the line or pulse repetition frequency. Thus, the closer the examined structures are to the transducer, the shorter the transit time of the ultrasonic pulse and the more rapidly pulses can be transmitted. Therefore, when examining structures that are relatively close to the transducer, both the transducer frequency and the line repetition frequency can be increased, thereby producing an image in the infant and the young child that is of higher overall quality than that generally obtainable in the adult.

The final consideration in transducer selection is focusing characteristics. In the single element mechanical or rotary systems, focusing is achieved by placing an acoustic lens over the front face of the transducer. This acoustic lens brings the beam to a focus within the near field of the transducer at a point that is determined by the radius of curvature of the lens. Increasing the size of the transducer increases the length of the near field and, hence, increases the depth at which the focus can be achieved. Once the radius of curvature of the lens is assigned, however, the focal length becomes fixed.

The possibility of achieving a variable focal length in a mechanical system by the use of an annular array of transducers has been suggested. In the annular array format, a series of concentrically oriented elements are used to transmit the interrogating pulse. As the pulse traverses the tissue, echoes arising from reflectors along the midportion of the beam strike each of the concentric rings in phase and, therefore, summate. Those arising from outside the central ray of the beam strike the concentric rings out-of-phase and, hence, tend to cancel each other. Optimizing the recording of reflectors along the central axis of the beam effectively focuses in both the Y or lateral and the X or thickness dimensions of the imaging plane.

In the phased array format, as discussed in Chapter 2, focusing can be achieved by three different methods: 1) An acoustic lens, 2) dynamic transmit and receive focusing, and 3) shading.

Initial Control Settings

Before beginning the cross-sectional examination, the instrument settings under operator control must be adjusted to permit initial image recording. These controls were discussed in Chapter 1 and include the system gain or coarse gain, which controls the amplitude of all echoes within the examining plane; the time-gain compensation or TGC, which selectively amplifies far-field echoes to correct for the normal loss of strength of the echo beam as it traverses the heart; the near gain, which controls the amplitude of echoes in close proximity to the transducer; the reject circuit, which selectively filters out all echoes below a certain predetermined amplitude; and the damping control, which adjusts the strength of the transmitted signal.

Specific control settings vary with different types of instrumentation and, as a result, must be individualized depending on the type of instrument used. In general, cross-sectional scanners, which have evolved from older M-mode echographs and utilize the original driving source, tend to be underpowered. The initial gain settings for these instruments are therefore higher than those required by instruments designed specifically for cross-sectional imaging. Ideal gain settings are deter-

mined by examining a number of representative patients with a particular instrument and recording the control settings at which optimal studies are recorded. A clinical range of gain requirements can be determined from these settings. The gain controls should be set initially in the higher portion of this clinical range and then adjusted downward if necessary. When the initial settings are too low, even though the sound beam traverses the heart along an appropriate path, no recognizable signals may be recorded, and the operator never achieves the initial structure recognition required to pursue the examination. When, in contrast, the gain settings are too high, even though the display scope may be cluttered with a large number of extraneous signals, primary structures can still be discerned. It is best, therefore, to err by setting the gain too high.

Relating these principles to specific control settings suggests that a strong or weakly damped signal should be transmitted initially. Thus, the damping control is set at only 10 to 20% of maximum to initiate the examination. Similarly, with the coarse gain function, one is attempting to amplify any signals returning from the heart at a reasonably high level in hopes of recording some recognizable echoes. Therefore, in addition to transmitting a strong pulse initially, the operator seeks to amplify the reflected signals highly. As a result, the coarse gain is initially set at 80 to 90% of maximum. When too many signals are recorded, one can easily decrease either their amplification or the strength of the interrogating beam. When few or no signals are recorded, the operator never knows whether the control settings are inappropriate or the heart has not been located.

The TGC amplifies the echoes from structures that lie at increasingly greater distances from the transducer. The structures of greatest interest in clinical echocardiography lie at the level of the left ventricle. It has become customary, therefore, to amplify maximally all echoes from the proximal boundary of the left ventricle (the interventricular septum) distally. This amplification is achieved by initially placing the distal portion of the ramp of the TGC circuit at a depth that corresponds to the average distance of the interventricular septum from the chest wall. In the adult, the septum is usually between 5 and 8 centimeters from the anterior chest wall, most typically at approximately 6.5 centimeters. Most cross-sectional instruments have an additional display scope that can be used to view signals in an A-mode format. The A-mode best displays the effects of the TGC and, thus, permits a precise definition of its location.

The echoes that originate from structures close to the transducer generally have high amplitude and, therefore, require less amplification than those returning from deeper in the heart. The near gain controls the amplitude of all echoes from structures proximal to the ramp of the TGC. Because these echoes require less amplification, the setting of the near gain control is normally 20 to 40% of maximum.

Finally, the reject circuitry must be adjusted. The objectives here are similar to those for the other control settings. Again, removing echoes that clutter an image is easier than trying to imagine what the image might look like if additional echoes were present. Therefore, the reject control is normally set at a relatively low setting to allow the display of a wide range of signal amplitudes. When multiple low-intensity signals obscure the image or prevent clear definition of more important structures, the amount of reject can be increased. A reject setting of 20 to 40% of maximum is therefore usually appropriate for an initial setting.

The control settings that are used to begin the examination are rarely those that are required to record the optimal final image. They are merely a starting point and should provide the examiner with enough data for initial structure identification and plane orientation.

Examination Sequence

Locating the Heart

The first step in the actual cross-sectional examination is locating the heart. To locate the heart the examiner must be familiar with (1) the principal echocardiographic windows; (2) three-dimensional cardiac anatomy, particularly the relationship of individual structures within the heart to each of the standard echocardiographic windows; and (3) the general imaging plane orientations that best record areas of initial interest.

In its normal position, the heart is enclosed within the bony skeleton of the thorax and is covered over most of its external surface by lung. Because ultrasound is poorly transmitted through bone and is reflected almost entirely by air-filled lung, the examiner must find a continuous soft tissue path or "window" through which the sound beam can travel to and from the heart. Unimpeded access can usually be obtained through four primary paths or "windows." These windows are located to the immediate left of the sternum in the interspaces between the third, fourth, fifth, and sixth ribs (parasternal); in the region of the cardiac apex (apical); over the anterior abdominal wall immediately beneath the lowest ribs (subcostal); and in the suprasternal notch (suprasternal). When the transducer is positioned over one of these windows, it is in a parasternal, apical, subcostal, or suprasternal location.[17]

Figure 3–3 illustrates the usual position of these windows in relation to the anterior chest wall and cardiac silhouette. The window positions indicated in this diagram apply to the normally positioned heart. When the heart is malpositioned or transposed, window position must shift accordingly. The suprasternal and subcos-

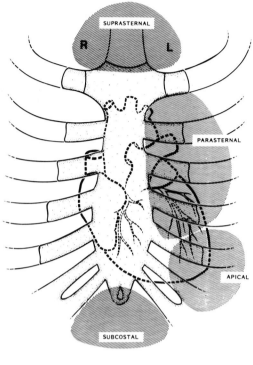

SUPRASTERNAL

R L

PARASTERNAL

APICAL

SUBCOSTAL

STANDARD TRANSDUCER LOCATIONS

Fig. 3–3. Diagram illustrates the position of the four primary echocardiographic windows in relation to the thoracic cage and underlying regions of the heart.

tal windows that lie in the midline of the body usually do not change despite changes in cardiac position. The apical and parasternal windows, however, shift in parallel with the heart. When the heart is normally oriented in the left chest, the terms apical and parasternal are used alone to designate these window positions. In unusual situations when the apex is palpated on the right chest, however, the terms "right apical" and "right parasternal" should be substituted.[17] Likewise, if the transducer must be shifted far from the midline in the subcostal location, the designation "right subcostal" or "left subcostal" should be used. The suprasternal notch is so small that variation in transducer position is impossible. When the transducer is shifted to the right or left of the corresponding sternocleidomastoid

muscle, it is referred to as in a right or left supraclavicular location.

The parasternal window is actually a series of small apertures that lie to the immediate left of the sternum at the level of the third, fourth, and fifth intercostal spaces. These windows are bordered medially by the left border of the sternum, superiorly and inferiorly by the contiguous ribs, and laterally by the lingula of the left lung. They directly overlie the base of the left ventricle and the mitral and aortic valves. The pulmonary and tricuspid valves are, as a rule, just beyond the margins of this composite window. All these important structures are closest to the transducer when it is in a parasternal location. In addition, their motion is largely perpendicular to the path of an imaging plane arising from the anterior chest wall, and hence, this motion is most appropriately assessed from this transducer location. The cross-sectional examination, therefore, is usually initiated and the majority of the study performed from a parasternal transducer location. Figure 3–4 illustrates the position of the cross-sectional probe when placed in a parasternal location.

The next most commonly utilized window is the cardiac apex. Apical position varies from patient to patient; consequently, the actual position of the cardiac apex must be located by palpation. Once the apex has been palpated, the transducer is placed directly over the apical impulse (Fig. 3–5). The apical impulse usually overlies a portion of the anterior left ventricular wall just proximal to the tip of the anatomic apex. From this position, the exploring plane can be directed either posteriorly (to record the apical region of the left ventricle) or superiorly and medially toward the right shoulder (to record structures at the base of the heart). The apical window has proved particularly useful because it is available in almost every case. In addition, the apical window is the *only* location from which all four cardiac cham-

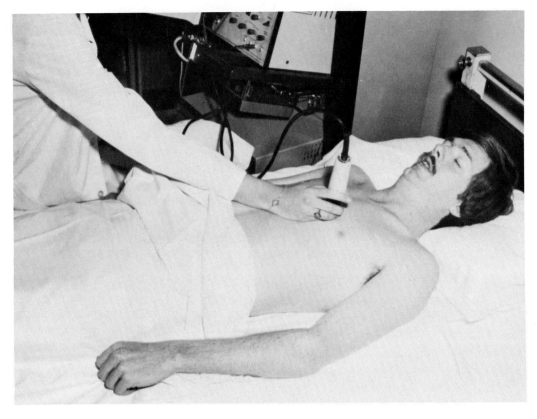

Fig. 3–4. Position of the cross-sectional probe on the anterior chest wall in the parasternal transducer location.

bers can be consistently recorded simultaneously in the adult.

The subcostal window,[17] also referred to as the subxiphoid window,[18] is located in the midline of the body immediately beneath the lowest ribs. When recording the heart from this location, the transducer is placed on the anterior abdominal wall and is pushed downward, depressing the skin until the transducer face lies beneath the plane of the anterior rib cage. The probe is then angled superiorly and leftward (toward the left shoulder) to direct the central ray of the examining plane toward the heart (Fig. 3–6). This window is particularly useful in patients with chronic obstructive lung disease and chest deformities in whom access to the heart through the anterior parasternal or apical windows may be restricted. The subcostal window also is useful in small children and neonates

because (as will be discussed later) it places the plane of the interventricular and interatrial septa perpendicular to the exploring sound beam and, hence, is optimally oriented to record these structures.

The suprasternal window is the last commonly employed transducer location. When utilizing this window, the exploring probe is placed directly in the suprasternal notch, and the sound beam is directed caudad, toward the left atrium (Fig. 3–7). From this location, the examining plane transects the aorta, the right pulmonary artery, and the left atrium in sequence as it penetrates into the chest. The aorta lies immediately beneath the suprasternal window. Little intervening tissue lies between the transducer face and the vessel. Thus, the sound beam readily passes into the aortic arch, thereby allowing this region to be recorded in almost every patient.

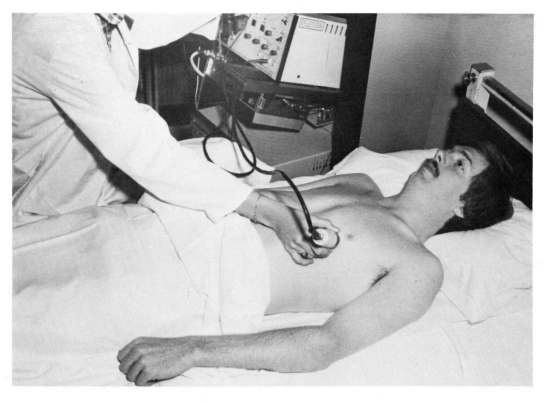

Fig. 3–5. Position of the cross-sectional probe at the cardiac apex. Although the patient in this illustration is supine, the apical window is frequently more accessible when the patient is in varying degrees of left lateral rotation.

Although these areas represent the most common transducer locations, the transducer can and should be placed at any point on the chest wall or elsewhere from which useful information can be obtained. One helpful method for locating other such potential windows is quickly palpating the chest wall over a region of interest. If an impulse from any underlying cardiac structure is palpated, the structure itself should lie immediately beneath the chest wall at that point. If the transducer is placed directly over this impulse, the sound beam should pass unimpeded into the structures below. A common example is the pulmonary artery, which characteristically dilates in a number of disease states. Pulmonary artery dilatation displaces the lung leftward and permits the transmission of the arterial impulse directly to the external surface of the chest. When this pulmonary artery pulsation is palpated and the exploring probe is placed directly over it, the pulmonary artery and pulmonary valves can be easily recorded.

A second technique that is helpful in locating alternative windows is simply to sweep the cross-sectional probe rapidly across the chest in a linear scan pattern. The large field of vision provided by this imaging format causes an image to flash on the display scope each time the sound beam finds access to the heart. Frequently, a number of unexpected windows are uncovered in this fashion. The procedure can be carried out rapidly with broad strokes and does not require the "hunt and peck" that is characteristic of the M-mode method. As soon as the heart is located, the scanning probe can be more carefully oriented. This type of searching process is especially useful when the cardiac silhouette is grossly distorted (e.g., by a large anterolateral aneurysm) and a portion of

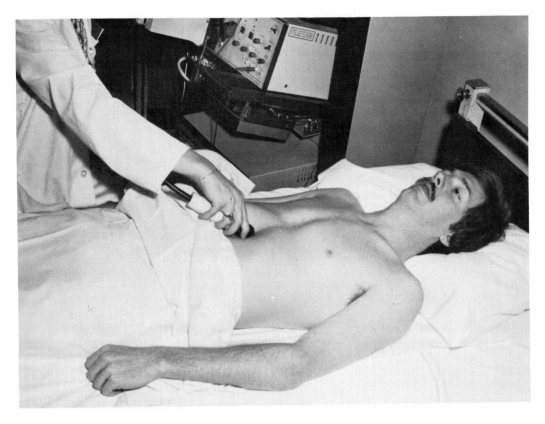

Fig. 3–6. Illustration of the cross-sectional probe in a subcostal location.

the heart underlies an unusual area of the chest (e.g., the midaxillary line). If the examiner does not scan outside the normal echocardiographic windows in such cases, significant disorders can be missed.

A number of factors influence the size of both the conventional and atypical echocardiographic windows and, as such, can facilitate or adversely affect the operator's initial search for the heart. Factors that increase window size are chamber dilatation, change in patient position, and decreased lung volume. Expanded lung volume or bone area generally decrease window size.

Increased window size due to chamber dilatation is most frequently noted in pathologic alterations of the right heart. In their normal orientations, the tricuspid valve and right ventricle lie beneath the sternum and, thus, may be difficult to re-

cord. As the right ventricle dilates, however, it expands leftward, shifting its position beneath and functionally enlarging the parasternal window. When right ventricular dilatation is combined with pulmonary artery dilatation, the area of the right heart that falls within the field of vision of the parasternal window may be vastly expanded.

Change in patient position may likewise increase window size or may shift structures into a position that facilitates viewing from a particular window. Rotating the patient from the supine to the left lateral position, for example, tends to shift the heart to the left. This change frequently moves the interventricular septum from beneath the sternum and permits its visualization from a parasternal transducer location. Positioning the patient on his left side also frequently increases the area of

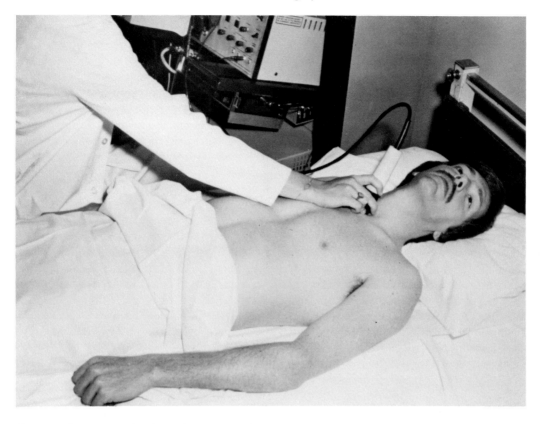

Fig. 3–7. Cross-sectional probe in the suprasternal transducer location. The patient's neck is slightly extended, and the head is rotated slightly to the left.

contact of the cardiac apex with the chest wall, thereby effectively expanding the apical window. Elevating the patient's head may also produce slight descent of mediastinal structures. Descent of the mitral or aortic valves may bring them out from under a rib and into a position where they can be recorded. Likewise, elevation of the head generally brings the heart closer to the subcostal window and decreases the penetration necessary to record structures from this location.

Increased bone density and lung volume occur most commonly in the elderly and combine to restrict access of the sound beam to the heart. In this population, calcification of the ribs narrows the intercostal spaces, while the expansion of the lungs commonly seen with chronic obstructive lung disease may totally obliterate the parasternal and apical windows. Other

transient causes of pulmonary hyperexpansion, such as Valsalva's maneuver or hyperventilation, can also restrict access of the exploring beam to the heart.

A decrease in lung volume can be achieved by asking the patient to hold his breath after deep expiration. This temporary maneuver is difficult but occasionally useful. An important exception to the rule that inspiration makes the echocardiographic study more difficult is found in the subcostal views. Here, deep-held *inspiration*, by shifting the heart closer to the transducer face, frequently improves visualization.

Three-Dimensional Cardiac Anatomy

The examiner must next consider the position of the principal cardiac structures within the chest and their relationship to the primary echocardiographic windows. Figure 3–8 diagrammatically illustrates the normal orientation of the primary structures sought by the examiner for initial recording and identification. The importance of these structures lies in: (1) their characteristic positions and motion patterns, which facilitate recognition; (2) their role as reference points for plane definition and fine plane positioning; and (3) their involvement in the more common cardiac disorders. The primary structures include the four cardiac valves, the apex, the papillary muscles, and the interventricular septum. When describing the relative positions of these structures within the chest, one should refer to those structures located toward the head or cranially as "superiorly oriented." Conversely, those positioned closer to the feet or caudally are referred to as "inferior." Structures located on the patient's right are designated as having a rightward orientation, whereas

those on the patient's left are leftward. Structures near the anterior chest wall are anterior, whereas those closer to the posterior wall of the chest are posterior. Rotation of structures is described as though the heart is viewed from below, looking upward *toward* the head.

The mitral valve, because of its central position within the heart, has historically formed the primary reference to which the position of other structures is related. As illustrated in Figure 3–8, the mitral valve is the most posteriorly positioned of the primary cardiac structures. It lies slightly to the left of the midline at the level of the fourth or fifth intercostal spaces. The tricuspid valve lies to the right of the mitral valve and is anterior and slightly inferior to the mitral valve. The aortic valve is superior to the mitral valve and is also anterior and slightly rightward in orientation. The pulmonary valve is the most superiorly positioned and is the most anterior of the structures at the base of the heart. It lies to the left of the aortic valve and almost directly superior to the mitral valve. The cardiac apex is the most inferior and leftward, as well as the most anterior, of the principal cardiac structures. The papillary muscles lie in the posterior hemisphere of the ventricle, parallel to the closure line of the mitral valve.

The examiner must be familiar not only with the position of these structures in the chest but also with their relationship to the primary echocardiographic windows. Figure 3–9 illustrates their positions in relation to the large parasternal window. The pulmonary valve lies at the left superior margin of this window and is the structure located most immediately beneath the window and, hence, closest to the transducer. The aortic valve is slightly more posterior and inferior and underlies the right-hand margin of the window along its right superior border. The tricuspid valve lies beneath the sternum just beyond the right-hand margin of the window, and at the annulus, its center is slightly inferior

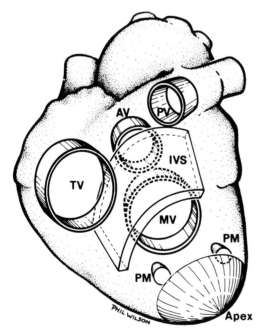

Fig. 3–8. Diagram depicts the normal orientation and relationship of the major cardiac structures within the chest. PV = pulmonary valve; AV = aortic valve; TV = tricuspid valve; MV = mitral valve; IVS = interventricular septum; PM = papillary muscle. (See text for further details.)

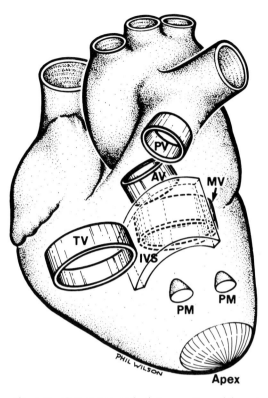

Fig. 3–9. Orientation and relative position of the primary echocardiographic structures when viewed from the parasternal transducer location. The center of this window normally overlies the medial third of the mitral valve. The abbreviations are similar to those in Figure 3–8. (See text for further details.)

to that of the aortic valve. When the right heart dilates, its position within the chest rotates clockwise, and the anteroposterior relationships of the tricuspid and aortic valves may reverse. The mitral valve lies beneath the center of the window and is the most posteriorly positioned of the four cardiac valves. The interventricular septum curves posterior from left to right in an arcuate fashion beneath this window. Its left-hand margin lies anteriorly almost immediately beneath the chest wall, whereas its right-sided boundary is posteriorly positioned at approximately the level of the coaptation line of the mitral leaflets. The anterior one third of the septum is almost perpendicular to the path of a sound beam emanating from the parasternal window and, hence, can be well

recorded, whereas the posterior one third of the septum is more parallel to the sound beam and is poorly visualized. The papillary muscles generally lie just beyond the left inferior border of the window and may be recorded by angling the imaging plane inferiorly and leftward. The cardiac apex, however, almost universally lies outside the parasternal window and cannot be visualized from this position.

Figure 3–10 illustrates the relative positions of these structures when viewed from a subcostal transducer location. From this vantage point, the tricuspid valve is positioned closest to the transducer. It is followed by the interventricular septum whose posteromedial surface is closest to the transducer and is oriented almost perpendicular to its face. The septum then curves superiorly and leftward away from the transducer such that the anterior portion of the septum lies parallel to the transducer. The mitral valve is slightly posterior and superior to the tricuspid valve. The papillary muscles and cardiac apex appear to the examiner's right and are situated farther from the transducer than is the mitral valve. The aortic valve lies at the same depth as the mitral valve and is slightly anterior, whereas the pulmonary valve is the farthest structure from this transducer location and, after the apex, is the most anteriorly situated.

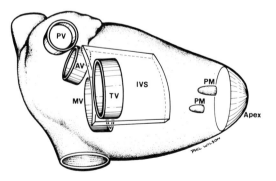

Fig. 3–10. Diagram depicts the relative locations of the primary cardiac structures when viewed from the subcostal transducer location. Abbreviations are similar to those in Figure 3–8. (See text for further details.)

Figure 3–11 illustrates the positions of these structures relative to the cardiac apex. From this viewpoint, the apex itself is most closely related to the transducer face. As the plane passes away from the transducer, it first encounters the papillary muscles, followed sequentially by the tricuspid and mitral valves. The tricuspid valve lies slightly closer to the transducer than does the mitral and is positioned anteriorly in the chest. The next structure encountered is the aortic valve which is still farther anterior. The pulmonary valve follows and, from this orientation, is the structure deepest to the transducer.

Finally, Figure 3–12 illustrates the orientation of the same structures viewed from the suprasternal notch. From this transducer location, the imaging plane must first pass through the aorta and right pulmonary artery before reaching the heart. Beneath the right pulmonary artery, the pulmonary valve lies closest to the transducer. This structure is followed sequentially by the aortic valve, the mitral valve, and the tricuspid valve. The papillary muscles and cardiac apex are too far from the transducer to be recorded in the normal situation.

The choice of a transducer location is ultimately determined by the orientation of the particular structure to be recorded relative to the available echocardiographic windows. As a rule, the transducer should be located in the position that places that structure as close as possible to the transducer face and in an orientation that is as perpendicular as possible to the path of the sound beam. After determining the appropriate transducer location, one must orient the imaging plane in the appropriate manner to best depict the specific features of the structures to be evaluated.

General Plane Orientation

General plane orientation is an attempt by the examiner to correctly align the imaging plane (based on external references or the expected position of intracardiac structures in the chest) such that it passes through the heart in a manner that records a desired structure, dimension, or axis. The

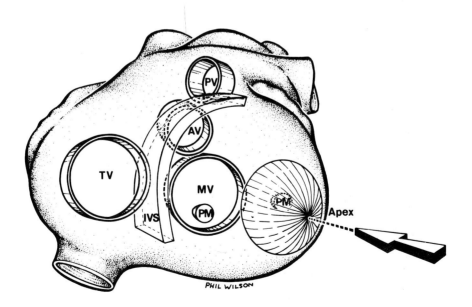

Fig. 3–11. Diagram illustrates the relative positions of the primary cardiac structures from the apical transducer location. Abbreviations are similar to those in Figure 3–8. (See text for further details.)

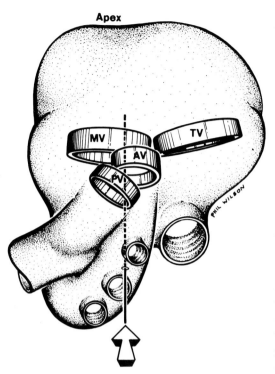

Apex

Fig. 3–12. Orientation of the primary cardiac structures from the suprasternal window. The arrow indicates the path along which the structures at the base of the heart are viewed from this location. Normally, the papillary muscles and apex cannot be recorded from this window. MV = mitral valve; TV = tricuspid valve; AV = aortic valve; PV = pulmonary valve.

orientation of any plane in space can be described by three non-colinear points. When the transducer's position can be defined, it can be used as one point. The examiner must then determine two other points to orient the imaging plane. Because two points describe a line, the plane can be oriented using the transducer location and either a real or imaginary line in space. The line that is most commonly used is one of the axes of the structure to be examined.

An axis, by definition, is a straight line about which a body or geometric figure may be supposed to rotate and with respect to which the body or figure is symmetric.[19] The long axis of any structure, therefore, is the longest linear dimension about which that structure is symmetric,

whereas the short axis is normally perpendicular to the long axis and is the shortest linear dimension about which that body would rotate in an orthogonal direction. Figure 3–13 illustrates the long and short axes of a series of simple geometric figures. Figure 3–14 depicts the long and short axes of the left ventricle. Because the borders of the left ventricle within any plane that includes the long axis are asymmetric, there is only one long axis of this chamber. Multiple planes, however, can pass through the ventricle parallel to and intersecting this long axis. In contrast, the borders of the ventricle are symmetric in a plane that intersects the short axis and is perpendicular to the long axis. A short axis, therefore, can be drawn between any two points along this 360-degree arc that can be connected by a line passing through the center of the ventricle. Thus, there are multiple short axes but only one plane that can intersect more than one of these axes simultaneously.

The long axis of the ventricle is also easier to define. It runs from the tip of the cardiac apex to the midpoint of the base of the ventricle. Any plane through this long axis should, therefore, bisect the ventricle into two equal halves. The true short axis lies in a plane that also bisects the ventricle into two halves with equal masses. The halves of the ventricle on either side of this plane, however, are not geometrically similar; consequently, the position of this plane cannot be determined visually and must be calculated. Because of the inherent difficulties in attempting to calculate the true short axis from the cross-sectional image. the short-axis views are generally considered as a family of planes oriented parallel to the true short-axis plane, rather than as a single plane passing through the short axis itself.

When recording most structures, the examiner seeks to align the Y or Z axis of the imaging plane (the X axis cannot be appreciated on the display and hence, is not

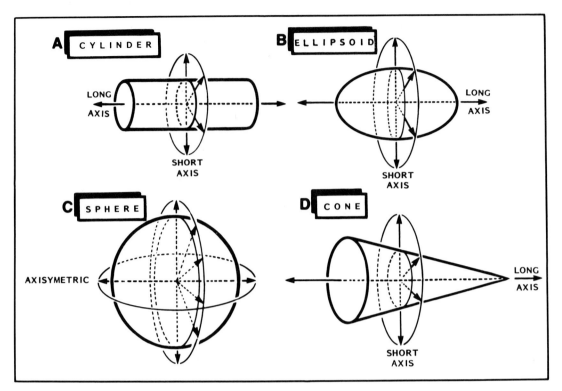

Fig. 3–13. Diagram illustrates the long and short axes of a series of simple geometric figures. The cylinder (*A*), ellipsoid (*B*), and cone (*D*) have only one long axis. There are, however, multiple short axes that can be drawn through the center of these figures and about which the figure is symmetric. Two or more of these short axes lie in a plane that is perpendicular to the long axis. In symmetric figures, such as the cylinder and the ellipsoid, the short axis can be measured directly. In more complicated figures, the short axis must generally be calculated. The sphere, in contrast to the other geometric figures, has no natural long or short axes and rotates about any line passing through its midpoint. Thus, the arbitrary long and short axes of a sphere must be assigned relative to some internal or external reference.

a useful reference) parallel to either the long or the short axis of the structure to be recorded. A long-axis view of the left ventricle, for example, is recorded by aligning the Y axis of the imaging plane parallel to the long axis of the ventricular chamber (Fig. 3–14, *B*). Both the X and Z axes of the imaging plane are thereby aligned perpendicular to the long axis. Because numerous planes may intersect the long axis of the left ventricle, the third point required to define the position of the particular plane in space must be provided either by the transducer location or by another reference that is either internal or external to the left ventricle. Ideally, a combination of both transducer location and additional reference points is used to

permit the most definitive determination of plane orientation. Thus, for example, a plane that passes through the long axis of the left ventricle from the anterior to the posterior surfaces of the heart (transducer in a parasternal location) and also passes between the papillary muscles without recording the echoes from either of these structures is defined within narrow limits.

Orienting the imaging plane relative to the short-axis plane of the left ventricle is achieved by aligning both the Y and Z axes of the imaging plane parallel to perpendicular short axes of the ventricle and orthogonal to the long axis (Fig. 3–14, *C*). The X axis in this format is parallel to the long axis. Internal references are then used to define the point at which a plane ori-

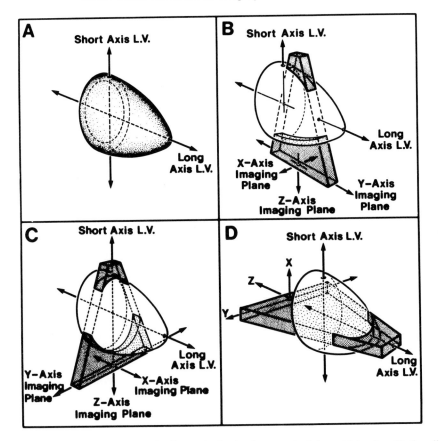

Fig. 3–14. *A,* The long and short axes of a figure similar in shape to the left ventricle. As with the ellipse, the cylinder, and the cone, the left ventricle has only one true long axis. Multiple planes rotated through a 360-degree arc, however, can pass through and can be parallel to this long axis. In addition, as with the cylinder, ellipse, and cone, multiple short axes of the left ventricle can be defined. However, only one plane can encompass more than one of these short axes. *B,* The relationship of the axes of a standard imaging plane to the axes of the left ventricle when the imaging plane is aligned parallel to the ventricular long axis and passes through it in an anteroposterior direction. *C,* The relationship of the axes of the imaging plane to those of the left ventricle when the imaging plane is aligned parallel to the ventricular short axis and is oriented in an anteroposterior direction. *D,* The relationship which would result if the imaging plane were directed from the left ventricular apex toward the base and if the plane included the ventricular long axis. (See text for further details.)

ented parallel to the short axis of the ventricle transects the ventricle. These references include the mitral valve and supporting apparatus, the papillary muscles, and the apical segment of the ventricle distal to the papillary muscles.

When viewing the ventricle from the cardiac apex, the examiner seeks to align the Z axis of the imaging plane along the long axis of the left ventricle. Both the X and Y axes are then parallel to the short-axis plane (Fig. 3–14, *D*). From this particular transducer position, the plane can be rotated 360 degrees without altering the

relationships of the axes of the imaging plane to those of the ventricle. The precise angle in which the imaging plane transects the ventricle, therefore, must be again determined by use of an external or internal reference.

Initiating the Examination

After the examiner and patient are appropriately positioned, the structures to be recorded and their orientation relative to the available echocardiographic windows are defined, and the ideal plane orientation to optimally view these structures is determined, the examiner is ready to begin the actual examination. The examination is initiated by placing the transducer in the selected location. The transducer face must then be coupled to the skin using an appropriate acoustic coupling gel. Coupling is important because it prevents air from entering between the transducer face and skin surface. Air in this location can produce a highly reflective interface and can cause significant loss in the acoustic energy available to penetrate the heart. When previously well-recorded structures begin to fade during the course of the examination, one can generally assume a loss of adequate coupling. This situation can be corrected by adding more gel.

When the transducer is appropriately positioned and coupled to the skin, the central ray of the imaging plane should be directed toward the structure of interest. This is achieved by angling the transducer in such a manner that an imaginary extension of the long axis of the probe would pass through the desired area. The imaging plane is then rotated to align its Y axis parallel to the appropriate axis of the structure to be recorded. When the imaging plane is properly oriented and gains access to the heart, an image should immediately appear on the display scope. When an image appears, the examiner must first identify the recorded structures to define the path of the imaging plane through the heart. When these structures are identified, they then form a reference for more precise alignment of the imaging plane or from which the plane position can be readjusted to record other structures of interest. If recognizable echoes do not appear, the imaging plane should be swept through the area where the heart is expected to lie until an identifiable image appears on the display scope.

The routine clinical examination is most frequently initiated by placing the transducer in a parasternal location at the level of the fourth or fifth intercostal spaces.

From this transducer location, the examiner normally seeks to record echoes from structures at the base of the heart (most particularly the mitral valve echo). The mitral valve is selected as a starting point because it lies most immediately beneath this window, is highly reflective, and has a characteristic motion pattern. Also, because of its central position within the heart, the mitral valve is a useful reference from which to locate other structures.

To record the mitral valve, the examiner directs the central ray of the imaging plane posteriorly and slightly leftward. The imaging plane is then rotated to align the Y-axis parallel to the long axis of the left ventricle and, hence, parallel to the path of the blood flow through the mitral leaflets. The long axis of the left ventricle runs roughly on a line from the cardiac apex to the right shoulder, or 30 to 45 degrees counterclockwise to the long axis of the body. In the majority of patients, when the transducer is oriented in this fashion the imaging plane should pass directly into the heart and should record echoes from the mitral valve, the left ventricular myocardium at the base of the heart, and a portion of the left atrium and proximal aortic root (Fig. 3–15). When any echoes from underlying structures appear on the display scope, the examiner is ready to advance to more precise structure identification and fine plane positioning.

If echoes are not recorded from this initial transducer location and image plane orientation, the examiner should then explore other portions of the parasternal window to find access to the heart. If this step is unsuccessful, the patient can be rotated into the left lateral position in an attempt to shift the heart slightly to the left and to expand the parasternal window. If this maneuver is also unsuccessful, the examiner may have to explore other transducer locations from which access to the heart can be obtained.

Structure Identification

Intracardiac structures are identified on the basis of one or more characteristics of

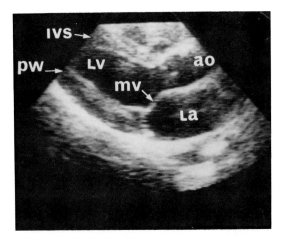

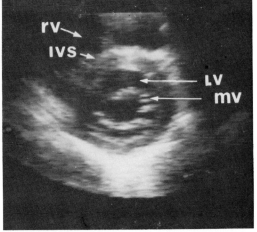

Fig. 3–15. Parasternal long-axis view of the left ventricle similar to that usually sought as a starting point for the cross-sectional examination. LV = left ventricle; La = left atrium; mv = mitral valve; ao = aorta, ivs = interventricular septum; pw = posterior wall. The apex in this orientation is to the viewer's left, and the aorta is to the viewer's right.

Fig. 3–16. Parasternal short-axis view of the left ventricle illustrates the expected relative positions of the right ventricle (rv), interventricular septum (ivs), left ventricular cavity (LV), and mitral valve (mv) in this image orientation.

their ultrasonic reflections. These characteristics include (1) positions within the chest, (2) general appearance, (3) motion patterns, (4) associations with other known structures, and (5) unique anatomic characteristics.

The most common and perhaps easiest approach to structure identification is based on the expected position of the larger cardiac structures within the chest. Figure 3–16 illustrates how this method can be employed. In this example, a transducer is placed on the anterior chest wall along the left sternal border, and the imaging plane is directed posteriorly into the chest parallel to the left ventricular short axis. If the heart is normally positioned, the first large echo-free spaced encountered by the sound beam should be the right ventricle. Moving echoes anterior to this space should then be reflected from the right ventricular free wall, whereas those beneath this space should arise from the interventricular septum. Assuming that this first group of structures is correctly identified, a second, large, echo-free space, lying beneath the septum, should represent the left ventricular cavity, whereas

moving echoes bordering this space posteriorly may presumably arise from the left ventricular posterior wall. Echoes within the left ventricular cavity should arise from the mitral valve. When the heart is normally positioned in the chest and the cardiac chambers are appropriately related, this approach usually leads to correct structure identification. When the heart is malpositioned or when chamber relationships are distorted, reliance on this approach has resulted in a surprising amount of confusion and has led to incorrect structure identification.

The second approach to structure identification is based on an analysis of the geometric configuration of the structure(s) being imaged. The chamber that has a circular configuration when viewed from the anterior chest wall in a plane parallel to its short axis and also is surrounded by a thick muscular wall is normally the left ventricle (see Fig. 3–16).

Exceptions to this kind of analysis also occur. In severe pulmonary hypertension and right ventricular volume overload, the right ventricle may become more circular than the left. Likewise, hypertrophy of a transposed right ventricle may prevent chamber identification on the basis of wall thickness.

Assessment of the motion patterns of intracardiac structures can be of particular value in structure identification. The broad amplitude and rapid motion of the cardiac valves serve to distinguish them from non-valvular structures. Additionally, the opening or closing of these valves in relation to the cardiac cycle allows separation of the atrioventricular (AV) from the semilunar valves. Although separation of valves into those regulating ventricular inflow and outflow may be relatively easy, specific identification of the individual AV and semilunar valves is frequently more complicated. Such complication occurs because valve motion is not an inherent feature of the valve leaflets, but is a passive function reflecting the pattern of blood flow through the valve and the relative pressure exerted on the opposing leaflet surfaces. Therefore, although the pattern and timing of valve motion may permit the identification of an atrioventricular valve, valve motion defines neither the number of leaflets the valve contains nor whether it lies in the mitral or tricuspid position. More precise valve identification must be gained through other means, such as comparing the relative position of these partially identified structures to one another or determining the number of leaflets the valve contains. The mitral valve inserts into the interventricular septum at a slightly more basal position than does the tricuspid valve when viewed from either the apical or subxiphoid window. Determination of the relative position of the valve leaflets as they insert into the septum, therefore, can permit differentiation of the AV valves. More simply, the mitral valve normally has two leaflets, and the tricuspid has three leaflets. Simply counting the number of leaflets in the AV valve may permit their separation.

Association with other structures of known identity is another method of iden-

tifying unknown areas of echo production. This method obviously requires the identification of the contiguous structures first, but has proven particularly useful in recognizing structures that are known to be present anatomically, but may not have previously been appreciated by the examiner or described by others. An example of this approach was the original identification of the linear band of echoes arising from the interatrial septum. Taken by themselves, these echoes would have had little meaning. When placed between the posteromedial border of the aorta and the posterior left atrial wall, however, their origin and significance became apparent.

Finally, a few structures have unique anatomic characteristics that can be used for definitive identification. For example, when the great vessels are malaligned, differentiation of the aorta and pulmonary artery at their origins may prove difficult. Determination of the paths and distribution of these vessels, however, permits positive identification based on their branching patterns. Thus, the artery that courses into the neck and gives off numerous large branches to the head and upper extremities is always the aorta. Conversely, the vessel that bifurcates into two branches of relatively equal size is always the pulmonary artery. Likewise, the valve at the origin of the pulmonary artery is always the pulmonary valve, and the valve at the base of the aorta is always the aortic valve. Although such unique structural configurations are rare, they are valuable in structure identification.

Ideally, a combination of all the available methods should be employed when attempting to identify any structure because the more characteristics of a particular structure that one can recognize, the more likely that the identification of the structure will be correct. For example, the determination that a structure that (1) lies approximately 6 cm beneath the anterior chest wall; (2) is characterized by two horizontal linear echoes when viewed with the scan plane parallel to its long axis and as a circle when viewed with the scan plane parallel to its short axis; (3) moves anteriorly during systole and posteriorly during diastole; (4) courses into the neck and gives off numerous large branches; (5) has an anterior border that is continuous with the interventricular septum and a posterior border that is continuous with the mitral valve; and (6) lies anterior to the left atrium and posterior to the right ventricular outflow tract, is the aorta is far more positive than an identification made on the basis of any one of these features alone. Although all structures are not as clearly defined as the aorta, an identification of a source of echoes is almost always possible if one carefully considers the location of a structure and its general configuration, motion patterns, and relationships to other known structures. Also, the identification of many structures independently is not necessary. If one or two structures can be identified, the other pieces of the puzzle can, as a rule, be easily fitted into place either by association or by exclusion.

Fine Plane Positioning

The final step in recording any cross-sectional image involves positioning the imaging plane as precisely as possible to appropriately display the desired features of a structure of interest. Precise plane positioning is determined from the recorded image itself and is independent of the position of the heart in the chest or of the relative positions of other cardiac structures. Precise plane positioning is essential because it determines the *reliability* of dimensions, appreciation of motion, and reproducibility of derived data.

A typical long-axis recording of the left ventricle can be used to illustrate how improper plane positioning adversely affects the data derived from the cross-sectional image. Figure 3–17, *A*, illustrates that when the imaging plane passes through

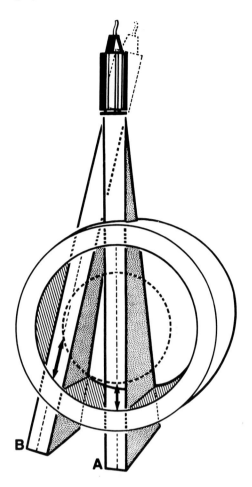

Fig. 3–17. Diagram illustrates the relative end-diastolic and end-systolic ventricular diameters and amplitudes of endocardial motion recorded in two different planes. Both planes are parallel to the ventricular long axis. Plane A passes through the center of the ventricle (long axis), recording a true ventricular diameter and appropriately depicting the amplitude of endocardial excursion. Plane B is eccentrically positioned and records a decreased ventricular diameter and an artifactually increased wall motion.

the long axis of the ventricle, the distance between contralateral points on the ventricular wall represents a true ventricular diameter. Additionally, motion of these points appropriately reflects actual left ventricular endocardial excursion. Conversely, as indicated in Figure 3–17, *B*, when the plane is angled so that it is parallel to, but passes to, one side of the long axis, the distance between points on the contralateral ventricular walls is less than a true diameter and motion is artifactually exaggerated.

If the examiner could see the structure to be recorded and the imaging plane simultaneously, it would be relatively simple to align the imaging plane parallel to any axis of the structure. Unfortunately, the examiner cannot directly visualize the structure to be recorded and must determine its shape, orientation, and position relative to the imaging plane from the image on the display scope. The probe must then be moved and the plane angled or rotated in an appropriate pattern to produce an optimal image based solely on the changes these movements produce in the image recorded. Fine plane positioning, therefore, requires the examiner's full understanding of the variations in the image that are produced by changes in plane positioning, the effects of improper plane orientation on image configuration, and the optimal structure configuration that can be recorded when the imaging plane is properly positioned.

To understand these concepts, one should consider the relationships of an imaging plane to a series of simple geometric figures. The simplest figure to consider is the cylinder. The cylinder has both a long axis and a short axis. Figure 3–18, A, illustrates that when an ultrasonic imaging plane transects the cylinder parallel to its long axis, two linear echoes, equally distant from each other at all points in the plane, are recorded. The effects of the improper transducer and, hence, plane positioning can be appreciated in panels B and C. When the plane is angled to the right or left of the long axis (B), the distance between the two echoes decreases. Thus, the plane passes through the long axis of the cylinder only where the separation of the two imaged echoes is the greatest. Likewise, when the transducer is rotated such that the plane is no longer parallel to, but crosses, the long axis at an angle, it cuts through the cylinder obliquely (C). When this occurs, the echoes

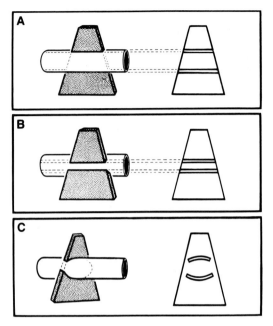

Fig. 3–18. *A,* Image recorded when a plane transects a cylinder along a path parallel to and intersecting its long axis. *B,* Image recorded when a plane transects a cylinder parallel to but to the left or right of its long axis. *C,* Image recorded when a plane transects the cylinder at an angle to its long axis. (See text for further details.)

at the two margins of the imaging plane begin to curve inward toward one another and continue to decrease as the imaging plane is rotated further from the true long axis. The diameter in the center of the scan remains maximal because the imaging plane passes through the long axis at this point. The plane is rotated parallel to the long axis of the cylinder then only when the diameter of the cylinder is equal at the center and both margins of the scan.

In this figure, the transducer is located over the middle of the cylinder. The transducer could obviously be moved either to the right or left without changing the recorded image. To determine the area of the cylinder transected by the plane, therefore, some external reference, such as the ends of the cylinder, is necessary.

Figure 3–19 contains three long-axis, cross-sectional scans of the cylindric aorta, which demonstrate these principles. In *A,* the scan is aligned parallel to the long axis

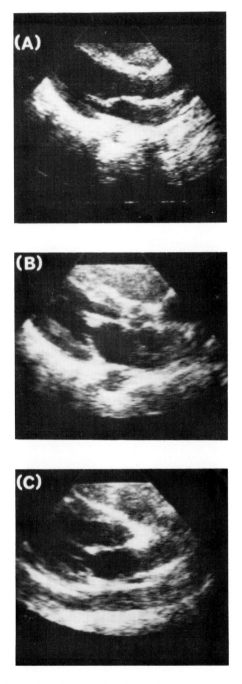

of the vessel, and the vessel walls are parallel and widely separated. In *B*, the transducer is angled improperly, and the vessel diameter decreases, whereas in panel *C*, the plane is rotated such that it cuts through the external margin of the vessel. When attempting to align the imaging plane parallel to the long axis of a cylindric structure, the examiner should rotate the transducer clockwise and then counterclockwise until the distance between the linear echoes at the margins of the scan plane are at their maximum. Then, by angling the plane back and forth across the cylinder until the separation of the echoes in the midportion and the margins of the recorded image is equidistant, the examiner can place the imaging plane not only parallel to but through the true long axis. Determination of transducer location depends on an external or internal reference.

Figure 3–20 illustrates the image produced when the imaging plane passes

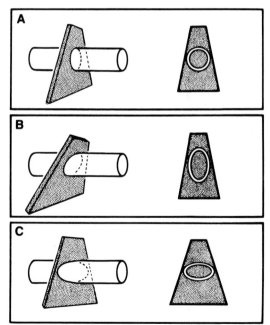

Fig. 3–19. Cross-sectional recordings illustrate the effects depicted diagrammatically in Figure 13–18. *A*, The scan plane passes through the aorta in an orientation that is parallel to and transects its long axis. *B*, The scan plane is angled to pass through the aorta parallel to but not through its long axis. The vessel, therefore, appears narrowed. *C*, The scan plane is rotated incorrectly and passes obliquely across the long axis of the aorta, thus transecting the lateral aortic wall.

Fig. 3–20. *A*, Circular image recorded when a plane transects a cylinder parallel to its short axis. *B*, Vertically elongated image recorded when a plane passes through a cylinder at an angle to its short axis. *C*, Horizontally elongated image recorded when a plane is abnormally rotated relative to the short axis of the cylinder.

through the short axis of the cylinder. In this example, the image appears circular, and its diameters are equal in all dimensions. When the examiner angles the transducer in either direction such that the imaging plane is no longer parallel to the vertical short axis of the cylinder, the vertical dimensions of the image gradually increase (Fig. 3–20, B). The horizontal dimension, however, remains constant. Thus, improper angulation relative to the short axis results in an increase in vertical obliquity of the image. Conversely, when the imaging plane is rotated either clockwise or counterclockwise from the true short-axis plane, the horizontal diameter of the image increases, and the vertical diameter remains the same (Fig. 3–20, C). Thus, improper angulation of the transducer relative to a true short-axis plane results in gradually increasing vertical obliquity, whereas improper rotation results in horizontal obliquity. To determine transducer position, one must again resort to some external reference.

Finally, Figure 3–21 illustrates the image recorded when the examining plane is directed through the cylinder from its left base. When the imaging plane is aligned along the long axis of the cylinder, the echoes from its margins are parallel to one another. Rotating the imaging plane does not alter the image, and hence, the degree of rotation of the plane must be determined from some external reference. Angling the plane, however, causes the echoes at the distal end of the image to curve inward toward one another, thereby indicating that the plane is no longer parallel to the long axis of the cylinder. Transducer position can be defined in this orientation by moving the transducer in an inferior-superior and medial-lateral direction until the distance between the echoes at the apex of the sector is as large as possible. When the distance between these echoes is the greatest, the transducer is lying over the true center of the base of the cylinder.

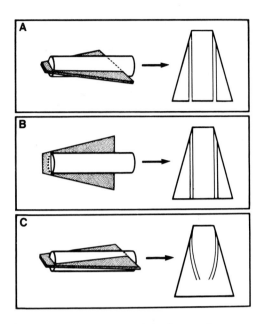

Fig. 3–21. *A,* Image recorded when a plane passes through a cylinder from apex to base through its long axis. *B,* The plane has been rotated; however, it remains parallel to the long axis, and therefore, the image is unchanged. *C,* The plane has been angled above the long axis, and the image from the margins of the cylinder at the base of the scan plane begin to taper inward.

To record an appropriate image in this transducer orientation, the examiner must initially define the transducer location and then must angle the plane in an inferior-superior orientation until the maximal diameter of the image at the base of the sector is recorded. The degree of rotation of the plane can only be determined from an external reference. In each of these examples, two of the three variables in image plane orientation can be determined directly from the image itself. In the first two examples (the long and the short axes), transducer location could not be defined from the image alone. In the apical view, the degree of plane rotation could not be determined.

When actually recording a cross-sectional study, transducer location can be determined in several ways (1) from the echocardiographic window over which the transducer is located and (2) from the image itself, by defining the orientation of recorded structures within the image or the position of the imaging plane relative to such anatomic references as the papillary muscles or mitral valve.

Figure 3–22 illustrates the images recorded when the scan plane transects a second simple geometric figure, the sphere. Because the sphere has neither true long nor short axes, the image produced is similar despite transducer location or degree of plane rotation. The only variable that can be directly determined from the image is the fact that the plane passes through the center of the sphere. If the plane is angled either to the left or the right of center, the diameters of the sphere gradually shrink. To determine that the plane is passing through the center of the sphere, therefore, the examiner should sweep the

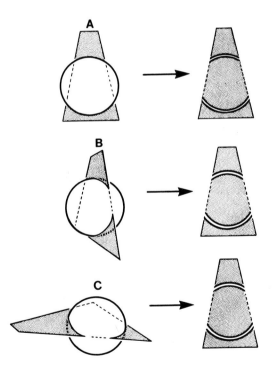

Fig. 3–22. Images obtained when a sphere is transected by a plane passing through its center. Because the sphere's axes are symmetric, variation in the direction, rotation, or angulation of the plane does not affect the recorded image as long as the plane passes through the center of the sphere. The only variable that can be determined directly from the image is whether the plane has intersected the true center. (See text for further details.)

plane from one side of the sphere to the other until the maximal diameter of the sphere is recorded. Both degree of plane rotation and transducer location must be defined by resorting to external references. Relating this illustration to the heart, the atria are relatively spheric structures without natural long or short axes. The long and short axes of the atria are therefore derived by relating them to the long and short axes of contiguous structures. Thus, the long axis of the left atrium is in a plane that is roughly parallel to the long axis of the left ventricle and the aorta. The same is true of the right atrium.

As structures become more complex, the orientation of the imaging plane becomes more difficult to define directly from the structure itself. In such cases, the examiner should seek to determine reproducible image orientation as an alternative to one that might be theoretically optimal. Figure 3–23 illustrates the relationship of an imaging plane to a pyramid with a triangular base. In Figure 3–23, A, the plane is aligned parallel to the long axis of the pyramid. The plane passes through the base parallel to the long axis at the point where the superior angle is most acute and the height of the base is shortest. Using this reference axis, when the plane is then swung back and forth across the more apical segment of the pyramid, it crosses the long axis at a point where the length at the left-hand margin of the sector is greatest. This type of orientation is difficult to achieve from the image itself, particularly when the structure is not perfectly symmetric.

Figure 3–23, B, illustrates a short-axis recording of the same structure. By assuming that the three sides of the figure form an equilateral triangle, appropriate angulation can be achieved by sweeping the plane from apex to base of the pyramid until the shortest length of the arms of the triangle is recorded. An appropriate degree of rotation can be defined by rotating the plane until the base of the triangle is

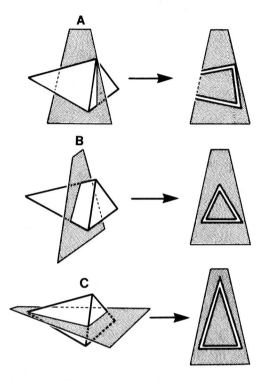

Fig. 3–23. Diagrams illustrate the relationships of a plane to a more complex figure—the pyramid with a triangular base. The difficulties in aligning the plane relative to such a figure are discussed in the text.

ternal or external references. For example, the right ventricle is a complicated structure. Aligning the transducer over the apex of the right ventricle is a relatively simple maneuver if one uses the principles previously indicated. Defining plane orientation as it passes through the right ventricle, however, is far easier if one uses the point of maximal tricuspid excursion to define the base of the long axis rather than attempting to determine plane orientation based on observed changes in right ventricular shape.

The use of internal or external references can be invaluable in fine plane positioning. Figure 3–24 illustrates how these references can be utilized to examine an irregularly shaped structure. The example

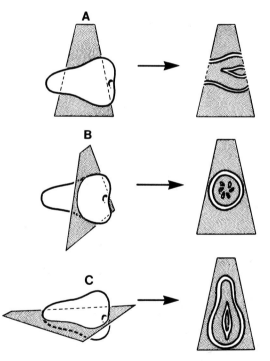

Fig. 3–24. Diagrams depict the images obtained when a plane passes through a structure with an internal reference—in this case, a pear with an internal seed pod. The single internal reference is invaluable because it permits one to define the position of the plane along the long axis (A), the orientation of the plane relative to the short axis, (B), and the elevation of the plane. When the position of the transducer is known and two internal or external references can be defined, the plane can be positioned precisely in space.

at its shortest length and is equal to the two arms. Here again, imaging plane position can be relatively assigned by moving the plane up and down the triangle and observing the changes in size.

Finally, in Figure 3–23, C, the imaging plane is directed from the apex of the triangle toward the base and parallel to the long axis. In this example, transducer position relative to the apex can be determined by moving the transducer location until the point where the angle between the two limbs of the triangle at the apex is most acute. Aligning the plane parallel to the long axis from this point, however, is more difficult.

The standardized recording of complex structures can therefore be achieved more easily by relating the orientation of the imaging plane to the axes of contiguous, more easily defined structures or by using in-used here is a pear-shaped structure with a seed pod in the center. Aligning the plane parallel to the long axis of the pear based on the distance between contralateral walls is helpful. Because of the irregularity of the structure, however, change in angle may not be reflected by large variations in dimension, and hence, lack of precision in position is possible. By aligning the plane such that it passes through both walls at a roughly maximal dimension and, at the same time, passes through the seed pod, one can obtain a precise, reproducible plane orientation. In addition, the irregularity of the figure helps to define transducer location because the area of the pear through which the imaging plane passes can be defined relative to the position of the seed pod.

Figure 3–24, *B*, illustrates a similar relationship for the short axis. Here, the short-axis orientation of the plane can be defined by angulation and rotation until the point of least horizontal and vertical obliquity is determined. Again, resorting to the position of the seed pod, the imaging plane can be easily determined to pass through the pear in a short-axis orientation at the level of, above, or below the seed pod, and hence, can be more precisely defined. Finally, relating this illustration to the apical view, the position of the seed pod presents a simple reference that is helpful in determining the degree of imaging-plane angulation required to transect the long axis. Here again, the degree of plane rotation cannot be assigned even using this centrally located transducer reference. If a second pear were placed next to the first and the imaging plane adjusted so that it passed through the seed pods of both pears, the position of the plane would be precisely defined. Although plane positioning can usually be achieved without resorting to internal or external references, such references make this process easier.

Figure 3–25 illustrates how these simple figures can be related to the individual cardiac structures. The pulmonary artery,

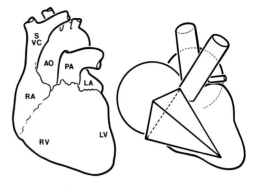

Fig. 3–25. Combination of simple figures represents the primary chambers and vessels of the heart. The principles utilized in recording the simple figures apply to the recording of each of the major areas of the heart. SVC = superior vena cava; AO = aorta; PA = pulmonary artery; LA = left atrium; RA = right atrium; RV = right ventricle; LV = left ventricle.

aorta, and left main coronary artery are all cylindric in configuration. When examining these structures, a long-axis view is customarily recorded first. This recording is achieved by (1) directing the central ray of the imaging plane toward the structure to be examined, (2) angling the imaging plane until the echoes from the anterior and posterior margins of the vessel are as parallel to one another as possible, and (3) sweeping the plane back and forth across the vessel, parallel to the long axis, until the distances separating the linear echoes at the margins of the scan are as large as possible. In this manner, the plane is initially directed toward the arterial vessel, aligned parallel to its long axis, and then angled so that it passes directly through the long axis. Transducer location can then be varied, and these steps can be repeated to orient the imaging plane relative to the particular area of the vessel desired. These principles are applicable whether the vessel is oriented directly perpendicular to the path of the imaging plane or placed at an angle to this plane.

The same principles apply when recording a short-axis view. The central ray is initially directed toward the structure. The imaging plane is then angled inferiorly to superiorly until the least vertical obliquity is recorded. It is then rotated in a clockwise to counterclockwise fashion until the least horizontal obliquity is achieved. The relationship of the plane to the short axis of the vessel is then defined by the use of internal or external references.

Similar principles can be applied to the examination of the left ventricle. The parasternal long axis is recorded when the ventricular dimensions at the left- and right-hand margins of the scan plane are the greatest and the plane has been angled back and forth across the ventricle to insure that it passes parallel to and through the long axis. The plane position can be confirmed by insuring that it passes through but does not record echoes from the papillary muscles and by optimizing it such that it passes through the mitral valve at the point of maximal mitral leaflet excursion, which should correspond to the midportion of the mitral valve. Short-axis views are again optimized by defining the plane position with the least horizontal or vertical obliquity and by orienting the position at which the plane passes through the ventricle by the use of internal references, such as the mitral valve apparatus, the papillary muscles, or the apical segment distal to the papillary muscles.

The apical view can be recorded using the same principles. The transducer location is first defined either by moving the probe about the apex until the point of most acute angulation of the myocardium is observed or by stepping the transducer down the short axis to a point where the circular ventricle disappears, which should represent the true anatomic apex, and then angling the central ray toward the base of the heart. Orientation of the plane parallel to the long axis can be confirmed by angling the beam in a superior-inferior direction until the diameter at the base of the ventricle is greatest. The rotation of the plane is defined using internal or external references, such as the combined mitral and tricuspid valves which,

in addition to the cardiac apex, form the three points necessary to orient the plane in space.

Utilizing these principles, one can reliably and reproducibly position the imaging plane such that chamber dimensions, wall motion, and structure abnormalities can be precisely recorded and their validity assured. The imaging plane can only be related to a specific structure of interest. Recording multiple structures optimally from the same plane position is difficult, if not impossible.

The foregoing discussion has been directed primarily to the steps involved in initiating the cross-sectional examination and recording the first imaging plane. The total examination is nothing more than a collection of images recorded from a family of imaging planes. The steps involved in recording each of these planes, from the first to the last, are identical, and the processes involved in recording each subsequent plane are similar to those involved in recording the initial image.

REFERENCES

1. Weyman, AE: Clinical application of cross-sectional echocardiography. *In* Handbook of Clinical Ultrasound. Edited by M deVlieger, et al. New York, John Wiley & Sons, 1978.
2. Kisslo, J, Von Ramm, OT, and Thurstone, FL: Cardiac imaging using a phased array ultrasound system. II. Clinical technique and application. Circulation, 53:262, 1976.
3. Sahn, DJ, et al.: The validity of structure identification for cross-sectional echocardiography. J Clin Ultrasound, 2:201, 1974.
4. Kotler, MN, Mintz, GS, Segal, BL, and Parry, WR: Clinical uses of two-dimensional echocardiography. Am J Cardiol, 45:1061, 1980.
5. Kloster, FE, et al.: Multiscan echocardiography. II. Technique and initial clinical results. Circulation, 48:1075, 1973.
6. Von Ramm, OT, and Thurstone, FL: Cardiac imaging using a phased array ultrasound system. I. System design. Circulation, 53:258, 1976.
7. Eggleton, RC, et al.: Visualization of cardiac dynamics with real-time, B-mode ultrasonic scanner. *In* Ultrasound in Medicine I. Edited by D. While. New York, Plenum Press, 1975.
8. Edler, I.: Ultrasound cardiogram in mitral valvular diseases. Acta Chir Scand, 111:230, 1956.
9. McDicken, WN, Bruff, K., and Paton, J: An ultrasonic instrument for rapid B-scanning of the heart. Ultrasonics, 13:269, 1974.

10. Bom, N, et al.: Ultrasonic viewer for cross-sectional analysis of moving cardiac structures. Biomed Engineering, 6:500, 1971.
11. Meyer, RA: Pediatric Echocardiography. Philadelphia, Lea & Febiger, 1977.
12. Goldberg, SJ, Allen, HD, and Sahn, DJ: Pediatric & Adolescent Echocardiography. Chicago, Year Book Medical Publishers, 1975.
13. Feigenbaum, H: Echocardiography. 2nd Ed. Philadelphia, Lea & Febiger, 1976.
14. Chang, S: M-mode Echocardiographic Techniques and Pattern Recognition. Philadelphia, Lea & Febiger, 1976.
15. Kossoff, G: The transducer. In Handbook of Clinical Ultrasound. Edited by M deVlieger. New York, John Wiley & Sons, 1978.
16. Somer, JC: Transducer arrays. In Handbook of Clinical Ultrasound. Edited by M deVlieger. New York, John Wiley & Sons, 1978.
17. Henry, WL, et al.: Report of the American Society of Echocardiography Committee on nomenclature and standards in two-dimensional echocardiography. Circulation, 62:212, 1980.
18. Chang, S, and Feigenbaum, H: Subxyphoid echocardiography. J Clin Ultrasound, 1:14, 1973.
19. Webster's New Collegiate Dictionary. Springfield, G & C Merriam Co., 1977.

Chapter 4

Standard Plane Positions—
Standard Imaging Planes

A small group from the almost limitless number of possible cross-sectional imaging planes and display formats has been used so commonly in clinical studies that it has become recognized as a standard.[1-10] The recognition and use of these standardized image formats have a number of advantages because they (1) facilitate communication among individual users and laboratories, (2) permit reproducible data recording for serial comparison of individual patients and/or groups of patients, (3) aid in structure recognition, and (4) provide a format that can be consistently and easily taught to experienced and inexperienced users. In addition, they contain the vast majority of data required in any echocardiographic examination and permit most important structures to be viewed from several different vantage points.

The standard imaging planes are designated on the basis of (1) transducer location; (2) spatial orientation of the imaging plane, which is a combination of both the angle and degree of rotation of the

plane; and (3) structure(s) recorded.[11] Thus, a plane recorded with the transducer in a parasternal location and the imaging plane orientation parallel to the long axis of the left ventricle would be termed a parasternal long-axis of the left ventricle.

When applied to individual planes, these descriptors may be fairly general. As a result, a family of planes, rather than a specific plane, can be included within one standard plane designation. For example, when the transducer is described as in a parasternal location, it may be positioned anywhere from the second to the sixth intercostal spaces and from the immediate left sternal border to the anterior axillary line. Even when the angle and degree of rotation of the plane are constant, movement of the probe within these broad boundaries can generate a large series of parallel planes that would fall within this category. The same latitude is present in the apical and subcostal locations. Because of the anatomic limitations of this window, only the suprasternal designation defines probe position more precisely.

The description of general plane orientation relative to a particular set of reference axes likewise contains considerable latitude. Plane orientation can first be described in relation to a number of references including (1) the anatomic planes of the body, (2) the heart as a whole, or (3) the individual structures within the heart. Each of these methods has advantages and disadvantages, and the relationships of the standard imaging planes to each of these references are considered in this chapter. However, because final precise plane position must be related to the particular structure of interest, I prefer to describe and name the standard planes in a similar fashion. In most instances, the axes of the individual cardiac structures are similar to those of the entire heart, and a description based on either standard would be the same. There are several exceptions to this rule (e.g., the right ventricular outflow tract and left main coronary artery) in which these axes are not the same. In these circumstances, plane orientation is related to the axes of the individual structure.

Planes that pass through any axis of a structure may intersect that axis from any direction through a full 360-degree arc. The addition of the transducer location defines this intersection more narrowly, but it can be positioned precisely only by relating plane position to specific internal references. As a result, a plane that passes through the left ventricular long axis from a parasternal transducer location is probably defined within only a 90-degree arc, whereas a parasternal plane that passes through the long axis of the left ventricle and splits the papillary muscles is defined within narrow limits. Finally, even the designation of the structure to be examined may be fairly general. Thus, a plane parallel to the short axis of the left ventricle may transect that chamber at any level from the apex to the base and, as in the aforementioned examples, must also

be more specifically defined by resorting to internal references. In this chapter, a method is described for precisely and reproducibly positioning each standard plane discussed.

The standard imaging planes described in this section are listed in Table 4–1. These planes are grouped initially by the transducer location from which they are recorded. They are then subgrouped on the basis of plane orientation and, finally, are related to the structure in question.

This listing of standard planes is not intended to be exhaustive. Other more inclusive systems have been devised, and

TABLE 4–1
STANDARD CROSS-SECTIONAL IMAGING PLANES

Parasternal
  A. Long axis
      1. Left heart
          a. Optimized for the aortic valve
          b. Optimized for the mitral valve and left ventricle
      2. Right ventricular inflow tract
      3. Right ventricular outflow tract
      4. Main pulmonary artery
      5. Cardiac apex
  B. Short axis
      6. Aortic valve and left atrium
      7. Left ventricle (mitral valve level)
      8. Left ventricle (papillary muscle level)
      9. Left ventricle (apex)
Apical
      10. Four chamber
      11. Five chamber
      12. Two chamber
      13. Long axis (left ventricle)
Subcostal
      14. Long axis of the heart
      15. Long axis of the right ventricular outflow tract
Suprasternal
      16. Long axis of the aortic arch
      17. Short axis of the aortic arch

---

additional planes have been described by individual authors.[1,2] This list does include, however, the planes that are most commonly utilized in routine clinical cross-sectional echocardiography and that contain the majority of the data required in any examination.

The concept used to describe each of these planes can be compared to photographing a ship on the horizon. When the ship is properly framed, the sea and sky are present in their proper proportions. Similarly, when the primary structures in each plane are correctly recorded, the other areas are naturally present and viewed in their proper perspective. In each series of figures, a reference mark (R) is included so that comparable points on the plane and the display can be related.

PARASTERNAL LONG-AXIS PLANES

Five long-axis planes are conventionally recorded from the parasternal transducer location. These planes include the long axis of the left heart, the right ventricular inflow tract, the right ventricular outflow tract, the main pulmonary artery, and the cardiac apex. Because of the large number of structures contained in the parasternal long axis of the left heart, it must frequently be specifically aligned to optimally record certain areas. The two most common subplanes are the parasternal long axis of the aortic root (left ventricular outflow tract) and the parasternal long axis of the mitral valve and left ventricle (left ventricular inflow tract).

The inclusion of the long axis of the cardiac apex in the parasternal group of planes might appear surprising because it is recorded with the transducer close to the cardiac apex. This is done for several reasons. First, the cardiac apex does not generally lie in the same plane as does the left ventricular outflow tract and, hence, is rarely recorded in a parasternal long-axis view of the left ventricle, which does include a well-recorded aortic root. When

an apparent apex appears, it generally has a rounded configuration and has been termed a "foreshortened apex." This configuration represents the passage of the imaging plane through the diaphragmatic surface of the left ventricle and does not convey information concerning either the structure or the function of the actual cardiac apex, which must be recorded separately.

Second, the parasternal long axis of the apex is recorded by placing the transducer over the anterior wall of the left ventricle slightly above the apical tip. Thus, the transducer is not positioned appropriately to use the apex as a "window." In addition, the central ray of the imaging plane is directed in an anteroposterior orientation, similar to that of the parasternal group, rather than upward toward the base of the heart, as occurs in the apical imaging planes. Finally, the apical plane is included as a separate entity to emphasize the importance of this region in patients with ischemic heart disease and to highlight the fact that apical structure and function are best recorded in an anteroposterior plane perpendicular to the long axis of this structure rather than in one of the apical views.

Parasternal Long Axis of the Left Side of the Heart

The parasternal long axis of the left heart is the most important and frequently recorded of the standard cross-sectional imaging planes. It encompasses most of the primary echocardiographic structures on the left side of the heart (the aortic valve, mitral valve, and interventricular septum) and is oriented such that these structures lie perpendicular to the path of the imaging planes, are optimally reflective, and are recorded using the axial resolution of the imaging system.

This imaging plane is recorded with the transducer placed in a parasternal location, usually in either the third, fourth, or fifth intercostal spaces to the immediate left of the sternum. The best initial point to position the transducer can usually be determined by running the fingertips along the lower left sternal edge until the widest and deepest interspace in this region is defined. The transducer is then placed in this interspace with the central ray of the imaging plane (which is an extension of the long axis of the transducer) directed posteriorly toward the dorsal surface of the thorax. The examining plane is then rotated to align its Y axis parallel to an imaginary line running from the right shoulder to the left flank. If the left ventricle is normally positioned, this plane orientation should align the imaging plane parallel to its long axis. Because the left ventricle is generally situated to the left of the sternum, a slight degree of leftward angulation (up to 30 degrees) of the plane (toward the left shoulder) is commonly necessary to direct it through the true long axis of the ventricular cavity. Figure 4–1, A, illustrates the characteristic spatial orientation of this imaging plane and the path along which it transects the left heart. When displayed, the tip of the sector, indicated by the reference mark (R), is positioned to the lower left on the viewing scope. The left heart therefore appears sectioned from apex to base and viewed from the left shoulder. In this orientation, the right ventricle, which is closest to the transducer, is displayed anteriorly, whereas the left ventricle and left atrium are posteriorly positioned. The apex is to the left, and the aorta is to the right.

Figure 4–1, B, diagrammatically depicts the relative positions of the primary and associated cardiac structures that are recorded in this view. Figure 4–1, C, is an actual parasternal long-axis recording. Beginning anteriorly at the apex of the sector, the chest-wall echoes, followed by the moving echoes from the anterior right ventricular wall, are initially recorded. Beneath the anterior right ventricular wall lies a portion of the right ventricular cav-

ity, which continues to the right as the infundibular portion of the right ventricular outflow tract. Continuing clockwise along the right-hand margin of the image, the aortic root and aortic leaflets can be seen. Moving leftward, the anterior margin of the aortic root becomes continuous with the membranous portion of the interventricular septum, whereas its posterior margin joins the anterior mitral leaflet at the anterior extreme of the left-sided atrioventricular ring. The left atrium lies behind the aortic root, and the posterior left atrial wall is the most posterior cardiac structure normally recorded in this view. Behind the left atrium, an oval, echo-free space is frequently noted. This space is produced by the descending aorta as it courses through the posterior thorax (see Chap. 7). The vessel typically appears oblong because this plane orientation is normally oblique to both its long and short axes. Continuing leftward, the left atrial posterior wall joins the left ventricular posterior wall at the posterior margin of the left-sided atrioventricular ring. In the groove between the atrial and ventricular walls, a circular echo-free space, representing the coronary sinus, is occasionally recorded (see Chap. 6). When the coronary sinus dilates, it may be confused with the larger descending aorta. They can be differentiated, however, by their motion patterns. The descending aorta is extracardiac and, therefore, does not move in concert with the heart, whereas the coronary sinus follows the motion pattern of the atrioventricular ring.

The left ventricular posterior wall extends leftward from the atrioventricular junction to the left-hand margin of the image and can generally be visualized to the level of the papillary muscles. By angling the plane toward the cardiac apex, the examiner may slightly increase the extent of the posterior wall that can be recorded; however, the left ventricular apex normally lies directly beneath the anterior chest wall, one or more interspaces below

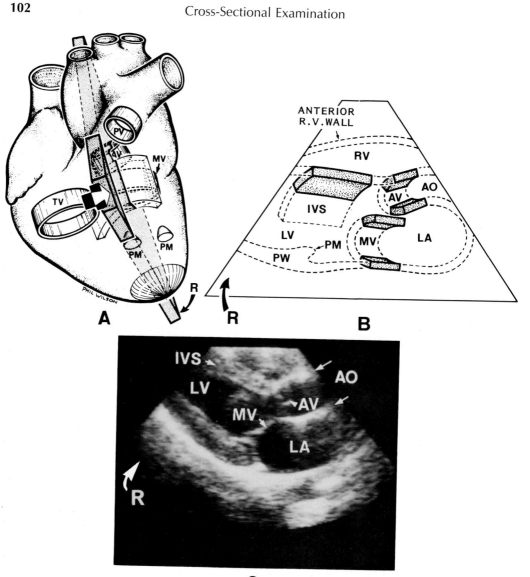

Fig. 4-1. *A,* Diagram illustrates the spatial orientation of the imaging plane in the parasternal long-axis view of the left heart and the path along which this plane intersects the principal echocardiographic structures in this area. The reference mark (R) indicates the side of the plane that is positioned in the lower left-hand corner of the display scope. PV = pulmonary valve; AV = aortic valve; MV = mitral valve; TV = tricuspid valve; PM = papillary muscles. *B,* Diagram illustrates the relative positions in which primary and adjacent structures recorded in the parasternal long-axis view of the left heart appear on the display scope. The reference mark (R) in this diagram corresponds to the point indicated by the corresponding reference mark in Figure 4-1, *A.* AO = aorta; RV = right ventricle; PW = posterior wall of the left ventricle; IVS = interventricular septum; LA = left atrium; AV = aortic valve; MV = mitral valve; LV = left ventricle; PM = papillary muscle. *C,* Parasternal long-axis recording of the base of the left heart. The labelling is similar to the preceding figures. (See text for further details.)

the transducer level commonly used to record the base of the heart. Thus, except in small hearts, the plane cannot be angled sharply enough to record the cardiac apex. The apex, therefore, must be visualized using a separate view (to be discussed later). Anterior to the posterior left ventricular wall is the large, echo-free left ventricular cavity, which is the largest single structure recorded. Within the left ventricular cavity, the full extent of the anterior and posterior mitral leaflets can be visualized with their chordal attachments to the papillary muscles. Anterior to the left ventricular cavity is the muscular interventricular septum. This structure can be recorded from its junction with the membranous septum directly inferior to the anterior aortic root to a point directly proximal to the cardiac apex.

The number and variety of structures contained within this imaging plane present several problems from both a recording and an interpretive standpoint. First, the examiner's eye cannot simultaneously look at all the moving structures in a 90-degree image critically. Therefore, in both recording and analysis, the images must be optimized to specific areas.

Secondly, the long axes of all the structures contained within this view do not normally lie in the same anatomic plane. The long axis of the aorta, for example, is normally oriented at approximately a 30-degree angle to the long axis of the left ventricle, and hence, plane positioning must be individualized to the particular area of interest to record precisely a true long axis of either of these structures.

Failure to recognize this fact has led to one of the most common errors encountered in cross-sectional imaging. This error arises because most examiners instinctively attempt to align the imaging plane to optimally record the valvular structures at the base of the heart, particularly the aortic valve and the aortic root. The plane must be parallel to the long axis of the aorta to achieve such a recording. Such placement displaces the plane to the right of the long axis of the left ventricle; consequently, the left-hand margin of the plane passes through the diaphragmatic surface of the left ventricle in the region of the posteromedial papillary muscle. The resulting image depicts the anterior and posterior walls of the ventricle curving toward each other and meeting at the left-hand margin of the scan. This pattern has

been referred to as a foreshortened apex or a truncated apex, but it clearly does not represent the true cardiac apex and may be displaced from it by a number of centimeters. Attempts to evaluate apical structure or wall motion or to derive a left ventricular long axis from this record are invalid.

Figure 4–1, C, which has been optimized to record the aortic valve, would probably result in such a foreshortened apex if continued to the left. Precise positioning of this plane, therefore, requires that the plane be individually optimized to record the most important structures it contains. Those of major interest include (1) the aortic valve and aortic root, (2) the mitral valve, and (3) the left ventricular chamber.

Precise positioning of the scan plane to record the aortic valve and aortic root is achieved by using the principles described in Chapter 3. First, the plane is rotated until the diameters of the vessel at the annulus and right-hand margin are maximal. This rotation aligns the plane parallel to the true long axis of the aorta. It is then swept across the vessel from the medial to lateral walls to assure maximal diameters at all points. As a result, the plane passes through the true long axis. This movement permits a quantitative determination of aortic root diameter at all levels and a comparison of diameters at individual levels. It also permits the recording of the maximal excursion of the aortic leaflets.

The long axis of the mitral valve is optimally recorded by angling the scan plane back and forth across the mitral leaflets to define the point of maximal leaflet opening amplitude. Because the valve, when fully opened, parallels the circumferential margin of the left ventricle, the peak amplitude of opening occurs in the midportion of the valve. The point of maximal leaflet opening should also correspond to the maximal left ventricular internal diameter at the base of the heart because the valve orifice is concentrically positioned within the left ventricular cavity.

Alignment of the plane parallel to the long axis of both the left ventricle and mitral valve requires that the internal diameters of the left ventricle be maximal at the mitral valve level and at the left-hand margin of the scan plane. To define its anteroposterior orientation more precisely, the left-hand margin of the plane should be aligned so that it passes between the two papillary muscles without recording echoes from either muscle. In this fashion, the plane passes through the true long axis of the left ventricle, and its anteroposterior position is defined within narrow limits. It should thus provide information that is both quantitative and reproducible.

The parasternal long axis of the left heart or one of its variations is ideally suited to evaluate the specific anatomic and functional characteristics of a number of structures, including:

1. The anterior right ventricular free wall and right ventricular cavity. Right ventricular free wall thickness, thickening, and excursion can be assessed. A right ventricular cavity dimension that correlates roughly with right ventricular size can also be obtained. This measurement, however, cannot be standardized, nor does it correspond to any natural right ventricular dimension. Although this measurement is comparable to the right ventricular dimension commonly recorded in M-mode studies, more representative right ventricular chamber measurements should be sought in other views (see Chap. 11).

2. The aortic root. Aortic root dimensions at multiple levels, from the aortic annulus to the proximal ascending aorta, can be visualized, and changes in aortic configuration characteristic of dilatation, aneurysms, or supravalvular stenotic lesions can be appreciated. This view is not particularly useful for detecting sinus of Valsalva aneurysms because each of the sinuses lies outside the scan plane. When sinus of Valsalva aneurysms are large they

may be evident in this view, but in general, they are better recorded by using a short-axis plane at the aortic root level (plane #6, see Chap. 7).

3. The aortic valve. Aortic leaflet thickening, calcification, reduced leaflet excursion due to anatomic restriction or disturbed transvalvular flow, doming of the congenitally stenotic valve, valvular vegetations, valvular motion relative to the aorta and left ventricular outflow tract, leaflet disruption, and prolapse can be recorded (see Chap. 7).

4. The left atrium. Left atrial anteroposterior and cranial-caudal dimensions, chamber area, phasic changes in chamber size, atrioventricular ring motion, and intracavitary masses, such as left atrial tumors and occasionally thrombi, can be appreciated (see Chap. 6).

5. The mitral valve. The systolic and diastolic configuration and motion patterns of the mitral leaflets, leaflet thickening, abnormalities of leaflet or chordal attachment, doming of the anterior mitral leaflet in mitral stenosis, the abnormal relationship of leaflet motion to the left ventricular and atrial chambers in anatomic mitral valve prolapse, mitral leaflet vegetations (see Chap. 5), and systolic anterior motion of the mitral valve such as occurs in idiopathic hypertrophic subaortic stenosis (IHSS) (see Chap. 7), can be visualized.

6. The anterobasal portion of the interventricular septum. Septal motion, thickness, systolic thickening, continuity with the anterior root of the aorta, location of the normal hinge point between systolic anterior motion of the basal septum in parallel with the aortic root and the posterior contractile movement of the body of the septum, and ventricular septal defects involving the membranous septum, particularly those associated with aortic overriding, can be appreciated. The ventricular septal defects that occur following acute myocardial infarction usually involve a more posterior portion of the apical sep-

tum and, hence, are not seen well in this view (see Chap. 12).

7. The left ventricle. This plane is optimally suited to record the anteroposterior or minor dimension of the left ventricle. This dimension can be optimized at the free edges of the mitral leaflets or a maximal dimension can be obtained. On occasion, the abnormal intracavitary echoes associated with left ventricular thrombi or tumors can be detected. The majority of thrombi, however, lie in the apical region and are best seen in the long axis of the cardiac apex or one of the apical views (see Chap. 8).

8. The posterior left ventricular wall. Posterior wall motion, thickness, and thickening can be determined (see Chap. 8).

9. The pericardium. The region immediately beneath the left ventricular posterior wall at the base of the AV ring represents the most common area for pericardial fluid accumulation. This region is also a common area for tumor infiltration of the pericardium. This view, therefore, is the most important initial imaging plane for evaluating pericardial integrity (see Chap. 15).

10. Mitral aortic continuity. Abnormal mitral aortic continuity, which occurs in double-outlet right ventricle (see Chap. 13), or the increase in mitral-aortic separation seen in various forms of fixed discrete subaortic stenosis can be appreciated (see Chap. 9).

11. Coronary sinus size and differentiation of many of the causes of coronary sinus enlargement (see Chap. 6).

Chamber measurements ideally recorded in this view are

1. The anteroposterior left ventricular internal dimension or short axis (see Chap. 8).

2. Aortic dimensions at any point from the aortic annulus to the farthest recordable extent of the ascending aorta. The diameter measured at the level of the sinuses of Valsalva, however, depends on the angle at which the plane intersects the sinuses and, hence, is neither as reproducible nor standardizable as are the other aortic dimensions (see Chap. 9).

3. Maximal aortic cusp separation. This dimension is recorded in both normal and stenotic aortic valves. Because the orifice may be eccentrically positioned in a stenotic valve, the maximal dimension may not correspond to the true long axis of the vessel and must be sought by scanning the imaging plane from the medial to the lateral walls of the aorta across the area of the stenotic valve (see Chap. 7).

4. The left atrial anteroposterior dimension. The left atrial superior-inferior dimension can also be obtained in this view. Recording this dimension may be easier, however, in an apical four-chamber view because the plane of the AV ring is more easily identified in that projection (see Chap. 6).

5. The atrioventricular ring diameter. This dimension is preferably recorded in this plane rather than in a short-axis view because the short-axis recording of the annulus is more difficult to standardize.

Measurements that generally cannot be recorded from this view are: (1) a long axis of the left ventricle, (2) a short axis of the right ventricle, and (3) a right ventricular outflow tract dimension.

Parasternal Long Axis of the Right Ventricular Inflow Tract

The parasternal long-axis view of the right ventricular inflow tract is intended to record the inferior portion of the right atrium, the tricuspid valve, and the basal two thirds of the right ventricle.

This view is recorded with the transducer in the parasternal location in either the third or the fourth intercostal spaces. As a rule, the transducer is moved laterally as far as possible from the sternum while still remaining within the parasternal window. The central ray is angled back beneath the sternum in the direction of the tricuspid valve. The transducer is then rotated approximately 15 to 30 degrees clockwise from the long axis of the left ventricle. This rotation aligns the Y axis of the imaging plane parallel to a line running from the right supraclavicular fossa to the left inguinal region. Figure 4–2, A, illustrates the spatial orientation of this plane. The only primary structure in this view is the tricuspid valve and the scan plane is typically positioned such that the tricuspid valve is in its center. Figure 4–2, B, diagrammatically depicts the path along which this plane transects the right ventricular inflow tract, and Figure 4–2, C, is an actual long-axis recording. In addition to the structures already mentioned, the proximal portion of the right ventricular outflow tract, bulging out from the anterior wall of the right ventricle above the anterior tricuspid leaflet, and the eustachian valve at the entrance of the inferior vena cava are also commonly recorded.

This plane is intended to record only the right ventricular inflow region, and the inclusion of any left-sided structures is inappropriate. The plane is optimized to record the right ventricle and tricuspid valve and is precisely positioned when both the anterior and posterior tricuspid leaflets are visualized at their point of maximal excursion and the right ventricular diameter at the left margin of the scan is maximal. When possible, following the tricuspid leaflets down to their insertion into the anterior and posterior right ventricular papillary muscles can be helpful because this should approximate the right ventricular long axis. Use of standard geometric reference figures to help to define precise positioning of this plane parallel to the right ventricular long axis is difficult because of the unusual shape of this chamber and the changes in its configuration that occur with dilatation. As a result, this plane is the most difficult to position precisely.

The parasternal long axis of the right ventricular inflow tract is the best view for evaluating tricuspid leaflet structure and function, particularly doming of the tricuspid valve in tricuspid stenosis and tricuspid vegetations. Prolapse of the anterior and posterior tricuspid leaflets can also be appreciated. This view is useful for detecting right atrial thrombi or tumors and intracavitary right ventricular masses. The right ventricular and right atrial dimensions recorded in this view are difficult to standardize, and hence, right ventricular chamber size is better evaluated in the apical or subcostal views. This view yields neither a true right ventricular long- nor short-axis dimension. The disorders recorded using this view are discussed in more detail in Chapter 9.

Parasternal Long Axis of the Right Ventricular Outflow Tract

The parasternal long-axis view of the right ventricular outflow tract is intended to record the infundibular portion of the right ventricle as it sweeps across the top of the aortic root, the pulmonary valve, and the proximal pulmonary artery. This view is recorded with the transducer placed in the parasternal window in the third or fourth intercostal spaces. It is best obtained with the transducer slightly below the true anatomic position of the right ventricular outflow tract and with the central ray of the imaging plane angled superiorly toward the right shoulder. The imaging plane is rotated approximately 30 to 45 degrees clockwise from the sagittal plane of the body. This rotation places the Y axis of the imaging plane parallel to a line running from the inner aspect of the left shoulder to the right flank.

Figure 4–3, A, illustrates the spatial orientation of this plane and the primary structure through which it passes. Figure 4–3, B, depicts diagrammatically the region of the heart transected by this plane, whereas Figure 4–3, C, is a representative

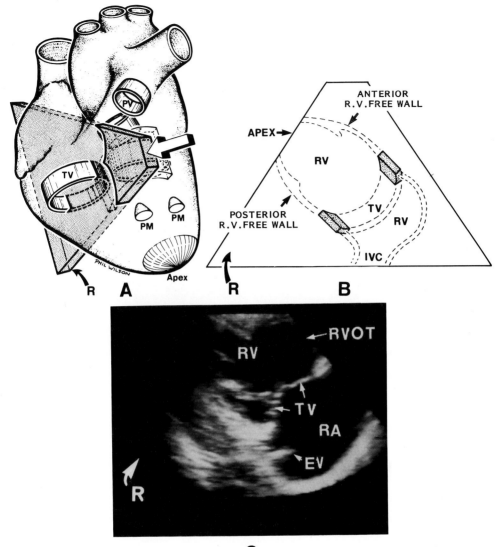

Fig. 4–2. *A,* Diagram illustrates the spatial orientation of the imaging plane in the parasternal long-axis view of the right ventricular inflow tract. The only primary structure transected by this plane is the tricuspid valve (TV), and the plane is oriented to pass through the center of the tricuspid orifice. R = reference mark; PV = pulmonary valve; PM = papillary muscle. *B,* Diagram depicts the relative positions on the display scope of the structures recorded in the parasternal long-axis view of the right ventricular inflow tract. R = reference mark; IVS = interventricular septum; RV = right ventricle; TV = tricuspid valve. *C,* Cross-sectional recording of the right ventricular inflow tract including the basal two thirds of the right ventricle (RV), two of the right ventricular papillary muscles, the anterior and posterior tricuspid valve (TV) leaflets, and the right atrium (RA). In addition, the eustachian valve (EV) and the proximal portion of the right ventricular outflow tract (RVOT), which bulges out from the anterior wall of the right ventricular cavity, can also be visualized. R = reference mark.

recording of this region. When appropriately positioned, the right ventricular outflow tract should appear on the display immediately beneath the chest wall. The pulmonary artery and pulmonary valve should be to the right, and the right ventricle should appear to the left. The aorta is transected obliquely and lies in the center of the scan, whereas the left atrium is posteriorly positioned. The plane is opti-

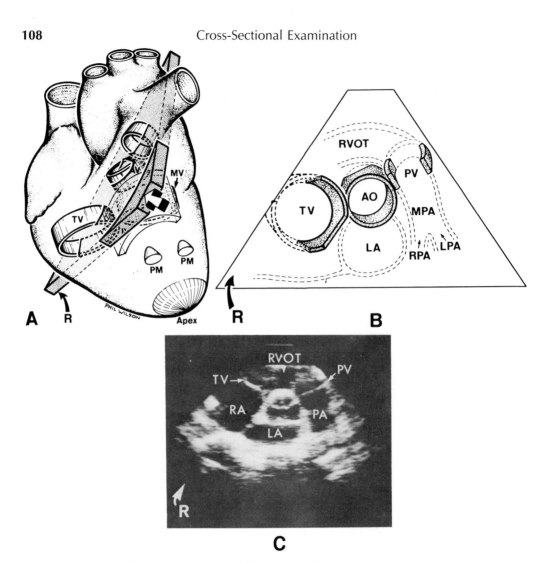

Fig. 4–3. *A,* Diagram illustrates the orientation of the imaging plane in the parasternal long-axis view of the right ventricular outflow tract. This plane transects the midportion of the pulmonary valve and passes obliquely through the aortic valve (AV) and anterior margin of the tricuspid valve (TV). MV = mitral valve; PM = papillary muscle; R = reference mark. *B,* Diagram illustrates the relative positions on the display scope of the primary and adjacent structures recorded in the parasternal long-axis view of the right ventricular outflow tract (RVOT). The stippled areas indicate the portions of the primary echocardiographic structures through which the imaging plane passes. Because the great vessels cross at their origins, the pulmonary valve (PV) is viewed in a plane that is parallel to its long axis, whereas the aorta (AO) and the tricuspid valve (TV) are imaged in a plane that is oblique to their short axes. R = reference mark; LA = left atrium; RPA = right pulmonary artery; LPA = left pulmonary artery; MPA = main pulmonary artery. *C,* Parasternal long-axis recording of the right ventricular outflow tract (RVOT). PV = pulmonary valve; PA = pulmonary artery; RA = right atrium; TV = tricuspid valve; LA = left atrium; R = reference mark. (See text for further details.)

mally recorded when the diameters of the right ventricular outflow tract are maximal at its proximal and distal extremes, the pulmonary valve is visible, and its motion is appreciated.

This plane is primarily used for assessing right ventricular outflow dimensions and is particularly useful in assessing infundibular diameter in patients with infundibular pulmonary stenosis and tetralogy of Fallot. It is also useful for recording pulmonary valve motion and configuration in patients with valvular pulmonary stenosis and pulmonary vegetations.

Parasternal Long Axis of the Main Pulmonary Artery

The parasternal long axis of the main pulmonary artery is recorded with the transducer in the third intercostal space and the central ray of the scan plane angled superiorly and rotated slightly clockwise relative to the parasternal long axis of the right ventricular outflow tract. This plane is utilized to evaluate the distal segment of the pulmonary infundibulum, the pulmonary valve, and the main pulmonary artery to its bifurcation. Figure 4–4, A, illustrates the spatial orientation of this plane relative to the pulmonary artery and valve. Figure 4–4, B, diagrammatically depicts the path along which this scan plane transects the distal right ventricular outflow tract and main pulmonary artery. Figure 4–4, C, is a representative recording of these structures. This plane orientation places the proximal portion of the pulmonary artery and the region of the pulmonary valve at the apex of the sector. The pulmonary artery then courses posteriorly along the right-hand margin of the display to its point of bifurcation into the right and left main pulmonary arteries. The pulmonary artery thus appears as if viewed from the cardiac apex. The aorta, which is transected obliquely, lies behind the proximal portion of this vessel and to its immediate left.

This imaging plane is appropriately recorded when the bifurcation of the main pulmonary artery into its two branches is well visualized, the diameter of the main pulmonary artery from the pulmonary valve to the point of bifurcation is maximal, and the walls of the vessel are parallel. This plane is particularly useful for recording abnormalities of the main pulmonary artery and, in certain cases, is helpful for confirming the diagnosis of valvular pulmonary stenosis.

Parasternal Long Axis of the Left Ventricular Apex

The parasternal long axis of the left ventricular apex is intended to record specifically the structural and functional characteristics of the apex. It is recorded with the transducer placed on the anterior chest wall above the apical impulse and the central ray directed toward the posterior thoracic wall. The imaging plane is then rotated to align its Y axis parallel to the long axis of the left ventricle.

Figure 4–5, A, illustrates the spatial orientation of this plane. The apical long axis can be located by: (1) aligning the imaging plane parallel to the short axis of the left ventricle at the apex (see plane 9, the parasternal short axis of the left ventricular apex), (2) placing the central ray of the imaging plane in the center of the ventricle, and then (3) rotating the plane 90 degrees about its Z axis. These steps should align the plane so that it is precisely parallel to the long axis of the ventricle and passes through the tip of the apex. Figure 4–5, B, diagrammatically depicts the path along which this plane transects the apex, whereas Figure 4–5, C, is a representative apical recording. The anatomic tip of the apex is displayed anteriorly and to the left. In addition to the apex, the anterior and posterior walls of the left ventricle to the level of the papillary muscles are recorded. This plane is precisely positioned by recording the most acute apical tip (the largest ventricular diameter at the right-hand margin of the scan) and positioning the plane such that it passes between the papillary muscles. Its position relative to the circumference of the ventricle can be cross-checked by rotating to the short axis without shifting the position of the Z axis or central ray.

This view is optimal for recording apical shape and wall motion. It is useful for detecting apical thrombi and intracavitary tumors involving the apex. However, its primary role is in the detection of apical dyskinesis[12] and aneurysms.[13]

PARASTERNAL SHORT-AXIS PLANES

Four standard planes are recorded from the parasternal location with the imaging

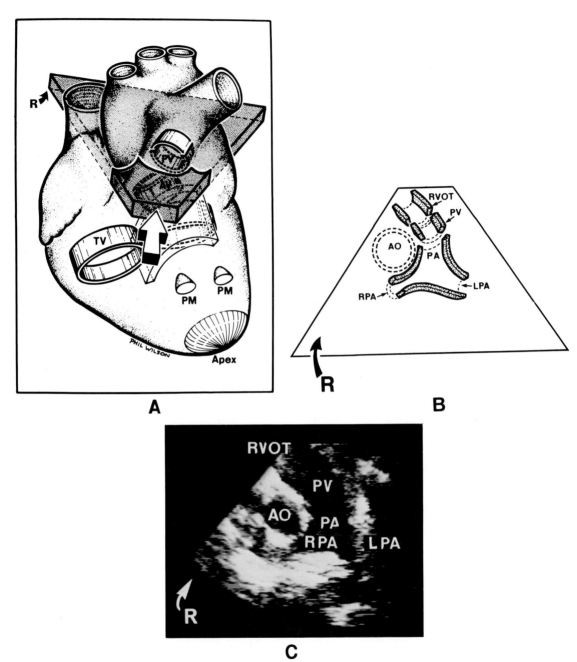

Fig. 4–4.   *A,* Diagram depicts the orientation of the imaging plane in the parasternal long-axis view of the main pulmonary artery. This plane transects the midportion of the pulmonary valve (PV) and continues through the pulmonary artery to its bifurcation. AV = aortic valve; TV = tricuspid valve; PM = papillary muscle. *B,* Diagram illustrates the relative positions of the pulmonary valve (PV) and adjacent structures as they appear on the display scope in the parasternal long-axis view of the main pulmonary artery (PA). The stippled areas indicate the portions of the vessels that are intersected by the imaging plane and, hence, are recorded on the final image. RVOT = right ventricular outflow tract; AO = aorta; LPA = left pulmonary artery; RPA = right pulmonary artery. *C,* Long-axis cross-sectional recording of the main pulmonary artery illustrates the proximal right ventricular outflow tract, the region of the pulmonary valve, the main pulmonary artery (PA), and its bifurcation into the right (R) and left (L) pulmonary arteries. The aorta, which is viewed in a plane oblique to its short axis, lies beneath the right ventricular outflow tract and to the left of the main pulmonary artery. R = reference point; AO = aorta.

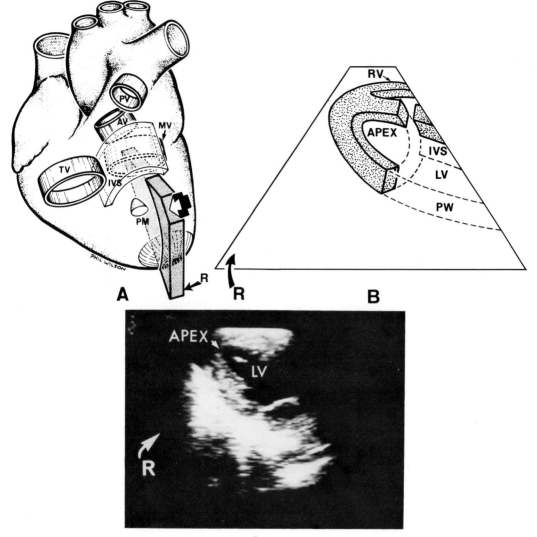

Fig. 4–5. *A,* Diagram illustrates the orientation of the imaging plane in the parasternal long-axis view of the cardiac apex. This plane passes through the tip of the left ventricular apex, intersects the long axis of the left ventricle, and passes between the two papillary muscles (PM). PV = pulmonary valve; AV = aortic valve; MV = mitral valve; TV = tricuspid valve; IVS = interventricular septum; R = reference mark. *B,* Diagram illustrates the relative positions of the structures recorded in the parasternal long axis of the cardiac apex on the display scope. The tip of the apex is displayed to the left. The apical portion of the interventricular septum (IVS) and posterior left ventricular walls (PW) courses to the right from the apical tip. RV = right ventricle; LV = left ventricle; R = reference mark. *C,* Long-axis parasternal recording of the left ventricular (LV) apex illustrates the normal apical configuration. R = reference mark.

plane aligned parallel to the short axes of the left ventricle or aorta. These planes are the parasternal short axis of the aorta and left atrium, the left ventricle at the mitral valve level, the left ventricle at the papillary muscle level, and the left ventricular apex. Each of the ventricular planes is oriented parallel to, rather than through, the true short axis of the left ventricle. Their specific point of intersection is designated on the basis of the structures the plane transects. Again, one might argue that the apical short axis view is not truly a para-sternal view, but rather an apical view. For reasons similar to those considered in the discussion of the apical long-axis view (standard plane #5), this apical short axis is considered a parasternal plane.

The four short-axis views are intended primarily to record the left heart. Although portions of right-sided structures are included in each of these views, the planes are not specifically oriented to record these structures optimally.

When the examiner wants to record any of the right-sided structures in their short-axis configuration, the transducer can be angled toward the right ventricle and the plane realigned (based on the principles described in Chap. 3) to optimally record the features of the area desired. To date, short-axis planes of right-sided structures have not been used frequently enough to be considered standard and, therefore, must be described individually.

Parasternal Short Axis of the Aortic Valve and Left Atrium

The parasternal short axis of the aortic valve and left atrium is recorded with the transducer in the third or fourth intercostal spaces to the immediate left of the sternum. The central ray of the imaging plane is directed either posteriorly toward the dorsal surface of the body or angled slightly rightward and superiorly toward the right shoulder. The plane is then rotated 90 degrees clockwise from a parasternal long-axis orientation at the aortic root level. This rotation places the Y axis of the imaging plane parallel to a line extending from slightly beneath the left shoulder to the right subcostal region. The spatial orientation of this plane and the path along which it intersects the primary structures at the base of the heart are illustrated in Figure 4–6, A. Figure 4–6, B, depicts diagrammatically the portion of these structures intersected by the plane and their relative positions on the display scope. The

right ventricular outflow tract is transected first and, thus, appears at the apex of the sector with the pulmonary valve to the right and the right ventricle to the left. The aorta appears circular and is positioned in the center of the scan with the left atrium posteriorly behind the aorta. The heart is thus displayed as if viewed from the apex. Figure 4–6, C, is an actual short-axis recording of the aortic root and surrounding structures. This imaging plane, although similar to that used in recording the long axis of the right ventricular outflow tract and the long axis of the left main coronary artery, lies midway between the two.

Recording of this plane is optimized to the short axis of the aortic root at the aortic valve level. Optimal alignment of this plane, as with other short-axis planes, is achieved by angling and rotating the transducer until the aortic root shows the least degree of vertical and horizontal obliquity and the aortic leaflets are recorded in as much detail as possible.

This imaging plane is best for recording specific features of (1) the aortic valve, including the aortic valve orifice, the number and orientation of the aortic leaflets, the position of the aortic commissures, the definition of aortic leaflet movement, and the degree of leaflet involvement with bacterial vegetations; (2) the aortic root, specifically the determination of the size of sinuses of Valsalva and the presence or absence of aneurysms (it may also be helpful in detecting aortic dissection); (3) the left atrium, including atrial tumors or thrombi; an anteroposterior atrial diameter, which can be correlated with the anteroposterior dimension recorded in the long-axis view; a medial-lateral dimension; and a long axis of the coronary sinus; and (4) the interatrial septum. Although the interatrial septum was first recorded and described using this view,[13,14] better visualization of the septum is obtained using either the apical four-chamber[9] or the subxiphoid planes.[7,8] The parasternal

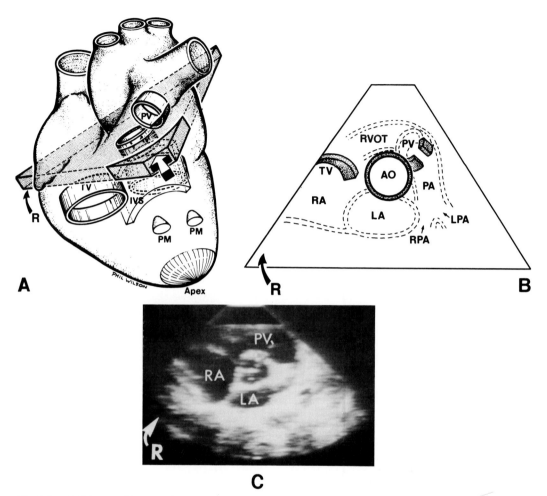

Fig. 4–6. *A,* Diagram illustrates the spatial orientation of the imaging plane in the parasternal short-axis view of the aortic root and the left atrium. This plane passes through the aortic valve (AV) parallel to its short axis and passes obliquely through the inferior margin of the pulmonary valve (PV). The point of the sector indicated by the reference mark (R) is displayed at the lower left-hand margin of the display scope. Structures recorded in this plane are therefore displayed as though viewed from the cardiac apex. TV = tricuspid valve; IVS = interventricular septum; PM = papillary muscle. *B,* Diagram illustrates the primary and adjacent cardiac structures that are recorded in the parasternal short-axis view of the aortic root (AO) and left atrium (LA). Their relative positions on the final display are also evident. R = reference mark; RA = right atrium; TV = tricuspid valve; RVOT = right ventricular outflow tract; PV = pulmonary valve; PA = main pulmonary artery; LPA = left pulmonary artery; RPA = right pulmonary artery. *C,* Parasternal short-axis recording of the aorta and left atrium. The aorta, which is transected parallel to its short axis, appears as a circular structure in the center of the scan. The left atrium (LA) lies directly behind the aorta, and the right ventricular outflow tract crosses above the aorta from left to right. A portion of the tricuspid annulus is recorded separating the right ventricle and atrium, whereas the interatrial septum, stretching posteriorly and to the left from the posteromedial border of the aorta, separates the left (LA) and the right atria (RA). PV = pulmonary valve; R = reference mark.

short axis is useful, however, for recording changes in anteroposterior atrial septal position and orientation in both left and right atrial enlargement. It can also be used to detect ostium primum and ostium secundum atrial septal defects and to observe contrast flow along the septum; however, it is not optimal for either of these tasks.

The parasternal short axis is also the primary view for assessing the relative position of the great vessels at the base of the heart and the number and orientation of the great vessels in the transposition complexes and truncus arteriosus.

Parasternal Short Axis of the Left Ventricle (Mitral Valve Level)

The parasternal short axis of the left ventricle at the mitral valve level is recorded with the transducer placed in a parasternal location in the third, fourth, or fifth intercostal spaces. The central ray of the scan plane is directed posteriorly or posteriorly and slightly leftward, and the imaging plane is rotated 90 degrees from the long axis of the left ventricle so that it is aligned parallel to the ventricular short axis. This plane orientation is roughly parallel to a line running from the left shoulder to the right flank.

Figure 4–7, A, illustrates the typical spatial orientation of this plane. It encompasses the entire left ventricle, the mitral valve, and the medial portion of the tricuspid valve. Figure 4–7, B, diagrammatically depicts the path along which the plane intersects the primary structures at the base of the heart. The relative orientation of the primary structures on the display scope is also shown. The anterior portion of the right ventricle is recorded first and is displayed anteriorly and to the left. Fragments of the tricuspid valve are commonly visible and are recorded along the left margin of the scan. The interventricular septum separating the right and left ventricles lies beneath the right ventricle, is normally concave toward the left ventricle, and anatomically forms a portion of the left ventricular wall. The left ventricle, which appears circular when viewed in short axis, is posterior and to the left. The mitral leaflets are recorded in the center of the left ventricle. The left ventricle, therefore, is displayed as if viewed from the cardiac apex. Figure 4–7, C, is a representative short-axis recording that illustrates the normal appearance and relative positions of these structures.

This plane is optimally recorded when both the anterior and posterior mitral leaflets are well visualized and when the left ventricular cavity shows the least vertical or horizontal obliquity. It is ideal for directly recording the mitral valve orifice and is used clinically to determine mitral valve area in mitral stenosis (see Chap. 5). This view is also useful for examining mitral leaflet redundancy in mitral valve prolapse, detecting the circumferential location of mitral vegetations, visualizing leaflet motion patterns in aortic insufficiency, and viewing incomplete leaflet closure in rheumatic mitral regurgitation.

The total circumference of the left ventricle can also be well recorded, and the absolute and relative patterns and amplitudes of left ventricular wall motion and thickening can be assessed. This plane is also used to detect distortions in left ventricular shape, specifically anterolateral aneurysms and abnormalities of interventricular septal position and motion. It is the primary plane used for assessing abnormalities in septal configuration in patients with right ventricular volume and pressure overload because the greatest degree of septal deformity and, thus, of left ventricular eccentricity is apparent in this view (see Chaps. 8 and 12).

Difficulties arise in attempting to visualize the anteromedial and anterolateral walls of the left ventricle. These two regions lie parallel to the ultrasonic beam, and the endocardial and epicardial targets in these areas are difficult to record. Both ventricular hypertrophy and increased endocardial infolding during systole make these targets easier to visualize. In many instances, however, the high lateral wall of the left ventricle cannot be recorded in this view, thereby making assessment of wall motion in this region impossible.

Parasternal Short Axis of the Left Ventricle (Papillary Muscle Level)

The parasternal short axis of the left ventricle at the papillary muscle level is recorded with the transducer in the fourth

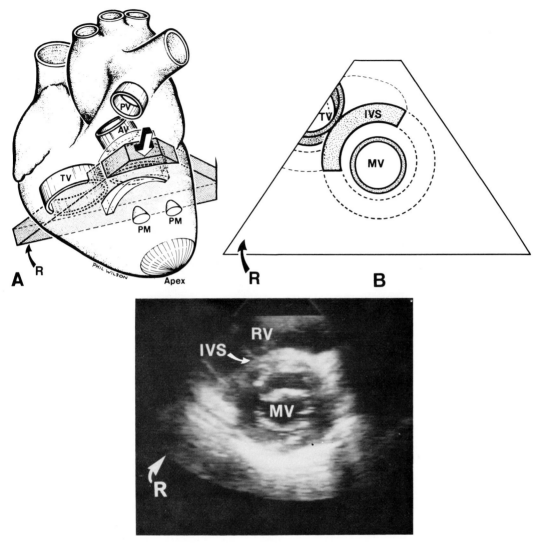

Fig. 4–7. *A,* Diagram illustrates the orientation of the imaging plane in the parasternal short-axis view of the left ventricle at the mitral valve level. This plane transects the mitral valve in a path parallel to its short axis, the base of the interventricular septum, and the medial portion of the tricuspid valve (TV). R = reference mark; PM = papillary muscle; AV = aortic valve; PV = pulmonary valve. *B,* Diagram illustrates the relative positions on the display scope of the primary and adjacent structures recorded in the parasternal short-axis view of the left ventricle at the mitral valve (MV) level. The medial portion of the tricuspid valve (TV) appears anterior and to the left immediately above the interventricular septum (IVS). The septum is to the left of center; the mitral valve is in the central portion of the scan. The medial anterior and posterior right ventricular walls and the entire circumference of the left ventricle at the base of the heart are also recorded in this view. R = reference mark. *C,* Parasternal short-axis recording of the left ventricle at the mitral valve (MV) level. This frame is recorded during diastole, and the mitral valve orifice surrounded by the curvilinear anterior and posterior mitral leaflets can be appreciated. The mitral valve lies within the left ventricular cavity, which appears circular in this orientation. The medial portion of the right ventricle (RV) and the interventricular septum (IVS) are also evident. R = reference mark.

or fifth intercostal spaces to the immediate left of the sternum. Transducer position is generally similar to that used to record the short-axis of the left ventricle at the mitral valve level. The papillary muscles can be recorded from this location by either angling the scan plane toward the cardiac apex or moving the transducer down one interspace. Plane rotation is identical to that used in recording the short axis of the left ventricle at the mitral valve level.

Figure 4–8, A, illustrates the orientation of this plane in space. Figure 4–8, B, diagrammatically depicts the path along which this plane intersects the papillary muscles and adjacent left ventricle. It typically encompasses the entire left ventricular cavity as well as the apical segment of the right ventricle. In this orientation, the right ventricle is displayed anteriorly and to the left. The interventricular septum is beneath the right ventricle, and the left ventricle is posterior. The papillary muscles are recorded along the medial and lateral walls of the left ventricular cavity. The posteromedial papillary muscle is displayed to the left, and the anterolateral papillary muscle is to the right. This plane, like all other short-axis planes, is displayed as if viewed from the apex. Again, as with other short-axis planes, fine plane positioning is achieved by alternately angling and rotating the plane until the least degree of horizontal and vertical obliquity is achieved. Both papillary muscles must be recorded because they are the internal reference that defines the final position of the plane. Figure 4–8, C, is an example of a parasternal short-axis recording of the left ventricle.

This imaging plane is optimally suited for recording left ventricular cavity size and myocardial function at the level of the papillary muscles. Assessment of the contractile pattern of the left ventricle at this level is of major importance in patients with ischemic heart disease. In addition, an association has been demonstrated between left ventricular dyskinesis at the base of the papillary muscle and the clinical syndrome of papillary muscle dysfunction due to incomplete mitral valve closure. This relationship is discussed in detail in Chapter 5.

Parasternal Short Axis of the Left Ventricle (Apical Level)

The parasternal short axis of the left ventricle at the cardiac apex is recorded with the transducer located on the anterior chest wall above or just proximal to the apical impulse. This location is usually at least one interspace lower than that used to record the papillary muscles. The central ray of the examining plane is directed posteriorly, and the plane rotated parallel to the orientation used to record the short-axis views at the mitral valve and papillary muscle levels.

The spatial orientation of this plane is illustrated in Figure 4–9, A. The plane normally transects the left ventricle just proximal to the apex and encompasses the entire circumference of the ventricle at a point midway between the papillary muscles and the apical tip. The only structures recorded at this level are the left ventricular cavity and the surrounding myocardium. A small segment of right ventricle is occasionally observed anteriorly. The position of this plane is defined by the absence of papillary muscles or apical endocardium. As depicted in Figure 4–9, B, only the left ventricular wall is typically recorded. Figure 4–9, C, is a normal apical short axis. As with the other short-axis views, precise plane position is achieved by angling and rotating the transducer until the least degree of horizontal or vertical obliquity of the left ventricle is obtained.

This imaging plane is primarily used in conjunction with the long-axis and apical views to assess the magnitude and extent of regional dyssynergy. It can also be helpful in detecting apical thrombi and in assessing the degree of circumferential involvement of the apex when an apical aneurysm is present.

APICAL VIEWS

There are four primary apical views: the apical four chamber, the apical five cham-

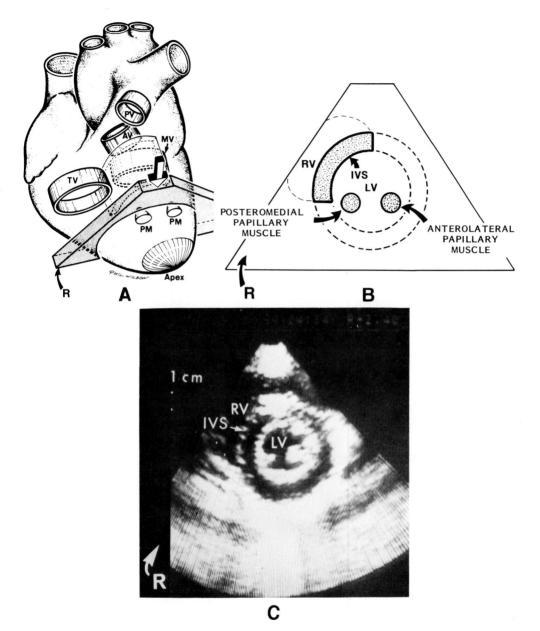

Fig. 4–8. *A,* Diagram illustrates the imaging plane orientation in the parasternal short-axis view of the left ventricle at the papillary muscle (PM) level. This plane transects the entire circumference of the left ventricle, the apical portion of the right ventricle, and by definition, includes both the anterolateral and posteromedial papillary muscles. R = reference mark; TV = tricuspid valve; MV = mitral valve; AV = aortic valve; PV = pulmonary valve. *B,* Diagram illustrates the relative positions of the primary and adjacent echocardiographic structures recorded in the parasternal long-axis view of the left ventricle (LV) as they appear on the display scope. The apical portion of the right ventricle (RV) is anterior and to the left, whereas the circular left ventricular cavity is in the center of the scan plane. The interventricular septum (IVS), which is concave toward the left ventricle, separates the right and left ventricular chambers. The posteromedial papillary muscle is displayed to the left, and the anterolateral papillary muscle is shown to the right. R = reference mark. *C,* Parasternal short-axis recording of the left ventricle (LV) at the papillary muscle level. The circular left ventricle is apparent in the center of the scan plane. The right ventricle (RV) is anterior and to the left. The anterolateral and posteromedial papillary muscles can be visualized arising from the endocardial surface of the left ventricular cavity. R = reference mark; IVS = interventricular septum.

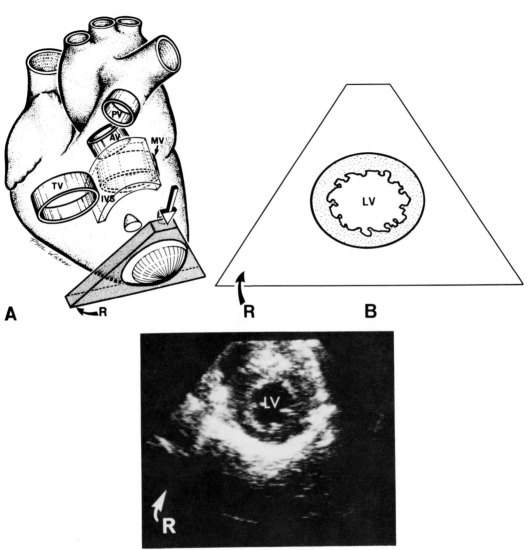

Fig. 4–9. *A,* Diagram illustrates the orientation of the imaging plane in the parasternal short-axis view of the cardiac apex. This plane transects the ventricle midway between the papillary muscles and the tip of the anatomic apex. On occasion, a small portion of the apical segment of the right ventricle and the apical extreme of the interventricular septum (IVS) are also included. R = reference mark; PV = pulmonary valve; AV = aortic valve; MV = mitral valve; TV = tricuspid valve. *B,* Diagram illustrates the circular short-axis appearance of the left ventricle (LV) at the apical level. This plane is defined by an absence of recognizable landmarks, and neither papillary muscles nor apical endocardium should be included. R = reference mark. *C,* Parasternal short-axis recording of the left ventricular apex. The circular left ventricle (LV) is recorded in the center of the sector, and a small portion of the right ventricle is evident anteriorly and to the left. There is some irregularity of the ventricular wall, but no clearly defined papillary muscles are evident. R = reference mark.

ber, the apical two chamber, and the apical long axis of the left ventricle. Each of these views is recorded with the transducer located directly over the anatomic tip of the cardiac apex and the central ray of the im-

aging plane directed toward the base of the heart. The apex can be located in two ways. The first method involves simply palpating the apical impulse and placing the transducer directly over the region of apical activity. Unfortunately, the apical impulse frequently does not overlie the true anatomic apex, but is produced by an adjacent area of the anterior left ventricular wall. In other cases, the apex may be distorted or its normal position occupied by structures other than the left ventricle. In these situations, the anatomic apex can be located by sequentially stepping the transducer down the short axis of the left ventricle. As the scan plane approaches the apex, the left ventricular cavity area gradually decreases, and the cavity is finally obliterated at the apical tip. This maneuver localizes the tip of the apex, and the apical views can then be recorded by angling the scan plane back toward the base of the heart. When the apical transducer position has been identified, all the apical views can be recorded from the same transducer location.

The Apical Four-Chamber View

The apical four-chamber view is recorded with the transducer located directly over the anatomic cardiac apex and the central ray of the scan plane directed superiorly and rightward toward the tip of the right scapula. The central ray is then angled to pass through the crux of the heart, and the plane is rotated until the full excursion of both the mitral and tricuspid valve leaflets are recorded. The spatial orientation of this plane is depicted in Figure 4–10, A. The position of the plane in space is fixed by three specific points: the cardiac apex, the mitral valve, and the tricuspid valve. When positioned in this fashion, the plane encompasses the left ventricle and atrium, right ventricle and atrium, the two atrioventricular valves, and the interventricular and interatrial septa. Motion of the right ventricular free wall and septum relative to the right and left ventricular cavities can also be visualized.

The resultant image is displayed such that the left ventricular apex is positioned at the apex of the sector (Fig. 4–10, B). The left ventricular cavity is anterior and to the right, and the left atrium is posterior and to the right behind the left ventricle. The right ventricle is anterior and to the left, and the right atrium is posterior along the left-hand margin of the display. The septa course vertically down the midline, and the apical extreme of the interventricular septum is closest to the apex of the sector. The atrioventricular valves are positioned horizontally and swing toward the apex of the sector during diastolic opening. Figure 4–10, C, is a representative recording of these structures.

Ideal positioning of this plane is achieved by placing the transducer over the precise anatomic cardiac apex and recording the maximal opening amplitude of both the mitral and tricuspid leaflets. Because the midpoint of the fully opened AV valves normally approximates the center of the corresponding ventricle, the valve orifices in the region of maximal leaflet opening should be intersected by the ventricular long axes. Because the long axis also passes through the apex, this plane alignment, when correctly positioned, should include the long axes of both ventricular chambers. Variations in plane angle may be utilized to record particular structures, such as the superior portion of the interatrial septum and the right and left inferior pulmonary veins. These variations are displaced from the ventricular long axis, are difficult to standardize, and, thus, are useful only for imaging the particular area of interest.

The apical four-chamber view is one of the most important standard planes because it encompasses both ventricles and atria simultaneously, thereby permitting the evaluation of their relative sizes, orientation, and structural integrity.

The left ventricle is transected from apex to base in a plane extending from the medial portion of the interventricular septum to the free lateral wall (or roughly from the 10 to the 4 o'clock positions of the corresponding short-axis planes). A ventricular

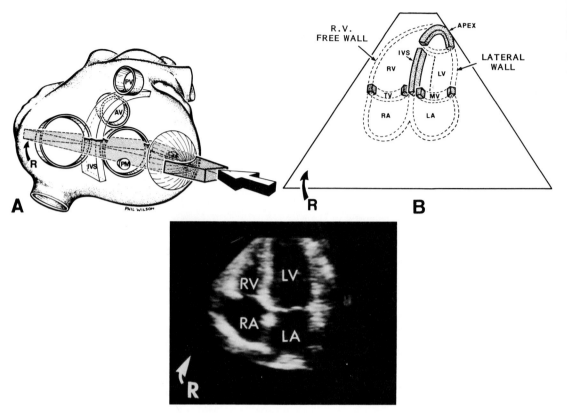

Fig. 4–10. *A,* Diagram illustrates the orientation of the imaging plane in the apical four-chamber view. This plane transects the heart from the tip of the cardiac apex to its superior border and passes through the center of both the mitral and tricuspid orifices. The point of the sector indicated by the reference mark (R) is displayed at the lower left of the display scope or as though viewed from beneath the heart. This plane transects the cardiac apex, the mitral and tricuspid valves, and the interventricular septum (IVS). It also encompasses both atria and ventricles and the interatrial septum. PM = papillary muscle; AV = aortic valve, PV = pulmonary valve. *B,* Diagram illustrates the orientation of the primary and adjacent cardiac structures as they appear on the display scope in the apical four-chamber view. IVS = interventricular septum; RV = right ventricle; LV = left ventricle; RA = right atrium; LA = left atrium; R = reference mark. *C,* Cross-sectional recording of the heart using the apical four-chamber view. The cardiac apex appears at the apex of the sector; the left ventricle (LV) is to the right and the right ventricle (RV) is to the left. The interventricular septum dividing these two chambers courses posteriorly through the midportion of the scan. The mitral and tricuspid valves are in their systolic position and, thus, are oriented perpendicular to the scan plane. Behind the AV valves, the left atrium (LA) positioned to the right, and the right atrium (RA) positioned to the left, are evident. Portions of the interatrial septum separating these two chambers can be visualized. R = reference mark.

area, long axis from the apical tip to the mitral annulus and short axis or minor dimension at any point along the long axis, can be measured (see Chap. 8). Endocardial targets along the medial and lateral walls unfortunately are recorded using the lateral resolution of the system and, therefore, are widened by the point-spread function of the beam at that level. This situation results in circumferential en-

croachment on the actual cavity area and in an underestimation of ventricular volumes and dimensions when the inner margins of the echoes are used to represent endocardial position. Motion of the septum and lateral wall can likewise be visualized, but is recorded as movement across data lines rather than along the beam axis and, thus, is not optimally displayed. This view, therefore, is more useful for assessing differences in motion at individual points along the ventricular walls than for measuring absolute excursion at any point.

The left ventricular apex must, by definition, be recorded in this and all the apical views. The tip of the apical endocardium unfortunately lies close to the transducer face, and the proximal ventricular walls curve away from the transducer in an arc that roughly parallels the path of the sound beam. The apical endocardium and ventricular wall motion in the apical region are therefore frequently not well recorded. Apparent apical motion can also be varied greatly by small changes in transducer position. For example, slight transducer displacement up the anterior ventricular wall causes the apex to appear rounded, dilated, and artifactually hypokinetic. Apical function, therefore, is better recorded in the parasternal long-axis view of the apex. The apical four-chamber view, however, is more useful for defining the apical intercept of the left ventricular long axis, detecting apical masses and thrombi, and recording gross distortions in apical geometry.

The right ventricle is likewise transected from apex to base in a plane extending from the midportion of the free lateral wall to the middle third of the interventricular septum. A right ventricular long axis, minor dimension at any point along the long axis, and right ventricular area can be determined (see Chap. 11). Motion of the right ventricular free wall and septum relative to the right and left ventricular cavities can also be visualized. The same limitations noted in attempting to record left ventricular medial and lateral wall endocardium are also encountered in the right ventricle. In addition, the right ventricular lateral wall is more difficult to record than is the left. Because the standard plane is optimized to record the left ventricular apex, slight adjustment of plane position may be required when attempting to record the right ventricular

long axis to ensure that the right ventricular apex is also included.

The left atrium is visualized in a plane extending from the AV ring to the superior atrial wall and from the interatrial septum to the free lateral border. Cranial-caudal and medial-lateral left atrial dimension, as well as an atrial area, can be obtained. Masses in the left atrium are well visualized, and their point of attachment to the atrial walls can frequently be assessed (see Chap. 6).

The pulmonary veins can often be visualized entering the superolateral and medial walls of the left atrium. Anomalies of pulmonary venous insertion can also be detected. The right atrium is recorded in a plane similar to that in which the left atrium is recorded, and comparable atrial dimensions and area measurements can be obtained (see Chap. 9). Intracavitary right atrial masses can frequently be visualized in this view, which forms an excellent complement to the parasternal long axis of the right ventricular inflow tract and subcostal long axis for demonstrating these lesions.

The entire extent of the midportion of the interventricular septum from the cardiac apex to the crux of the heart is displayed. Both acquired and congenital ventricular septal defects, particularly those of the ostium primum and AV canal varieties, are well visualized in this view. This apical view is particularly useful for recording the acquired ventricular septal defects that develop as a complication of acute myocardial infarction. These lesions are most commonly noted in the apical portion of the septum posteriorly, which is a well-visualized area (see Chap. 8).

The relationship of the interventricular and interatrial septa can also be defined. Normally, the ventricular and atrial septa do not lie along a straight line from apex to base, and the atrial septum is displaced slightly to the left of the ventricular septum.[1]* Right and left atrial volume and pressure overloads may alter these rela-

---

*Toward the left atrium rather than toward the viewer's left

tionships, and their presence can be inferred from the changes in atrial septal position they produce.

Finally, the relative systolic and diastolic positions, motion, and structural integrity of the mitral and tricuspid valves can be readily appreciated. The anterior mitral leaflet arises medially from the interventricular septum; the posterior leaflet arises from the lateral margin of the left-sided AV ring. The septal leaflet of the tricuspid valve likewise inserts medially, whereas the large anterior tricuspid leaflet arises from the lateral ring margin. The posterior tricuspid leaflet is not recorded in this plane. The anterior leaflet of the mitral valve normally inserts into the left atrioventricular ring at the superior end of the membranous septum. The septal leaflet of the tricuspid valve, in contrast, inserts into the midportion of the membranous septum and, therefore, is displaced toward the cardiac apex approximately 5 to 10 mm relative to the anterior mitral leaflet.[1] This anatomic distinction is important because it permits identification of the AV valves and accompanying ventricular chamber.

During systole, the leaflets of both AV valves are positioned so that they are parallel to the plane of their respective atrioventricular rings and perpendicular to the path of the scan plane. This orientation permits optimal leaflet visualization, and hence, this view is ideal for detecting abnormalities characterized by abnormal systolic position of the leaflets relative to the AV ring such as mitral and tricuspid valve prolapse, flail leaflets, and incomplete leaflet closure, which typically occurs with papillary muscle dysfunction. During diastole, the open leaflets point toward the apex, are oriented parallel to the path of the ultrasonic beam, and, as a result, are less well visualized. Some diastolic abnormalities, such as valve doming with stenotic lesions, can be recorded, but in general, less useful information is available during this portion of the cardiac cycle.

The Apical Five-Chamber View

The apical five-chamber view is recorded using a transducer position and plane orientation similar to those used to obtain the four-chamber view. From this position, the plane is angled slightly anterior toward the anterior chest wall. As the plane is shifted, the area occupied by the crux of the heart in the four-chamber view is replaced by the left ventricular outflow tract and proximal aorta. Figure 4–11, A, illustrates the spatial position of this plane. Using this plane orientation, in addition to the original four chambers, the aortic valve and the aortic root or a fifth chamber can be visualized.

The image orientation is similar to that for the four-chamber view with the apex positioned at the peak of the sector, the two ventricular chambers located anteriorly, and the two atrial chambers located posteriorly (Fig. 4–11, B). The left ventricle and left atrium are located to the right, and the right ventricle and right atrium are to the left. The fifth or aortic chamber lies posteriorly between the two atria. Figure 4–11, C, is an example of the five-chamber view. In this figure, the proximal portion of the outflow tract originates from the medial portion of the left ventricle at the base of the heart. The ventricular portion of the outflow tract is bounded medially by the interventricular septum, which continues distally as the medial border of the aortic root, and laterally by the anterior mitral leaflet and the base of the left ventricle, which are continuous with the lateral aortic root. The aortic leaflets can be seen in the proximal aorta.

This plane has limited utility beyond the assessment of the proximal portion of the left ventricular outflow tract and, as

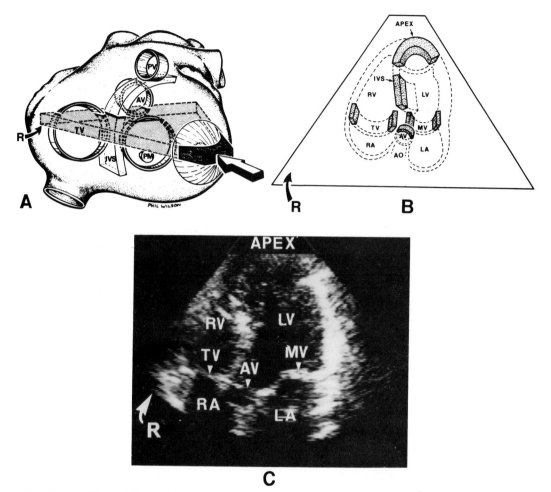

Fig. 4–11. *A,* Diagram illustrates the orientation of the imaging plane in the apical five-chamber view. This plane passes through the anatomic tip of the cardiac apex and is oriented to transect the superior margin of the mitral valve, the tricuspid valve (TV) and the inferior border of the aortic valve (AV). R = reference mark; PM = papillary muscle; IVS = interventricular septum; PV = pulmonary valve. *B,* Diagram illustrates the relative position of the major and adjacent cardiac structures recorded in the apical five-chamber view as they appear on the display scope. IVS = interventricular septum; RV = right ventricle; LV = left ventricle; TV = tricuspid valve; MV = mitral valve; AV = aortic valve; RA = right atrium; LV = left atrium, AO = aorta, R = reference mark. *C,* Cross-sectional recording of the heart obtained using the apical five-chamber view. As in the apical four-chamber view, the cardiac apex appears at the tip of the sector. The left ventricle (LV) and left atrium (LA) are displayed to the right, and the corresponding right-sided chambers are to the left. Portions of the mitral (MV) and tricuspid valves (TV) are evident. The left ventricular outflow tract appears posteriorly in the midportion of the scan. Aortic leaflets are apparent in the outflow tract. RV = right ventricle; AV = aortic valve; RA = right atrium; R = reference mark.

such, is optimally oriented when this region can be clearly visualized. Its major role is to assess left ventricular outflow disorders, specifically subvalvular membranous obstruction, subvalvular tunnels, and the relationship of interventricular septal hypertrophy to the left ventricular outflow tract.

The Apical Two-Chamber View

The apical two-chamber view is intended to record only the left ventricle and atrium with the interposed mitral valve. In contrast to other standard imaging planes with orientations defined by the structures they include, the apical two-chamber view is positioned on the basis of structures (specifically the right side of the heart) that are not included. In recording this plane, the transducer is again positioned directly over the cardiac apex. The central ray of the scan plane is directed parallel to the long axis of the left ventricle. This position shifts the central ray slightly to the left of its position in the four-chamber view. The scan plane is then rotated until right-sided cardiac structures cannot be visualized. Because the right ventricle overlies between one third and two fifths of the circumference of the left ventricle at the base (see the *Parasternal Short Axis at the Mitral Valve Level*), the area of the left ventricular free wall through which a plane can pass, which includes the long axis of the left ventricle and excludes the right ventricle is limited. When one includes the thickness of the scan plane, this area becomes more limited.

Figure 4–12, A, diagrammatically illustrates the orientation of this plane and its relationship to the interventricular septum and other right-sided structures. When displayed (Fig. 4–12, B), the image shows the left ventricular apex slightly to the left of the apex of the sector with the anterior left ventricular wall to the right and the posterior left ventricular wall to the left. The mitral valve is posterior, slightly to the right of center, with the anterior leaflet to the right and the posterior to the left. The left atrium is positioned posteriorly and to the right. Figure 4–12, C, is an example of a two-chamber view of the heart.

The apical two-chamber view is optimally recorded when the transducer is located over the true anatomic apex of the ventricle and the left ventricular diameter at the base of the ventricle is at its maximum. This indicates that the plane is positioned perpendicular to the maximal short axis and parallel to the true long axis of the ventricle. Right ventricular structures are completely excluded.

This imaging plane is orthogonal to the four-chamber view and, as such, should be useful for biplane cross-sectional imaging of the left ventricle. The plane provides a long axis to the left ventricle, which can be correlated with the long axis obtained in the four-chamber view, and a short axis in an orthogonal plane to the four-chamber short axis. The two-chamber view records the anterior and posterior wall endocardium in an orientation that is parallel to the beam axis and, hence, does not provide optimal visualization. This particular imaging plane has no unique value and is used primarily in conjunction with the apical four-chamber view to generate biplane data.

The Apical Long Axis of the Left Ventricle

The apical long-axis view of the left ventricle is similar in orientation to the parasternal long axis of the left ventricle. The only difference is transducer location. To record the apical view, the transducer is placed directly over the cardiac apex, and the central ray of the imaging plane is aligned parallel to the long axis of the left ventricle. The path of the central ray is similar to that used in the apical two-chamber view. The transducer is then rotated to position the Y axis of the scan plane such that it passes through the midportion of the aortic and mitral valves and includes the ventricular long axis (Fig. 4–13, A). This position generally requires a 30-degree counterclockwise rotation from a true anteroposterior orientation. In addition to the apex and the mitral and aortic valves, the transducer encompasses the anterior portion of the interventricular septum, the posterior ventricular wall from apex to mitral annulus, the left atrium, and the proximal aortic root.

When displayed (Fig. 4–13, B), the cardiac apex appears at the tip of the sector with the right ventricle to the right and the left ventricular posterior wall to the left. The aorta is posterior and to the right, and the left atrium is posterior and to the left.

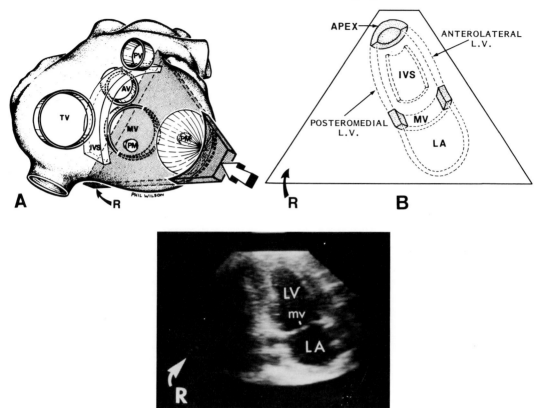

Fig. 4–12. *A,* Diagram illustrates the orientation of the imaging plane in the apical two-chamber view of the left heart. This plane transects the cardiac apex and passes through the midportion of the mitral valve (MV). The orientation of this plane is defined by the fact that no interventricular septum (IVS) or right ventricle is recorded. PV = pulmonary valve; AV = aortic valve; TV = tricuspid valve; PM = papillary muscle; R = reference mark. *B,* Diagram illustrates the relative positions of the primary and adjacent cardiac structures when displayed in the apical two-chamber view of the left ventricle (LV). IVS = interventricular septum; MV = mitral valve; LA = left atrium; R = reference mark. *C,* Cross-sectional recording of the left ventricle using the apical two-chamber view. The apex of the ventricle appears to the left and anteriorly in the sector. The anterior wall of the left ventricle is to the right, and the posteromedial wall is to the left. The mitral leaflets separating the left ventricle (LV) and left atrium (LA) are apparent posteriorly and to the right. The left atrium is behind the mitral valve (MV). R = reference mark.

Figure 4–13, *C,* is a representative recording of the apical long-axis view of the left ventricle.

Fine plane positioning is defined by recording the cardiac apex and the maximal excursion of the mitral valve and aortic leaflets. In addition to recording these three points, the plane should be aligned such that the maximum short-axis diameter of the ventricle at the base is recorded. This diameter should correspond to the point of peak mitral excursion and should fix the plane in a standardized and reproducible fashion.

This particular imaging plane provides little additional information when all the other examining planes are available. It is a reasonable alternative, however, to the parasternal long-axis view and is used primarily to record the aortic valve and ventricular walls in a plane that corresponds to the parasternal long axis when the parasternal window is unavailable. Each of these areas, unfortunately, is less than optimally recorded. The aortic valve lies in the far field of the scan and is difficult to record in detail. The anterior septum courses directly under the chest wall.

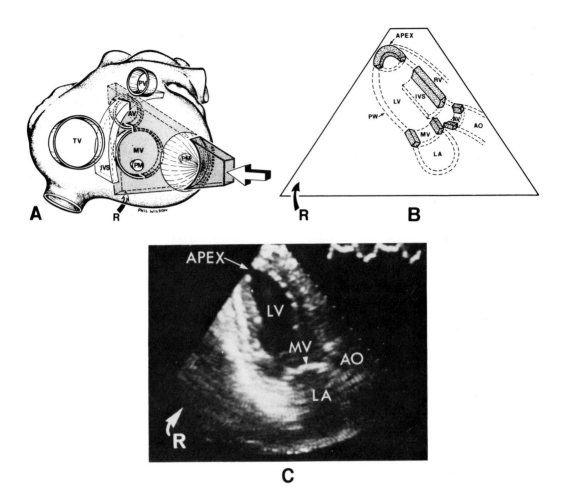

Fig. 4–13. *A,* Diagram illustrates the orientation of the imaging plane in the apical long-axis view of the left ventricle. This plane passes through the tip of the cardiac apex, the center of the mitral valve (MV), and the midportion of the aortic valve (AV). It also transects the anterior portion of the interventricular septum (IVS) along a line stretching from the cardiac apex to the junction of the interventricular septum with the anterior aortic root. PV = pulmonary valve; TV = tricuspid valve; PM = papillary muscle; R = reference mark. *B,* Diagram illustrates the relative positions of the primary and adjacent cardiac structures as they appear on the display scope in the apical long-axis view. RV = right ventricle; LV = left ventricle; IVS = interventricular septum; PW = posterior wall; AV = aortic valve; MV = mitral valve; AO = aorta; LA = left atrium; R = reference mark. *C,* Apical long-axis recording of the left ventricle (LV), aortic valve, and mitral valve (MV). These structures are displayed in a fashion similar to their appearance in the parasternal long-axis view of the left heart or as though viewed from the left shoulder. AO = aorta; LA = left atrium; R = reference mark.

Often, the lateral extent of the imaging plane cannot be directed underneath the rib cage to record the distal one third to one half of this region. In addition, the anterior and posterior walls of the ventricle are oriented parallel to the beam axis. Endocardial resolution, therefore, is poor, and any assessment of the amplitude of wall motion is limited.

SUBCOSTAL EXAMINATION

Echocardiographic recording of the heart from the subxiphoid or subcostal region developed initially as an alternative to parasternal recording in patients with chronic obstructive lung disease.[15] In these patients, the parasternal window was frequently obliterated by the hyperinflated lung, and the heart shifted medially and inferiorly toward the subxiphoid region. The frequency with which the cardiac impulse could be palpated in this region suggested that intracardiac structures might be recorded by directly placing the transducer in the subxiphoid area. Further experience with the cross-sectional technique has demonstrated that cardiac structures can be recorded in the majority of adult and virtually all pediatric patients from this transducer position and that a number of cardiac structures are optimally visualized in this particular orientation.[7,8,15] The two primary subcostal views are the subcostal long axis of the heart and the subcostal long axis of the right ventricular outflow tract.

Subcostal Long Axis of the Heart

The subcostal long axis is recorded with the transducer placed in the subcostal window and the central ray directed superiorly and leftward toward the left clavicle. The transducer is then rotated to align the Y axis of the imaging plane parallel to the long axis of the left ventricle. This view is comparable to the apical four-chamber view in that it permits visualization of the right and left ventricles, the right and left atria, and both atrioventricular valves. The Z axis of the imaging plane, however, is orthogonal to that of the apical view and, hence, permits enhanced visualization of structures that are aligned parallel to the central ray of the scan plane in the apical position. Figure 4–14, A, illustrates the relative orientation of this plane.

The resulting image shows the right-sided cardiac structures, which are closest to the transducer, positioned anteriorly in the sector and the left-sided structures positioned posteriorly (Fig. 4–14, B) The left and right ventricles are displayed to the viewer's right and the left and right atria to the viewer's left. The heart is therefore displayed as if viewed from beneath the plane. Figure 4–14, C, is a cross-sectional

recording of a subcostal long axis and illustrates the typical appearance of these structures.

Fine plane positioning is achieved by angling the scan plane along a dorsal-to-ventral path to record the maximal amplitude of mitral and tricuspid valve motion combined with a maximal minor diameter of the left ventricle and left and right atria. When all these criteria cannot be achieved in one orientation, the examiner may have to align the plane to best record the individual area of interest. The right ventricular minor dimension varies greatly with plane angulation and hence, does not aid in plane alignment.

This image orientation permits a long axis of both the left and right ventricles to be visualized. Also, a short axis of both ventricular chambers drawn from the medial to lateral walls can be seen. Left ventricular free wall motion should be well visualized, as should motion of the posterolateral free wall of the right ventricle. The entire sweep of the interventricular and interatrial septa can be recorded in a plane that is perpendicular to the path of the sound beam. The left and right atria can be visualized, as can the insertion of the inferior vena cava into the right atrium.

This plane position best records the interventricular and interatrial septa, permits analysis of the relative positions of insertion of the septal leaflet of the tricuspid valve and the anterior leaflet of the mitral valve, and should theoretically be the best view for recording the character and amplitude of motion of the free right ventricular wall and free lateral left ventricular wall. It is the optimal view for assessing the integrity of the interatrial septum and for analyzing atrial septal motion.

Difficulties in recording this view relate to problems in defining transducer position and the initial orientation of the central ray. Because the subcostal window is broad and has no specific landmarks, the operator may sometimes have difficulty in precisely defining where the transducer

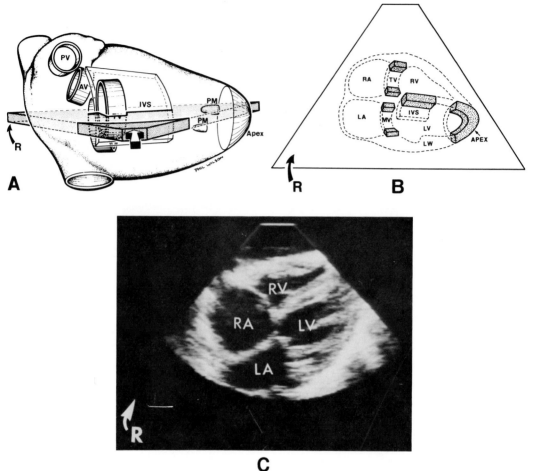

Fig. 4–14. *A,* Diagram illustrates the orientation of the imaging plane in the subcostal long-axis view of the heart. This plane initially transects the lateral wall of the right ventricle; consequently, the tricuspid valve (TV) is recorded first, followed by the interventricular septum (IVS) and mitral valve. When displayed, the point of the sector indicated by the reference mark (R) is positioned at the lower left-hand corner of the display scope. The resultant image, therefore, is displayed as though the structures were viewed from beneath the heart. PV = pulmonary valve; AV = aortic valve; PM = papillary muscle. *B,* Diagram illustrates the relative positions of the primary and adjacent structures recorded in the subcostal long-axis view on the display scope. The apex in this orientation is positioned to the right and posteriorly. The right ventricle (RV), tricuspid valve (TV), and right atrium (RA) are closest to the apex of the sector. LW = lateral wall of the left ventricle; LA = left atrium; MV = mitral valve; IVS = interventricular septum; LV = left ventricle; R = reference mark. *C,* Subcostal long-axis recording of the heart. RA = right atrium; RV = right ventricle; LA = left atrium; LV = left ventricle.

should initially be placed. Further, the degree of transducer angulation in this particular view is greater than that of any of the other views, and hence, there is a tendency not to angle the beam deeply enough and, as a result, not to transect the heart. In addition, in many cases, the heart may lie deep to the transducer and may thus fall in an area of diminished lateral resolution. This situation may make the recording of laterally oriented structures

more difficult. Despite these problems, the subcostal long-axis view is useful in all patients and, in infants, may be the best view for evaluating relative chamber size, septal integrity, and AV valve position and integrity.

Subcostal Long Axis of the Right Ventricular Outflow Tract

The subcostal long axis of the right ventricular outflow tract is recorded from the same transducer location used to record the subcostal long axis of the heart. The central ray is initially oriented to pass through the base of the mitral leaflets. From this position, the central ray is directed cephalad toward the left clavicle, and the scan plane is rotated clockwise approximately 90 degrees to align it parallel to the long axis of the right ventricular outflow tract. In this orientation, the imaging plane transects the right ventricular outflow tract parallel to its long axis from the tricuspid valve orifice to the main pulmonary artery. Figure 4–15, A, illustrates this plane orientation.

On the display scope, the heart appears inverted with the right ventricular inflow region at the apex of the sector, the outflow tract along the right-hand margin of the screen, and the left ventricle viewed in short axis along the left-hand margin. Figure 4–15, B, diagrammatically depicts the structures recorded in this imaging plane, while Figure 4–15, C, is an example of a subcostal long-axis recording of the right ventricular outflow tract.

This view is primarily intended to record the full sweep of the right ventricular outflow tract and, as such, is optimally recorded when the maximal transverse diameters of the inflow and outflow areas are simultaneously visualized with the pulmonary leaflets. The subcostal view offers an alternative to the parasternal short-axis view for recording the tricuspid valve orifice and may prove useful in tricuspid stenosis. It might also be anticipated that, in valvular pulmonary stenosis, systolic doming of the pulmonary leaflets could be best appreciated in this view because the domed leaflets should be oriented perpendicular to the imaging plane. The parasternal long axis of the right ventricular outflow tract, however, remains the view of choice for detecting valvular pulmonary stenosis because of the greater ease of the pulmonary valve recording and the favorable position of the valve in the near field of the scan plane.

This image orientation can be used as a starting point from which the transducer can be angled either superiorly toward the cranial margins of the atria or inferiorly toward the cardiac apex. This flexibility offers the potential to record multiple short axes of these chambers in an orientation that is orthogonal to the parasternal views. To date, however, these views are not sufficiently popular to be considered routine or standard.

Noncardiac Structures That Can Be Examined from the Subcostal Location

A number of extracardiac vascular structures can be easily recorded from the subcostal region. These structures include the hepatic veins and their connection with the inferior vena cava, the inferior vena cava itself and its junction with the right atrium, and the abdominal aorta. There is potential for recording inferior vena caval obstruction and dilatation, detecting backflow of contrast from the right atrium into the inferior vena cava and hepatic veins in instances of tricuspid regurgitation, and viewing tumor migration up the inferior vena cava in patients with metastatic abdominal malignancies. The abdominal aorta can also be traced from its origin beneath the diaphragm to its bifurcation into the iliac arteries. The anterior abdominal wall provides an uninterrupted window for the exploring transducer, and hence, multiple long- or short-axis recordings of these vessels are available.

SUPRASTERNAL VIEWS

The suprasternal views are used to examine the great vessels as they course cephalad from the heart. Structures that can be recorded from this transducer location include the aortic arch and its primary branches to the head and upper extremities, the proximal descending thoracic aorta, the primary branches of the pulmonary artery, and the major veins drain-

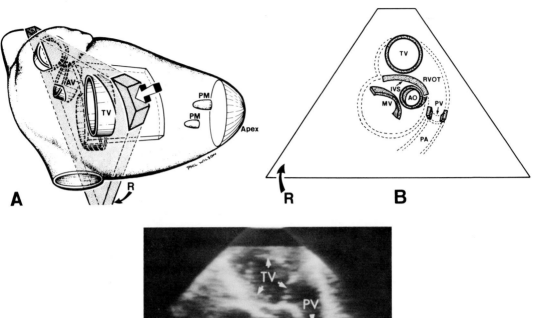

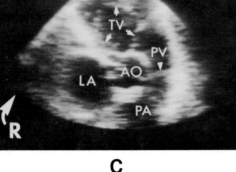

Fig. 4–15. *A,* Diagram illustrates the orientation of the imaging plane in the subcostal long-axis view of the right ventricular outflow tract. In this orientation, the plane initially transects the tricuspid valve (TV), then the basal segment of the interventricular septum, a fragment of the mitral valve, the aortic valve (AV), and finally the pulmonary valve. R = reference mark; PM = papillary muscle. *B,* Diagram illustrates the relative positions of the primary and adjacent structures recorded in the subcostal long-axis view of the right ventricular outflow tract on the display scope. The tricuspid valve (TV) is positioned anteriorly at the apex of the sector. The right ventricular outflow tract courses posteriorly along the right-hand border of the sector. The pulmonary valve (PV) is the most posterior of the primary structures and, likewise, the farthest to the right on the display. RVOT = right ventricular outflow tract; IVS = interventricular septum; MV = mitral valve; AO = aorta; PA = pulmonary artery; R = reference mark. *C,* Cross-sectional recording of the right ventricular outflow tract from the subcostal transducer location. The entire sweep of the right ventricular outflow tract from the tricuspid valve (TV) level, through the pulmonary infundibulum and the pulmonary valve (PV), to the main pulmonary artery is evident. The aorta (AO), which is transected somewhat obliquely to its short axis, appears relatively circular and lies in the center of the scan. The structures are displayed as though viewed from the cardiac apex. R = reference mark.

ing into the right atrium. The examination of this region is performed with the transducer placed directly in the suprasternal notch. To facilitate transducer placement, the patient should be positioned in a manner that makes the suprasternal notch as accessible as possible. The head should be in a neutral position and the chin angled either to the left or right at about 45 degrees. When performing these maneuvers, the examiner tries to relax the sternoclei-

domastoid muscles as well as the skin in the suprasternal region to permit the transducer head to be positioned beneath the sternum. When this position is achieved, the aorta lies almost immediately beneath the transducer face, and access to the arch vessels can be achieved in almost every case. Two primary views have been described using the suprasternal transducer position—the suprasternal long and short axes of the aortic arch.

Suprasternal Long Axis of the Aortic Arch

The suprasternal long axis of the aortic arch is recorded with the transducer directly in the suprasternal notch and the central ray of the scan plane directed inferiorly and posteriorly. The transducer is then rotated until the scan plane is oriented approximately midway between the coronal and sagittal planes of the body. When oriented in this manner, the imaging plane should pass directly into the aortic arch allowing the arch, the arterial branches to the upper extremities and the distal portions of the ascending aorta, and the proximal descending aorta to be visualized. Figure 4–16, A, illustrates this plane position.

When displayed on the viewing scope (FIg. 4–16, B), the aortic arch should be anterior at the apex of the sector with the descending aorta along the right-hand margin and the ascending aorta along the left-hand margin of the screen. The left atrium lies posteriorly. In some patients, the 90-degree scan is not wide enough in the near field to encompass the ascending and descending portions of the aorta in the same scan plane. In such patients, the transducer must be angled leftward to record specifically the descending thoracic aorta or rightward to record the ascending aorta. As a rule, the degree of transducer rotation is constant. Figure 4–16, C, is an example of a suprasternal long-axis recording of the aortic arch that illustrates the typical appearance of the structures in this area.

This view is intended to record the aortic arch with as much of the ascending and descending aorta included as possible. The aortic arch is optimally recorded when the diameter of the aorta is at its maximum throughout the scan plane. Identification of the branches of the aorta is determined relative to the left carotid artery. This artery is readily recorded, and its identity can be determined by following its course into the neck. When this vessel is identified, the innominate and subclavian branches can be identified by their proximal and distal relationships. The suprasternal long-axis view is optimally suited for recording dilatation or aneurysm formation in the aortic arch, coarctation of the aorta, patent ductus arteriosus in infants, evaluation of the size of the right pulmonary artery, and potentially for assessing ascending aorta to right pulmonary artery anastomoses.

Suprasternal Short Axis of the Aortic Arch

The suprasternal short axis of the aortic arch is obtained with the transducer in the suprasternal notch and the central ray directed inferiorly and slightly posteriorly. The short axis is recorded by rotating the transducer 90 degrees from the long axis. In this orientation, the scan plane passes through the aorta in short axis, through a portion of the superior vena cava, through the right pulmonary artery parallel to its long axis, and through the left atrium. Figure 4–17, A, illustrates the orientation of this imaging plane.

On the display scope, the ascending aorta is positioned superiorly and slightly to the right (with the long axis of the pulmonary artery coursing from right to left in the midportion of the screen), and the left atrium is positioned posteriorly (Fig. 4–17, B). The bifurcation of the right pulmonary artery is visualized on occasion to the left of the image. The superior vena cava is recorded to the left and anteriorly. Figure 4–17, C, is an example of a short-axis view of the aorta from the suprasternal transducer location.

Optimal orientation of this view must be individualized depending on the structure the examiner wishes to visualize primarily. When one is interested in the short axis of the aorta, the image is optimally recorded when the least horizontal or vertical obliquity of the vessel is noted. When

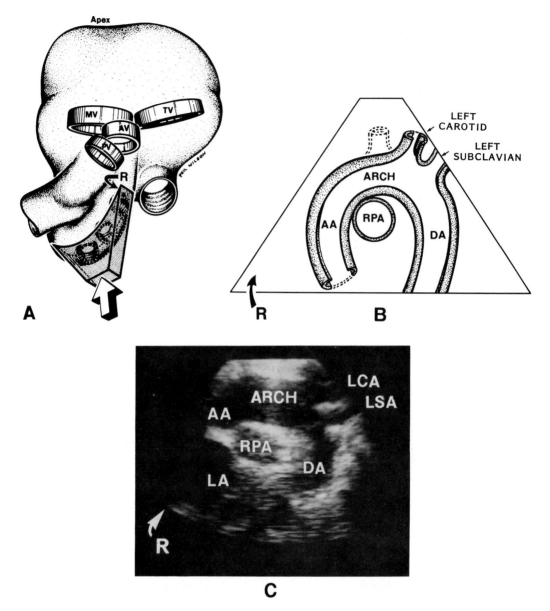

Fig. 4–16. *A,* Diagram illustrates the orientation of the imaging plane in the suprasternal long-axis view of the aortic arch. As illustrated by the reference mark (R), the plane is displayed as though viewed from the anterior chest wall with the ascending aorta to the left and the descending aorta to the right. MV = mitral valve; TV = tricuspid valve; AV = aortic valve; PV = pulmonary valve. *B,* Diagram illustrates the relative positions of the structures recorded in the suprasternal long-axis view of the aorta on the display scope. The ascending aorta (AA) is positioned to the left, the aortic arch is at the apex of the sector, and the descending aorta (DA) is to the right. The right pulmonary artery (RPA) is transected in a plane oblique to its short axis and appears relatively circular beneath the aortic arch. The left carotid artery is the first arterial vessel branching from the arch to the left of the apex of the sector and is used as a reference mark for identifying the other arterial branches. R = reference mark. *C,* Suprasternal long-axis recording of the aortic arch with the ascending portion of the aorta (AA), the arch, and the descending aorta (DA) demonstrated. The left carotid (LCA) and left subclavian (LSA) branches of the aortic arch are also visible. The left atrium (LA) is behind the right pulmonary artery (RPA) and appears as the most posterior structure in the scan. The right pulmonary artery is oblong because it is transected in a plane oblique to its short axis. R = reference mark.

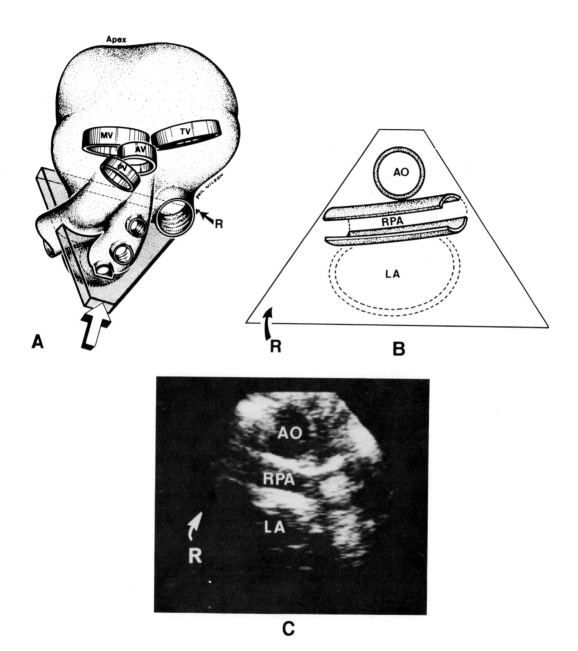

Fig. 4–17. *A,* Diagram illustrates the orientation of the imaging plane in the suprasternal short-axis view of the aortic arch. MV = mitral valve; TV = tricuspid valve; AV = aortic valve; PV = pulmonary valve; R = reference mark. *B,* Diagram illustrates the relative positions of the structures recorded in the suprasternal short-axis view of the aortic arch on the display scope. The aorta (AO), which is recorded in a plane parallel to its short axis, appears circular. The right pulmonary artery (RPA), which is transected in a plane that is roughly parallel to its long axis and thus appears as a cylindric structure, is beneath the aorta. The left atrium (LA), which is imaged in a superior-inferior orientation, is behind the right pulmonary artery. R = reference mark. *C,* Suprasternal short-axis recording of the aortic arch illustrates the circular configuration of the aorta (AO), the linear echoes from the margins of the right pulmonary artery (RPA) and the left atrial (LA) superior segment behind the right pulmonary artery. R = reference mark.

the right pulmonary artery is the structure of interest, the maximal diameter at the proximal and distal ends of the artery should be recorded. When one is interested in the superior vena cava, the plane must be angled toward the maximal expanse of this structure. Recording the entire long axis of the superior vena cava requires counterclockwise rotation and anterior angulation of the transducer. This plane orientation might be refined to a point where the superior vena cava can be visualized to join in the right atrium.[1] The overall clinical role of this plane, however, remains to be defined.

M-MODE COMPONENT OF A CROSS-SECTIONAL EXAMINATION

M-mode recordings, when required, can be obtained from specific areas of the cross-sectional image to add temporally unique or more easily analyzed quantitative data to the cross-sectional study. Most cross-sectional echographs permit M-mode recordings to be obtained using the same transducer and basic instrumentation as that employed in the cross-sectional studies. Mechanical scanning instruments require the transducer to stop at a specific point in the sector to display data lines in the M-mode format. Phased array systems are advantageous because every second or third data line can be obtained from a particular transducer orientation and displayed as an M-mode recording while the remainder of the data lines remain available to record a simultaneous two-dimensional image. Because the two-dimensional scan can be recorded simultaneously with the M-mode, the position of M-mode sampling can be more precisely maintained. In addition, using a phased array system, two or more separate B-mode lines can be selected and recorded as simultaneous M-modes while still preserving a sufficiently high line density in the cross-sectional mode to record a recognizable image.

The M-mode record is an invaluable adjunct to the cross-sectional technique because of inherent features. First, M-mode permits enhanced recording of individual targets. This enhancement occurs for several reasons that can be best understood by considering the echocardiographic visualization of the left ventricular endocardium. The left ventricular endocardium is used as an example because it must be clearly displayed before any quantitative evaluation of left ventricular volume or function is possible. When attempting to record the endocardium, the M-mode beam must be optimized to record only two points, one from the endocardial surface of the interventricular septum and the other from the endocardial surface of the posterior wall. At standard recording speeds, the M-mode lines are so densely packed together that if only 50% or less of the individual pulses actually generated echoes from the endocardial interfaces, the endocardium would still appear continuous on the graphic record. In contrast, in each cross-sectional image more than 100 data lines must be positioned such that they intersect the left ventricular endocardium at an appropriate angle to generate a recordable echo. Inability to achieve this positioning frequently causes one segment of the ventricular endocardium to be well recorded and other areas to be poorly visualized. In this case, if 50% or less of the cross-sectional lines actually contained endocardial reflections, a poor-quality image would result. Also, in the M-mode format, a much larger number of pulses is transmitted toward a specific small area of the ventricle, thereby increasing the chances that some endocardial reflections from this area will be recorded. The cross-sectional sound energy, in contrast, is spread over a wide area of the ventricle, thereby decreasing the chances that any particular area will be intersected at an ideal orientation. For these reasons, optimizing the single M-mode beam to generate an endocardial echo is easier than recording the endocardium throughout an entire cross-sectional scan plane. In the future, the cross-sectional technique may be utilized to determine the spatial configuration of the left ventricle and to align the M-mode beam such that it transects an area of interest. Linear distances along this line and regional amplitude and rate of motion, however, will be derived from the M-mode or comparable recording system.

Second, the M-mode record has a much higher effective sampling rate and, hence, is far better for timing intracardiac events. Most dedicated M-mode instruments have a pulse repetition frequency of 1000 per second, whereas the M-mode derived from cross-sectional instruments may have a pulse repetition frequency of 3000 to 4000 per second. Such frequency permits exquisite timing of cardiac valvular and wall motion and, hence, is an optimal method for defining the rate and timing of structure movement. In contrast, the cross-sectional instruments examine a particular area at a rate that corresponds to the frame rate of the imaging system. Maximal frame rates in current use vary from 15 to 60 frames or fields per second, and hence, timing of motion is much less precise.

Finally, the M-mode record is generated in an easily analyzed graphic format. Records can be examined quickly, areas of the record can be selected for more detailed examination, and measurements can be easily accomplished from the graphic record. In comparison, a cross-sectional examination lasting 5 minutes yields 18,000 individual fields of data. Analyzing these fields individually represents an enormous task. Furthermore, comparing data in one area of the video record with those in another area to select the optimal segment for analysis is difficult. Finally, making direct measurements from the video screen is difficult because of the curvature of the image, and at present, some form of graphic record must be produced, which requires additional time. Although a variety of recent computer analysis systems have simplified the processes, it is still easier to make simple measurements from an M-mode source.

Therefore, the cross-sectional examination is anticipated to proceed much like a microscopic examination. The cross-sectional study is analogous to the low-power examination,in which the overall configuration of a particular area is determined and areas of greater interest selected. The study may then move to a higher-power or M-mode examination in which specific areas can be subjected to a more rigorous examination. The more detailed data can then be used for precise timing of events, quantitative measurement of interface positions at preselected areas of the heart, and providing a more readily measureable graphic record.

Even more detailed and "higher power" information may become available in the future through the use of advanced signal analysis technique; however, this type of data must await future development.

REFERENCES

1. Tajik, AJ, et al.: Two-dimensional real-time ultrasonic imaging of the heart and great vessels. Mayo Clin Proc, 53:271, 1978.
2. Bansal, RC, et al.: Feasibility of detailed two-dimensional echocardiographic examination in adults. Prospective study of 200 patients. Mayo Clin Proc, 55:291, 1980.
3. Kloster, FE, et al.: Multiscan echocardiography II. Technique and initial clinical results. Circulation, 48:1975, 1973.
4. Kisslo, J, Von Ramm, OT, and Thurstone, FL: Cardiac imaging using a phased array ultrasound system. Clinical technique and application. Circulation, 53:262, 1976.
5. Griffith, JM, and Henry, WL: A sector scanner for real-time two-dimensional echocardiography. Circulation, 49:1147, 1974.
6. Henry, WL, et al.: Measurement of mitral valve orifice area in patients with mitral valve disease by real-time two-dimensional echocardiography. Circulation, 51:827, 1975.
7. Lange, LW, Sahn, DJ, Allen, HD, and Goldberg, SJ: Subxyphoid echocardiography in infants and children with congenital heart disease. Circulation, 59:513, 1979.
8. Bierman, FZ, and Williams, RG: Subxyphoid two-dimensional imaging of the interatrial septum in

infants and neonates with congenital heart disease. Circulation, *60*:80, 1979.

9. Silverman, NH, and Schiller, NB: Apex echocardiography: a two-dimensional technique for evaluating congenital heart disease. Circulation, *57*:503, 1978.

10. Eggleton, RC, et al.: Visualization of cardiac dynamics with real-time B-mode ultrasonic scanners. *In* Ultrasound Medicine. Edited by D White. New York, Plenum Press, 1975.

11. Report of the American Society of Echocardiography Committee on Nomenclature and Standards in Two-Dimensional Imaging. Circulation *62*:212, 1980.

12. Hickman, H.O., et al.: Cross-sectional echocardiography of the cardiac apex. Circulation II, *56*:589, 1977.

13. Weyman, AE, et al.: Detection of left ventricular aneurysms by cross-sectional echocardiography. Circulation, *54*:936, 1976.

14. Dillon, JC, et al.: Cross-sectional echocardiographic examination of the interatrial septum. Circulation, *55*:115, 1977.

15. Schapira, JN, Martin, RP, Fowles, RE, and Popp, RL: Single and two-dimensional echocardiographic features of the interatrial septum in normal subjects and patients with an atrial septal defect. Am J Cardiol, *43*:816, 1979.

16. Chang, S, Feigenbaum, H, and Dillon, J: Subxyphoid echocardiography. Chest, *68*:233, 1975.

Section 3

Clinical Applications of Cross-Sectional Echocardiography

Chapter 5

Left Ventricular Inflow Tract, Part 1: The Mitral Valve

The left ventricular inflow tract has three major components: the mitral valve and supporting apparatus, the left atrium, and the pulmonary veins (Fig. 5–1). This portion of the heart collects oxygenated blood from the pulmonary vascular bed, stores the blood transiently, and then transports it to the left ventricle for subsequent ejection into the systemic circulation. The mitral valve, in addition to permitting unimpeded flow into the left ventricle during diastole, prevents systolic regurgitation into the left atrium and helps to funnel blood into the aorta.

The coronary sinus is also included in this section. This structure, although contributing to right ventricular inflow, lies immediately beneath and is consistently recorded with the left atrium. Consequently, the coronary sinus is discussed with this region.

THE MITRAL VALVE

The mitral valve has historically been a structure of principal echocardiographic interest. The pioneering studies of Edler and Hertz on the role of pulsed reflected ultrasound in cardiac diagnosis dealt primarily with the identification and analysis of the echoes returning from the mitral valve.[1,2] Likewise, the changes in the motion pattern of the mtral valve echo in mitral stenosis, which were observed by these investigators, represent the first clinical application of the echocardiographic technique and continue to remain the cornerstone of echocardiographic diagnosis.[2–4]

The early interest in the mitral valve occurred because of its high reflectivity, characteristic motion pattern, and location directly beneath the parasternal echocardiographic window, which combined to facilitate its location and recording. Additional features that have contributed to the continued echocardiographic importance of the mitral valve are its central position within the heart (which makes the mitral valve an ideal landmark from which to locate other structures) and its frequent involvement in a variety of disorders that

139

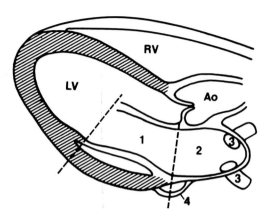

Fig. 5–1. Diagram of the left ventricular inflow tract. The mitral valve region (1) includes the area from the tips of the papillary muscles to the mitral annulus. The left atrial chamber (2) extends from the mitral annulus to the superior atrial wall. Two pairs of pulmonary veins, the right and left superior and inferior veins (3), insert into the corresponding superior medial and lateral walls of the left atrium. The coronary sinus (4) is anatomically incorporated into the posterior wall of the left atrium beneath the atrioventricular groove. The coronary sinus appears circular because it is transected parallel to its short axis. AO = aorta; LV = left ventricle; RV = right ventricle.

affect the structure and function of the left side of the heart.

Anatomy

Anatomically, the mitral valve is a complex structure composed of the mitral leaflet tissue, chordae tendineae, papillary muscles, left ventricular myocardium subjacent to the papillary muscles, and fibromuscular mitral annulus.[5–9] Functional integrity of the valve requires that each of these components performs appropriately and acts in concert with its other members. The mitral leaflets actually represent a continuous veil of fibrous tissue whose base is attached around the entire circumference of the mitral orifice to the fibromuscular ring, the mitral annulus. The free edges of the leaflet veil show several indentations. Two of these indentations, the anterolateral and posteromedial mitral commissures, are regularly placed and

permit the mitral valve's division into the anterior and posterior leaflets.[10] A line drawn between these two commissures runs parallel to the coaptation line of the mitral leaflets and likewise parallels a line drawn between the tips of the two papillary muscles. The anterior mitral leaflet is a relatively long, semicircular or triangular structure, whereas the posterior leaflet, although shorter, has a more extensive area of attachment to the mitral annulus. The distal third of both leaflets is roughened and opaque, whereas the proximal two thirds are smooth and clear.[8] The roughened area is important because it receives the insertions of the chordae tendineae on its ventricular surface. A ridge at the superior margin of this roughened area marks the line of coaptation of the anterior and posterior leaflets.[9]

The anterior mitral leaflet has a common point of attachment to the fibrous skeleton of the heart with the left coronary cusp and half of the noncoronary cusp of the aortic valve.[10]

The chordae tendineae arise from the tips of the anterolateral and posteromedial papillary muscles and course superiorly to insert into the mitral leaflets at both the free leaflet edges and superior margins of the roughened area. The chordae from the posteromedial papillary muscle supply the medial half of both the anterior and posterior mitral leaflets, whereas those from the anterolateral papillary muscles supply the lateral half of both leaflets.[10]

Although the left ventricular papillary muscles are anatomically termed anterolateral and posteromedial, both of these muscle groups, from an echocardiographic standpoint, lie in the posterior hemisphere of the ventricle with their tips oriented parallel to the closure line of the mitral leaflets. For this reason, the terms "anterior" and "posterior" appear unnecessary, and hence, they are referred to throughout this book as the medial and lateral papillary muscles. Either papillary muscle group may have one or more distinct "bellies of muscle." They may, likewise, arise as separate finger-like projections from the left ventricular myocardium or may be more intimately involved with the left ventricular trabeculae.[11] The papillary muscles move in concert with the subjacent left ventricular myocardium during systolic ventricular contraction. Dysfunction of the papillary muscles appears to be related to concomitant dysfunction of the myocardium at their base.[12,13]

METHODS OF CROSS-SECTIONAL EXAMINATION

The mitral valve is examined using three primary imaging planes. These include (1) *the parasternal long axis of the left ventricle at the mitral valve level,* (2) *the parasternal short axis of the left ventricle at the mitral valve level,* and (3) *the apical four-chamber view.* The mitral valve can also be recorded, albeit less optimally, in a variety of other planes, including the apical two-chamber, five-chamber, and long-axis views, and the subcostal long axis of the left ventricle. A portion of the mitral valve is frequently recorded in the subcostal long axis of the right ventricular outflow tract, and a subcostal short axis of the left ventricle at the mitral valve level can be recorded if necessary. To determine the contractile function of the left ventricular myocardium at the base of the papillary muscles (which may affect normal mitral closure), one must also record a short-axis view of the left ventricle at the papillary muscle level.

The primary view for recording the mitral valve is the parasternal long axis (Fig. 5–2, A).[14] This imaging plane transects the midportion of the bodies of both the anterior and posterior mitral leaflets from their points of insertion into the mitral annulus to their free edges. It also includes the anterior and posterior extremes of the mitral annulus and some of the chordae

tendineae. The precise point at which the free edge of the mitral leaflets joins the chordae is difficult, if not impossible, to define. They therefore usually appear as one continuous structure.[15] When appropriately aligned parallel to the long axis of the left ventricle, this plane should pass between but fail to record the two papillary muscles. The plane, however, can be angled in a medial or lateral direction to record either of the papillary muscles if desired. This imaging plane records the motion of both mitral leaflets in an anteroposterior direction, their systolic and diastolic positions and spatial configurations (Figs. 5–2, B and C), the anteroposterior mitral annular diameter, the motion pattern of the mitral annulus in both a superoinferior and anteroposterior direction, and the temporal and spatial positions of the mitral leaflets in relation to the left ventricular cavity, annulus, and atrium.

The parasternal short axis of the left ventricle at the mitral valve level is depicted in Figure 5–3. This view is important because it permits direct visualization of the mitral valve orifice.[16] It is the primary plane for recording mitral valve orifice area and for assessing the location and extent of involvement for the mitral valve orifice in focal disorders. It encompasses the entire circumferential area of both the anterior and posterior mitral valve leaflets and can be positioned to record these leaflets at any level from the free edges to the point of annular insertion.

The apical four-chamber view passes through the mitral leaflets obliquely at approximately a 30-degree angle to the line of leaflet coaptation (Fig. 5–4).[17] Because the coaptation line of the leaflets is ordinarily displaced toward the posterior portion of the ventricle, this oblique orientation causes the plane to transect more of the anterior mitral leaflet than of the posterior. The anterior leaflet is displayed medially and the posterior leaflet laterally. This plane orientation is ideal for determining the position of the atrioventricular

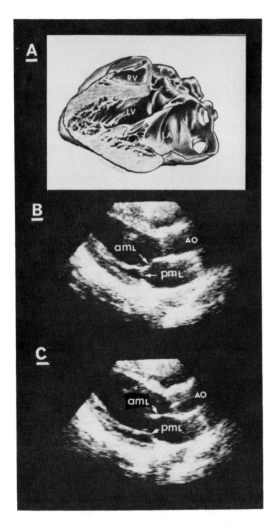

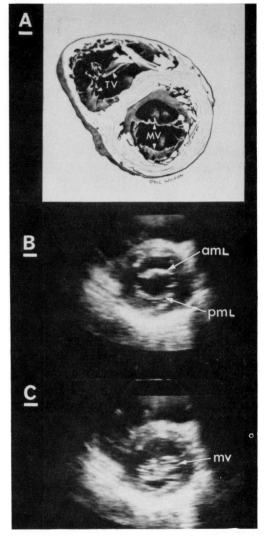

Fig. 5–2. *A,* Diagram depicting an anatomic section through the left ventricle (LV), mitral valve, and left atrium (LA) corresponding to the path of the imaging plane in the parasternal long-axis view of the left ventricular inflow tract. *B,* Systolic configuration of the mitral valve and adjacent structures in this long-axis plane. The anterior (AML) and posterior mitral leaflets (PML), their coaptation point, and the chordae tendineae, stretching from the region of leaflet coaptation toward the papillary muscles, are recorded. *C,* Diastolic frame demonstrates the open mitral valve. The anterior mitral leaflet (AML) and the full extent of the posterior mitral leaflet (PML) and its chordal extension to the papillary muscles can be visualized. AO = aorta; RV = right ventricle; LV = left ventricle.

Fig. 5–3. *A,* An anatomic section through the right and left ventricles at the free edges of the mitral leaflets corresponding to the region recorded in the parasternal short-axis view of the mitral valve (MV). *B,* Diastolic frame illustrates the seperated anterior (AML) and posterior mitral leaflets (PML) surronding the mitral valve orifice. The normal circular diastolic configuration of the left ventricle in short axis is evident. *C,* Systolic frame illustrates the coapted mitral leaflets. The left ventricular cavity area is decreased, and the circular left ventricular walls are thicker than those in the comparable diastolic recording. TV = tricuspid valve.

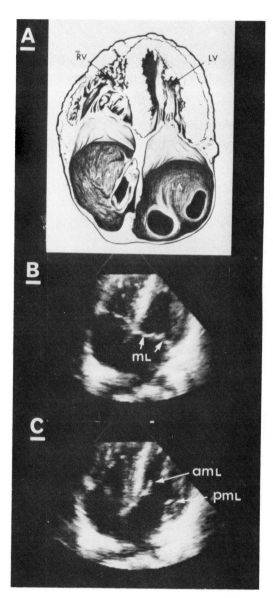

Fig. 5–4. Apical four-chamber view of the mitral valve. *A,* An anatomic section through the left (LV) and right (RV) ventricles and left (LA) and right (RA) atria. The diagram corresponds to the path of the imaging plane in this view. *B,* Systolic frame illustrates the coapted mitral leaflets (ML). The anterior mitral leaflet arises at the superior margin of the interventricular septum and extends laterally perpendicular to the septum. The posterior leaflet arises from the lateral margin of the atrioventricular ring and extends medially to join the anterior leaflet. *C,* Diastolic frame with the (medial) anterior (AML) and (lateral) posterior (PML) mitral leaflets widely separated and pointing toward the apex of the left ventricle.

ring and for defining the point of leaflet closure relative to this anatomic landmark. It is also useful for defining the point of mitral leaflet insertion into the interventricular septum and for relating it to the level of insertion of the tricuspid leaflet.

Normal Mitral Leaflet Motion— Long-Axis View

The normal mitral leaflets are thin, pliable structures that move freely in response to the relative forces acting on their surfaces. The diastolic motion of these leaflets is a combination of both independent leaflet motion in response to blood flow through the valve orifice and motion of the mitral annulus to which the leaflets are attached. Systolic motion of the coapted leaflets, in contrast, passively follows that of the mitral annulus and papillary muscles.

The normal pattern of mitral leaflet motion recorded in the long-axis, cross-sectional view is depicted and described in Figures 5–5, *A* through *H*. At the onset of ventricular systole (*A*), the left ventricle is maximally dilated, and the coapted mitral leaflets and mitral annulus are in their most posterior and cephalad position. At this point, the leaflets appear as a horizontally placed, narrow-based funnel. The base of this funnel is formed by the mitral annulus, the curvilinear sides by the basal two thirds of the mitral leaflets, and the spout by the distal third of the leaflets and the chordae tendineae. As systole progresses (*B*), the mitral valve and annulus are drawn anteriorly and toward the cardiac apex so that, by end-systole, the valve is in its most anterior and apical position. Left atrial filling during this period elevates the posterior aortic root and increases the diameter of the mitral annulus. This increase in annular diameter separates the basal attachment points of the mitral leaflets and causes them to become more vertically oriented in the ventricle.

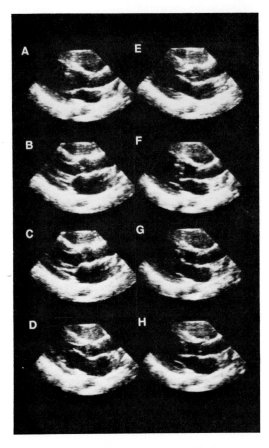

Fig. 5–5.   The normal sequence of mitral leaflet motion in the parasternal long-axis view. (See text for details.)

During isovolumic relaxation (C), the leaflets shift downward toward the left ventricular cavity.

At the onset of diastolic inflow, the leaflet tips fly rapidly apart (D) and continue this motion until they approach the endocardial surfaces of the ventricle. At the point of peak leaflet separation, the distance between the leaflets exceeds the mitral annular diameter, and the annulus thus represents the area of anatomic limitation to left ventricular inflow. Having reached the point of peak opening, the leaflets almost immediately begin to reclose (E). Downward or closing motion of the anterior leaflet is initiated by downward movement of the posterior aortic root in response to left atrial emptying. The leaflets then swing inward toward each other and,

during the slow phase of ventricular filling, assume a neutral or floating position within the left ventricular cavity (F). Following atrial systole (G), the leaflets reopen. Final leaflet closure is initiated by atrial relaxation (H) and is completed by ventricular systole.

Normal Mitral Leaflet Motion— Short-Axis View

The short-axis projection is ideally suited to evaluate the changes that mitral leaflet motion produces on the configuration of the mitral orifice and on the relationship of the ventricular surface of the leaflets to the endocardial margins of the ventricle at sequential points during the diastolic filling period. The normal pattern of mitral leaflet motion in the short-axis view is depicted in Figures 5–6, A through H. Beginning at end-systole (A), the coapted mitral leaflets are positioned posteriorly in the ventricle in a line that roughly parallels the anterior chest wall. At the onset of diastole (B), an initial anterior movement of the coapted leaflets is followed almost immediately by the onset of rapid valve opening. During the rapid opening phase (C), the leaflets initially separate evenly along the entire width of the closure line. This separation causes the orifice to appear transiently more rectangular than circular. As motion of a central portion of the leaflets continues, however, they become more parallel to the circular endocardial margin of the ventricle, and the orifice assumes a circular configuration (D). Almost immediately after reaching the point of peak opening (E), the leaflets begin to move inward toward the center of the ventricle. Movement at the center of the leaflets is greater than at the margins, and the orifice, therefore, becomes more oval in configuration.

During the slow phase of ventricular filling, the leaflets assume a floating position within the ventricular chamber (F), and the orifice assumes a consistent oval ap-

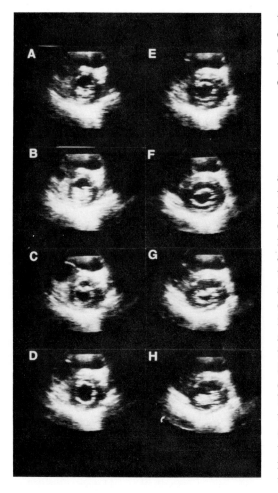

Fig. 5–6. Normal pattern of mitral leaflet motion in the parasternal short-axis view. (See text for details.)

pearance. At the onset of atrial systole, the leaflets separate again, the orifice becomes more circular, and the orifice area increases. With atrial relaxation, the leaflets move toward a closed position (G). This motion is primarily caused by downward movement of the anterior leaflet, which may actually assume an orientation that is convex anteriorly prior to final systolic closure. At the point of leaflet coaptation (H), the anterior and posterior leaflets with their chordal attachments appear as a linear band or mass of echoes horizontally positioned in the posterior portion of the ventricle. During systole, the coapted leaflets move anteriorly in concert with

the anterior motion of the posterior wall of the ventricle and, as the ventricular area decreases, become more closely associated with the posterior-wall endocardial echoes.

Normal Mitral Leaflet Motion— Apical Four-Chamber View

Mitral leaflet motion is more difficult to analyze in the apical four-chamber view than in either the long- or short-axis views for two reasons. First, in the four-chamber orientation, the imaging plane transects the mitral valve along a line that passes just above the medial commissure and below the lateral commissure. As noted in the section on short-axis motion, movement of the leaflets is lesser in these areas than in their midportions. As a result, more subtle changes in the pattern of leaflet motion may be more difficult to appreciate. Secondly, although the leaflets are oriented parallel to the path of the ultrasonic beam during systole and, hence, are well visualized, the opened leaflets during diastole point almost directly toward the transducer and thus become far more difficult to record. The apical four-chamber view, therefore, is better for analyzing the configuration and motion patterns of the mitral leaflets during systole than during diastole.

Figure 5–7, A through H, depicts the motion pattern of the mitral leaflets in this view. At end-systole (A), the mitral leaflets are coapted and lie in the plane of the mitral annulus. At the onset of diastole (B), the leaflets initially bow outward toward the cardiac apex. As the rapid phase of leaflet opening continues, the leaflet tips swing freely from about their insertion points into the anteromedial and posterolateral margins of the mitral annulus until they lie parallel to the septum and the lateral walls of the ventricle, respectively (C). When the leaflets are fully open, one can frequently record the entire sweep of the chordae, from the anterior leaflet to the

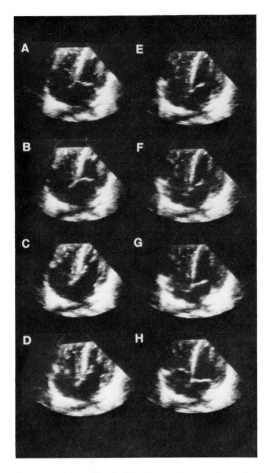

Fig. 5–7. Normal mitral leaflet motion in the apical four-chamber view. (See text for details.)

lateral papillary muscle, as they arc through the ventricular chamber. After reaching full excursion, the leaflets almost immediately separate from the ventricular walls (*D*) and move slightly inward toward the center of the ventricle. This inward motion continues until a mid-diastolic resting or floating position in the ventricular chamber is reached (*E*). Atrial contraction is accompanied by variable leaflet reopening (*F*). As the atrium relaxes, there is corresponding movement inward toward the mitral annulus (*G*), and a fully closed position. When closed, the leaflets are positioned parallel to the plane of the mitral annulus and perpendicular to the long axis of the left ventricle. During ventricular systole (Fig. 5–7, *H*), the annulus

moves upward toward the cardiac apex. As annular movement progresses, the coapted leaflets sink slightly posteriorly and appear to "set" within the annulus prior to reopening during the next diastolic period. Normally, the leaflets do not break the plane of the mitral annulus during this systolic segment.

Factors Affecting Timing, Amplitude, and Rate of Mitral Leaflet Motion

Mitral leaflet motion is influenced by a variety of factors including (1) the relative pressures in the left atrium and left ventricle,[18–21] (2) the velocity and volume of blood flow through the mitral orifice,[18,20,22–24] (3) motion of the points of leaflet attachment at the mitral annulus[25] and papillary muscles, (4) left ventricular diastolic compliance,[26] and (5) the systolic performance of the left ventricle.[27] Figure 5–8 diagrammatically depicts the relationships of the left atrial and left ventricular pressures and mitral valve flow to mitral leaflet motion. Beginning at the point of aortic valve closure, left ventricular pressure falls rapidly. As ventricular pressure approaches left atrial pressure, the mitral leaflets shift downward into the ventricle (see Figs. 5–5, *B* and *C*). This motion is associated with a low rate and volume of flow recorded at the mitral annulus, but not with actual leaflet opening.[18] Following the intersection of the left ventricular and left atrial pressure curves, a positive left atrial—left ventricular gradient develops, the mitral leaflets fly open, and the flow through the valve rapidly accelerates.[18,23,28] The rate of leaflet opening (D–E slope) appears directly related to flow into the left ventricle[29] and inversely related to initial diastolic left ventricular pressure.[19] The degree of leaflet separation at peak diastolic opening can likewise be related to transmitral flow at low flow rates.[29] At higher flow rates, leaflet separation is limited by the endocardial surface of the ventricle, and this relationship can no longer exist.[23]

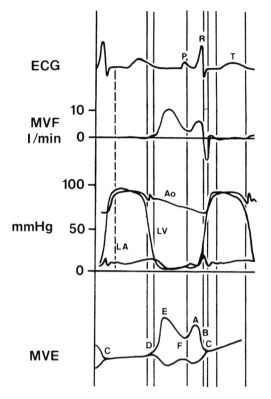

ECG

MVF
l/min

10

0

100

mmHg 50

0

Ao

LV

LA

R

P

T

E

A

B

C

D

F

C

MVE

Fig. 5–8. Diagram comparing the temporal sequence and relative magnitudes of mitral valve flow (MVF) in liters per minute (1/min); the aortic (AO), left ventricular (LV), and left atrial (LA) pressure curves in millimeters of mercury (mm Hg), and the motion pattern of the mitral valve echo (MVE). The mitral valve echo depicted here corresponds to a typical M-mode recording of mitral leaflet motion at the free edges of the valve leaflets. The D point is the position of the leaflets at the onset of diastolic opening. The E point represents the point of peak leaflet opening. The E-F slope represents the initial diastolic closing motion of the valve leaflets, and the A wave represents leaflet reopening in response to atrial systole. The A-C slope corresponds to end-diastolic leaflet closure, and the C point reflects final leaflet coaptation. Point B is the position of the mitral leaflets at the onset of ventricular systole. Normally, leaflet closure is initiated by atrial relaxation and completed by the systolic rise in left ventricular pressure. Relating the points on the mitral valve echogram to the long-axis cross-sectional recording in Figure 5–5, the C point of the mitral valve echogram corresponds to the leaflet position in panel A. The D point corresponds to panel B, whereas panel C occurs slightly after the D point (just as the leaflets are beginning to open). The E point of the mitral valve echogram corresponds to panel D. Downward motion following the E point is reflected in panel E. The F point of the mitral valve echogram corresponds to panel F, whereas the A-wave corresponds to panel G. Panel H then corresponds to the B point of the mitral valve echogram. (See text for further details.) (Adapted from Nolan, SP: Patterns of instantaneous mitral valve flow and the atrial contribution to ventricular filling in the mitral valve. *IN* The Mitral Valve: A Pluridisciplinary Approach. Edited by D. Kalmanson. Littleton, MA, Publishing Sciences Group, 1976.)

Upon reaching their full excursion, the leaflets immediately begin to reclose.[30] The point of peak leaflet excursion (E point) is reached before peak flow velocity is recorded, and the leaflets begin their downward motion (E–F slope) while flow is still accelerating.[18,23]

The factors that influence the pattern and rate of initial diastolic closure are complex. Several mechanisms have been proposed to explain this dissociation between transmitral flow and leaflet motion. It was initially felt that, as the leaflets opened, tension was produced because of chordal stretching with resultant recoil of the leaflets as they reached their point of peak opening.[31] In contrast, early echocardiographic data suggested that the initial downward motion of the leaflets occurred as a result of posterior motion of the mitral annulus.[21,23] More recently, it has been postulated that flow through the mitral orifice causes tip vortices to form at the leaflet edges, which initiate leaflet closure.[22,32] Analysis of leaflet motion in cross-sectional studies supports the early M-mode observations that the initial downward motion of the anterior mitral leaflet occurs in response to downward displacement of the mitral annulus and posterior wall of the aortic root (see Fig. 5–5, *E*).

The greater portion of the leaflet closure (E–F slope), however, results from free motion of the leaflets about their point of annular attachment. This motion has been attributed to the formation of a ring vortex system within the ventricle.[22,30,32,33] These vortices begin immediately after valve opening with the formation of small tip vortices at the free margins of the cusps and continue to expand as the in-rushing blood strikes the cardiac apex, spreads out, and flows back up along the walls of the ventricle. The vortices then turn back behind the leaflets toward the apex, thereby forming the ring vortex system. Because of the configuration of the ventricle, the main strength of this vortex system is concentrated behind the anterior leaflet. The strength of these vortices is related to flow into the ventricle, and the rate of leaflet closure should also be related to the rate and volume of diastolic inflow.

In support of these concepts, clinical studies have shown a direct correlation between the percent ventricular inflow during the first third of diastole and early diastolic mitral closing velocity (E–F slope, Fig. 5–8, MVE).[24] In contrast, a decrease in initial diastolic closing rate has been observed in patients with increased left ventricular initial diastolic volume or decreased compliance, which are both associated with a shift in percent ventricular filling toward the latter third of diastole.[24]

During atrial contraction, the left atrial—left ventricular pressure gradient increases as does the flow velocity through the mitral valve.[18] As the atrium relaxes, there is a decrease or even reversal in this gradient as well as in mitral valve flow. This change is accompanied by movement of the leaflets toward a closed position (A–C slope).[34] With ventricular systole, the left ventricular and left atrial pressure cross and valve closure is completed.[18] Note, however, that flow through the valve may continue after atrial and ventricular pressures have intersected, thereby reflecting the higher pressure required to stem the established flow through the valve leaflets.[18]

Several conditions may alter the normal pattern of late diastolic mitral leaflet closure (A–C slope, Fig. 5–8). The most noteworthy of these are (1) an increase in PR interval and (2) a rapid rise in left ventricular diastolic pressures (e.g., with aortic insufficiency). Prolongation of the PR interval causes atrial contraction to occur earlier in diastole. As the atrium relaxes, the atrioventricular pressure gradient reverses and the mitral valve flow decelerates rapidly.[23] These changes are followed by premature apposition of the valve cusp.

In patients with severe aortic insufficiency, the rapid rise in ventricular dia-

stolic pressure may also reverse the atrioventricular pressure gradient and cause premature closure of the valve leaflets.[35–37] This early closure may be protective because it prevents the left atrium and pulmonary circuit from exposure to the inordinately high end-diastolic pressures in the left ventricle.

Effects of Abnormal Pressure and Flow on Mitral Valve Motion

Marked reduction in flow through the mitral valve reduces maximal leaflet-opening amplitude and the rate of leaflet movement. The diminished mitral leaflet opening increases the separation between the ventricular surface of the leaflets at peak opening and the ventricular endocardium [E-point septal separation] (Fig. 5–9, B and D). M-mode studies have demonstrated that an increased distance between the anterior leaflet and the septum (greater than 5 mm) at peak leaflet opening is associated with a reduced ejection fraction (less than 50%).[27] This relationship is based on the assumption that the volume of blood entering the ventricle during diastole is directly related to the percent ejected during the preceding systole. These relationships are also noted in the cross-sectional format and form a useful basis for roughly estimating left ventricular performance in a manner that is independent of ventricular geometry.

In the short-axis view, the reduced leaflet motion caused by diminished transmitral flow is reflected by a decrease in the mitral valve orifice area. Figure 5–9, D illustrates this reduction in absolute orifice area at peak leaflet opening. The maximal orifice area that occurs in response to mitral valve flow is termed the functional mitral valve area. This area is in contrast to the anatomic orifice area, which is the maximal allowable anatomic separation of the leaflets. The relationship of these two areas becomes important when considering stenotic values because flow can be

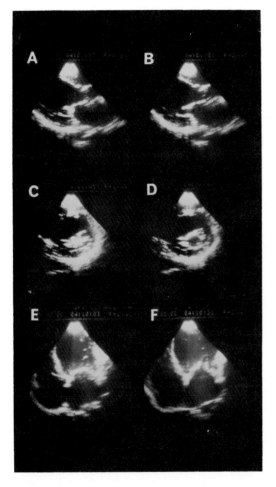

Fig. 5–9. Cross-sectional echogram from a patient with severe cardiomyopathy, left atrial and ventricular dilatation, and a marked reduction in left ventricular stroke volume and ejection fraction. *A* and *B,* Systolic and diastolic long-axis recordings of the mitral valve illustrate a decrease in diastolic mitral leaflet separation and an increase in distance between the ventricular surface of the anterior mitral leaflet and the endocardium of the interventricular septum at peak leaflet excursion (E point septal separation). *C* and *D,* Systolic and diastolic short-axis recordings illustrate the reduction in mitral valve orifice area at peak diastolic opening in relation to the left ventricular cavity size. *E* and *F,* Systolic and diastolic frames recorded in the apical four-chamber view again illustrate the reduction in diastolic mitral leaflet separation. During systole (*E*), the coapted leaflets fail to reach the plane of the mitral annulus during peak systolic closure. This failure results in the displacement of the leaflets into the left ventricular cavity and has been associated with the clinical syndrome of papillary muscle dysfunction (see section on papillary muscle dysfunction).

reduced to a point where an orifice that is anatomically reduced is no longer functionally restrictive. Likewise, at high flow rates, a deformed orifice, which is within the normal absolute range for valve areas, may be functionally restrictive because it is still smaller than the separation that would be achieved by the leaflets if anatomic restriction were not present. For these reasons, absolute values for orifice area must be treated with caution. An orifice that is restrictive in one flow setting may be more than adequate to accept the reduced flow volume in another setting.

In the apical four-chamber view, the decrease in rate and amplitude of leaflet motion is again noted. As illustrated in Figure 5–9, *F,* this decrease is characterized by failure of the leaflet tips to approach the lateral margins of the ventricular wall at peak diastolic separation. Also, in this case there is displacement of the leaflets downward into the ventricular cavity during systole (Fig. 5–9E) (see Papillary Muscle Dysfunction later in this chapter).

Although precise measurement of rate and timing of leaflet motion is better recorded in the M-mode format, decrease in amplitude of leaflet excursion, increase in separation between the leaflets and ventricular walls, and decrease in or distortion of the mitral orifice area are readily appreciated on the cross-sectional record.

ABNORMAL MITRAL VALVE ECHOGRAM

Proper function of the mitral valve requires unimpeded passage of blood from the left atrium into the left ventricle during diastole and the prevention of backflow into the left atrium during systole. On the basis of these functional requirements, mitral valve disorders can be divided into (1) those that restrict diastolic flow into the left ventricle and are characterized echocardiographically by a decrease in orifice size or distortion in orifice configuration, (2) those that primarily affect the systolic competence of the valve and are associated with abnormalities of the leaflet closure, (3) structural abnormalities of the valve leaflets or supporting structures, which may occur with or without disruption of valvular function, and (4) prosthetic mitral valves.

Abnormalities Associated with Restricted Left Ventricular Inflow

Valvular lesions that primarily obstruct left ventricular inflow are rheumatic mitral stenosis, mitral stenosis and insufficiency, congenital mitral stenosis, and parachute mitral valve. The mitral valve orifice is also frequently distorted in aortic insufficiency, and inflow may be disturbed in this condition. A variety of other structural disorders of the mitral valve and left atrium may also impede left ventricular inflow; however, these are discussed in the appropriate sections.

Rheumatic Mitral Stenosis

Rheumatic mitral stenosis is the classic lesion that produces obstruction to left ventricular inflow. This acquired form of chronic valvular heart disease is characterized by a diffuse thickening of the mitral leaflets, fusion of the commissures, and shortening and fusion of the chordae tendineae. These abnormalities combine to decrease the size of the mitral valve orifice, thereby restricting the flow of blood into the left ventricle.[38]

Mitral stenosis is characterized echocardiographically by (1) an increase in echo production from the thickened, deformed mitral leaflets, (2) abnormal diastolic leaflet motion, and (3) a reduction in mitral valve orifice area.[16,39–43]

Increased echo production from the deformed mitral leaflets can be observed in almost every instance of rheumatic mitral stenosis.[37,41] This increased reflectivity may involve either the anterior or posterior leaflets and is most prominent at the margins of the valve orifice and along the line of commissural fusion.[41] As leaflet de-

formity becomes more severe, the area of increased reflectivity expands superiorly toward the mitral annulus. Calcification of the rheumatic valve also begins at the tips of the leaflets and spreads upward toward the annulus. This pattern is in contrast to the distribution of calcification and the corresponding area of increased echo production noted in mitral annular calcification, where initial involvement occurs at the annulus and subvalvular region and spreads downward toward the leaflet tips.[44]

Abnormal mitral leaflet motion may be evident throughout diastole or only during the initial phase. It is best recorded in the parasternal long-axis view. Changes in anterior leaflet motion are most evident.[16,39] The abnormal motion is characterized by (1) restricted excursion of the leaflet tips,[16,39–42] (2) prominent diastolic doming of the anterior leaflet into the left ventricular outflow tract,[16,39,41] and (3) decrease in, or total loss of, the normal initial diastolic closing motion of the anterior mitral leaflet (E–F slope, see Fig. 5–8).[39]

The initial diastolic motion abnormalities occur in the following sequence. At end-systole, the leaflets are coapted, the posterior leaflet is frequently more prominent and erect than normal, and its body is oriented in a convex arc toward the left atrium.[39] Immediately prior to valve opening, the leaflets shift downward toward the left ventricular cavity. The posterior leaflet reverses its position and becomes concave toward the left atrium, and the anterior leaflet bows inward toward the left ventricle.[39] Almost immediately, the leaflets initiate their rapid opening sequence, and the leaflet tips separate. Motion of the tip of the anterior leaflet, however, is quickly arrested because of the commissural fusion.[16,39,41] The body of the leaflet, in contrast, continues anteriorly and, in the absence of corresponding motion of the leaflet tip, produces an abrupt knee-like bend in the midportion of the anterior leaflet (convex toward the septum). Continued distention of the body of the anterior leaflet pulls the anterior and posterior leaflet tips farther anteriorly. The leaflet tips, however, remain in close apposition, thereby resulting in an obvious decrease in orifice diameter. Figure 5–10 is an example of a domed stenotic mitral valve at the point of peak leaflet excursion and illustrates these features.

The body of the leaflet must be pliable for diastolic doming of the anterior leaflet to occur. When the leaflet is extensively fibrosed or calcified, doming may not be evident. In these instances, real-time analysis of leaflet motion shows the anterior leaflet moving stiffly and stopping abruptly, as though suddenly restrained at its point of maximal excursion. This action is in contrast to the free motion and smooth acceleration and deceleration of normal valve leaflets and indicates that stenosis is present.

Although diastolic doming is a relatively specific characteristic of mitral stenosis, there are at least three situations in which apparent doming of the valve may occur in the absence of stenosis. The most common situations are the redundant floppy valves sometimes seen in mitral valve prolapse syndrome and mass lesions or vegetations involving the free edge of the anterior mitral leaflet.

Figure 5–11, A, is an example of a patient with both mitral valve prolapse and an apparent mass lesion on the free edge of the anterior mitral leaflet. The abrupt, nearly right-angle curve of the anterior leaflet in this example is similar to the type of doming seen in mitral stenosis. The free unrestricted motion of these leaflets and a normal mitral valve orifice diameter, however, differentiate the apparent stenotic valves from the truly stenotic valves. Finally, in normal persons, when the full extent of the mitral valve leaflets and chordae are recorded, a gradual arc is inscribed, extending from the aortic root to the papillary muscle tips (Fig. 5–11, B). This arc has been confused with valvular doming and stenosis. It can be readily differentiated from true mitral stenosis, however, by the smooth deceleration of the normal anterior leaflet as it reaches complete excursion; the position of the apical tip of the arc at the level of the papillary muscles rather than at the free edges of the mitral leaflets; and the normal mitral valve orifice diameter.

After reaching full excursion, the domed anterior leaflet of mitral stenosis either may be held in this fully distended position throughout diastole or may gradually begin to reclose. The rate of diastolic leaflet closure (E–F slope) depends on the du-

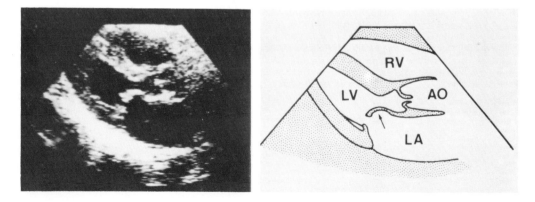

Fig. 5–10.   Parasternal long-axis recording of a domed, stenotic, mitral valve. The posterior mitral leaflet is more erect than normal. The anterior mitral leaflet domes prominently into the left ventricular outflow tract (vertical arrow), and the mitral valve orifice diameter is reduced. Left atrial dilatation is also evident. RV = right ventricle; AO = aorta; LV = left ventricle; LA = left atrium.

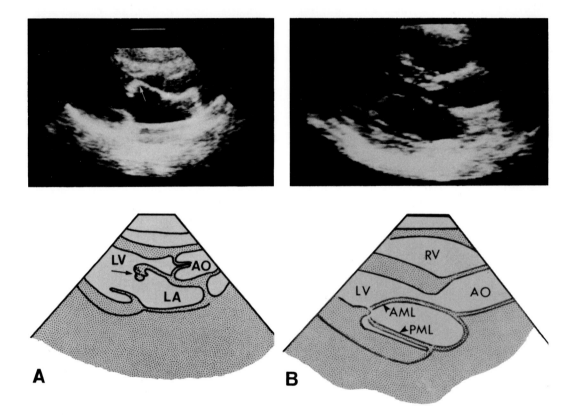

Fig. 5–11. *A,* Top, Diastolic recording from a patient with mitral valve prolapse and an apparent mass lesion involving the free edge of the anterior mitral leaflet. An abrupt, almost right-angle bend in the midportion of the anterior leaflet simulates the doming seen in mitral stenosis (arrow). Bottom, The increased echo density at the tip of the anterior leaflet is indicated by the horizontal arrow. LV = left ventricle; AO = aorta; LA = left atrium. *B,* Parasternal long-axis view of the mitral valve from a normal patient, in whom the full extent of the anterior mitral leaflet is recorded (from the anterior point of insertion into the mitral annulus to the papillary muscles). This gives the valve the appearance of an elongated dome and has been confused with mitral stenosis. This configuration is usually produced by either abnormal medial or lateral angulation of the transducer and can readily be differentiated from true mitral stenosis by the position of the tip of the arc at the level of the papillary muscles and by the smooth acceleration and deceleration of the anterior leaflet in real time. RV = right ventricle; LV = left ventricle; AO = aorta; AML = anterior mitral leaflet; PML = posterior mitral leaflet.

ration of the distending pressure against the atrial surface of the valve. With moderate or severe stenosis, the pressure gradient may persist throughout diastole, thereby maintaining the leaflets in their fully distended position and preventing diastolic closure. In this setting, the only independent leaflet motion occurs during initial diastolic valve opening and with systolic closure.[39] Any movement of the leaflets during this period, therefore, is caused by motion of the mitral annulus, which is displaced superiorly and posteriorly as the ventricle fills. The leaflets are displaced in the same manner. With less severe obstruction, the pressure gradient across the valve may dissipate during the latter portion of diastole, thereby allowing the anterior leaflet to gradually fall back toward a closed position. When sinus rhythm is present, reopening may occur in response to atrial systole.

Many attempts have been made to relate the rate of diastolic leaflet closure (E–F slope) to severity of stenosis.[2,24,45–48] Although a rough correlation should exist between this closure rate and the duration of the pressure gradient across the valve, the E–F slope is affected by factors other than mitral valve orifice size, such as the severity of fibrosis or calcification of the leaflets, compliance of the left ventricle,[26] rate and volume of flow through the mitral orifice,[22,23,24,29] and diastolic motion of the mitral annulus.[25,39] Consequently, in individual cases, attempts to estimate severity of stenosis from rate of leaflet closure alone may be misleading.[49]

Anatomic reduction in mitral orifice area is the hallmark of mitral stenosis, and assessment of severity of stenosis is based on direct measurement of the degree of orifice area reduction.[16,39–42] The mitral valve orifice is best visualized in the parasternal short-axis view with the scan plane positioned such that it is parallel to and passes directly through the valve orifice.[16] This positioning is most easily achieved by first determining the location of the mitral valve orifice in the parasternal long-axis view. If the orifice is then placed in the center of the scan plane, the rotation of the transducer 90 degrees should align the scan plane directly across the valve orifice. The limiting orifice can be recorded by angling the scan plane in a superior-inferior arc until the smallest anatomic valve orifice recorded during maximal initial diastolic leaflet distention is visualized.

The characteristic features of the stenotic mitral valve in the short-axis projection are illustrated in Figure 5–12.[16] The stenotic valve shows a general increase in reflectivity from the orifice margins, limitation of leaflet separation at the commissures, and a marked decrease in orifice area. The orifice typically has a fish-mouthed shape, is longer in its horizontal than vertical dimension, and tapers smoothly at each lateral margin.

The true mitral valve orifice can be measured as soon as it has been properly imaged. Measurement can be accomplished by transferring the image to some form of hard copy for manual measurement or by use of one of the many computer devices now available for measuring areas directly from the video screen. When a manual approach is used, the inner margin of the valve orifice is outlined as illustrated in Figure 5–13. The area contained within this outline can be either planimetered or, more simply, placed over a piece of calibrated graph paper. The millimeter squares enclosed within the outline of the valve orifice are related to the number of squares contained in a square centimeter as determined from the image calibration marks. We have found the latter method to be the quickest of the manual approaches and associated with the least interobserver error.[42]

Reported success rates for recording a measurable mitral valve orifice vary from 83[39] to 100%.[41] Figure 5–14 illustrates the success rates for mitral valve orifice recording from the Indiana laboratory for the

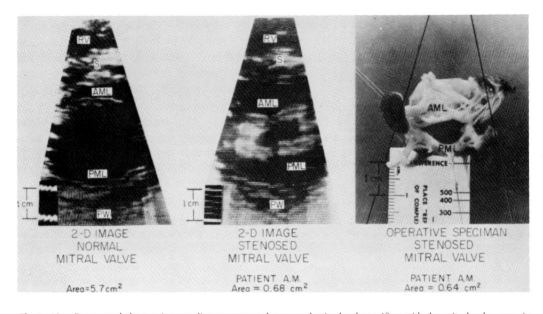

Fig. 5–12. Parasternal short-axis recording compares the normal mitral valve orifice with the mitral valve seen in rheumatic mitral stenosis. The left-hand panel illustrates the normal mitral valve. The leaflets are thin and, at peak diastolic opening, separate widely and lie parallel to the circumferential margin of the left ventricular endocardium. The center panel is a stenotic mitral valve. The margins of the orifice are thickened, the commissures are fused, and the orifice area is decreased. The right-hand panel is an anatomic specimen from the same patient illustrating the similarity in both orifice configuration and size between the echocardiographic image and the pathologic anatomy. RV = right ventricle; S = septum; AML = anterior mitral leaflet; PML = posterior mitral leaflet; PW = posterior wall. (From Henry WL, et al.: Measurement of mitral orifice area in patients with mitral valve disease by real-time two-dimensional echocardiography. Circulation, 51:827, 1975. Reproduced by permission of the American Heart Association.)

years 1974 to 1979 for patients undergoing hemodynamic studies. Although the over-all success rate for this group is only 87%, the results include studies performed during the earlier learning phase of this technique, and the success rate has improved to 96% for the years 1977 to 1979.

The accuracy of the echocardiographic measurement of the mitral valve orifice has been established by comparing this value to the mitral valve area measured directly at the time of surgery,[16] calculated from hemodynamic data,[39–43] and determined pathologically from excised specimens.[40,42] Figure 5–15 compares the mitral valve orifice measured by the cross-sectional echogram with that obtained at surgery in 14 patients. In 12 of these 14 instances, the two measurements were within 0.3 cm² of each other, and the echocardiogram tended to underestimate the surgical valve area. This underestimation

can be attributed to areas of dense fibrosis or calcification along the orifice margin, which increase the intensity of the returning echoes and thereby encroach on the orifice area.[16] In addition, targets at the lateral margins of the orifice are imaged by using the lateral resolution of the system. The echoes from these points, therefore, are widened by the point-spread function of the scanning beam and also encroach on the lumen. Fortunately, the stenotic valve orifice has a consistent fish-mouthed shape. Its long dimension is oriented perpendicular to the direction of propagation of the scan plane. Because of this orientation, the majority of the orifice is recorded using the axial resolution of the system, and the effects of decreased lateral resolution on orifice size are minimized.

Studies examining the relationship of the echocardiographic mitral valve orifice size and the mitral valve area calculated

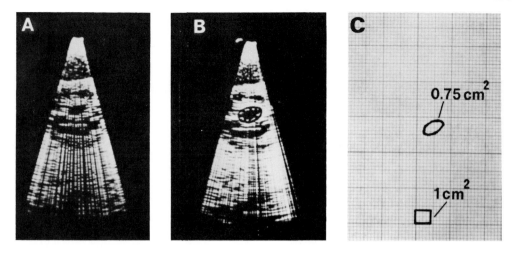

Fig. 5–13. Simplified method for mitral valve orifice measurement. *A,* A stenotic mitral valve at peak diastolic opening. *B,* The inner margin of the orifice has been outlined such that the inner border of the outlined area (interrupted line) corresponds to the inner margin of the orifice. *C,* This outline is then transferred to graph paper, and the area of the orifice is compared to a square centimeter as defined from the image calibration marks.

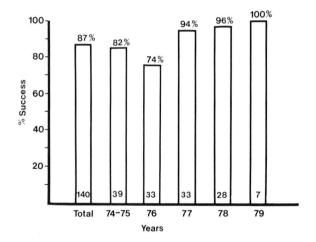

Fig. 5–14. Success rate for recording a measurable mitral valve orifice by cross-sectional echocardiography for the years 1974 to 1978 and the first quarter of 1979. (Data compiled from studies performed at the Indiana University Hospital laboratory.)

from hemodynamic data have also shown a good correlation when both measurements could be obtained.[39–43] Figure 5–16 compares the success rates of the echocardiographic and hemodynamic methods of determining mitral valve orifice area in a group of 140 consecutively examined patients.[42] In 19 of these 140 patients, the mitral valve orifice could not be recorded echocardiographically. In comparison, the mitral valve area could not be calculated from the available hemodynamic data in 21 of the 140 cases. This occurred primarily in patients with combined mitral stenosis and insufficiency and resulted from an inability to determine an angio-

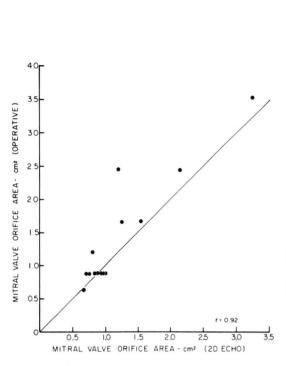

Fig. 5–15. Original comparison of the mitral valve orifice area measured by two-dimensional echocardiography with the area determined at surgery. (From Henry, WL, et al.: Measurement of mitral orifice area in patients with mitral valve disease by real-time two-dimensional echocardiography. Circulation, 51:827, 1975. Reproduced by permission of the American Heart Association.)

graphic cardiac output because of associated aortic insufficiency, arrhythmia, or incomplete opacification or visualization of the ventricle. Figure 5–17 illustrates the correlation between the echocardiographic and hemodynamic mitral valve areas in the 100 patients in whom both sets of data were available. Correlation is good through a wide range of orifice sizes in patients with both isolated mitral stenosis and mitral stenosis and insufficiency. The echocardiographic valve area in these cases tends to overestimate the hemodynamic area by approximately 0.3 cm². This overestimation occurs because the cross-sectional echogram records only the limiting orifice, whereas the transval-

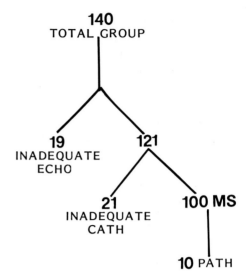

Fig. 5–16. Comparative success rates for echocardiographic and hemodynamic determinations of mitral valve orifice area in 140 consecutive patients examined by both techniques.

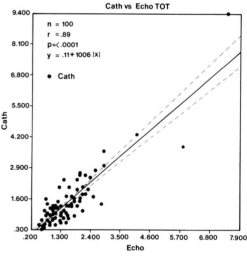

Fig. 5–17. Correlation between echocardiographic and hemodynamic measurements of mitral valve area for a total group of 100 patients with valvular mitral stenosis.

vular gradient is composed of all the factors that contribute to inflow obstruction; the funnel shape of the valve, the decrease in orifice size, and the resistance to ventricular inflow offered by the thickened, fused chordae.

When patients with isolated mitral stenosis are considered separately (Fig. 5–18), the correlation between echocardiographic and hemodynamic valve areas is not as good. In an attempt to explain the difference, we compared both of these parameters with direct pathologic measurement in 10 patients in whom the valves were excised en bloc at surgery. Figure 5–19 illustrates the correlation between the echocardiographic mitral valve area and the pathologic measurements, whereas Figure 5–20 illustrates the corresponding relationship of the hemodynamic valve areas with the same pathologic data. Although the correlation is good in both instances, the echocardiographic measurement of valve area correlates more closely with the pathologic measurement than does the hemodynamic estimate. The greatest variation in the echocardiographic data occurs at the smaller valve areas where the measurement error is greatest. The largest difference between the hemodynamic and pathologic data, in contrast, occurs at larger valve areas where a small change in measured transvalvular gradient results in a large variation in the

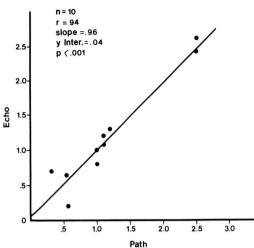

Fig. 5–19. Correlation between the echocardiographic measurement of mitral valve area and direct pathologic measurement of the excised valve. Correlation is excellent with a slight degree of scattering in the lower range.

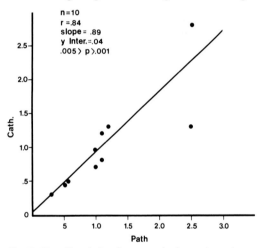

Fig. 5–20. Correlation between the hemodynamic estimate of mitral valve area and the directly measured mitral valve area for the 10 patients reviewed in Figure 5–19. Here, the correlation is not as good, and the scatter is greater at the larger valve areas.

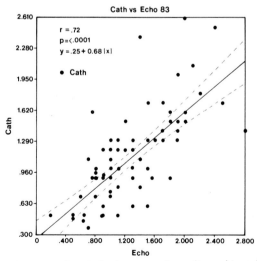

Fig. 5–18. Correlation between echocardiographic and hemodynamic estimates of mitral valve area only in patients with isolated mitral stenosis (N = 83). This correlation is not as good as that for the total group because of the narrowed range of valve areas included and the measurement errors inherent in both methods.

calculated valve area. Unfortunately, this type of correlation tends to select in favor of the echocardiogram because densely calcified or deformed valves, which are recorded least accurately by the echocardiogram, can rarely be removed intact and, hence, are not available for comparison.

Several factors may distort the echocardiographic appearance of the mitral valve orifice and thus affect the accuracy of orifice measurements. These include (1) improper imaging plane orientation relative to the valve orifice,[16] (2) inappropriate receiver gain settings,[39,41] (3) selecting an orifice for measurement that is recorded after valve closure has begun, and (4) confusing an extraneous echo-free area for the valve orifice.

Improper imaging plane orientation characteristically produces an orifice that appears larger than the true limiting orifice.[16] This enlargement can result from improper plane angulation, rotation, or placement relative to the tip of the dome. Each of these factors distorts the orifice in a different manner and can be recognized by the alterations they produce. Figure 5–21 contains a series of mitral valves recorded from the same patient that illustrate each of these distortions. Panel A contains the appropriately recorded, fish-mouth-shaped, stenotic orifice. In B, the same orifice is distorted in a vertical dimension. This distortion occurs because the imaging plane is angled improperly and enters the dome of the valve anteriorly above the level of the orifice and then passes through the valve obliquely to exit through the posterior tip of the orifice. This angle increases the vertical dimension of the orifice disproportionately to the horizontal dimension and enlarges the apparent valve area. In C, the orifice is elongated horizontally. This configuration is recorded when the plane is rotated improperly and passes through one of the lateral margins of the dome above the true orifice. In addition to increasing the horizontal dimension disproportionately to the vertical dimension, this pattern also causes the improperly recorded orifice margin to lose its normal tapered configuration and to become more rounded. Finally, in D, the imaging plane passes through the dome parallel to but above the true orifice. This orientation increases both the vertical and horizontal dimensions and causes both orifice margins to appear more rounded than tapered.

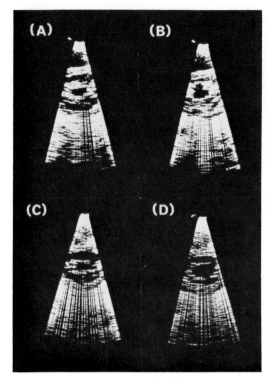

Fig. 5–21. Series of four mitral valve orifices recorded from the one patient with mitral stenosis. This figure illustrates the variations in orifice configuration that can be produced by improper plane angulation and/or rotation. A, The appropriately recorded valve orifice. B, The orifice is distorted vertically by improper angulation. C, The orifice is distorted horizontally by improper rotation. D, The orifice is enlarged in both dimensions by the improper placement of the imaging plane in relation to the valve orifice. (See text for further details.)

Inappropriate receiver gain settings can either enlarge or constrict the orifice.[39,41] If the gain is too low, echo dropout often occurs at the margins of the orifice. The echo dropout increases the apparent orifice area.[39] Conversely, abnormally high gain settings increase both the axial and the lateral echo width, consequently encroaching on the orifice and reducing its apparent area (Fig. 5–22).[41] This effect is greater in densely fibrotic or calcified valves where the echoes are stronger initially.[16]

Whenever possible, the mitral valve orifice should be recorded and measured during initial diastole when the valve is always maximally distended. In patients

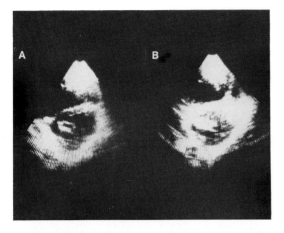

Fig. 5–22. Illustration of the effects of gain setting on mitral valve orifice size. *A,* The gain is appropriately set, and the mitral valve orifice is clearly visualized. *B,* The gain is inappropriately high and almost completely obliterates the orifice.

with more severe lesions, the time of measurement is less important because pressure is exerted against the valve throughout diastole, and little change in orifice area occurs. With less severe lesions, however, partial closure may occur as diastole progresses, and orifice measurements made later in the diastolic filling period may underestimate the maximal valve area. This possibility is particularly true with atrial fibrillation during long diastolic filling periods.

Movement of the valve in a direction perpendicular to or into the short-axis imaging plane may also affect the recorded size of the mitral valve orifice. This motion is due to the normal superior diastolic motion of the mitral annulus, which draws the distended mitral leaflets superiorly as the ventricle fills. Thus, when the imaging plane is positioned above the limiting orifice at initial diastole, the superior motion of the valve draws the dome through the imaging plane as diastole progresses, and the orifice decreases as it approaches the apex.

Occasionally, an echo-free area in the chordal-papillary muscle region or an apparent secondary orifice in the valve itself can be recorded. These areas generally

have indistinct margins and do not demonstrate the normal fish-mouthed configuration. Confusion concerning the location of the actual orifice can be resolved by returning to the long-axis view and defining the point of leaflet separation at the tip of the valve. Also, because the maximal leaflet separation in long axis should equal the vertical dimension of the orifice in short axis, comparison of these dimensions can help to define the true limiting orifice.

Finally, some valvular orifices are so densely calcified that the area of leaflet opening cannot be identified.[16] Figure 5–23 is an example of such a valve. Failure to record an orifice in a densely calcified valve usually indicates that severe stenosis is present.

Mitral Commissurotomy

When the decrease in the orifice area of the stenotic mitral valve reaches a critical level, surgical intervention is generally necessary. This procedure may involve either replacement of the diseased valve with a prosthesis or enlargement of the

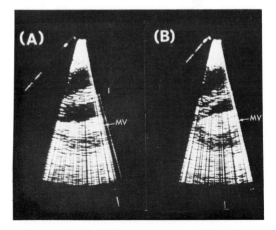

Fig. 5–23. Systolic and diastolic short-axis recordings from a patient with a densely calcified mitral valve. *A,* Recording during systole, the valve appears as a dense band of highly reflective echoes draped across the left ventricular chamber. *B,* In diastole, this band of echoes shifts somewhat anteriorly; however, no orifice can be visualized. MV = mitral valve.

valve orifice by means of a mitral commissurotomy. Commissurotomy, when possible, appears to be the procedure of choice because of its lower incidence of mortality, morbidity, and postoperative complications in comparison to valve replacement.[50]

Several reports have indicated that cross-sectional echocardiography is a useful technique for defining the structure and area of the mitral valve orifice following commissurotomy,[49,50] determining the increase in orifice size resulting from the surgical procedure,[43] assessing the long-term effects of the commissurotomy on valve area,[50] and potentially identifying suitable patients for this surgical procedure.[47] Commissurotomy characteristically alters the appearance of the mitral valve orifice in short axis by elongating the horizontal dimension of the orifice disproportionately to the vertical dimension. Vertical leaflet excursion typically remains restricted and stiff. In some instances, the enlargement of one commissure may be greater than that of the other, further distorting the postoperative orifice configuration. Figures 5–24, A and B, are recordings of the mitral valve orifice from the same patient taken before and after commissurotomy.

In a group of 10 patients studied by cross-sectional echocardiography and cardiac catheterization both prior to and 6 months after commissurotomy, a good correlation in the mitral valve area, determined by both techniques at both sampling periods, was demonstrated.[43] In the postoperative state, the echocardiogram again slightly overestimated the hemodynamic valve area (0.3 cm²), and the overall correlation (r = 0.84) was similar to that noted in uninstrumented valves.[43]

In addition to determining the short-term effects of commissurotomy, the echocardiographic method has also proven useful in determining the long-term influence of mitral commissurotomy on mitral valve area.[50] In a study of 18 patients ex-

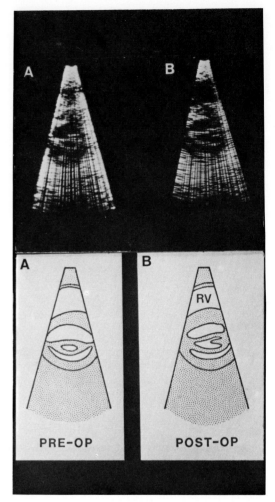

Fig. 5–24. Pre- and post-commissurotomy recordings of the mitral valve orifice from a patient with mitral stenosis. A, Before the operation the orifice is markedly decreased and has a fish-mouthed appearance. B, After the operation, an increase in valve area is most prominent in the lateral or horizontal dimension. In addition, separation of the valve leaflets is greater at the lateral commissure and there is a second lateral indentation in the anterior leaflet just above the native commissure.

amined 10 to 14 years after a documented successful commissurotomy (Fig. 5–25), no change in valve area was noted in 13 patients, whereas in 5 patients (28%), restenosis was evident. This method further helped to separate the patients with increasing symptoms who had evidence of restenosis (3) from those with recurrent symptoms but no change in valve area (3).

SERIAL CHANGE IN MITRAL VALVE AREA

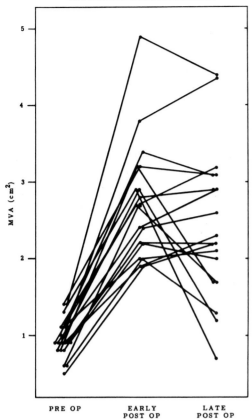

Fig. 5–25. Long-term changes in mitral valve area following successful commissurotomy. Both preoperative and early postoperative values for mitral valve area were determined hemodynamically. The late postoperative values were cross-sectional studies recorded 10 to 14 years after the documented successful commissurotomy. (From Heger, JJ, et al.: Long-term changes in mitral valve area after successful mitral commissurotomy. Circulation, 59:443, 1979. Reproduced by permission of the American Heart Association.)

Although precise correlation of symptoms with echocardiographic valve areas is not possible, it has been suggested that symptoms are commonly noted in patients with valve areas of less than 1.1 cm²/m² after commissurotomy and are less frequently observed in patients with larger postoperative valve areas.[43]

Finally, the echocardiographic method may be helpful in determining the suitability of a patient for commissurotomy.[43] Extensive fibrosis, calcification, and mitral insufficiency are considered at least as relative contraindications to commissurotomy. The echocardiographic method can clearly demonstrate significant calcification and distortion of the valve orifice and can evaluate leaflet pliability. Although mitral insufficiency cannot be directly assessed by the cross-sectional echogram, normal left ventricular size and stroke volume are a good indication that significant mitral regurgitation is not present. Thus, although precise criteria have not yet been established for selecting a patient for commissurotomy, the presence of a thin, freely mobile leaflet in the absence of dense fibrosis or calcification should indicate a good candidate for prospective commissurotomy.

Mitral Stenosis and Prolapse

Prolapse of the mitral valve is frequently noted in patients with mitral stenosis. An incidence of between 10[51] and 40%[39] has been reported. When prolapse does occur in association with mitral stenosis, it almost invariably involves the anterior mitral leaflet and is associated with extreme leaflet pliability and prominent diastolic doming. Figure 5–26 is a recording from a patient with mitral stenosis and prolapse that demonstrates both the marked diastolic doming and systolic prolapse of the anterior mitral leaflet.

The reason for this association is unclear. Both prolapse and mitral stenosis affect predominantly females and may therefore represent the chance association of the two relatively common disorders with the superimposition of the rheumatic process on a valve that is already predisposed to prolapse. Alternatively, the continued wear and tear on a pliable leaflet due to repeated diastolic distention might result in leaflet degeneration and/or stretching.

Posterior leaflet prolapse has, to date, been noted in only one case, where it followed mitral commissurotomy and an episode of subacute bacterial endocarditis.

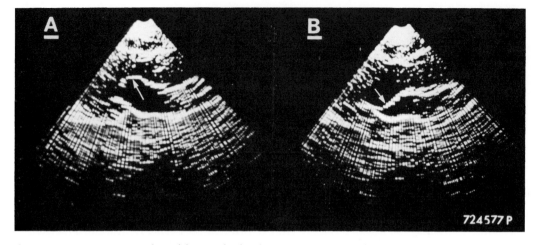

Fig. 5–26.   *A,* Long-axis recording of the mitral valve demonstrates both mitral stenosis and mitral valve prolapse. *A,* During diastole, there is diastolic doming of the anterior leaflet (arrow) with a reduction in mitral orifice diameter. *B,* Systolic prolapse of the anterior leaflet (arrow).

The almost exclusive involvement of the anterior leaflet and association with pronounced doming suggest that continued diastolic distention of the leaflet either is a direct cause or exaggerates an underlying predisposition.

Mitral Stenosis and Insufficiency

The combination of mitral stenosis and insufficiency includes a broad spectrum of valvular deformities ranging from the predominantly stenotic lesion with minimal valve leakage to the severely insufficient valve that offers only limited obstruction to left ventricular inflow. As with pure mitral stenosis, the stenotic component of the combined lesions is indicated by diastolic doming of the anterior mitral leaflet.[16,40] This finding is even more important in the combined lesion because, in many patients with predominant insufficiency, the absolute valve area may be within the normal range. The stenosis then becomes a relative phenomenon because the deformed orifice, although not reduced below the normal range, is inadequate to handle the combined forward and regurgitant volumes that must pass through the valve during diastole. This situation is evidenced, however, only by diastolic doming and not through the measurement of valve area. Figure 5–27 is a recording of the mitral valve of a patient with mitral stenosis and insufficiency that illustrates diastolic doming of the valve in the setting of a relatively large leaflet separation.

When the stenotic component of the combined lesion predominates, leaflet separation in long axis and valve orifice in short axis are reduced. Likewise, left ventricular size and stroke volume are usually normal. As the regurgitant component becomes more dominant, the mitral valve orifice, as a rule, becomes larger, as do left ventricular chamber size and stroke volume. In some patients with predominant mitral regurgitation, incomplete closure of the leaflets in the short axis may also be observed.[52] This phenomenon will be discussed further in the section on mitral insufficiency.

The correlation between echocardiographic and hemodynamic mitral valve area is better with combined lesions than with isolated stenosis (Fig. 5–28). This fact reflects the wider range of valve areas seen with combined lesions and the greater accuracy in the measurement of large echocardiographic valve orifices.

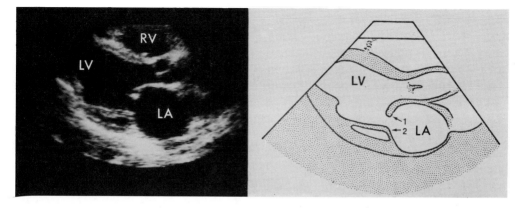

Fig. 5–27. Long-axis recording of the mitral valve, left ventricle (LV), and left atrium (LA) in a patient with mitral stenosis and mitral insufficiency. Diastolic doming of the anterior mitral leaflet is prominent, indicating that the valve is stenotic despite the reasonably large separation between the anterior and posterior borders of the mitral valve orifice (arrows 1 and 2 respectively). The posterior leaflet is stiff and immobile and stands erect during diastole. RV = right ventricle.

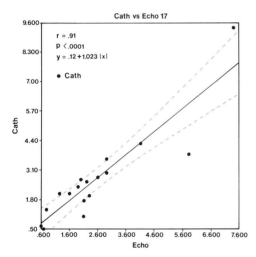

Fig. 5–28. Correlation between echocardiographic and hemodynamic estimates of mitral valve orifice area in patients with combined mitral stenosis and insufficiency. Hemodynamic values are derived using the Gorlin formula and angiographic cardiac output.

Also note that the rate of diastolic mitral valve closure or E–F slope correlates better with mitral valve area in patients with combined mitral stenosis and insufficiency than in those with mitral stenosis alone.[40] This improved correlation probably occurs because both the posterior motion of the annulus and the closure rate of the anterior leaflet bear a direct relationship to the rate of left ventricular inflow and an inverse relationship to mitral valve area. The high inflow rates of predominant mitral insufficiency, therefore, should increase both the annular and the leaflet components of the E–F slope and thus exaggerate the difference in initial diastolic leaflet closure rate when compared to the low inflow rates of predominant stenosis.

Congenital Mitral Stenosis

Congenital mitral stenosis is a rare disorder of the mitral valve and is characterized by variable and often extensive deformity of the valve apparatus. Such deformity may include thickening, fibrosis, and nodularity of the mitral leaflets; fused, rudimentary, or absent commissures; thickened, shortened, and intra-adherent chordae; and fibrotic papillary muscles. These lesions may combine to transform the valve into a thickened, funnel-shaped, flat or diaphragm-like structure that offers variable obstruction to left ventricular inflow.[53–57] Echocardiographically, the appearance of the valve depends on the degree of deformity. When the valve is more severely deformed, the leaflets appear highly reflective and thickened, leaflet motion is stiff and restricted, and diastolic leaflet excursion is reduced.[58] When the leaflets are more pliable, diastolic doming may be evident.

Figure 5–29 is a recording from a 6-month-old child with congenital mitral stenosis and illustrates diastolic mitral leaflet doming and systolic prolapse. In short axis, the mitral orifice was reduced in size, and two papillary muscles were recorded. Calcification of the valve is not typical. The left ventricle in such instances is normal in size, which serves to distinguish this lesion from mitral atresia. Diastolic vibration of the mitral leaflets was noted in one report;[58] however, the reason for its appearance is unclear because the area of turbulence should be distal to the valve. When obstruction is significant, the left atrium may dilate, and when long-standing pulmonary hypertension occurs, right-sided structures may also be enlarged. Although a large series is not available, measurement of valve area in the congenitally stenotic valve will presumably be similar to that in rheumatic mitral stenosis.

Parachute Mitral Valve

Parachute mitral valve is a congenital form of mitral stenosis characterized by a single, large, papillary muscle originating from the floor of the left ventricle. The leaflets and chordae are typically normal. The chordae, however, converge to insert into the single papillary muscle, causing blood to flow through the intrachordal spaces to reach the left ventricle. When these spaces are narrowed, mitral stenosis results.[59,60] Echocardiographically, the long-axis mitral valve configuration shows an increase in reflectivity and a reduction in leaflet motion.[58] The characteristic feature of this disorder, however, is the recording in short axis of a single, large, papillary muscle that is positioned posteriorly

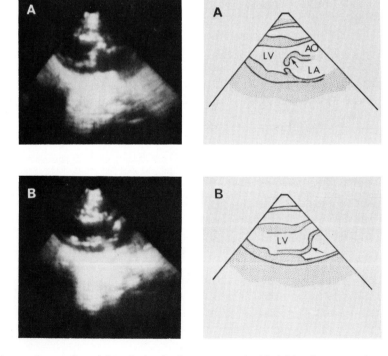

Fig. 5–29. Long-axis recording of the mitral valve from a 6-month-old child with congenital mitral stenosis and systolic prolapse. *A,* The diastolic doming of the pliable stenotic anterior leaflet. The point of peak doming is indicated by the oblique arrow in the accompanying diagram. *B,* A systolic recording illustrates the pronounced systolic prolapse. The region of prolapse is indicated by the arrow in the accompanying diagram. AO = aorta; LV = left ventricle; LA = left atrium.

in the center of the left ventricle.[58] Figure 5–30 illustrates this large, single, papillary muscle.

Supravalvular Mitral Ring

Another form of congenital, left ventricular inflow obstruction is the supravalvular mitral ring. The supravalvular ring or membrane is composed of connective tissue, arises from the base of the atrial aspects of mitral leaflets, and extends inward to encroach on the mitral inlet. It can be distinguished from cor triatriatum by its location below the left atrial appendage and foramen ovale. The valve leaflets and supporting structures are typically normal.[61–63] These rings appear on the cross-sectional echogram as an anomalous band of echoes stretching across the left atrium at the level of the mitral annulus.[58] This band of echoes typically moves inward toward the mitral valve in diastole and superiorly away from the mitral valve in systole.[58]

Figure 5–31 illustrates a supravalvular ring recorded in the apical four-chamber view. This plane is ideal for recording these rings because it places them perpendicular to the path of the scan plane. The ring in this case appears as two bands of linear echoes arising from the medial and lateral margins of the mitral annulus and extending inward to partially obstruct the mitral inflow area. The mitral leaflets that lie in the region of the turbulence beyond the area of obstruction vibrate during diastolic inflow.[58]

The Mitral Valve in Aortic Insufficiency

Mitral valve motion and diastolic orifice configuration may be altered in aortic insufficiency. These abnormalities involve primarily the anterior leaflet and are characterized by (1) a decrease in the opening amplitude of the anterior leaflet in long and short axis; (2) an abnormal short-axis mitral orifice configuration; and (3) diastolic leaflet oscillation.[64] The reduced amplitude of anterior leaflet excursion is apparently caused by the regurgitant stream of blood from the aorta that strikes the leaflet and impedes its normal opening

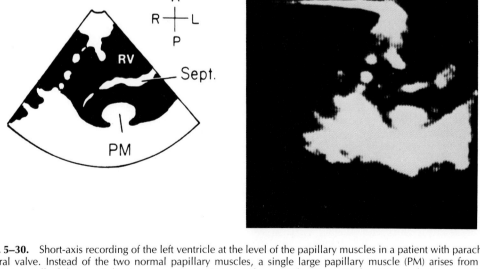

Fig. 5–30. Short-axis recording of the left ventricle at the level of the papillary muscles in a patient with parachute mitral valve. Instead of the two normal papillary muscles, a single large papillary muscle (PM) arises from the posterior wall of the ventricle. Sept. = septum; RV = right ventricle. (From Snider, RA, et al.: Congenital left ventricular inflow obstruction evaluated by two-dimensional echocardiography. Circulation, 61:848, 1980. Reproduced by permission of the American Heart Association.)

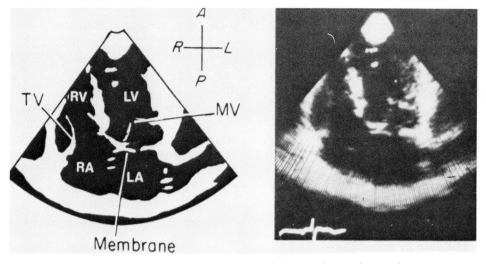

Fig. 5–31. Apical four-chamber view demonstrates a supravalvular mitral ring. The mitral ring appears as a pair of linear echoes arising from the medial and lateral margins of the mitral annulus and extending inward, thereby partially obstructing the left ventricular inlet. Normal mitral leaflet tissue is apparent in the ventricle beneath the obstructing ring. Appropriate structures are labelled in the accompanying diagram. TV = tricuspid valve; RV = right ventricle; LV = left ventricle; RA = right atrium; LA = left atrium; MV = mitral valve. (From Snider, RA, et al.: Congenital left ventricular inflow obstruction evaluated by two-dimensional echocardiography. Circulation, 61:848, 1980. Reproduced by permission of the American Heart Association.)

pattern. This reduction in leaflet opening is most prominent in mid- and late diastole; however, even the initial portions of diastolic opening may be impaired in more severe cases.

The valve orifice in short axis is deformed because the restriction in anterior leaflet excursion is most pronounced in the center of the leaflet, where peak vertical separation normally occurs. This restriction causes the anterior leaflet to appear flattened rather than convex anteriorly, and in severe cases, it may actually be concave toward the left ventricular outflow tract. As diastole progresses, the deformity generally becomes more pronounced. Figures 5–32, A and B, are short-axis recordings of the mitral valve orifice from two patients with aortic insufficiency and illustrate this pattern.

In these instances, the curvature of the anterior leaflet parallels that of the posterior leaflet, and the mitral orifice assumes the curved slit appearance rather than the normal circular or oval pattern. Once this abnormal configuration is assumed, it is generally maintained through-

out the remainder of the diastolic filling period. Atrial systole may cause the anterior leaflet to move anteriorly; however, as a rule, the movement is not sufficient to restore the orifice to a normal configuration. Although this deformity of the mitral valve orifice has not been related to the Austin Flint murmur, it does occur most prominently during the phase of diastole in which this murmur is recorded.[65–67] It also is consistent with intracardiac phonocardiographic evidence suggesting that the murmur arises from the left ventricular inflow tract.[68]

The abnormal pattern of mitral leaflet diastolic motion and the orifice configuration, although characteristic of aortic insufficiency, are not seen in all cases and, therefore, are not sensitive indicators of this disorder. This atypical orifice configuration, however, has not been observed in other disorders and, hence, appears to be fairly specific. A similar pattern can be seen in normal patients in the frame or frames immediately preceding valve closure; however, this pattern occurs late in the diastolic cycle and is associated with

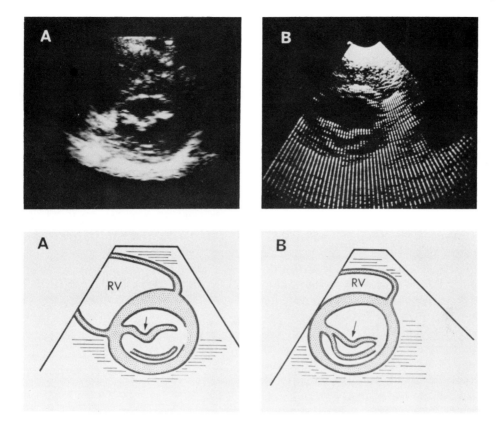

Fig. 5–32. Short-axis recordings of the mitral valve orifice in mid-diastole from two patients with aortic insufficiency. In each case, the midportion of the anterior mitral leaflet is inverted. The leaflet is, therefore, concave toward the left ventricular outflow tract in contrast to its normal convex orientation. The area of peak concavity is indicated in each case by the vertical arrow in the accompanying diagram. RV = right ventricle.

otherwise normal leaflet motion. As such, it should offer no confusion.

Abnormalities Associated with Mitral Insufficiency

Normal systolic closure of the mitral valve depends on the integrated function of the mitral leaflets, chordae tendineae, papillary muscles, and subjacent left ventricular myocardium. Failure of any of these components to function normally may result in improper leaflet closure and valvular insufficiency.[7,69] Echocardiography has not proved to be a sensitive or specific method for directly detecting insufficiency of the mitral valve. Although a number of abnormal leaflet closure patterns that are highly associated with val-vular insufficiency have been described, a diagnosis of mitral insufficiency based on the echogram alone is rarely possible.[52] The major role of cross-sectional echocardiography in mitral insufficiency has been in determining the cause of the valvular abnormality in patients with recognized valvular leakage.[70] Thus, patterns of abnormal systolic leaflet closure or motion have been described in rheumatic mitral insufficiency, mitral valve prolapse, ruptured chordae tendineae and flail mitral leaflets, papillary muscle dysfunction, and cleft mitral valve. Structural changes in the valve leaflets and supporting apparatus have also been noted in other disorders that may be associated with mitral insufficiency, such as bacterial endocarditis, mitral annular calcification, and left atrial myxoma.

Rheumatic Mitral Regurgitation

Rheumatic mitral regurgitation is characterized pathologically by loss of leaflet tissue from fibrosis and contraction, and by thickening, and fibrosis of the chordae tendineae.[71] Commissural fusion is not evident in pure mitral insufficiency, and this characteristic differentiates pure mitral insufficiency from combined lesions. In some instances, the fibrosis and chordal fusion may primarily affect the posterior leaflet with little or no anterior leaflet involvement.[72] Pure mitral regurgitation occurs in approximately 10% of patients with rheumatic mitral valve disease.[73]

Echocardiographically, rheumatic mitral insufficiency is characterized by an increase in echo production from the thickened deformed leaflets primarily in the region of the leaflet tips.[52,70] Long-axis motion of the anterior leaflet is unrestricted, and in the absence of associated mitral stenosis, leaflet doming is not evident. The posterior leaflet is frequently more erect than normal and may be so deformed that motion is not evident. In one series, anterior leaflet prolapse was noted in 3 of 10 patients with pure rheumatic mitral insufficiency.[70]

In short axis, the orifice area is typically normal in size, and the leaflet edges are thickened. No commissural fusion is evident. Incomplete leaflet coaptation can be noted during early systole in some instances and can be related to the severity of the insufficiency (Fig. 5–33).[52] This incomplete closure is usually seen at one of the commissural margins, but it may also involve the central portion of the coaptation line. When the area of incomplete closure involves only one leaflet margin, regurgitation is usually mild. When both margins or the entire closure line are involved, regurgitation tends to be more severe (Fig. 5–34).[52] This sign appears fairly

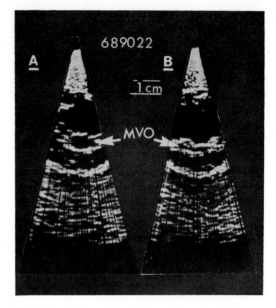

Fig. 5–33. Short-axis recordings of the mitral valve orifice during diastole and systole from a patient with rheumatic mitral stenosis and insufficiency. A, The diminished mitral valve orifice (MVO) of mitral stenosis is evident. B, Incomplete systolic mitral coaptation with an extensive slit-like opening between the anterior and posterior leaflets can be visualized. This failure of the leaflets to coapt has been associated with mitral regurgitation in rheumatic mitral valve disease.

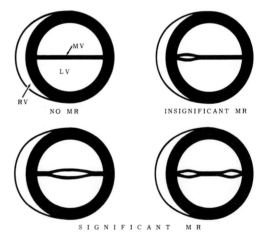

Fig. 5–34. Diagram illustrates the various patterns of incomplete mitral closure that have been observed and their qualitative relationship to the severity of mitral regurgitation (MR). MV = mitral valve; LV = left ventricle; RV = right ventricle.

specific; however, it is insensitive, and its absence cannot be used to exclude regurgitation. Additional attempts have been made to quantitate these regurgitant orifices; however, the role and accuracy of this type of measurement remain to be established.[74]

Mitral Valve Prolapse

Mitral valve prolapse is an anatomic and functional cardiac disorder characterized by displacement of all or part of one or both mitral leaflets superiorly into the left atrium during ventricular systole.[75] Whereas prolapse of other organs is usually downward because of the pull of gravity, the prolapsing mitral valve is thrust superiorly by systolic pressure in the left ventricle. Mitral prolapse has been associated with a variety of seemingly unrelated cardiac disorders, and to date, no single cause has been defined.[76–85]

In general, prolapse results from a disproportion either between the mitral leaflets and the orifice they occlude or between the leaflets and their myocardial-papillary muscle-chordal support system, which restrains them in the ventricular cavity during systole.[86] This disproportion may arise as a result of (1) stretching, elongation, or redundancy of the mitral leaflets themselves; (2) abnormalities of ventricular size, function, or geometry that distort or shorten the ventricular support base for the leaflets; or (3) partial loss of systolic chordal support. From an anatomic standpoint, however, true prolapse relates only to the abnormal leaflet position and does not, of itself, imply any underlying mechanism or clinical syndrome.

Mitral prolapse is suggested clinically by the presence of a midsystolic click and/or late systolic murmur.[75,87,88] This association, unfortunately, is not uniform. Patients with clicks and murmurs may not have angiographic evidence of prolapse, whereas others with angiographically well-documented prolapse have been clinically silent. Until recently, objective documentation of leaflet prolapse has therefore re-

quired angiographic demonstration of leaflet billowing into the left atrium during systole. Even the role of this "gold standard" has been questioned because of the wide interobserver variability noted in identifying prolapse and because of the difficulties in visualizing the anterior mitral leaflet angiographically.[89] In addition, the lack of symptoms in most patients with prolapse makes untenable the routine use of an invasive procedure to document its presence.

Early M-mode reports suggested that mitral prolapse was associated with a characteristic pattern of prominent midsystolic posterior displacement of the mitral leaflet echo.[90–92] This possibility raised the hope that M-mode echocardiography might offer a simple, reliable, noninvasive method of objectively defining the presence of this abnormality. Unfortunately, with increased experience, questions concerning the appropriate diagnostic criteria and resulting sensitivity and specificity of this technique have arisen.[93,94] Consequently, such basic questions as the incidence of prolapse have been impossible to resolve.[94–96] Careful analysis of the pattern of mitral leaflet motion relative to the M-mode beam has given insight into many of these difficulties and has suggested that the systolic motion and orientation of the prolapsing mitral leaflets are such that the M-mode method is poorly suited to record faithfully the true pattern of leaflet motion.[97] Because mitral valve prolapse has been associated with a number of ominous complications, such as sudden death, subacute bacterial endocarditis, intractable congestive heart failure, and left ventricular tachyarrhythmias, we must, if at all possible, clearly define the patient group with this disorder.

Cross-sectional echocardiography offers a convenient noninvasive method for recording the motion and position of both mitral leaflets throughout the cardiac cycle in relation to each other, to external reference points, to surrounding cardiac structures, and to time.[97–100] This motion can be analyzed not only in the resting state but also under conditions of physiologic stress or pharmacologic intervention. For these reasons, the cross-sectional technique is theoretically the ideal method for evaluating mitral leaflet motion and detecting anatomic mitral prolapse.

The cross-sectional diagnosis of mitral valve prolapse rests on the demonstration of abnormal superior motion or arcing of one or both mitral leaflets above the level of the mitral valve annulus into the left atrium.[97–99] The mitral annulus is selected as the reference plane to separate prolapsing from nonprolapsing leaflets for two reasons: (1) in the absence of the mitral valve, this plane anatomically separates the left ventricle from the left atrium; and (2) it offers a clearly definable echocardiographic reference to which leaflet motion and position can be continuously related throughout the cardiac cycle.

In the majority of studies to date, the parasternal long-axis view of the mitral valve has been used to analyze mitral leaflet motion and annular position.[97–101] In this plane, the mitral annulus is considered to extend from the insertion point of the anterior mitral leaflet to the junction of the left atrial and left ventricular walls posteriorly. Figures 5–35, A through D, demonstrate the patterns seen with prolapse of the anterior, posterior, and combined mitral leaflets. In each instance, the leaflets are displaced into the left atrium above the plane of the mitral annulus. The motion of the leaflets required to reach this point represents the combined effects of superior motion of the valve leaflet(s) and apical motion of the mitral annulus. Because the maximum extent of these oppositely directed movements occurs at end-systole, the most pronounced degree of prolapse is also evident at this point of the cardiac cycle. Despite this abnormal motion, the leaflets retain a normal, convex, systolic orientation toward the left ventricular cavity. When the orientation is

reversed and the leaflet(s) becomes convex toward the left atrium, a diagnosis of flail mitral leaflet is more appropriate.

The apical four-chamber view has recently been reported as more sensitive than the parasternal long-axis view for detecting prolapse.[102] This improved sensitivity is greater for anterior than for posterior leaflet prolapse and is more evident in patients with mild or moderate prolapse.[102] The diagnosis of prolapse in the four-chamber view is similar to that in the parasternal long axis and consists of superior arcing of the leaflets beyond the plane of the mitral annulus. The mitral annular plane in this view is taken from the point of insertion of the interatrial septum into the left ventricular myocardium medially to the corresponding atrioventricular junction laterally. The improved sensitivity of this view relates to better visualization of the leaflets during systole and greater ease in defining the annulus. Figure 5–36 illustrates the appearance of prolapsing mitral leaflets in this plane.

Additional echocardiographic features reported in mitral valve prolapse include (1) exaggerated motion of the posterior mitral ring,[70,98,101] (2) abnormal contraction of the interventricular septum,[102] (3) displacement of the mitral coaptation point,[70,98] and (4) morphologic changes of the leaflets themselves.[103] The exaggerated motion of the posterior mitral annulus is characterized by an increase in the apical or inferior component of annular motion without a corresponding increase in the normally associated anterior motion. This phenomenon has been noted in just fewer than 75% of cases, is usually associated with posterior leaflet prolapse, and produces an apparent undermining of the posterior leaflet as it arcs back into the left atrium.[98,102] Corresponding motion of the anterior border of the mitral annulus is not present, and this disparity between the motion of the anterior and posterior margins of the annulus accounts for the

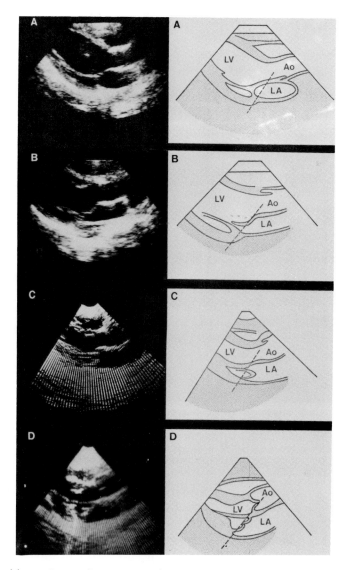

Fig. 5–35. Parasternal long-axis recordings compare the normal pattern of mitral leaflet systolic coaptation (*A*) with that seen with anterior (*B*), posterior (*C*) and combined (*D*) mitral leaflet prolapse. In each case, the prolapsing leaflet(s) extends superior to the plane of the atrioventricular ring (indicated by the interrupted line in the accompanying diagram) and, thus, arcs or bows into the left atrium during systole. LV = left ventricle; AO = aorta; LA = left atrium.

relatively easy visual recognition of this phenomenon.

Abnormal ventricular motion in the four-chamber view characterized by disproportionate contraction of the medial annular margin and an inward bend of the interventricular septum in the papillary muscle region has likewise been observed.[102] This abnormal motion occurs in a smaller percentage of patients with mitral prolapse (30%), and its significance remains to be defined.

Displacement of the mitral leaflet coaptation point has been described in two studies. Disagreement exists, however, regarding the direction of this displacement. In one report, the displacement was described as anterior,[70] whereas the second

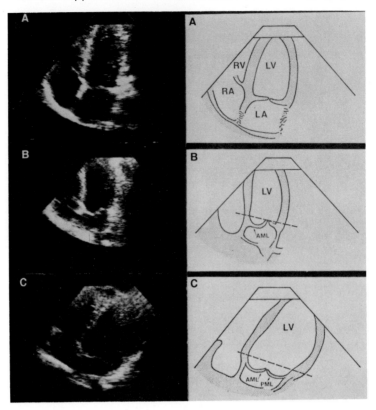

Fig. 5–36. Apical four-chamber recordings from a normal patient (*A*), an anterior mitral leaflet prolapse (*B*), and a combined anterior and posterior mitral leaflet prolapse (*C*). In the normal example, the coapted leaflets lie parallel to, but do not break, the plane of the mitral annulus at the point of peak systolic posterior displacement. In *B* and *C*, the prolapsing leaflets can be appreciated to arc beyond the plane of the mitral annulus (indicated by the dashed line in the diagrams to the right). RV = right ventricle; LV = left ventricle; RA = right atrium; LA = left atrium.

report suggested that the leaflets coapted in an abnormally posterior position.[98] Abnormal posterior displacement of the mitral leaflet coaptation point does occur in a number of patients with mitral valve prolapse. Such displacement may be seen in other conditions, however, and, by itself, cannot be considered diagnostic of prolapse.

Finally, a number of morphologic changes in the mitral leaflets have been noted, including an increase in posterior leaflet size and length relative to the anterior leaflet; thickening of the anterior leaflet and chordae tendineae, and, in some cases, marked leaflet redundancy and infolding.[103] Figure 5–37 illustrates a redundant floppy mitral leaflet in the short-axis view.

Despite these associated findings, the diagnosis of the anatomic mitral leaflet prolapse rests on the demonstration of superior arcing or billowing of the leaflet(s) beyond the plane of the mitral annulus in either the parasternal long-axis or apical four-chamber views. Observed abnormalities of left ventricular motion and/or leaflet structure may aid in this diagnosis; however, such abnormalities are adjunctive and none can be considered, by themselves, as diagnostic of mitral prolapse.

When mitral prolapse is observed on two-dimensional echocardiography, it most frequently appears to involve both leaflets. In three series involving a total of 180 patients,[70,98,101] prolapse of both leaflets was noted in 75 to 90% of cases. Isolated prolapse of the posterior leaflet was

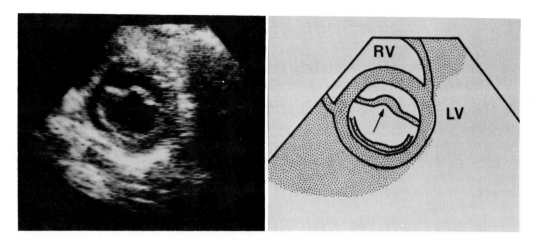

Fig. 5–37. Short-axis recording of the mitral valve orifice from a patient with mitral valve prolapse illustrates the floppy, redundant, thickened nature of the anterior leaflet that is sometimes noted in these cases. RV = right ventricle; LV = left ventricle.

the next most common occurrence (10 to 20%), whereas anterior leaflet prolapse was infrequently seen (3 to 5%).

To date, no connection has been found between the severity of symptoms and the pattern or severity of mitral leaflet prolapse.[70,97] Likewise, although the majority of patients studied have had either a midsystolic click, a late systolic murmur, or a click and murmur, it should be expected that anatomic mitral valve prolpase and the clinical click-murmur syndrome, although associated, will not prove to be uniformly related.

Studies comparing the sensitivity and specificity of cross-sectional and M-mode echocardiography in detecting mitral valve prolapse have been inconsistent. In one series, 10% of patients with prolapse in two-dimensional studies were shown as normal by M-mode echocardiography.[101] In a second study, 7 of 29 patients with both echocardiographic and angiographic prolapse were likewise shown as normal by M-mode echocardiography.[98] Conversely, in a third report of 41 patients with clinical and M-mode echocardiographic evidence of prolapse, only 29 showed leaflet arcing into the left atrium

on two-dimensional echo.[104] Although many of these discrepancies can be related to the criteria used in the initial diagnosis of prolapse, the relative roles of these two techniques remain to be established. Theoretic considerations, however, support the primacy of the two-dimensional echocardiogram in this area because it eliminates the problem of describing two-dimensional leaflet motion relative to a single, fixed, spatial reference.[97]

Comparison of the two-dimensional, echocardiographic, and angiographic visualization of prolapse suggests a good correlation. Of 34 patients with angiographic evidence of prolapse, only 30 demonstrated prolapse when studied by cross-sectional echocardiography.[98] In nine patients, however, anterior leaflet prolapse was noted on the two-dimensional studies and was not appreciated by angiography.[98] Because these studies were not recorded simultaneously and reflected different physiologic states, some variation was expected. The cross-sectional method, however, does appear superior for recording the anterior leaflet prolapse.

Severity of Mitral Valve Prolapse

Assessment on cross-sectional studies of the severity of mitral prolapse has, in general, been based on a visual appreciation of the magnitude of leaflet displacement into the left atrium. Comparison of the severity of prolapse between patients or patient groups or of the effectiveness of physiologic, pharmacologic, or surgical interventions on the severity of prolapse, however, requires some method for quantitating this disorder. Figure 5–38 illustrates a method that has been devised to provide this type of quantitation.[99] This method has been applied to long-axis recordings only; however, it could easily be adapted to the apical four-chamber view.[99]

Because the prolapsing motion of the mitral leaflets is defined in relation to the plane of the mitral ring, one must first define this plane. Although the mitral valve ring is orthogonal to the parasternal long-axis imaging plane, its position can be de-

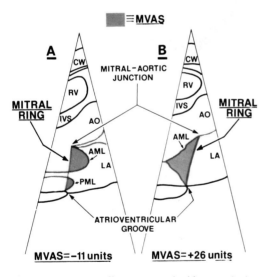

Fig. 5–38. Diagram illustrates a method for quantitating the tendency of the mitral leaflets to prolapse. *A,* The amount of prolapse is equal to the area of the leaflets above the plane of the mitral ring (shaded area) and is assigned a negative value. *B,* The nonprolapsing segment is the normal area between the leaflets and the mitral ring (shaded area) and is arbitrarily designated as positive. When part of the valve prolapses and part is normal, the overall tendency of the leaflets to prolapse is the sum of the positive and negative areas. The MVAS units (mitral valve area subtended by the coapted leaflets) are arbitrary. CW = chest wall; RV = right ventricle; IVS = interventricular septum; AO = aorta; AML = anterior mitral leaflet; LA = left atrium; PML = posterior mitral leaflet.

scribed by a line that connects the mitral aortic junction anteriorly and the atrioventricular groove at the insertion of the posterior mitral leaflet posteriorly. The mitral annular dimension is then determined as the length of this line. To quantitatively assess the systolic geometry of the mitral valve with respect to the mitral ring, the area enclosed or subtended by the coapted mitral leaflets with respect to the mitral ring is then determined. To denote this parameter, the acronym MVAS (mitral valve area subtended) has been introduced.[99]

The shaded areas in Figure 5–38 correspond to this MVAS measurement in a normal patient and in a patient with mitral valve prolapse. To differentiate subtended areas on the ventricular and atrial side of the ring, mitral valve segments on the ventricular side are designated as positive and those on the atrial side as negative. Prolapse is then defined as present if and when any point of the mitral valve in systole is situated on the atrial side of the mitral ring. The area subtended by the prolapsing segment with respect to the ring is then considered as negative. The total MVAS, in any case, is equal to the sum of the area subtended by the nonprolapsing segments (positive) and the prolapsing segments (negative). When the area of the nonprolapsing segment exceeds that of the prolapsing segment, the MVAS is positive. However, mitral valve prolapse nonetheless exists. As the degree of prolapse increases, MVAS approaches zero, and when the area subtended by the prolapsing segment exceeds that of the nonprolapsing segment, MVAS becomes negative. MVAS, therefore, does not define the presence or absence of prolapse but indicates the tendency of the mitral leaflets to prolapse.

We have, to date, used these quantitative methods to examine two clinical questions. In one study, the degree of prolapse was related to the severity of left ventricular deformity in patients with atrial septal defect prior to and following defect repair. We noted that as left ventricular geometry normalized after the operation, the tendency of the mitral leaflets to prolapse decreased.[99] In a second preliminary study, the presence of ventricular tachyarrhythmias in patients with the clinical click-murmur syndrome was related to the MVAS on cross-sectional study.[105] When patients with clinical evidence of mitral valve prolapse syndrome with ventricular tachyarrhythmias were compared with a comparable group without ventricular tachycardia, no difference in MVAS was noted.

Cross-sectional echocardiography, therefore, appears to be an ideal method for examining mitral leaflet motion both alone and in relationship to surrounding structures. The noninvasive nature of this modality and its potential for quantitation make cross-sectional echocardiography particularly applicable to a commonly encountered but largely asymptomatic population, such as the mitral valve prolapse group. Anatomic mitral leaflet prolapse should not be expected to equate with the clinical click-murmur syndrome. In interpreting clinical studies, I indicate this distinction by using the term, "anatomic mitral valve prolapse." Other features may be described that can relate more closely to the clinical syndrome. This should not be the goal of the cross-sectional echogram, however. If these clinical signs, by themselves, represent an adequate "gold standard," nothing else is necessary. When objective evidence of anatomic prolapse is desired or a method for determining the severity of this disorder is required, the cross-sectional echogram is available to the clinician.

Ruptured Chordae Tendineae

The most common cause of acute severe mitral insufficiency is ruptured chordae tendineae. Chordal rupture may occur in the absence of underlying disease or may be secondary to rheumatic heart disease,

bacterial endocarditis, mitral valve prolapse, connective tissue disorders, myocardial infarction, IHSS, and trauma. Patients with spontaneous rupture most often have posterior leaflet involvement, whereas chordal rupture secondary to other disorders apparently involves the anterior and posterior leaflets equally.[106-108]

The echocardiographic pattern of chordal rupture varies depending on the degree of loss of leaflet support. In mild cases, this pattern may take the form of exaggerated mitral prolapse, whereas in more severe cases, flail mitral leaflet may be present.[70,109,110] In some instances, the chordae themselves can be seen flying wildly about the left ventricular cavity. When the disrupted chordae cannot be visualized directly, the diagnosis rests on the pattern of leaflet motion. Marked leaflet abnormalities, such as the flail leaflet (see below), imply chordal or papillary muscle rupture. Less dramatic leaflet abnormalities, however, such as the development or extension of mitral prolapse, require that the presence of chordal rupture be inferred from the clinical situation. When chordal rupture is associated with marked insufficiency of the mitral valve, the associated increase in heart rate and left ventricular stroke volume also draw attention to the leaflet abnormality.

Flail Mitral Leaflet

Flail mitral leaflet is the most severe form of mitral leaflet motion disturbance that results from disruption of the supporting apparatus (chordae tendineae and papillary muscles). The flail motion of the mitral leaflets is most prominent in a plane parallel to the long axis of the left ventricle and left atrium and, thus, can be best visualized in either the parasternal long-axis or the apical four-chamber view. Because only a portion of the mitral leaflet may be flail, the scan plane must be swept from one margin of the mitral orifice to the other so that a localized area of distorted leaflet motion is not overlooked.

A flail valve is characterized by a whipping motion of the tip of the affected leaflet through a 180-degree or greater arc about its point of annular attachment.[109,110] This motion has been compared to that of a detached sail in the wind. During diastole, the leaflet tip points into the left ventricular cavity, and the leaflet body is concave toward the left ventricle. With the onset of systole, the leaflet is thrust upward into the left atrium. The leaflet tip completely reverses its direction and points toward the left atrium. The body of the leaflet, therefore, is concave toward the left atrium or superiorly. This pattern is in contrast to the prolapsing leaflet in which the leaflet body always remains concave toward the left ventricle. Normal systolic coaptation of the anterior and posterior leaflets is lost, and a clearly defined separation between these leaflets in both the parasternal long-axis and apical four-chamber views can usually be determined.

When the loss of leaflet support is caused by bacterial endocarditis, an increase in echo production from the free edges of the ruptured chordae and leaflet tips is frequently noted. Figures 5–39 and 5–40 are examples of flail anterior and posterior mitral leaflets, respectively. The range of motion of the anterior leaflet is normally greater than that of the posterior leaflet. This range is exaggerated when the leaflets become flail, and as indicated in Figure 5–39, the anterior leaflet may actually arc upwards into the left ventricular outflow tract during diastole. When such movement occurs, the leaflet swings through more than 270 degrees from full diastolic to full systolic excursion. The posterior leaflet, in contrast, is limited in its motion by the posterior wall of the left ventricle and normally cannot arc through more than 180 degrees.

Papillary Muscle Dysfunction

The papillary muscles and subjacent left ventricular myocardium provide the foundation that supports the mitral leaflets during ventricular systole. Abnormal function of the papillary muscles has been associated with improper leaflet closure and resultant valvular insufficiency.[111–115]

Papillary muscle dysfunction is most commonly associated with ischemic heart disease; however, other causes, such as cardiomyopathy, left ventricular dilatation, trauma, and a variety of disorders of the endocardium and myocardium that disturb function in the region of the papillary muscles, have been implicated.[70] The presence of this disorder has been most commonly established on clinical grounds by the occurrence of a new murmur of mitral insufficiency in a setting consistent with dysfunction of the papillary muscles.

Recent cross-sectional studies have demonstrated abnormalities of both leaflet motion and systolic leaflet position in patients with clinical evidence of papillary muscle dysfunction.[116,117] These leaflet abnormalities are almost invariably associated with left ventricular dysfunction at the base of one or both papillary muscles and/or with apparent calcification or fibrosis of the papillary muscles themselves.[116,117] The most common pattern of abnormal leaflet motion is characterized by the apparent failure of one or both mitral leaflets to reach the normal peak systolic position relative to the mitral annulus.[116] This pattern is best recorded and has been most extensively studied in the apical four-chamber view.[116] It has also been referred to as incomplete leaflet closure; however, the leaflet tips may actually coapt.

Figure 5–41 is an example of this phenomenon. In this figure, the anterior mitral leaflet is restrained more deeply than normal in the left ventricular cavity, and the posterior leaflet assumes a relatively normal position in relation to the mitral annulus. The leaflets do not appear to coapt, and there is an abrupt bend in the midportion of the anterior mitral leaflet with the tip curving inward toward the center

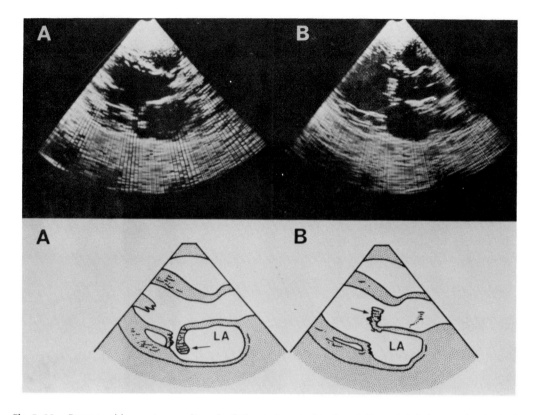

Fig. 5–39. Parasternal long-axis recording of a flail anterior mitral leaflet. *A,* Recorded during systole, the leaflet arcs backward into the left atrium (LA). The body of the leaflet is concave toward the atrial chamber or superiorly. *B,* During diastole, the freely mobile leaflet is thrust upward into the left ventricular outflow tract and swings wildly in an arc about its point of attachment. This patient also has bacterial endocarditis, and the mass of echoes at the tip of the flail leaflet presumably represents vegetative material. (See horizontal arrows in the diagrams.)

of the left ventricular cavity at approximately a 30-degree angle to the base of the leaflet. This pattern has been reported in a high percentage (91%) of patients with ischemic heart disease and clinical evidence of papillary muscle dysfunction.[116] It is rarely noted in patients with ischemic disease without clinical evidence of papillary muscle dysfunction (8%) and is never seen in normal patients. The anterior leaflet is always involved, and incomplete posterior leaflet closure occurs much less frequently (12%). When this phenomenon occurs, it almost invariably is associated with dyskinesis at the base of one papillary muscle (96%); however, the leaflet pattern is the same regardless of the papillary muscle involved.[116]

Long-axis studies have likewise shown that the leaflets are tethered more deeply in the left ventricular cavity during systole.[117] This tethered configuration is characterized by apical displacement of the coaptation point in both early and late systole and by outward bowing of the lower third of the bodies of the leaflets with increased convexity toward the left ventricular cavity.

Figures 5–42 and 5–43 explain diagrammatically (1) the forces that produce the type of incomplete closure noted in Figure 5–41, (2) the reason for the universal involvement of the anterior mitral leaflet, and (3) the observation that the leaflet pattern is the same regardless of which papillary muscle is involved. As illustrated in these diagrams, each papillary muscle

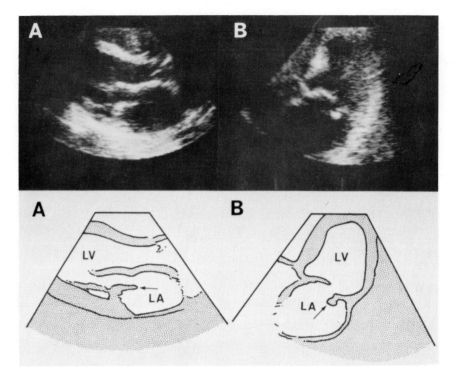

Fig. 5–40. Parasternal long-axis and apical four-chamber systolic recordings from a patient with a flail posterior mitral leaflet. In each of these views, the free leaflet tip is directed toward the left atrium (LA) and the body of the leaflet is concave superiorly toward the atrium. The leaflet tip is indicated by the arrows in each diagram. LV = left ventricle.

gives off chordal attachments to both the anterior and posterior mitral leaflets equally. These chordae attach to both the free edges and bodies of the leaflets. Presumably, the chordal length is such that tension is normally equally distributed during systole. Echocardiographically, both papillary muscles lie in the posterior half of the left ventricle. A line, which joins their tips, runs parallel to the coaptation line of the mitral leaflets. When dyskinesis occurs at the base of either papillary muscle, the papillary muscle is displaced posteriorly relative to the coaptation line of the mitral leaflets and medially or laterally relative to the midportion of the leaflet body. As illustrated in Figure 5–42, the posterior displacement increases the distance from the tip of the papillary muscle to the body of the anterior leaflet, thereby resulting in increased tension in this region. The corresponding distance from the

papillary muscle tip to the body of the posterior leaflet should remain relatively unchanged until the dyskinesis becomes profound. Thus, the anterior leaflet should selectively be pulled toward the cardiac apex, and its complete systolic closure should be prevented. In contrast, little additional tension is exerted on the posterior leaflet, and its closure pattern should remain relatively normal.

Applying the same reasoning to the medial or lateral component of the dyskinetic process, Figure 5–43 suggests that the maximum tension should be exerted in the central portion of the mitral leaflet. When both of these components are combined, the maximum tension should occur in the midportion of the anterior leaflet. The degree of abnormal tension in the midportion of the anterior leaflet should depend on the presence and degree of dyskinesis and should be relatively independent of

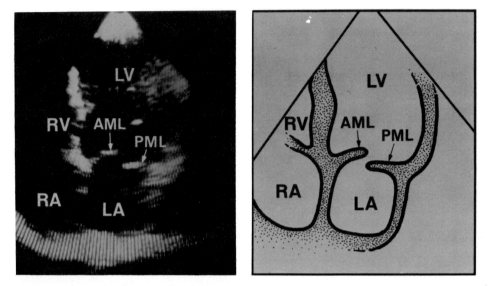

Fig. 5–41. Apical four-chamber recording from a patient with ischemic heart disease and clinical evidence of papillary muscle dysfunction. The anterior mitral leaflet (AML) is tethered within the cavity of the left ventricle (LV) and fails to reach the plane of the mitral annulus at the point of peak systolic closure. The posterior mitral leaflet (PML), in contrast, appears to close normally, giving the appearance of leaflet malapposition. RV = right ventricle; RA = right atrium; LA = left atrium.

the papillary muscle involved. Because of the uneven tension exerted on the anterior and posterior leaflets, the anterior mitral leaflet should be involved uniformly, whereas posterior leaflet involvement is expected only with more severe degrees of dyskinesis. With generalized left ventricular dilatation, symmetric and additive pull on both leaflets may displace them into the left ventricular cavity (Fig. 5–44); however, any disproportion in tension always affects the anterior leaflet preferentially.

The relationship of mitral valve prolapse to papillary muscle dysfunction has been more difficult to define. In one series that specifically excluded patients with any evidence of prolapse prior to their ischemic event, prolapse did not arise de novo after infarction.[116] In a second, smaller study of a more heterogeneous population, prolapse was noted in 5 of 14 patients with papillary muscle dysfunction and, in each case, was associated with increased reflectivity of a papillary muscle suggestive of fibrosis or calcification.[117]

Cleft Mitral Valve

Clefts in the anterior mitral leaflet occur in association with other defects in the endocardial cushions or as isolated lesions.[118] The anterior leaflet may be partially or completely cleft. Accessory chordae, not found in a normal heart, characteristically arise from the interventricular septum and attach to the margins of the cleft. These chordae tend to hold the leaflets anteriorly in the outflow tract during systole and frequently provide inadequate leaflet support. Valvular insufficiency results. Although the major functional abnormality occurs during systole, the cleft valves are most easily detected during diastole.

Figure 5–45 is an example of one of these valves. The cleft is best visualized in the short axis at the free edges of the leaflet and is characterized by a separation between the medial and lateral leaflet halves, which move independently.[70] The cleft mitral valve may be confused with an anatomic tricuspid valve. They can be dif-

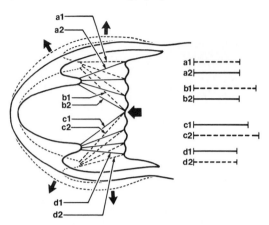

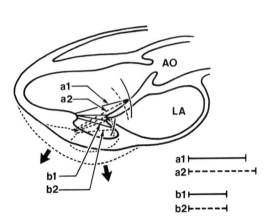

Fig. 5–42. Diagram illustrates the relative effects of the posterior component of the dyskinetic motion of the left ventricle at the base of the papillary muscles on the anterior and posterior mitral leaflets. The solid lines illustrate the normal relationship of the papillary muscles and chordae to the leaflets. The interrupted lines illustrate the relationship occurring with dyskinesis. The distance from the papillary muscle to the body of the anterior leaflet (a1 vs a2) increases more than the distance to either the tip or body of the posterior leaflet (b1 vs b2). AO = aorta; LA = left atrium.

Fig. 5–43. Diagrammatic representation of the two papillary muscles and a mitral leaflet viewed from above. This diagram illustrates the effects of the medial or lateral component of dyskinesis at the base of either papillary muscle on the mitral leaflet. The solid lines illustrate the normal papillary muscle-chordal-leaflet orientation, whereas the interrupted lines illustrate the dyskinetic orientation. Dyskinesis of either papillary muscle results in the exertion of maximum tension in the midportion of the mitral leaflet (b1 vs b2 and c1 vs c2). The lateral margins of the leaflet, in contrast, are subjected to little increase in tension (a1 vs a2 and d1 vs d2). This medial lateral component, combined with the posterior component described in Figure 5–42, suggests that the increased tension produced by the dyskinetic process, irrespective of the papillary muscle involved, should always effect the midportion of the body of the anterior mitral leaflet.

ferentiated, however, by the appearance of only two points of leaflet attachment in the cleft mitral valve.

At the base of the valve, anterior displacement of the medial insertion point may also be noted, and in the long axis, the leaflets are frequently thickened.

Structural Abnormalities of Leaflets or Supporting Structures

Mitral Annular Calcification

Mitral annular calcification is a degenerative disorder that occurs in elderly people and is characterized by calcium deposition in the mitral annular region or in the angular space between the posterior mitral leaflet and the subjacent left ventricular posterior wall. This disorder may be associated with mitral insufficiency, conduction abnormalities, congestive

heart failure, and, when extremely severe, obstruction to left ventricular inflow.[119–123] Cross-sectional echocardiography appears to be a sensitive method for detecting the presence of calcium in the region of the mitral annulus and may be more specific than radiographic studies in differentiating this type of calcification from that involving the mitral leaflets.[124] Although the term, mitral annulus calcification, is commonly used, one cannot differentiate true calcification from dense sclerosis by echocardiography.

The presence of mitral annular calcification is indicated on the echogram by a dense localized, highly reflective area at the base of the posterior mitral leaflet.[124] This echogenic area may be small and discrete or may extend to involve the entire annular region and posterior mitral leaflet, thereby making discrete leaflet visualiza-

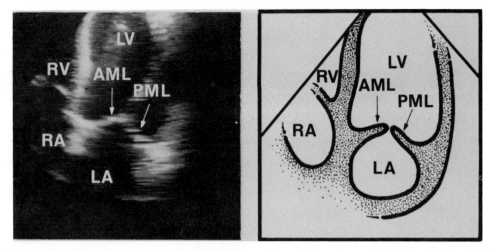

Fig. 5–44. Apical four-chamber view from a patient with cardiomyopathy and generalized left ventricular dilatation. In this case, tension on both the anterior (AML) and posterior mitral leaflets (PML) is increased because of a generalized increase in chordal-leaflet separation. This generalized increase in tension on both leaflets results in failure of either leaflet to reach the plane of the mitral annulus during systole. LV = left ventricle; RV = right ventricle; RA = right atrium; LA = left atrium.

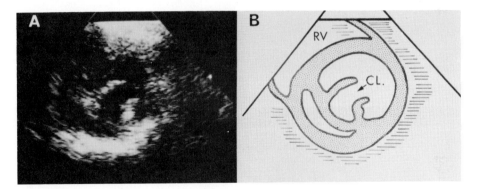

Fig. 5–45. Short-axis recording of a cleft mitral valve. The cleft occurs in the midportion of the anterior leaflet and is evident during diastolic opening. CL = cleft; RV = right ventricle.

tion impossible. Calcification of the posterior mitral annulus occurs approximately five times as frequently as calcification of the anterior portion of the annulus.[124] Annular calcification, when present, may be combined with aortic annular calcification. Isolated calcification of the anterior margin of the annulus is rarely observed. Figure 5–46, A, is a recording of a patient with calcification of the posterior margin of the mitral annulus. This area of increased reflectivity can be observed on each of the standard views and is confined to the posterior margins of the annulus at approximately the 6 o'clock position. Figure 5–46, B, in contrast, is a recording of a patient with massive calcification involving both the anterior and posterior margins of the mitral annulus and the aortic root. In this example, visualization of the mitral leaflets is difficult.

Mitral Valve Vegetations

Valvular vegetations are the characteristic lesions of bacterial endocarditis. These vegetations are friable, verrucous masses composed of clumps of bacteria or fungi, platelets, fibrin, white blood cells,

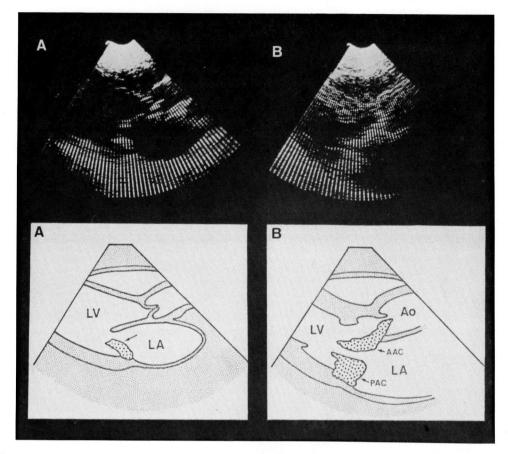

Fig. 5–46. Parasternal long-axis recordings from two patients with mitral annular calcification. *A,* A small degree of calcification is confined to the posterior margin of the annulus and the base of the posterior leaflet. *B,* Massive calcification involves both the posterior and anterior mitral annular segments. The area of calcification is indicated by the stipple in the diagram below. AAC = anterior annular calcification; PAC = posterior annular calcification; LV = left ventricle; LA = left atrium; AO = aorta.

red blood cells, and varying amounts of necrotic tissue. They are usually located in areas previously altered by rheumatic, congenital, or syphilitic cardiac lesions but may be found on apparently normal surfaces. The vegetative lesion is usually attached to a broad-based area of degenerated valvular tissue. Vegetations may assume a variety of sizes and shapes, varying from small, flat, granular lesions to large, fungating, friable masses. Vegetations may erode and disrupt the valve leaflets and adjacent structures or, when large, may obstruct flow through the valve. Pieces of the vegetation may dislodge, resulting in peripheral emboli. Healing is in-

itiated by the invasion of polymorphonuclear leukocytes, and eventually, the infecting organisms disappear. Fibroblasts infiltrate the area and the vegetations may become hyalinized and may even calcify. The remnant of the vegetation is then finally covered with a layer of endothelium.[125]

Vegetations appear on the echogram as an irregular mass of echoes that is usually attached to a valve leaflet and moves in concert with that leaflet.[126-136] When the vegetations are small, they may appear as no more than an irregular lump or bump in the leaflet, most commonly toward the tip. Figure 5–47 is a long-axis, cross-sectional recording of a patient with verru-

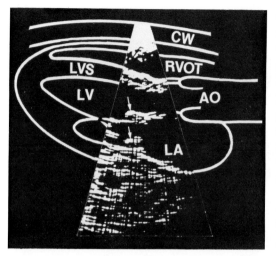

Fig. 5–47. Long-axis parasternal recording of the mitral leaflets from a patient with verrucous endocarditis (Libman-Sacks endocarditis). The vegetations appear as focal accumulations of echoes on the ventricular surfaces of the anterior and posterior leaflets (vertical arrows). CW = chest wall; RVOT = right ventricular outflow tract; IVS = interventricular septum; LV = left ventricle; AO = aorta; LA = left atrium.

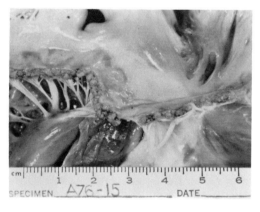

Fig. 5–48. Gross specimen from the same patient indicates the small, warty vegetations along the margins of the leaflets.

cous endocarditis with a rim of small vegetations along the ventricular margins of both the anterior and posterior mitral leaflets. These vegetations appear as a focal accumulation of echoes along the leaflet margins (vertical arrows).

Figure 5–48 is a pathologic specimen from the same patient illustrating the gross appearance of these vegetations and the correspondence of their location to the in-

crease in echo production in the clinical recording. In other patients, the vegetations may be attached to the leaflet by a stalk, or a portion of the vegetation may be more loosely supported and more freely moving. When such situations occur, the corresponding echoes are highly mobile and more easily identified because of this mobility. Vegetations are more prominent when they are large or associated with damage to the valvular structures.

Figure 5–49 is a recording from a patient with a massive vegetation involving the base of the mitral annulus posteriorly and extending up the medial and lateral walls of the mitral ring. This vegetation produces almost complete occlusion of the mitral valve orifice and offers obstruction to left ventricular inflow. Figure 5–50 is an example of a more extensive vegetative lesion. In this example, the pathologic process has resulted in perforation of the body of the posterior mitral leaflet. In both the long- and short-axis views, the fenestration in the leaflet can be visualized, as can the vegetation itself on the tip of the posterior leaflet.

The sensitivity of M-mode echocardiography in detecting bacterial vegetations has been reported to range from 34[133] to 55%.[134] Recording of vegetations generally requires that they be 2 mm or greater in diameter.[126] The cross-sectional echogram has variously been reported to have a sensitivity equal to[137] or superior to that of the M-mode method.[136] Although the relative sensitivities of these techniques appear roughly comparable, the cross-sectional echogram is accepted as a preferable means for defining vegetation size, location relative to other cardiac structures, and motion pattern.[136] In addition, when vegetations involve prosthetic valves, they may be difficult to separate from the dense echoes of the prosthesis. In these instances, the spatial orientation of the two-dimensional echogram makes it the procedure of choice.

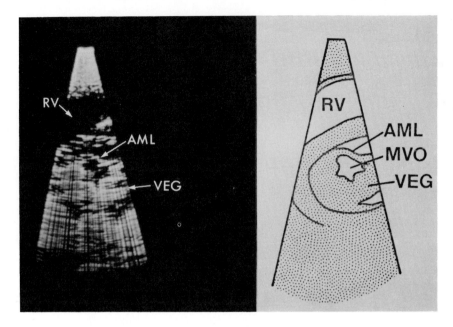

Fig. 5–49. Short-axis recording of the mitral valve orifice (MVO) demonstrates a massive vegetation (VEG) involving the base of the mitral annulus posteriorly and extending up the medial and lateral walls of the mitral ring. The vegetation produces almost complete occlusion of the mitral orifice. RV = right ventricle; AML = anterior mitral leaflet.

Earlier M-mode studies have suggested that, when vegetations are recorded, the clinical prognosis is poor, and many of these patients require valve replacement or expire.[133] Although the outlook may not be as ominous as originally suggested, the majority of patients with vegetations on the echocardiogram still eventually develop a major complication of their disease. This fact is supported by the high incidence of surgical or pathologic confirmation of echocardiographically identified vegetations in studies to date.[136–138]

Little is known about the natural history of bacterial vegetations on two-dimensional echocardiography. In a study of 6 patients, followed for an average of 50 weeks, the vegetations became smaller and more echo dense with time.[127] In two patients, vegetation size decreased dramatically, and in both of these patients, the decrease in size was associated with peripheral embolization. Vegetations do not appear to change size quickly in the absence of embolization, and a decrease in size cannot be regarded as an indication of success or failure of antibiotic therapy. Likewise, little is known about the relationship of vegetation size and/or mobility to their tendency to embolize. Although large, mobile, vegetations would be expected to have a greater tendency toward embolization, this expectation has not been confirmed to date.

In addition to direct visualization of vegetations, the cross-sectional echogram plays a major role in detecting such complications of mitral valve vegetations as flail mitral leaflets, ruptured chordae tendineae, and mitral prolapse. Although the echogram presents anatomic and functional data, it does not provide histologic or bacteriologic information. Thus, although a particular echocardiographic pattern or complication can be consistent with bacterial endocarditis, this association rarely can be stated absolutely from the echogram alone.

Prosthetic Mitral Valves

Prosthetic mitral valves can be divided into the bioprostheses, or tissue valves, and

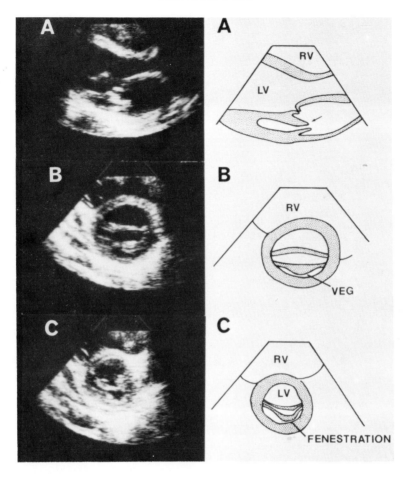

Fig. 5–50. *A,* Parasternal long-axis recording of a vegetative lesion of the posterior mitral leaflet with a fenestration in the leaflet body (horizontal arrow in accompanying diagram). *B,* Short-axis recording with the circumferential location of the vegetation (VEG) indicated at the tip of the arrow in the diagram. *C,* Short-axis systolic recording illustrates the fenestration through the valve leaflet caused by the disruptive infectious process. RV = right ventricle; LV = left ventricle.

the mechanical valves. The bioprostheses are more easily visualized echocardiographically because the leaflets, which are the functional components of the valve, have a reflectivity and motion pattern similar to native valves. In contrast, mechanical valves are composed of highly reflective materials which, at normal gain settings, tend to oversaturate the recording system and, thus, are less well defined.

The most common bioprosthesis in current use is the formaldehyde fixed porcine xenograft. This valve is composed of a three-leaflet porcine aortic valve attached to a sewing ring with three struts that support and shield the valve. Figure 5–51 illustrates the appearance of a porcine valve in each of the three standard recording planes. The sewing ring, which surrounds the base of the valve, is visible in all three planes. In the long-axis and apical four-chamber views, two margins of the ring are recorded. These margins lie in the plane of the mitral annulus and appear separate from the annular margins. Because the struts are oriented 120 degrees from each other around the circumference of the sewing ring, only two can be recorded in a plane that passes through the long axis of the valve. In the short-axis

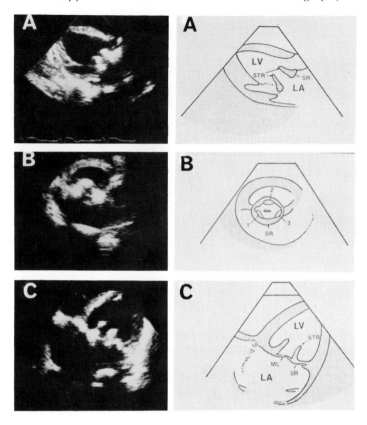

Fig. 5–51. *A,* Long-axis recording of a porcine mitral valve. The tips of the valve struts (STR) and the sewing ring at the base of the valve (SR) are indicated in the diagram to the right. *B,* The short-axis recording of the porcine valve indicates the bright reflective characteristics of the three struts (labelled 1, 2, and 3 in the diagram to the right). A leaflet commissure is also evident in the center of the valve orifice. *C,* An apical four-chamber recording from the same patient. Again, two of the three valves struts, the valve leaflets (ML), and the sewing ring are evident. LA = left atrium; LV = left ventricle.

view, all three struts and the sewing ring can be seen simultaneously.

The valve leaflets lie within the circular orifice. Although anatomically a semilunar aortic valve, the pattern of leaflet motion follows the pattern of blood flow through the mitral orifice and may have an aortic or mitral configuration, depending on the relationship of the valve orifice to transmitral flow. When the valve is restrictive, flow continues throughout diastole, and the leaflets initially open widely and remain fully open. This pattern is similar to that seen with a normal aortic or stenotic mitral valve. When the valve is large relative to the flow through the orifice, a normal period of reduced mid-di-

astolic flow occurs, and the leaflets move toward a closed position during this period corresponding to the normal mitral pattern.

The normal porcine valve has a smooth contour with no focal irregularities.[138] The sewing ring moves in concert with the mitral annulus, and although the precise degree of valve motion relative to the annulus depends on the manner of implantation, there is normally no independent motion of the prosthesis.[139] The valve leaflets appear thin and discrete. Normal leaflet thickness is 3 mm or less.[139] Success in recording these bioprosthetic valves has been good. A 97% success rate has been reported in one series.[139]

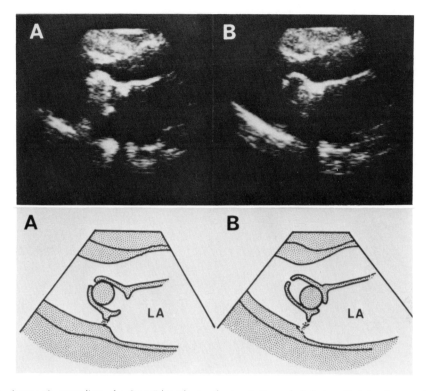

Fig. 5–52. Long-axis recording of a Starr-Edwards prosthesis. *A,* Recorded during diastole; *B,* recorded during systole. In *A,* the ball moves forward or apically into the cage, whereas during systolic closure (*B*), the ball is seated at the base of the sewing ring. LA = left atrium.

The normal appearance and/or motion of the porcine valve may be altered in a variety of disorders, including bacterial endocarditis, leaflet degeneration, thickening and stenosis, or disruption. Characteristic echocardiographic abnormalities of the bioprosthetic valve include increased leaflet thickness, a focal mass or masses of echoes attached to the valve leaflets, excessive rocking or erratic motion of the valves, and systolic displacement of leaflet echoes into the left atrium.[139,140] Leaflet thickening has been associated with both infectious endocarditis and valvular stenosis and disruption. It has also been noted in patients with peripheral embolization. Increased rocking or erratic motion of the valve occurs with valvular dehiscence, and a focal mass on the bioprosthetic valve has been associated, in all instances to date, with infectious endocarditis. When valve leaflet echoes are

recorded in the left atrium, leaflet disruption is usually present.

The evaluation of mechanical prostheses has proved more difficult. The inert materials used in constructing these valves are highly reflective, and although the valves themselves are easily recognized, detailed visualization of their components is difficult to obtain. At normal gain settings, echoes from individual targets on the valve surface are grossly distorted in the lateral dimension. The areas behind these strong reflections may be poorly recorded because of acoustic shadowing, and multiple reverberation from the valve structure may further distort the image. At lower gain settings, the valves are better visualized, but the surrounding, less highly reflective tissue may not be recorded. Figures 5–52 and 5–53 are examples of a Starr-Edwards valve recorded in both the long-axis and the apical view. The gain setting

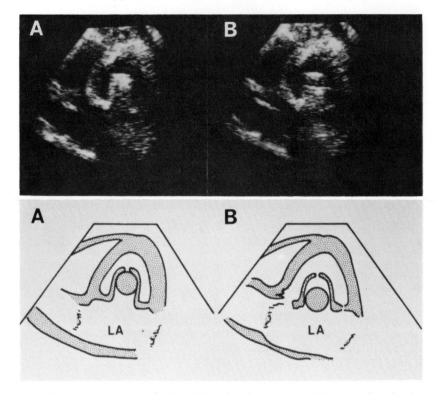

Fig. 5–53. Apical four-chamber view of a Starr-Edwards valve. *A,* Recorded during diastole, this view again illustrates the ball positioned at the tip of the cage. *B,* The ball is in its closed systolic position. LA = left atrium.

is low to permit definition of the ball and cage; consequently, background structures are poorly visualized. Despite these recording limitations, one can still evaluate gross valve component contours, overall valve motion, and ball displacement and detect discrete or mobile masses attached to or surrounding the valve.

REFERENCES

1. Edler, I, and Hertz, C: Use of ultrasonic reflectoscope for the continuous recording of movements of heart walls. Kung Fysiograf Sallsk Lund Fordhandl, *24:*40, 1954.
2. Edler, I: The diagnostic use of ultrasound in heart disease. Acta Med Scand [Suppl], *308:*32, 1955.
3. Edler, I: Ultrasound cardiogram in mitral valve disease. Acta Chir Scand, *3:*230, 1956.
4. Edler, I, and Gustafson, A: Ultrasonic cardiogram in mitral stenosis. Acta Med Scand, *159:*85, 1957.
5. Rusted, IE, Schiefley, CH, and Edwards, JE: Studies of the mitral valve: I. Anatomic features of the normal mitral valve and associated structures. Circulation, *6:*825, 1952.
6. Chiechi, MA, Lees, WM, and Thompson, R: Functional anatomy of the normal mitral valve. J Thorac Surg, *32:*378, 1956.
7. Silverman, ME, and Hurst, JW: The mitral complex. Am Heart J, *76:*399, 1968.
8. Lam, JHC, Ranganathan, N, Wigle, ED, and Silver, MD: Morphology of the human mitral valve: I. Chordae tendineae: a new classification. Circulation, *41:*449, 1970.
9. Ranganathan, N, Lam, JHC, Wigle, ED, and Silver, MD: Morphology of the human mitral valve: II. The valve leaflets. Circulation, *41:*459, 1970.
10. Ranganathan, N, Silver, MD, and Wigle, ED: Recent knowledge of the anatomy of the mitral valve. *In* The Mitral Valve. Edited by D Kalmanson. Acton, MA, Publishing Sciences Group, 1976.
11. Ranganathan, N, and Burch, GE: Gross morphology and arterial supply of the papillary muscles of the left ventricle of man. Am Heart J, *77:*506, 1969.
12. Rider, CF, Taylor, DEM, and Wade, JD: The effect of papillary muscle damage on atrioventricular valve function in the left heart. Q J Exp Physiol, *50:*15, 1965.
13. Tsakiris, AG, Rastelli, GC, and Amorim, D: Effects of experimental papillary muscle damage on mitral valve closure in intact anesthetized dogs. Mayo Clin Proc, *45:*275, 1970.
14. Griffith, JM, and Henry, WL: A sector scanner for real-time two-dimensional echocardiography. Circulation, *49:*1147, 1974.

15. Roelandt, J, et al.: Ultrasonic two-dimensional analysis of the mitral valve. In The Mitral Valve. Edited by D Kalmanson. Acton, MA, Publishing Sciences Group, 1976.

16. Henry, WL, et al.: Measurement of mitral orifice area in patients with mitral valve disease by real-time two-dimensional echocardiography. Circulation, 51:827, 1975.

17. Silverman, NH, and Schiller, NB: Apex echocardiography: a two-dimensional technique for evaluating congenital heart disease. Circulation, 57:503, 1978.

18. Nolan, SP: The normal mitral valve. Patterns of instantaneous mitral valve flow and the atrial contribution to ventricular filling. In The Mitral Valve. Edited by D Kalmanson. Acton, MA, Publishing Sciences Group, 1976.

19. Konecke, L, Feigenbaum, H, and Chang, S: Abnormal mitral valve motion in patients with elevated left ventricular end diastolic pressure. Circulation, 47:989, 1973.

20. Lewis, JR, Parker, JO, and Burggraf, GW: Mitral valve motion and changes in left ventricular end-diastolic pressure: a correlative study of the PR-AC interval. Am J Cardiol, 42:383, 1978.

21. Zaky, A, Nasser, WK, and Feigenbaum, H: A study of mitral action recorded by reflected ultrasound and its application in the diagnosis of mitral stenosis. Circulation, 37:789, 1968.

22. Bellhouse, BJ: Fluid mechanics of a model mitral valve and left ventricle. Cardiovasc Res, 6:199, 1972.

23. Laniado, S, et al.: A study of the dynamic relations between the mitral valve echogram and phasic mitral flow. Circulation, 51:104, 1975.

24. DeMaria, AN, et al.: Mitral valve early diastolic closing velocity in the echocardiogram: relation to sequential diastolic flow and ventricular compliance. Am J Cardiol, 37:693, 1976.

25. Zaky, A, Grabhorn, L, and Feigenbaum, H: Movement of the mitral ring. A study of ultrasound cardiography. Cardiovasc Res, 1:121, 1967.

26. Quinones, MA, Gaasch, WH, Waisser, E, and Alexander, J: Reduction in the rate of diastolic descent of the mitral valve echogram in patients with altered left ventricular diastolic pressure-volume relations. Circulation, 49:246, 1974.

27. Massie, BM, Schiller, NB, Ratshin, RA, and Parmley, WW: Mitral-septal separation: new echocardiographic index of left ventricular function. Am J Cardiol, 39:1008, 1977.

28. Pohost, GM, et al.: The echocardiogram of the anterior leaflet of the mitral valve: correlation with hemodynamic and cineroentgenographic studies in dogs. Circulation, 51:88, 1975.

29. Rasmussen, S, et al.: Stroke volume calculated from the mitral valve echogram in patients with and without ventricular dyssynergy. Circulation, 58:125, 1978.

30. Tsakiris, AG, Gordon, DA, Mathieu, Y, and Lipton, I: Motion of both mitral valve leaflets: a cineroentgenographic study in intact dogs. J Appl Physiol, 39:359, 1975.

31. Rushmer, RF, Finlayson, BL, and Nash, AA: Movements of the mitral valve. Circ Res, 4:337, 1956.

32. Taylor, DE, and Wade, JE: The pattern of flow around the atrioventricular valves during diastolic ventricular filling. J Physiol, 207:71, 1970.

33. Taylor, DE, and Wade, JE: Patterns of blood flow within the heart: a stable system. Cardiovasc Res, 7:14, 1973.

34. Zaky, A, Steinmetz, E., and Feigenbaum, H: Role of the atrium in closure of mitral valve in man. Am J Physiol, 217:1652, 1969.

35. Pridie, RB, Beham, R, and Oakley, CM: Echocardiography of the mitral valve in aortic valve disease. Br Heart J, 33:296, 1971.

36. Mann, T, McLaurin, L, Grossman, W, and Craige, E: Assessing the hemodynamic severity of acute aortic regurgitation due to infective endocarditis. N Engl J Med, 293:108, 1975.

37. Botvinick, EH, et al.: Echocardiographic demonstration of early mitral valve closure in severe aortic insufficiency. Its clinical implications. Circulation, 51:836, 1975.

38. Pomerance, A, and Davies, MJ: The Pathology of the Heart. London, Blackwell Scientific Publications, 1975.

39. Nichol, PM, Gilbert, BW, and Kisslo, JA: Two-dimensional echocardiographic assessment of mitral stenosis. Circulation, 55:120, 1977.

40. Wann, LS, et al.: Determination of mitral valve area by cross-sectional echocardiography. Ann Intern Med, 88:337, 1978.

41. Martin, RP, et al.: Reliability and reproducibility of two-dimensional echocardiographic measurement of the stenotic mitral valve orifice area. Am J Cardiol, 43:560, 1979.

42. Weyman, AE, et al.: Five-year experience in correlating cross-sectional echocardiographic assessment of the mitral valve area with hemodynamic valve area determinations. Am J Cardiol, 43:386, 1979. (Abstract)

43. Henry, WL, and Kastl, DG: Echocardiographic evaluation of patients with mitral stenosis. Am J Med, 62:813, 1977.

44. D'Cruz, I, Panetta, F, Cohen, H, and Glick, G; Submitral calcification or sclerosis in elderly patients: M-mode and two-dimensional echocardiography in "mitral annulus calcification." Am J Cardiol, 44:31, 1979.

45. Segal, B, Likoff, W, and Kingsly, B: Echocardiography. Clinical application in mitral stenosis. JAMA, 195:99, 1966.

46. Gustafson, A: The correlation between ultrasound cardiography, hemodynamics and surgical findings in mitral stenosis. Am J Cardiol, 19:32, 1967.

47. Winters, WL, et al.: Reflected ultrasound as a diagnostic instrument in study of mitral disease. Br Heart J, 29:188, 1967.

48. Wharton, CFP, and Lopez-Bescos, L: Mitral valve movement. A study using an ultrasound technique. Br Heart J, 32:344, 1970.

49. Cope, GD, et al.: A reassessment of the echocardiogram in mitral stenosis. Circulation, 52:664, 1975.

50. Heger, JJ, et al.: Long-term changes in mitral valve area after successful mitral commissurotomy. Circulation, 59:443, 1979.
51. Beasley, B, and Kerber, R: Does mitral prolapse occur in mitral stenosis? Am J Cardiol, 43:367, 1979.
52. Wann, LS, Feigenbaum, H, Weyman, AE, and Dillon, JC: Cross-sectional echocardiographic detection of rheumatic mitral regurgitation. Am J Cardiol, 41:1258, 1978.
53. Bernstein, A, Weiss, F, and Gilbert, L: Uncomplicated congenital mitral stenosis. Am J Cardiol, 2:102, 1958.
54. Daoud, G, et al.: Congenital mitral stenosis. Circulation, 27:185, 1963.
55. Ferencz, C, Johnson, AL, and Wiglesworth, FW: Congenital mitral stenosis. Circulation, 9:161, 1954.
56. Singh, SP, et al.: Congenital mitral stenosis. Br Heart J, 29:83, 1967.
57. van der Horst, RL, and Hastreiter, AR: Congenital mitral stenosis. Am J Cardiol, 20:773, 1967.
58. Snider, RA, Roge, CL, Schiller, NB, and Silverman, NH: Congenital left ventricular inflow obstruction evaluated by two-dimensional echocardiography. Circulation, 61:848, 1980.
59. Shone, JD, et al.: The developmental complex of "parachute mitral valve," supravalvular ring of left atrium, subaortic stenosis, and coarctation of aorta. Am J Cardiol, 11:714, 1963.
60. Simon, AL, Friedman, WF, and Roberts, WC: The angiographic features of a case of parachute mitral valve. Am Heart J, 77:809, 1969.
61. Perloff, JK: Congenital mitral stenosis. In The Clinical Recognition of Congenital Heart Disease. Philadelphia, Saunders, 1970.
62. Johnson, NJ, and Dodd, K: Obstruction to left atrial outflow by a supravalvular stenosing ring. J Pediatr, 51:190, 1957.
63. Rogers, HM, Waldron, BR, Murphey, DFH, and Edwards, JE: Supravalvular stenosing ring of left atrium in association with endocardial sclerosis (endocardial fibroelastosis) and mitral insufficiency. Am Heart J, 50:777, 1955.
64. Feigenbaum, H: Echocardiography. 3rd Ed. Philadelphia, Lea & Febiger, 1981.
65. Flint, A: On cardiac murmurs. Am J Med Sci, 44:29, 1862.
66. White, PD: A note on the differentiation of the diastolic murmur of aortic regurgitation and of mitral stenosis. Boston Med Surg J, 195:1146, 1926.
67. Segal, JP, Harvey, WP, and Corrado, MA: The Austin-Flint murmur: its differentiation from the murmur of rheumatic mitral stenosis. Circulation, 18:1205, 1958.
68. Reddy, SP, et al.: Pressure correlates of the Austin-Flint murmur. An intracardiac sound study. Circulation, 53:210, 1976.
69. Roberts, WC, and Perloff, JK: Mitral valve disease: a clinicopathologic survey of the conditions causing the mitral valve to function abnormally. Ann Intern Med, 77:939, 1972.
70. Mintz, GS, Kotler, MN, Segal, BL, and Parry, WR: Two-dimensional echocardiographic evaluation of patients with mitral insufficiency. Am J Cardiol, 44:670, 1979.
71. Levy, MJ, and Edwards, JE: Anatomy of mitral insufficiency. Prog Cardiovasc Dis, 5:119, 1962.
72. Nixon, PG, Woller, GH, and Radigan, LR: Mitral incompetence caused by disease of the mural cusp. Circulation, 19:839, 1959.
73. Selzer, A, and Katayama, F: Mitral regurgitation: clinical patterns pathophysiology and natural history. Medicine, 51:337, 1972.
74. Wann, LS, et al.: Cross-sectional echocardiographic orientation of regurgitant valve area in patients with rheumatic mitral valve disease. Clin Res, 26:278A, 1978.
75. Criley, JM, et al.: Prolapse of the mitral valve: clinical and cineangiographic findings. Br Heart J, 28:488, 1966.
76. Betriu, A, et al.: Prolapse of the posterior leaflet of the mitral valve associated with secundum atrial septal defect. Am J Cardiol, 35:363, 1975.
77. Salomon, J, Shah, PM, and Heinle, RA: Thoracic skeletal abnormalities in idiopathic mitral valve prolapse. Am J Cardiol, 36:32, 1975.
78. Bon Tempo, CP, et al.: Radiographic appearance of the thorax in systolic click-late systolic murmur syndrome. Am J Cardiol, 36:27, 1975.
79. Brown, OR, et al.: Aortic root dilatation and mitral valve prolapse in Marfan's syndrome: an echocardiographic study. Circulation, 52:651, 1975.
80. Gooch, AS, et al.: Prolapse of both mitral and tricuspid leaflets in systolic murmur-click syndrome. N Engl J Med, 287:1218, 1972.
81. Winkle, RA, et al.: Arrhythmias in patients with mitral valve prolapse. Circulation, 52:73, 1975.
82. Jeresaty, RM: Sudden death in the mitral valve prolapse-click syndrome. Am J Cardiol, 37:317, 1976.
83. Allen, H, Harris, A, and Leatham, A: Significance and prognosis of an isolated late systolic murmur: a 9- to 22-year follow-up. Br Heart J, 36:525, 1974.
84. Barlow, JB, et al.: Late systolic murmurs and nonejection ("mid-late") systolic clicks: an analysis of 90 patients. Br Heart J, 30:203, 1968.
85. Gulotta, SJ, et al.: The syndrome of systolic click, murmur and mitral valve prolapse: a cardiomyopathy? Circulation, 49:717, 1974.
86. Criley, JM, and Kissel, GL: Prolapse of the mitral valve: the click and late systolic murmur syndrome. In Progress in Cardiology. Vol 4. Edited by J Goodwin and PF Yu. Philadelphia, Lea & Febiger, 1976.
87. Barlow, JB, et al.: The significance of late systolic murmurs. Am Heart J, 66:443, 1963.
88. Reid, JVO: Mid-systolic clicks. S Afr Med J, 35:353, 1961.
89. DeMaria, AN, Neumann, A, Lee, G, and Mason, DT: Echocardiographic identification of the mitral valve prolapse syndrome. Am J Med. 62:819, 1977.
90. Dillon, JC, Haine, CL, Chang, S, and Feigenbaum, H: Use of echocardiography in patients with prolapsed mitral valve. Circulation, 43:503, 1971.

91. Kerber, RE, Isaeff, DM, and Hancock, EW: Echocardiographic patterns in patients with the syndrome of systolic click and late systolic murmur. N Engl J Med, 284:691, 1971.

92. Popp, RL, Brown, OR, Silverman, JF, and Harrison, DE: Echocardiographic abnormalities in mitral valve prolapse syndrome. Circulation, 49:428, 1974.

93. DeMaria, AN, et al.: The variable spectrum of echocardiographic manifestations of the mitral valve prolapse syndrome. Circulation, 50:33, 1974.

94. Markiewicz, W, et al.: Mitral valve prolapse in one-hundred presumably healthy young females. Circulation, 53:464, 1976.

95. Brown, OR, Kloster, FE, and DeMots, H: Incidence of mitral valve prolapse in the asymptomatic normal. Circulation (Suppl II), 52:II-27, 1975.

96. Procacci, PM, Savran, SV, Schreiter, SL, and Bryson, AL: Prevalence of clinical mitral valve prolapse in 1169 young women. N Engl J Med, 294:1086, 1976.

97. Sahn, DJ, Allen, HD, Goldberg, SJ, and Friedman, WF: Mitral valve prolapse in children. A problem defined by real-time cross-sectional echocardiography. Circulation, 53:65, 1976.

98. Gilbert, BW, et al.: Mitral valve prolapse two-dimensional echocardiographic and angiographic correlation. Circulation, 54:716, 1976.

99. Schreiber, TL, Feigenbaum, H, Weyman, AE, and Stewart, J: Effects of atrial septal defect repair on left ventricular geometry and degree of mitral valve prolapse. Circulation, 61:888, 1980.

100. Weyman, AE: Clinical applications of cross-sectional echocardiography. In Handbook of Clinical Ultrasound. Edited by M deVlieger. New York, Wiley, 1978.

101. Mardelli, TJ, Morganroth, J, Chen, CC, and Naito, M: Apical cross-sectional echocardiography: the standard for the diagnosis of mitral valve prolapse. Circulation, 60:11, 1979. (Abstract)

102. D'Cruz, I, Shah, S, Hirsch, L, and Goldberg, A: Abnormal systolic motion of the posterolateral basal left ventricle in mitral valve prolapse: a new cross-sectional echocardiographic sign. Am J Cardiol, 45:434, 1980. (Abstract)

103. DeMaria, AN, et al.: Abnormalities of cardiac structure in mitral prolapse syndrome: evaluation by cross-sectional echocardiography. Circulation (Suppl. III), 56:111, 1977. (Abstract)

104. Rakowski, H, Martin, RP, and Popp, RL: Two-dimensional echocardiographic findings in mitral valve prolapse. Circulation, 55 & 56:1, 1977. (Abstract)

105. Friedman, A.: Unpublished data.

106. Sanders, CA, et al.: Diagnosis and surgical treatment of mitral regurgitation secondary to ruptured chordae tendineae. N Engl J Med, 276:943, 1967.

107. Luther, RR, and Meyers, SN: Acute mitral insufficiency secondary to ruptured chordae tendineae. Arch Intern Med, 134:568, 1974.

108. Sanders, CA, Armstrong, PW, Wilkerson, JT, and Dinsmore, RE: Etiology and differential diagnosis of acute mitral regurgitation. Prog Cardiovasc Dis, 14:129, 1971.

109. Child, JS, et al.: M-mode and cross-sectional echocardiographic features of flail posterior mitral leaflets. Am J Cardiol, 44:1383, 1979.

110. Mintz, GS, Kotler, MN, Segal, BL, and Parry, WR: Two-dimensional echocardiographic recognition of ruptured chordae tendineae. Circulation, 57:244, 1978.

111. Wiggers, C, and Feil, H: The cardiodynamics of mitral insufficiency. Heart, 1:149, 1922.

112. Levy, MJ, and Edwards, JE: Anatomy of mitral insufficiency. Prog Cardiovasc Dis, 5:119, 1962.

113. Perloff, JK, and Roberts, WC: The mitral apparatus. Functional anatomy of mitral regurgitation. Circulation, 46:227, 1972.

114. Burch, GE, DePasquale, NP, and Phillips, JH: Clinical manifestations of papillary muscle dysfunction. Arch Intern Med, 112:112, 1963.

115. Burch, GE, DePasquale, NP, and Phillips, JH: The syndrome of papillary muscle dysfunction. Am Heart J, 75:399, 1968.

116. Godley, RW, et al.: Incomplete mitral leaflet closure in patients with papillary muscle dysfunction: 2-D echo and papillary muscle dysfunction. Circulation, 63:565, 1981.

117. Ogawa, S, Hubbard, FE, Mardelli, TJ, and Dreifus, LS: Cross-sectional echocardiographic spectrum of papillary muscle dysfunction. Am Heart J, 97:312, 1979.

118. Perloff, JK: The Clinical Recognition of Congenital Heart Disease. Philadelphia, Saunders, 1970.

119. Roberts, WC, and Perloff, JK: Mitral valvular disease: a clinicopathological survey of the conditions causing the mitral valve to function abnormally. Ann Intern Med, 77:939, 1972.

120. Geill, T: Calcification of the left annulus fibrosus (230 cases). Acta Med Scand, 239:153, 1950.

121. Simon, MA, and Liu, SF: Calcification of the mitral valve annulus and its relation to functional valvular disturbance. Am Heart J, 48:497, 1954.

122. Kirk, RS, and Russell, JGB: Subvalvular calcification of mitral valve. Br Heart J, 31:684, 1969.

123. Pomerance, A: Pathological and clinical study of calcification of the mitral valve ring. J Clin Pathol, 23:354, 1970.

124. D'Cruz, I, Panetta, F, Cohen, H., and Glick, G: Submitral calcification or sclerosis in elderly patients: M-mode and two-dimensional echocardiography in "mitral annulus calcification." Am J Cardiol, 44:31, 1979.

125. Friedberg, CL: Diseases of the Heart. Philadelphia, Saunders, 1966.

126. Dillon, JC, et al.: Echocardiographic manifestations of valvular vegetations. Am Heart J, 86:698, 1973.

127. Spangler, RD, Johnston, ML, and Holmes, JH: Echocardiographic demonstration of bacterial vegetations in active infective endocarditis. J Clin Ultrasound, 1:126, 1973.

128. Martinez, EC, Burch, GE, and Giles, TD: Echocardiographic diagnosis of bacterial endocarditis. Am J Cardiol, 34:845, 1974.

129. Lee, CC, Ganguly, SN, Magnisalis, K, and Robin, E: Detection of tricuspid valve vegetations by echocardiography. Chest, 66:432, 1974.

130. Wray, TM: The variable echocardiographic features of aortic valve endocarditis. Circulation, 52:658, 1975.

131. Wray, TM: Echocardiographic manifestations of flail aortic valve leaflets in bacterial endocarditis. Circulation, 51:832, 1975.

132. Roy, P, et al.: Spectrum of echocardiographic findings in bacterial endocarditis. Circulation, 53:474, 1976.

133. Wann, LS, Dillon, JC, Weyman, AE, and Feigenbaum, H: Echocardiography in bacterial endocarditis. N Engl J Med, 295:135, 1976.

134. Thompson, KR, Nanda, NC, and Gramiak, R: Reliability of echocardiography in the diagnosis of infectious endocarditis. Radiology, 125:473, 1977.

135. Kisslo, J, et al.: Echocardiographic evaluation of tricuspid valve endocarditis: an M-mode and two-dimensional study. Am J Cardiol, 38:502, 1976.

136. Gilbert, BW, et al.: Two-dimensional echocardiographic assessment of vegetative endocarditis. Circulation, 55:346, 1977.

137. Mintz, GS, Kotler, MN, Segal, BL, and Parry, WR: Comparison of two-dimensional and M-mode echocardiography in the evaluation of patients with infective endocarditis. Am J Cardiol, 43:738, 1979.

138. Stafford, A, et al.: Serial echocardiographic appearance of healing bacterial vegetations. Am J Cardiol, 44:754, 1979.

139. Schapira, JN, et al.: Two-dimensional echocardiographic assessment of patients with bioprosthetic valves. Am J Cardiol, 43:510, 1979.

140. Alam, M, Madrazo, AC, Magilligan, DJ, and Goldstein, S: M-mode and two-dimensional echocardiographic features of porcine valve dysfunction. Am J Cardiol, 43:502, 1979.

Chapter 6

Left Ventricular Inflow Tract, Part 2: Left Atrium, Pulmonary Veins, and Coronary Sinus

LEFT ATRIUM

Anatomy

The left atrium is a thin-walled, ovoid chamber that lies directly beneath the aorta and, with the right atrium, is the most posteriorly positioned cardiac structure.[1,2] This chamber is bordered inferiorly by the mitral annulus and medially by the interatrial septum. The posterior, lateral, and superior walls are not typically in contact with other cardiac structures; however, the right pulmonary artery and pulmonary veins may frequently be recorded along the superior margin of the left atrium, and the descending aorta is seen commonly beneath its posterior wall. The endocardial surface of the left atrial wall is normally smooth and continuous and is interrupted only by the insertions of the right and left pulmonary veins superiorly, by the orifice of the atrial appendage anterolaterally, and by the mitral orifice inferiorly. An addi-tional depression in the midportion of the interatrial septum represents the position of the foramen ovale.

Examining Planes and Linear Dimensions

The left atrium is imaged using the parasternal long-axis, short-axis, and apical four-chamber views.[3,4] Because of its spherical or ovoid shape, the left atrium has no natural long or short axis. The axes of the left atrium, therefore, are defined echocardiographically relative to those of the major adjacent structures. Thus, the echocardiographic long axis of the left atrium lies in the same plane as the long axis of the aorta and left ventricle. Likewise, the short axis of this chamber corresponds to the short axes of these adjacent structures. The longest dimension of the atrium, however, may not lie in the long-axis plane.[3] An additional plane, the subcostal long axis, is particularly useful for recording the interatrial septum (see

Chap. 12). The subcostal long axis is the only standard plane in which this structure is perpendicular to the path of the ultrasonic scan. It may also be useful for detecting left atrial disorders, particularly in children.[4–6]

Figure 6–1 illustrates the parasternal long-axis view of the left atrium. This plane passes through the atrium in an antero-posterior direction. The Y axis of the imaging plane is oriented parallel to a line running from the midportion of the superior atrial border to the midportion of the mitral annulus. This plane should pass between but should not record the ostia of the pulmonary veins.

Two linear dimensions can be derived from the parasternal long-axis view: an anteroposterior dimension (d_1) and a superior-inferior dimension (d_2). The antero-

posterior dimension is taken as the distance between the posterior root of the aorta and the posterior left atrial wall at the level of the aortic valve. This line should pass through and be perpendicular to the superior-inferior axis and should approximate the longest anteroposterior dimension of the atrium at any level in this plane.

The superior-inferior dimension (d_2) is measured from the superior atrial wall to the plane of the mitral annulus through a point that roughly bisects the anteroposterior dimension. The plane of the mitral annulus (rather than the atrial surface of the mitral leaflets) is used as the inferior boundary of this dimension because it is a constant reference in both systole and diastole. Measurements are taken from the inner border of the endocardial echoes of

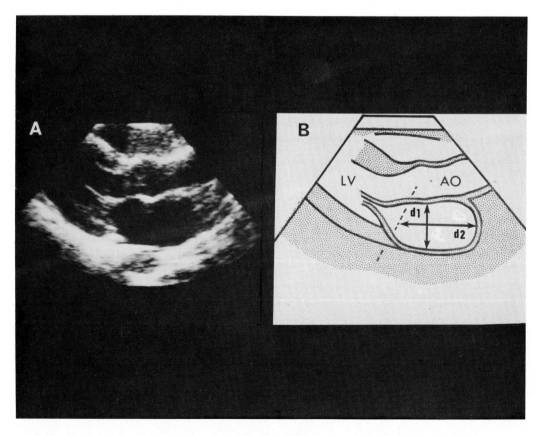

Fig. 6–1. Parasternal long-axis recording of the left atrium. The anteroposterior dimension (d_1) and the superior-inferior dimension (d_2) are indicated in the accompanying diagram. AO = aorta; LV = left ventricle.

the chamber walls. This procedure is in contrast to M-mode dimensions where the leading-edge method has been recommended.[7] In the cross-sectional format, however, the inner-edge method appears preferable because these points are also included in area measurements. In addition, these points permit consistency because the leading edge of the superior margin of the atrium is frequently not visualized.

The superior border of the atrium may be difficult to record in the parasternal long-axis view because it lies parallel to the path of the imaging plane. This border should normally arise from the posterior aortic root at the level of the superior margin of the left coronary sinus. When the superior border is not visualized at this level, one can assume that it has not been adequately recorded and that d_2 is artifactually long. In addition, when the imaging plane is angled too far laterally or medially, it may pass through the orifice of one of the pulmonary veins, again causing loss of definition of the superior border of the atrium.

In the parasternal short-axis view of the left atrium (Fig. 6–2), the imaging plane passes through this chamber from the anterior to the posterior borders. The Y axis of the imaging plane is oriented parallel to a line running from its medial to lateral margins. This plane may transect the atrium at any point along its long axis from the annulus to the superior border; however, for purposes of measurement, the plane should be positioned at the level of the aortic leaflets. Two linear dimensions can also be derived from this plane: an anteroposterior dimension (d_{1s})* and a medial-lateral dimension (d_{3s}). The anteroposterior dimension is taken as the length of a line drawn from the midportion of the posterior aortic root anteriorly to the posterior atrial wall. If properly recorded, the length of this line should correspond to the anteroposterior dimension recorded in the long-axis view (d_1). The medial-lateral dimension (d_{3s}) then is the distance between the endocardial intercepts of a line that is perpendicular to and bisects the anteroposterior dimension. The medial and lateral borders of the atrium may be difficult to record in this view because they are oriented parallel to the imaging plane. In addition, targets along these walls are recorded using the lateral resolution of the system. These targets are consequently

---

*Because the same dimension may be recorded in two or more planes, the subscript (s) for short axis and (a) for apical four chamber are used in the text to denote dimensions recorded in those planes. When a subscript is not present, the reader can presume that the dimension is recorded in a parasternal long axis. Subscripts are not included in the figures because the reference plane itself is always provided.

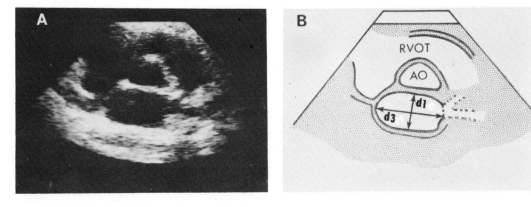

Fig. 6–2. Parasternal short-axis view of the left atrium. The anteroposterior dimension recorded in this plane (d_1) and the medial-lateral dimension (d_3) are indicated in the accompanying diagram. AO = aorta; RVOT = right ventricular outflow tract.

widened by the point-spread function of the beam, thus encroaching on the chamber lumen.

The apical four-chamber view transects the atrium from the mitral annulus to its superior wall (Fig. 6–3). In this orientation, the Y axis of the imaging plane is slightly oblique to a true transverse plane of the atrium and, thus, is parallel to a line that is rotated between 15 and 30 degrees clockwise from the true medial-lateral dimension of this chamber. The linear dimensions derived from this plane are a superior-inferior dimension (d_{2a}) and a medial-lateral dimension (d_{3a}). The superior-inferior dimension is taken from the midpoint of the mitral annular plane to the center of the superior atrial wall. The medial-lateral dimension is taken as the length of a line from the interatrial septum to the free lateral wall that bisects d_{2a}.

The optimal plane for recording each of the atrial dimensions is determined (1) by the orientation relative to the scan plane of the endocardial surfaces that define the limits of that measurement, (2) by the proximity of these surfaces to the transducer, and (3) by the ease of defining plane angulation and rotation. Although correlation between similar dimensions derived from each of the different views has

been good, differences have been noted that can be related to the imaging difficulties inherent in each plane.[3] Analysis of these differences suggests the appropriate plane for recording each dimension. Thus, in a large group of patients with atria of varying sizes, the anteroposterior dimension (d_1) was noted as generally longer when recorded in the short-axis than when recorded in the long-axis view.[3] This discrepancy probably reflects the difficulties in defining plane angulation in the short axis because improper angulation elongates the vertical or anteroposterior dimension and suggests that the long-axis plane is preferable for recording this measurement.

Likewise, the medial-lateral dimension (d_3) was noted as consistently shorter in the apical four-chamber view in both normal patients and patients with dilated atria when compared with the corresponding dimension in the short axis.[3] Here again, this discrepancy can be explained by the imaging characteristics of the system. In both views, the walls are parallel to the scan plane. However, in the apical view, the walls are farther from the focal zone and, hence, the point-spread function is greater, thereby leading to greater encroachment of the endocardial targets on

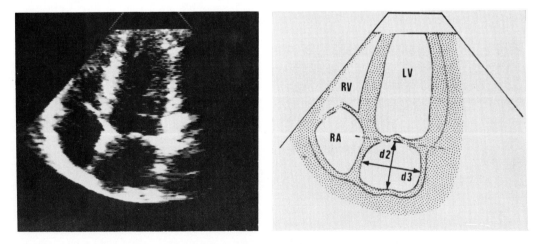

Fig. 6–3. Left atrial recording in the apical four-chamber view. The linear dimensions obtainable from this view are indicated in the diagram to the right. A superior-inferior dimension (d_2) and a medial-lateral dimension (d_3) can be derived as indicated. LV = left ventricle; RV = right ventricle; RA = right atrium.

the atrial lumen. Consequently, the short-axis view should be preferable for recording this dimension.

The superior-inferior dimension, in contrast, appears comparable when recorded in both the four-chamber and long-axis views.[3] The four-chamber view may prove to be preferable, however, because the plane of the mitral annulus is generally more easily defined in this orientation.

The anteroposterior dimension (d_1) has been the basis for estimating left atrial size in M-mode studies[8,9] and correlates well with the angiographic anteroposterior minor axis of the atrium.[10,11] This dimension also correlates with the angiographic area of the left atrium recorded in the right anterior oblique projection[9,12] and with bi-plane angiographic volumes.[11]

Normal Cyclic Variations in Left Atrial Dimensions

The size of the atrium normally changes throughout the cardiac cycle, as does the normal relationship of its dimensions. During left ventricular systole, the atrium serves as a reservoir for blood flowing from the pulmonary veins and, as a result, gradually increases in size from end-diastole to end-systole.[13]

Figures 6–4 and 6–5 illustrate this change in atrial size as well as the corresponding change in the linear dimensions. As these recordings demonstrate, the atrium expands primarily by elongating in anteroposterior and superoinferior directions. This expansion is accompanied by elevation of the aortic root and inferior motion of the mitral annulus. The medial-lateral dimension does not change markedly because these walls are pulled in the same direction as the aortic root moves anteriorly. The atrium, therefore, is more spherical at end-systole than at end-diastole.

The atrial dimensions are most often measured at end-ventricular systole (just prior to mitral valve opening) because the atrial volume is greatest at this point.[7,10]

Fortunately, as illustrated in Figures 6–4 and 6–5, the atrium is also most spherical at this point and thus, a single dimension is most representative of chamber volume.

The left atrium dilates in a variety of pathologic states, including chronic mitral valve disease, left ventricular failure, and such left-to-right shunts as patent ductus arteriosus[14–16] and ventricular septal defect.[17] When the left atrium dilates, all end-systolic dimensions appear to increase symmetrically,[3] the medial and lateral walls bow outward, and the atrium becomes more spherical. The configuration of the dilated left atrium is illustrated in Figure 6–6.

Because the single anteroposterior, end-systolic dimension has proved representative of left atrial size, it has not been necessary to calculate echocardiographic left atrial volumes. If calculation should prove desirable, however, data are available for volume determination using the area-length method (assuming the ellipsoid model as is done angiographically) or Simpson's rule.

Left atrial enlargement can also be detected by relating the echocardiographic end-systolic, anteroposterior diameter of the atrium to the aortic root diameter at the same point in the cardiac cycle. In normal persons, the left atrial aortic root ratio should be equal to or less than 1.1.[18] This relationship assumes that the aortic root is neither dilated nor hypoplastic. In the majority of cases, this assumption is valid, and an increase in this ratio can be used as a ready visual reference to indicate the presence of left atrial enlargement (see Figs. 6–6, A and B).

The left atrium may be smaller than normal in several situations. This typically occurs with

1. Left-to-right shunting at the atrial level, which partially or completely bypasses the left atrium, as in total or partial anomalous pulmonary venous connection[19] or atrial septal defect with partial

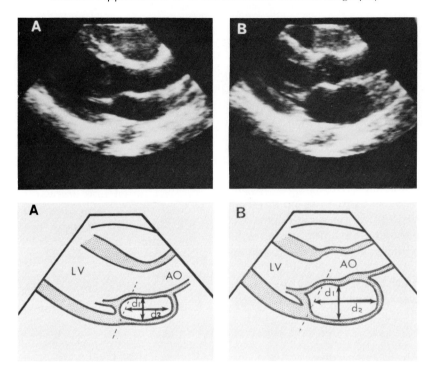

Fig. 6–4.   Parasternal long-axis recordings of the left atrium at end-diastole (A) and at end-systole (B). In this plane, the atrium expands by both elevation of the aortic root with an increase in d_1 and expansion in a superior-inferior direction with an increase in d_2. LV = left ventricle; AO = aorta.

anomalous pulmonary venous drainage. On occasion, a large atrial septal defect may result in extreme right atrial dilatation and clockwise rotation of the structures at the base of the heart. Such rotation shifts the aortic root to the left and posteriorly, thereby compressing the left atrium.

2. Marked dilatation of the aortic root (e.g., Marfan's syndrome, sinus of Valsalva aneurysms and aortic dissection) may encroach on the left atrium.

3. Extracardiac masses, which elevate the atrial floor.

4. Hypoplasia of the left heart.

Left Atrial Tumors

Tumors involving the left atrium may be intracavitary, mural, or extracardiac. The most common intracavitary tumor is the left atrial myxoma. These myxomata are gelatinous, friable masses that commonly arise on a pedicle from the rim of the interatrial septum in the region of the fossa ovalis. Myxomata vary in size and may become large enough to fill the left atrium almost completely and to obstruct the mitral valve orifice. When obstructive, they may present clinically with signs and symptoms suggestive of mitral stenosis. Alternatively, the continual pounding of the tumor against the mitral valve may disrupt the valve apparatus producing mitral insufficiency.[20] They may also produce constitutional symptoms that mimic bacterial endocarditis, and portions of the tumor may break off, releasing embolic material into the systemic circulation.[21] Because of the variable manifestations of these tumors, they are rarely detected clinically, and patients are usually referred for echocardiographic evaluation with a suspected diagnosis of rheumatic mitral valve disease.

Atrial myxomata appear echocardiographically as mobile, well-circumscribed

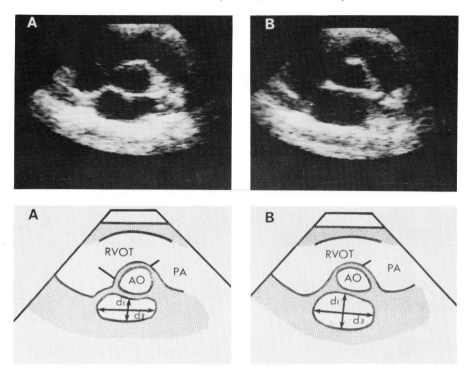

Fig. 6–5. Parasternal short-axis recordings of the left atrium at end-diastole and end-systole. The primary direction of atrial expansion in this plane is in the anteroposterior dimension. There is little change in the medial-lateral dimension (d_3). The atrium, therefore, shifts in configuration from a flattened oval shape at end-diastole to a more circular configuration at end-systole.

masses of echoes within the cavity of the left atrium. Because of the histologic composition of the tumors, there are multiple reflective interfaces within the interior, which result in an internal speckled pattern and make the body of the tumor as reflective as its margins. These tumors are typically mobile, prolapse through the mitral valve orifice during diastole, and are thrust back into the left atrial cavity during systolic ejection.

Figure 6–7 is an example of a large prolapsing myxoma recorded in long axis, and Figures 6–8 and 6–9 are examples of another myxoma in both the long-axis and the apical four-chamber view. Motion of the tumor generally trails slightly behind that of the mitral valve. As a result, the valve usually opens fully before the tumor swings into the valve orifice. When the tumor obstructs the mitral orifice during diastole, the mitral valve is held open both

by the tumor itself and by flow through the orifice around the tumor. No diastolic closing motion (E–F slope) is noted. These tumors, on occasion, may not move, and when this lack of motion occurs, the diagnosis is more difficult.

Atrial myxomata may become secondarily infected. If so, the patient's complaints may relate to the tumor itself or to the infectious process.[22] Figure 6–10, A is an example of a large atrial mass discovered unexpectedly in a patient with disseminated histoplasmosis. Histologically, a small nidus of myxomatous tissue was present; however, the majority of the mass was composed of vegetative material and fungi. The similarity between this mass and those previously illustrated emphasizes again that, although the echogram can detect the presence of intracardiac masses, it cannot define their histologic composition.

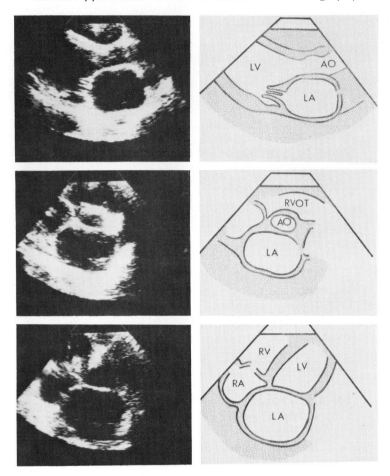

Fig. 6–6. Long-axis, short-axis and apical four-chamber views from a patient with marked left atrial dilatation. The atrium expands in all dimensions and becomes more spherical as it dilates. LV = left ventricle; AO = aorta; LA = left atrium; RVOT = right ventricular outflow tract; RV = right ventricle; RA = right atrium.

Metastatic tumors may also extend into the left atrium and can simulate an atrial myxoma. Figure 6–10, *B*, is an example of a large intra-atrial tumor that was noted in a patient with metastatic osteogenic sarcoma. This tumor mass can be distinguished from the typical myxoma because it involves the lateral portion of the atrium and arises from a broad base along the posterior atrial floor, rather than from the interatrial septum.

Mural tumors are detected by irregularities they produce in the atrial wall, by infringement on the cavity of the atrium, or by calcification of the tumor. In contrast to intracavitary masses, mural tumors are typically immobile. Figure 6–11 is an example of a calcified fibroma that produces an irregularity along the inferior-posterior border of the atrium. This tumor actually arises from the myocardium at the base of the left ventricle, but has expanded into the cavity of the left atrium above the mitral annulus. This mass is highly reflective and suggests calcification within the tumor. During the pathologic examination, both fibrous encapsulation and calcification of the tumor were noted.

Tumors located in the posterior mediastinum may also enlarge to compress the left atrium from behind.[23] Figure 6–12 illustrates a large, small-cell carcinoma

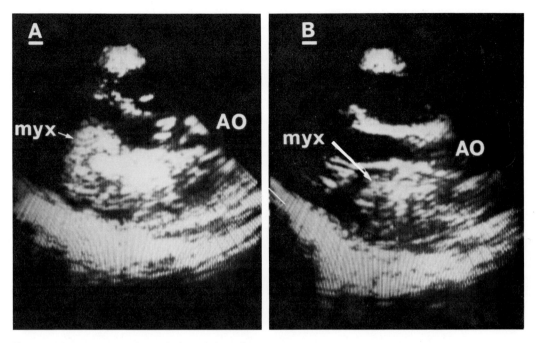

Fig. 6–7. Long-axis recordings of a large left atrial myxoma (MYX) during diastole (*A*) and systole (*B*). The tumor appears as a large, circular, echo-producing mass that can be visualized within the confines of the left atrial cavity during systole. During diastole, however, the tumor shifts into the mitral valve orifice almost totally filling the orifice. AO = aorta.

originating from the posterior mediastinum and extending anteriorly to distort the posterior atrial wall and to compress the atrial cavity.

Left Atrial Thrombi

Left atrial thrombi typically develop when blood stagnates within the atrium or the integrity of the endocardial surface is interrupted. These situations may occur with left atrial dilatation, atrial arrhythmias with resultant loss of normal coordinate atrial contraction, mitral valve disorders, or following mitral valve replacement. The sensitivity of the cross-sectional echogram in detecting left atrial thrombi has not been examined; however, several dramatic cases have been reported in which this technique identified thrombi prior to the development of major complications. When thrombi are detected echocardiographically, they appear as well-demarcated masses of echoes within the left atrial cavity that can be seen in multiple views.[24] The borders of these masses are generally well defined and may change with time.[24] The thrombi may be attached at varying points along the atrial walls and generally show some mobility, which is usually evidenced by motion toward the mitral valve orifice during diastole.

Figure 6–13, *A* is an example of a large and globular mass of echoes in the posterior region of the left atrium produced by one of these atrial thrombi. Visualization of small thrombi, flat mural thrombi, and thrombi in the region of the left atrial appendage has not been reported. To date, experience suggests that, despite the individual instances that have been described, the frequency with which atrial thrombi are detected echocardiographically is far below that noted surgically or pathologically. This experience suggests that the echocardiogram is not a sensitive method for visualizing these lesions.

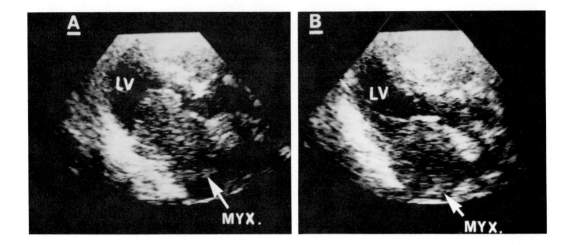

Fig. 6–8. Long-axis recording illustrates another atrial myxoma (MYX). Again, the large tumor appears as a circular mass of echoes within the confines of the left atrial cavity during systole (B). During diastole (A), the tumor prolapses through the mitral valve orifice into the left ventricular (LV) cavity, completely filling the orifice.

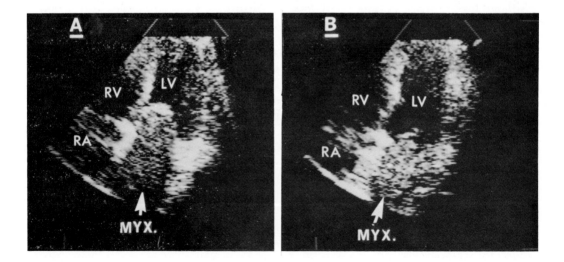

Fig. 6–9. Apical four-chamber view of the tumor demonstrated in Figure 6–8. A, Diastolic frame. B, Recorded just after the onset of ventricular systole. This figure illustrates the anterior mitral leaflet closing behind the tumor as the tumor shifts into the left atrium. RV = right ventricle; LV = left ventricle; RA = right atrium; MYX = myxoma.

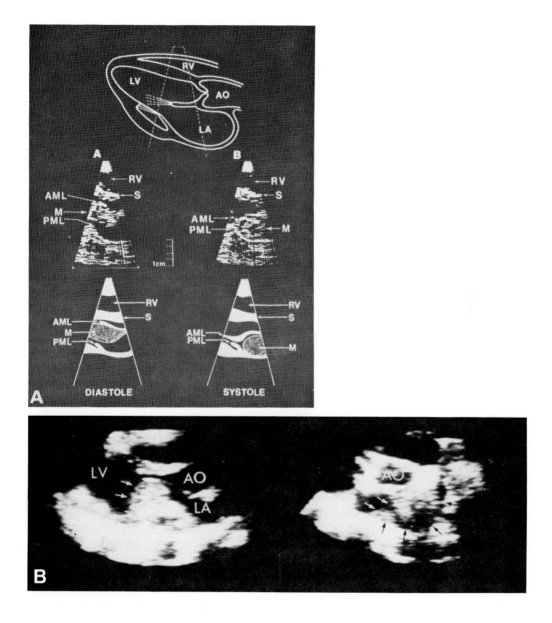

Fig. 6–10. *A,* Long-axis recording from a patient with disseminated histoplasmosis and a secondarily infected left atrial myxoma. The diastolic frame illustrates the tumor prolapsing through the mitral valve orifice. During systole, the tumor lies within the left atrial cavity. RV = right ventricle; LV = left ventricle; AO = aorta; LA = left atrium; AML = anterior mitral leaflet; M = mass; PML = posterior mitral leaflet; S = septum. (From Rogers, EW, Weyman, AE, Noble, RJ, and Bruins, SG: Left atrial myxoma infected with histoplasma capsulatum. Am J Med, 64:683, 1978.) *B,* Parasternal long- and short-axis recordings from a patient with metastatic osteogenic sarcoma and a large intra-atrial tumor mass. During diastole (left), the tumor prolapses throughout the mitral valve orifice; however, its attachment by a broad base to the left atrial floor is still apparent. The short-axis recording (right) demonstrates that the tumor is confined to the central and lateral portions of the left atrium and appears to obstruct the pulmonary veins. The tumor is clearly separated from the interatrial septum, and its position within the atrium helps to differentiate its appearance from that of the typical myxoma. AO = aorta; LV = left ventricular; LA = left atrium.

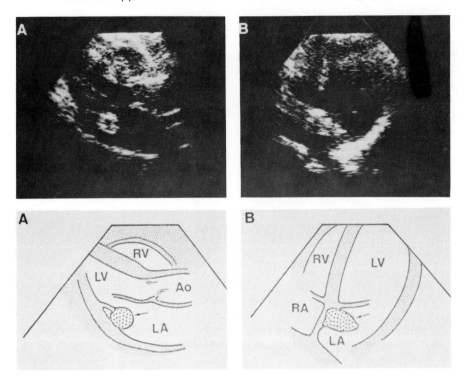

Fig. 6–11. Calcified, encapsulated fibroma of the left ventricular wall at the base of the atrioventricular ring, which has expanded superiorly into the left atrial cavity. *A,* A long-axis view; *B,* an apical four-chamber view. In each case, the gain has been reduced to allow the calcification within the tumor to stand out in contrast to the reduced background echoes. RV = right ventricle; LV = left ventricle; LA = left atrium; AO = aorta; RA = right atrium.

Congenital Aneurysms of the Left Atrium

Isolated aneurysms of the left atrium in the absence of mitral valve or left ventricular disease are rare. These aneurysms, although considered to be congenital in origin, are usually clinically silent until the second to fourth decade. They may involve the wall of the body of the atrium; however, they are more frequently confined to the left atrial appendage. Congenital aneurysms are associated with systemic embolization and/or recurrent supraventricular tachyarrhythmias, and when present, aneurysectomy is usually recommended.[25]

Figure 6–13, *B,* is an example of a congenital aneurysm of the left atrial appendage. The aneurysm appears as an echo-free space along the lateral margins of the left atrium and the basal half of the left ventricle, which indents the wall of the left ventricular chamber. The aneurysm communicates with the left atrial cavity through a broad neck. This aneurysm was an unsuspected finding in a patient who was referred for echocardiographic study following a systemic embolic event.

Cor Triatriatum

Cor triatriatum is characterized by partition of the left atrium into two discrete chambers by a fibrous or fibromuscular diaphragm. This diaphragm typically divides the atria above the atrial appendage and fossa ovalis. Such a location serves to differentiate the membrane of cor triatriatum from the supravalvular mitral ring. One or more openings in the fibrous membrane may permit flow of blood from the pulmonary venous system into the true left atrium.[26,27] The size of these openings determines the degree of left atrial obstruc-

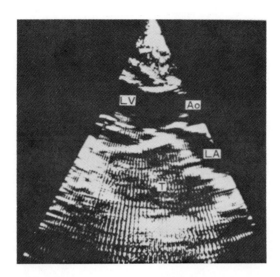

Fig. 6–12. Long-axis recording of the left atrium demonstrates a large small-cell carcinoma of the posterior mediastinum that has expanded anteriorly, thereby displacing the left atrial wall and compressing the left atrial cavity from below. LA = left atrium; LV = left ventricle; T = tumor; AO = aorta. (From Yoshikawa, J, et al.: Cross-sectional echocardiographic diagnosis of large left atrial tumor and extra-cardiac tumor compressing the left atrium. Am J Cardiol, 42:853, 1978.)

tion. The obstructing membrane of cor triatriatum appears echocardiographically as an anomalous band of echoes stretching across the chamber at a level midway between the mitral ring and the superior atrial border.[28,29] This membrane shows phasic motion and is displaced inferiorly toward the mitral orifice during diastole and superiorly toward the superior left atrial border during systole.[28] Although these membranes can be viewed in either the parasternal long-axis, the subcostal long-axis, or the apical four-chamber views,[28,29] the latter view appears preferable because it places the membrane perpendicular to the path of the imaging plane.

Figure 6–14 is a recording from a patient with cor triatriatum. In this patient, the membrane appears as a pair of thin, elongated linear echoes originating from the medial and lateral margins of the atrium and stretching downward toward the mitral orifice. A central perforation is evident in the membrane, which permits blood

flow into the small residual left atrial chamber and left ventricle.

PULMONARY VEINS

Normal Appearance

Normally, four separate veins connect the pulmonary vascular bed with the left atrium. The upper and lower veins from the right lung enter the superior-medial border of the left atrium, and the corresponding pair from the left lung insert into the superior-lateral border. The position and orientation of the pulmonary veins make them difficult to visualize echocardiographically. Although segments of one or more pulmonary veins can be recorded in each of the standard atrial imaging planes, recording of all the venous connections in any single view is generally not possible.

Figure 6–15, A, is a long-axis recording that illustrates the right upper and lower pulmonary veins as they enter the superior-medial border of the left atrium. When viewed in this orientation, the veins lie

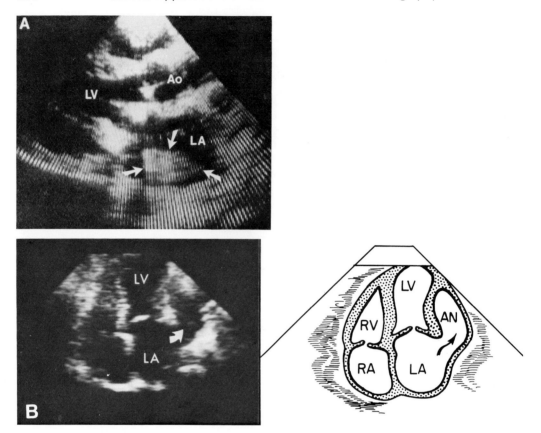

Fig. 6–13. *A,* Long-axis recording of a large left atrial thrombus arising in a patient with a prosthetic mitral valve. The thrombus appears as a relatively homogeneous, large, echo-producing mass within the posterior left atrial cavity (indicated by the arrows). (From Mikell, FL, et al.: Two-dimensional echocardiographic demonstration of left atrial thrombi in patients with prosthetic mitral valves. Circulation, *60*(3):1183, 1979. Reproduced by permission of the American Heart Association.) *B,* Apical four-chamber recording illustrates a congenital aneurysm of the left atrial appendage. The aneurysm (AN) has dissected along the lateral wall of the left ventricle (LV) and distorts the shape of the base of the left ventricle. It is connected to the left atrial cavity (LA) by a large neck. The entrance to the aneurysm is indicated by the curved arrow. RV = right ventricle; RA = right atrium.

next to one another. Their long axes are oriented parallel to that of the aorta. Figure 6–15, *B,* is a short-axis recording that illustrates the left upper and left lower pulmonary veins as they enter the lateral border of the left atrium. In this view, the veins separate at a slight angle as they course leftward from the atrial wall. Figure 6–15, *C,* demonstrates the venous connections in the four-chamber view. From this vantage point, both the medial and lateral venous insertions of three (two lateral and one medial) of the pulmonary veins can be visualized.

To date, success rates for pulmonary venous visualization have been reported only in infants.[30] In one study, at least one pulmonary vein was recorded in 94% of infants with a variety of congenital cardiac disorders. Two veins were visualized less frequently (77%). The best single view for recording the pulmonary veins proved to be the apical four-chamber view (86% of infants had at least one vein recorded in this view alone). The most consistently imaged vein was the left upper pulmonary vein, noted in 54% of cases.

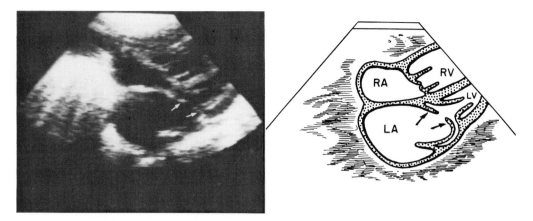

Fig. 6–14. Subcostal long-axis recording from a patient with cor triatriatum. The transatrial membrane (arrowheads) is elongated and, during diastole, lies just above the mitral inlet. Its origin, however, is above the left atrial appendage. The atrium above the membrane is markedly dilated. RA = right atrium; RV = right ventricle; LV = left ventricle; LA = left atrium.

Total Anomalous Pulmonary Venous Return

Abnormalities of the pulmonary venous system are many and varied. Two general terms are used to describe these abnormalities: (1) anomalous pulmonary venous connection, which indicates that all (total) or part (partial) of the pulmonary venous system is connected to the right atrium either directly or via one of its tributary veins, and (2) anomalous pulmonary venous drainage, which is a functional term and implies that one or more of the pulmonary veins is directed so that its flow passes preferentially into the right atrium usually by way of an associated atrial septal defect.[31]

When anomalous pulmonary venous connection is total, the pulmonary veins may connect with the right atrium separately or, more often, may combine into a venous chamber behind the left atrium. A separate vascular channel then arises from this accessory chamber to connect with the right atrium or one of its tributaries. Common sites of connection include the coronary sinus, innominate vein, superior vena cava, and right atrium directly. A number of echocardiographic findings, which although not specific for total anomalous pulmonary venous connec-

tion, are uniformly associated with this disorder. These nonspecific features, in general, are easily defined and must be present before the diagnosis can be entertained. They include (1) a right ventricular volume overload pattern and (2) an atrial septal defect with obligatory right-to-left shunting. The right ventricular volume overload pattern occurs because both systemic and pulmonary venous blood enters the right atrium, and the majority of this increased volume must be borne by the right ventricle. The volume overload pattern is characterized by an increase in right ventricular chamber size, displacement of the interventricular septum toward the left ventricle, and paradoxic septal motion. The atrial septal defect is necessary for survival because, without it, blood cannot reach the left side of the heart. The defect can be visualized directly in the short-axis, four-chamber, or subcostal long-axis views and can be confirmed by peripheral contrast injection with the demonstration of a right-to-left shunt at the atrial level. In addition, the left atrium is usually smaller than normal because of the reduced inflow into the chamber; however, this finding by itself is not of diagnostic value.[5]

Specific echocardiographic characteristics of total anomalous pulmonary ve-

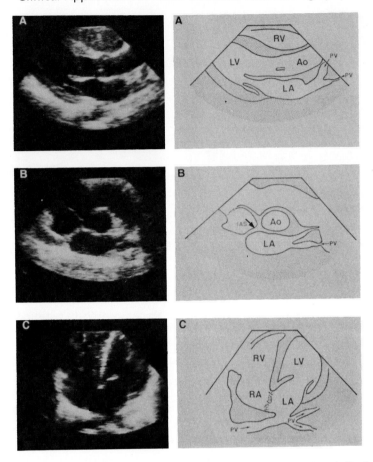

Fig. 6–15. *A,* Long-axis recording of the left atrium (LA) with the transducer angled medially illustrates the right superior and inferior pulmonary veins (PV) inserting into the superior border of the left atrium. *B,* Short-axis recording of the left atrium (LA) illustrates the superior and inferior left pulmonary veins (PV) inserting into the lateral wall of the atrial chamber. *C,* Apical four-chamber view illustrates the insertion of two of the three pulmonary veins (PV) (two lateral; and one medial). AO = aorta; IAS = interatrial septum; RV = right ventricle; LV = left ventricle; RA = right atrium; LA = left atrium.

nous return relate to the direct demonstration of the venous chamber behind the left atrium and of additional changes that may be recorded in the tributary veins to which this chamber is connected.[19,29] The common ventricular chamber appears as an echo-free space that is best visualized on the apical and subxiphoid views, is separated from the atria by a linear band of echoes, and, thus, appears as a subdivision behind the true left atrium. The position of this chamber may vary, depending on the site of connection of the anomalous pulmonary venous inflow into the right heart.[30] These changes in posi-

tion, however, appear subtle and may be difficult to appreciate.

It has also been reported that the level of entry of the anomalous venous connection into the systemic circulation can be detected based on the visualization of an accessory venous pattern and/or dilatation of the tributary vein receiving the anomalous pulmonary venous flow.[19] The easiest abnormal tributary vein to record is the coronary sinus. When the anomalous pulmonary veins connect with the coronary sinus, the coronary sinus typically dilates. When coronary sinus dilatation is combined with an anomalous chamber be-

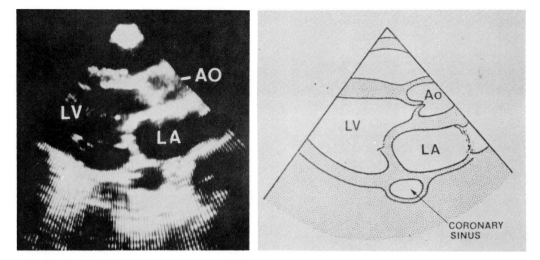

Fig. 6–16. Long-axis recording of the left atrium (LA) and left ventricle (LV) illustrates a dilated coronary sinus lying posterior to the left atrium in the region of the atrioventricular groove. The dilated coronary sinus appears circular because this plane transects the vessel parallel to its short axis. This recording was obtained in a patient with a severe biventricular failure and right atrial hypertension. The fact that this vessel represents the coronary sinus and not the descending aorta can be confirmed by its motion, which is parallel with that of the atrioventricular ring. AO = aorta.

hind the left atrial wall, a right ventricular volume overload pattern, and an atrial septal defect with right-to-left shunting, total anomalous pulmonary venous return to the coronary sinus is strongly suggested.

The patterns of flow in anomalous pulmonary venous drainage have not yet been defined echocardiographically. It has been observed during cardiac catheterization, however, that if a catheter is placed in the pulmonary veins and echocardiographic contrast is injected, the resulting pattern of venous blood flow can be defined from the distribution of contrast within the left and right sides of the heart.[32] This procedure may be adjunctive when the angiographic definition of venous flow patterns proves difficult.

CORONARY SINUS

The coronary sinus is located in the atrioventricular groove along the posterior surface of the heart. It is covered by a layer of muscle fibers from the left atrial wall and by the pericardium and, therefore, is partially incorporated into the atrial wall.

Echocardiographically, the coronary sinus is best visualized in the parasternal long-axis view. When recorded, it appears as a circular echo-free space lying posterior to the left atrial wall just superior to the atrioventricular junction. This echo-free space characteristically moves in concert with the atrioventricular ring. This motion pattern differentiates the coronary sinus, particularly when dilated, from the descending aorta, which may likewise appear circular and lie behind the left atrial wall. The aorta, however, is independent of the heart, and therefore, its motion pattern does not follow that of the atrioventricular ring. The normal coronary sinus is visualized relatively infrequently in adults and rarely, if at all, in children.[33]

Dilatation of the coronary sinus is frequently noted in patients with right ventricular dysfunction and right atrial hypertension (Fig. 6–16). Marked coronary sinus dilatation also occurs owing to increased volume flow into this structure from anomalous venous communications.[34] Three patterns of anomalous venous drainage into the coronary sinus have

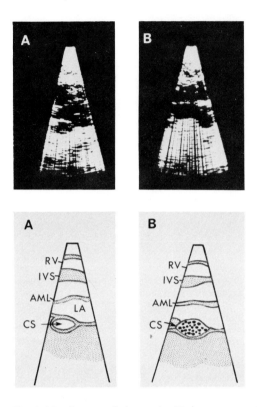

Fig. 6–17. Parasternal, long-axis, 30-degree scans of the coronary sinus (CS) from a patient with persistent left superior vena cava. *A,* The dilated coronary sinus is indicated. *B,* Indocyanine green (Cardio-green) dye has been injected into the left basilic vein and courses into the right atrium through the dilated coronary sinus, which becomes opaque. RV = right ventricle; IVS = interventricular septum; AML = anterior mitral leaflet; LA = left atrium.

been characterized echocardiographically.[33] These include (1) persistent left superior vena cava with drainage into the coronary sinus, (2) total anomalous pulmonary venous return with coronary sinus drainage, and (3) coronary AV fistula with drainage into the coronary sinus. Persistent left superior vena cava is a fairly common congenital anomaly that is found in 0.5%[35,36] of normal patients and in from 3 to 10% of patients with congenital heart disease.[34] This diagnosis is suspected whenever the coronary sinus is dilated and can be confirmed by injection of echocardiographic contrast into the left basilic vein. When injected into the left arm, con-

trast should flow through the persistent left superior vena cava into the coronary sinus, thereby opacifying this dilated chamber.

Figure 6–17 is an example of a patient with a persistent left superior vena cava recorded prior to and after contrast injection. In the left-hand panel, the dilated echo-free coronary sinus is illustrated at the base of the atrioventricular ring. Following contrast injection into the left arm, this entire area is opacified, thereby confirming this diagnosis. Contrast injected into the right basilic vein conversely flows normally through the right superior vena cava into the right atrium. The coronary sinus remains echo-free. When the persistent left superior vena cava communicates with the left atrium rather than with the coronary sinus, this chamber is opacified following left-arm injection.[37]

Coronary sinus dilatation due to total anomalous pulmonary venous connection is detected by the associated presence of a right ventricular volume overload pattern, an atrial septal defect with a mandatory right-to-left shunt, and the demonstration of a common venous chamber behind the left atrium. Contrast injection in either the right or the left basilic vein results in total opacification of both the left and right sides of the heart, and the contrast fails to enter the dilated coronary sinus.

A coronary AV fistula with drainage into the coronary sinus produces a high-pressure shunt and, in addition to coronary sinus dilatation, should be associated with obvious dilatation of the coronary artery involved.

REFERENCES

1. Hurst, JW: The Heart. New York, McGraw-Hill, 1974.
2. Gray, H: Gray's Anatomy. Edited by CM Goss. Philadelphia, Lea & Febiger, 1959.
3. Schabelman, SE, et al.: Comparison of four two-dimensional echocardiographic views for measuring left atrial size. Am J Cardiol, 41:391, 1978.
4. Tajik, AJ, et al.: Two-dimensional real-time ultrasonic imaging of the heart and great vessels.

Technique, image orientation, structure identification and evaluation. Mayo Clin Proc, 53:281, 1978.

5. Bierman, FZ, and Williams, RG: Subxiphoid two-dimensional imaging of the atrial septum. Am J Cardiol, 41:354, 1978.

6. Lange, LW, Sahn, DJ, Allen, HD, and Goldberg, SJ: Subxiphoid cross-sectional echocardiography in infants and children with congenital heart disease. Circulation, 59:513, 1979.

7. Sahn, DJ, DeMaria, A, Kisslo, J, and Weyman, AE: Recommendations regarding quantitation in M-mode echocardiography: results of a survey of echocardiographic measurements. Circulation, 58:1072, 1978.

8. Feigenbaum, H: Echocardiography. 2nd ed., Philadelphia, Lea & Febiger, 1976.

9. Hirata, T, et al.: Estimation of left atrial size using ultrasound. Am Heart J, 78:43, 1969.

10. Lundstrom, NR, and Mortensson, W: Clinical applications of echocardiography in infants and children. II. Acta Paediatr Scand, 63:33, 1974.

11. Yabeb, SM, et al.: Echocardiographic determination of left atrial volumes in children with congenital heart disease. Circulation, 53:268, 1976.

12. tenCate, FJ, et al.: Dimensions and volumes of left atrium and ventricle determined by single beam echocardiography. Br Heart J, 36:737, 1974.

13. Murray, JA, Kennedy, JW, and Figley, MM: Quantitative angiocardiography. II. The normal left atrial volume in man. Circulation, 37:800, 1968.

14. Silverman, NH, Lewis, AB, Heymann, MA, and Rudolph, AM: Echocardiographic assessment of ductus arteriosus in premature infants. Circulation, 50:821, 1974.

15. Baylen, B, Meyer, RA, and Kaplan, S: Echocardiographic assessment of patent ductus arteriosus in prematures with respiratory distress. Circulation (Suppl. III), 50:16, 1974. (Abstract)

16. Goldberg, SJ, et al.: A prospective 2½ year experience wtih echocardiographic evaluation of prematures with patent ductus arteriosus (PDA) and respiratory distress syndrome (RDS). Am J Cardiol, 35:139, 1975. (Abstract)

17. Carter, WH, and Bowman, CR: Estimation of shunt flow in isolated ventricular septal defect by echocardiogram. Circulation (Suppl IV), 48:64, 1973. (Abstract)

18. Brown, OR, Harrison, DC, and Popp, RL: An improved method for echographic detection of left atrial enlargement. Circulation, 50:58, 1974.

19. Bierman, FZ, and Williams, RG: Subxiphoid two-dimensional echocardiographic diagnosis of total anomalous pulmonary venous return in infants. Am J Cardiol, 43:401, 1979. (Abstract)

20. Nasser, WK, et al.: Atrial myxoma. I: Clinical and pathologic features in nine cases. Am Heart J, 83:694, 1972.

21. Greenwood, WF: Profile of atrial myxoma. Am J Cardiol, 21:367, 1968.

22. Rogers, EW, Weyman, AE, Noble, RJ, and Bruins, SG: Left atrial myxoma infected with histoplasma capsulatum. Am J Med, 64:683, 1978.

23. Yoshikawa, J, et al.: Cross-sectional echocardiographic diagnosis of large left atrial tumor and extracardiac tumor compressing the left atrium. Am J Cardiol, 42:853, 1978.

24. Mikell, FL, et al.: Two-dimensional echocardiographic demonstration of left atrial thrombi in patients with prosthetic mitral valves. Circulation, 60(5):1183, 1979.

25. Bramlet, DA, and Edwards, JE: Congenital aneurysm of left atrial appendage. Br Heart J, 45:97, 1980.

26. Lucas, RV, et al.: Congenital causes of pulmonary venous obstruction. Pediatr Clin North Am, 10:781, 1963.

27. Niwayama, G: Cor triatriatum. Am Heart J, 59:291, 1960.

28. Snider, AR, Roge, CH, Schiller, NB, and Silverman, NH: Congenital left ventricular inflow obstruction evaluated by two-dimensional echocardiography. Circulation, 61:848, 1980.

29. Breitweser, JA, and Meyer, RA: Use of echocardiography to evaluate structure and function in congenital heart disease. In Progress in Cardiology. Edited by PN Yu and JN Goodwin. Philadelphia, Lea & Febiger, 1979.

30. Sahn, DJ, Allen, HD, Lange, LW, and Goldberg, SJ: Cross-sectional echocardiographic diagnosis of the sites of total anomalous pulmonary venous drainage. Circulation, 60:1317, 1979.

31. Perloff, JN: The clinical recognition of congenital heart disease. Philadelphia, Saunders, 1970.

32. Danilowicz, D, and Kronzon, I: Use of contrast echocardiography in the diagnosis of partial anomalous pulmonary venous connection. Am J Cardiol, 43:248, 1979.

33. Snider, AR, Ports, TA, and Silverman, NH: Venous anomalies of the coronary sinus: detection by M-mode, two dimensional and contrast echocardiography. Circulation, 60:721, 1979.

34. Mantini, E, Grondin, CM, Lillehei, CW, and Edwards, JE: Congenital anomalies involving the coronary sinus. Circulation, 33:317, 1966.

35. Fraser, RS, Dvorkin, J, Rossall, RE, and Eidem, R: Left superior vena cava: A review of associated congenital heart lesions. catheterization data and roentgenologic findings. Am J Med, 31:711, 1961.

36. Cha, EM, and Khoury, GH: Persistent left superior vena cava. Radiology, 103:375, 1972.

37. Foale, RA, Bourdillon, PD, Somerville, J, and Rickards, AF: Cross-sectional echocardiographic features of anomalous systemic and coronary venous return. Am J Cardiol, 43:385, 1979. (Abstract)

Chapter 7

Left Ventricular Outflow Tract

The left ventricular outflow tract can be considered to extend from the free edges of the mitral leaflets to the aortic bifurcation. It can be conveniently divided at the aortic valve into three primary segments: (1) the aortic valve and supporting structures, (2) the cylindric aorta, and (3) the funnel-shaped subvalvular region. The outflow tract courses in a wide arc through the thorax and abdomen. It begins within the left ventricular cavity in the midportion of the left chest and sweeps cephalad toward the neck. It then arcs posteriorly and caudad passing behind the posterior border of the left pulmonary artery and left ventricle before penetrating the diaphragm and continuing along the midline of the abdomen.[1] Such an extensive area obviously cannot be examined from a single transducer location, and as a result, the outflow tract must be imaged from a number of different vantage points to determine its overall integrity.

The precise methods for examining the individual segments of the outflow tract are discussed in the appropriate section. In general, however, the subvalvular portion, which lies within the left ventricular cavity, is examined from a low parasternal transducer location; the supravalvular region and ascending aorta are examined from a slightly higher precordial location; and the transverse aortic arch (with the contiguous portions of the ascending and descending aorta) are viewed from the suprasternal notch. The descending thoracic aorta is frequently observed passing behind the left atrium or left ventricle, whereas the abdominal aorta from the diaphragm to the bifurcation can readily be recorded from the anterior abdominal wall. Despite these multiple areas of access, a small portion of the ascending aorta and a more extensive area of the descending thoracic aorta from the level of the left pulmonary artery to the diaphragm remain difficult to visualize. Fortunately, isolated lesions in these areas are rare, and with these exceptions, the outflow tract can be examined with relative ease in the majority of patients.[2,3]

Because the left ventricular outflow tract is a cylindric or tubular structure, it is optimally recorded with the scan plane aligned parallel to its long axis (see Chap. 3). This alignment permits the diameter of

212

the vessel within the entire scan area to be visualized and local areas of narrowing or dilatation to be appreciated. Scans across the short axis of the outflow tract can be obtained at multiple levels; however, with the exception of the aortic valve and root and the proximal inflow region, these views have not added significant additional information.

THE AORTIC VALVE

Normal Anatomy

The aortic valve is both clinically and echocardiographically the most important single component of the left ventricular outflow tract. Anatomically, the aortic valve is composed of three symmetric, semilunar or pie-shaped cusps. These cusps are designed to permit free egress of blood from the left ventricle during systole and to prevent backflow during diastole. The tricuspid configuration is theoretically optimal because two cusps of equal size can close tightly but cannot open completely without considerable elastic stretch. Four or more cusps, in contrast, could open fully but would lack sufficient basal support relative to the leaflet area to maintain diastolic competence. Three cusps can open to the full dimensions of the valve ring and still produce a perfect seal when closed.[4]

The aortic cusps attach at their base to a fibrous ring, the aortic annulus. Three outpouchings of the aortic wall, the sinuses of Valsalva, are positioned behind the aortic cusps when the valve is opened. The right coronary artery arises from the sinus that is positioned to the right and anteriorly, whereas the left coronary artery arises from the left posterior sinus. The third sinus, positioned to the right and posteriorly, does not give rise to a coronary artery and is therefore termed the noncoronary sinus. The aortic leaflets take their names from the sinuses with which they are associated and, thus, are termed the right, left, and noncoronary leaflets. The sinuses are anatomically configured such that, in addition to giving rise to the coronary arteries, they also protect the coronary ostia. During systole, the open aortic leaflets, which lie in front of the coronary ostia, shield the ostia from the main force of the ejected blood. The separation of the leaflets from the ostia provided by the sinuses also prevents coronary occlusion because if a leaflet were to come into direct contract with the coronary orifice, it would shut off flow from the aorta. The coronary pressure would then fall rapidly as blood left the distal coronary arterial system, and the leaflet would be held against the orifice by the high differential pressure. This catastrophe is presumably prevented by the presence of adequate space behind the open valve cusps.[4]

Examining Planes

The aortic valve is examined echocardiographically in two primary imaging planes: (1) the parasternal long axis and (2) the parasternal short axis at the aortic valve level. The valve can likewise be recorded in the apical five-chamber view, which is orthogonal to the long- and short-axis planes, and in both a long- and short-axis projection from the subcostal transducer location.[5-8]

In the parasternal long-axis view, the imaging plane transects the aortic valve in an anteroposterior direction, and its Y axis is aligned parallel to the long axis of the aorta. Because the aorta is normally to the right of the transducer when it is in the parasternal location, the long-axis plane is usually angled such that it passes through the right and noncoronary aortic leaflets.

Figure 7–1 is an example of a normal aortic valve recorded in the parasternal long-axis view. During diastole (A), a thin linear echo is recorded in the midportion of the aortic root. This echo is produced by the coapted free edges of the aortic cusps, which are oriented perpendicular

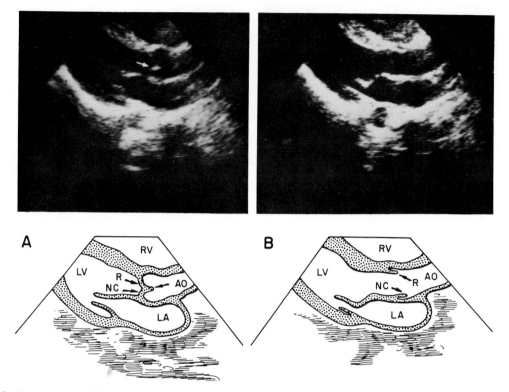

Fig. 7–1. Parasternal long-axis recording of a normal aortic valve. The positions of the right (R) and noncoronary (NC) aortic leaflets during diastole (A) and systole (B) are illustrated. The single linear echo arising from the coapted aortic leaflets is indicated by the horizontal arrow (A). RV = right ventricle; LV = left ventricle; AO = aorta; LA = left atrium.

to the path of the imaging plane. The bodies of the thin, smooth leaflets, in contrast, are oriented parallel to the imaging plane and, thus, are less well visualized. In B, recorded during systole, the leaflet echoes are separated and lie in close apposition to the walls of the aorta. The right coronary leaflet is anterior, and the noncoronary leaflet is posterior. At peak systolic opening, the aortic cusps normally parallel the inner margins of the aortic annulus.

The parasternal short-axis view of the aortic valve is recorded with the imaging plane aligned parallel to the short axis of the aortic root at or just superior to the level of the aortic annulus. Ideally, the commissures separating the three aortic leaflets should be visualized during diastole, and the open aortic leaflets should be seen during systole. In routine clinical studies, however, the aortic commissures

can be clearly visualized in only about 73% of cases.[3]

Figure 7–2 illustrates the normal short-axis appearance of a tricuspid aortic valve during diastole (A) and systole (B). In the diastolic recording, the three aortic commissures are evident and outline the position of the aortic leaflets. The right coronary leaflet (R) is positioned anterior and leftward, the left coronary leaflet (L) is to the right and posterior, and the noncoronary leaflet is to the left and posterior.* This normal short-axis configuration of the tricuspid aortic valve has been likened to the Mercedes-Benz emblem lying on its side. Panel B illustrates the systolic con-

---

*Because the leaflets are displayed as if viewed from below their right-left orientation in the image is the opposite of their anatomic orientation, i.e., the right coronary leaflet, which is positioned to the patient's right, appears on the left side of the recorded image and thus to the viewer's left.

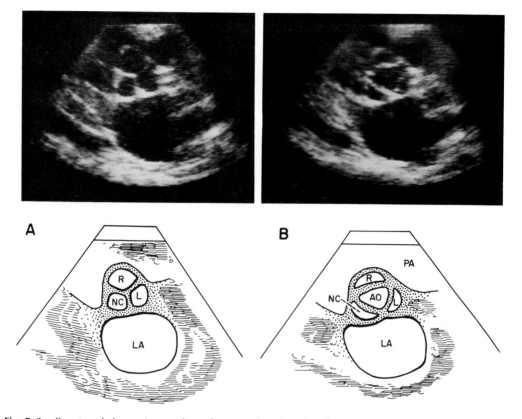

Fig. 7–2. Parasternal short-axis recording of a normal aortic valve during diastole (*A*) and systole (*B*). During systole, the commissures of the trileaflet valve outline the positions of the right (R), noncoronary (NC), and left (L) coronary leaflets. During systole, the leaflets separate widely producing an orifice that appears as a triangle with curved sides. LA = left atrium; PA = pulmonary artery.

figuration of the aortic leaflets and their relationship to the semicircular sinuses of Valsalva. In this example, the aortic orifice appears as a triangle with curved sides.

The short-axis view is ideal for recording the aortic orifice and for defining the location of focal aortic valve abnormalities. It is also useful for evaluating disorders of the aortic root, such as sinus of Valsalva aneurysms and aortic root dissection. When recording this view, remember that the aortic root normally moves in a superior-inferior direction with cardiac contraction and relaxation. At the onset of ventricular systole, the aortic root is in its most superior position. As the ventricle contracts, the aortic root and valve are drawn in an apical or inferior direction. Consequently, a stationary imaging

plane records a more superior portion of the aortic valve at end-systole than at end-diastole. This motion of the valve through the imaging plane creates particular problems when trying to visualize the valve orifice in valvular aortic stenosis because the position of the orifice continuously shifts relative to the examining plane.

In the apical five-chamber view, the imaging plane is oriented such that it passes through the open aortic valve from the point of basal attachment to the leaflet tips. The five-chamber view is more difficult to obtain than are the parasternal views and has limited clinical applicability. It may be useful, however, in demonstrating the domed, stenotic valve of congenital aortic stenosis or the presence of subvalvular membranes. In these instances, the lesions are placed perpendicular to the path of the imaging plane, and their visualization may be facilitated.

Relationship of Aortic Leaflet Motion to Cardiac Output and Transvalvular Flow Patterns

Normal aortic leaflet motion depends on both the volume and the character of flow through the aortic valve. A marked reduction in forward cardiac output may decrease both the rate and the amplitude of aortic leaflet opening. Such a reduction may also result in valve closure beginning prior to the end of mechanical systole.[9,10] A decrease in amplitude of aortic leaflet motion is associated with a corresponding decrease in systolic aortic valve area. When valve closure begins prior to the end of systole, a further decrease in valve area may be noted. Figure 7–3 is a short-axis aortic valve recording from a patient with congestive cardiomyopathy and illustrates the reduced aortic valve opening that can occur in low flow states. In any measurement of aortic valve area, therefore, one must remember that reduced flow through

the valve may reduce the valve area independent of any leaflet disorder or may exaggerate the anatomic decrease in valve area in patients with aortic stenosis.

Obstructive lesions located beneath the valve also characteristically affect aortic leaflet motion by changing either the character or the cross-sectional area of the stream of blood passing through the valve orifice. Turbulent flow typically induces high-frequency vibrations in the poorly supported leaflets, whereas a transient reduction in systolic outflow or a decrease in the cross-sectional area of the flow jet may cause the leaflets to move toward a closed position prior to end-systole. Thus, in a discrete subaortic stenosis, initial leaflet opening is typically normal, i.e., to the margins of the aortic annulus. Once flow is established, however, the reduced cross-sectional area of the flow stream caused by the subvalvular lesion results in diminished leaflet separation as the leaflets fall back to parallel the margins of the flow jet.[11,12] In idiopathic hypertrophic subaortic stenosis, the midsystolic decrease in forward cardiac output caused by the functional subvalvular obstruction pro-

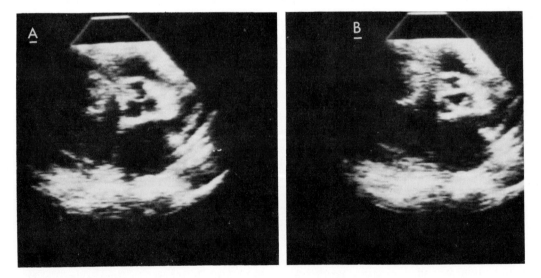

Fig. 7–3. Parasternal short-axis recording of the aortic valve illustrates the effects of reduced cardiac output on the systolic aortic valve orifice configuration. *A*, During diastole, the normal trileaflet aortic configuration is evident. *B*, During systole, there is a reduction in leaflet separation and a corresponding decrease in aortic valve orifice area at peak opening.

duces a corresponding midsystolic closing movement of the aortic leaflets with subsequent reopening when forward flow is re-established at end-systole.[13,14] Although these abnormalities of aortic leaflet motion are best demonstrated with an M-mode recording, they can clearly be seen during the cross-sectional study, and their presence frequently draws attention to the subvalvular lesion.

The Abnormal Aortic Valve Echogram

Aortic valve disorders can be separated echocardiographically into those that (1) restrict aortic valve opening and thus inhibit systolic outflow, (2) prevent normal diastolic leaflet coaptation, or (3) are characterized by structural changes in the aortic valve or root but are not uniformly associated with stenosis or insufficiency.

Valvular Aortic Stenosis

Valvular aortic stenosis is the most common cause of left ventricular outflow obstruction.[15] It may be acquired or congenital. Acquired valvular aortic stenosis is usually a result of rheumatic endocarditis, which causes adhesion of the leaflet commissures and leaflet thickening and/or retraction. The severity of the valvular stenosis depends on the number of commissures that are adherent. When only one commissure is involved, the normal tricuspid aortic valve is converted to a bicuspid valve with little resulting obstruction. When two or more commissures are fused, the degree of valve opening lessens progressively, and the leaflets likewise tend to be more deformed and thickened. Secondary calcification is common and further restricts leaflet motion and distorts the valve orifice.[16]

Congenital aortic stenosis is characterized by a dome-like deformity of the valve with a perforation at the apex similar to that seen with congenital pulmonary stenosis. The congenitally stenotic valve may have a single cusp and commissure (uni-commissural unicuspid aortic stenosis) or, more commonly, may be bicuspid with two distinct leaflets and commissures. The congenitally stenotic aortic valve also tends to calcify with advancing age. When calcification occurs, mobility of the valve is limited, and severity of stenosis may increase. When calcification is severe, the differentiation of a congenitally deformed valve from acquired stenosis may be difficult.[16]

Congenital, rather than acquired, abnormalities of leaflet structure appear to underlie the majority of cases of adult calcific aortic stenosis. In one series of 105 patients with isolated aortic stenosis, for example, 51% had bicuspid, 31% tricuspid, and 12% unicuspid valves.[17] This combined predominance of bicuspid and unicuspid valves, which can be presumed to represent congenital deformities, underscores the significance of these lesions in the late development of clinically important aortic stenosis.

Aortic stenosis is defined echocardiographically as any abnormality of the aortic valve in which the leaflets physically encroach on the lumen of the outflow tract. Stenotic valves are divided echocardiographically, as they are anatomically, into the more densely fibrotic, calcified valve usually seen in the adult and the pliable, domed, congenitally stenotic valve of the child. There is, however, no precise age at which this transition occurs and it is not uncommon to see a freely doming stenotic valve into the fourth decade and beyond.

Adult Calcific Aortic Stenosis

The calcified, stenotic aortic valve of the adult is characterized by an increase in echo production from the thickened, deformed valve cusps, by decreased mobility of the leaflets, and by an absolute decrease in maximal leaflet separation and/or orifice size.[6,18,19]

Normally, the thin, smooth aortic cusps

are poorly visualized during diastole in the parasternal views because they are aligned parallel to the path of the scan plane. When the leaflets become fibrotic or calcified, the cusp tissue becomes increasingly reflective, and leaflet visualization improves. When fibrosis or calcification is severe, the leaflets may be more highly reflective than surrounding structures and may stand out in sharp contrast to the less dominant background.

Calcification typically begins at the base of the involved leaflet(s) and progresses toward the free edge(s). The right coronary cusp appears by far the most commonly affected. Commissural fusion, likewise, is most frequently noted between the right and noncoronary leaflets. The left coronary cusp, in contrast, shows the least tendency for deformity and calcification.

Systolic leaflet motion is characteristically reduced. In contrast to the normal full excursion of the leaflets to the margins of the aortic annulus, all or a portion of the leaflet(s) become fixed, thereby limiting motion. This may involve only a portion of one leaflet or may progress to a point where the entire valve is fixed and immobile. The pattern of leaflet fixation follows that of calcification and fibrosis—beginning at the base of the involved leaflet and progressing toward the free edge. It is not uncommon to see a leaflet whose base is fixed and calcified, although the free edge remains thin and mobile.

The restricted motion reduces the absolute separation between the leaflets and thereby narrows the aortic orifice. Although the maximum leaflet separation may vary depending on the portion of the valve examined, peak separation has been shown to be roughly related to severity of stenosis.[6,18,19] Figure 7–4 illustrates the long- and short-axis appearance of a severely stenotic aortic valve.

Detection. The echocardiographic detection of valvular aortic stenosis has been excellent, with success rates of 100% being reported in two large series.[18,19] In each of these studies, however, normal persons were compared with patients with hemodynamically significant valvular aortic stenosis. Because the valve orifice must be decreased by roughly 75% before a significant gradient develops, major anatomic deformity must have been present in the majority of the aortic stenosis group, and this sensitivity is therefore not unexpected.[20] The overall sensitivity of the echogram in detecting lesser degrees of anatomic deformity has not been determined. Many patients are examined in whom there is basal thickening and decreased motion of one or more leaflets, but also in whom the decrease in orifice area is less than critical. Although a systolic ejection murmur typically prompts the clinical examination, these patients are generally not surgical candidates, and confirmation of the limitation in orifice area has not been obtained to date. Despite this lack of surgical or postmortem confirmation, the uniform association of leaflet thickening and decreased motion with significant valvular aortic stenosis and its absence in normal persons suggests that the echogram is a sensitive method for visualizing leaflet deformity of lesser degrees than can be detected hemodynamically. Although these valves do not impose a hemodynamic burden on the left ventricle, their detection is clinically important, because they place the patient at risk for the development of more severe stenosis as well as for other complications, such as bacterial endocarditis.

Estimation of the severity. Two methods have been described for estimating the severity of aortic stenosis directly from the cross-sectional echogram. These include (1) measurement of the maximum, long-axis, aortic cusp separation (MACS) and (2) direct short-axis measurement of the aortic valve area. In addition, qualitative information is frequently available from the short-axis evaluation of leaflet motion (even when the orifice itself cannot be fully recorded). Such information permits either

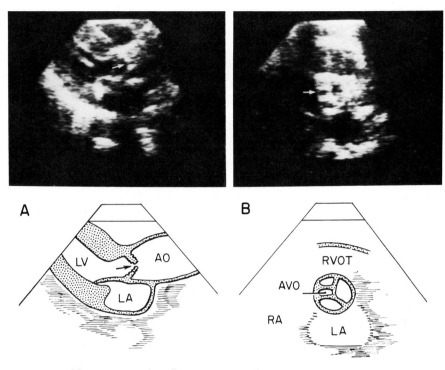

Fig. 7–4. *A,* Parasternal long-axis recording illustrates severe valvular aortic stenosis. The valve leaflets are more highly reflective than normal and dome slightly during systolic opening. Leaflet separation at the valve orifice is reduced (horizontal arrow). There is concentric hypertrophy of the left ventricle (LV). *B,* Parasternal short-axis recording illustrates the decreased aortic valve orifice area with cusp separation occurring only in the commissure between the right and noncoronary leaflets. The horizontal arrow points to the valve orifice (AVO). AO = aorta; RVOT = right ventricular outflow tract; RA = right atrium; LA = left atrium.

direct estimation of severity or modification of the data derived from the MACS measurement. Indirect estimation of the peak systolic aortic valve gradient can also be derived from the left ventricular systolic wall thickness and cavity dimension using the constant wall-stress hypothesis.

Maximal aortic cusp separation. The initial method for estimating severity of aortic stenosis was based on an observed relationship between the degree of restriction of aortic leaflet motion (maximal aortic cusp separation) and the hemodynamic severity of the stenotic lesion.[6,18,19]

The maximal aortic cusp separation (MACS) is determined by sweeping the scan plane across the valve from the medial to the lateral walls of the aorta until the region of maximal leaflet excursion is recorded. This maneuver must be repeated until all areas of the valve are clearly vis-

ualized because the point of maximal leaflet separation may be eccentrically positioned and more difficult to record than areas of the valve that are more severely deformed. Once the area of maximal excursion is visualized, the cusp separation is measured from the inner margins of the anterior to the inner margins of the posterior cusp echo. The measurement of maximal cusp separation is illustrated in Figure 7–10.

The MACS clearly separates normal persons from patients with critical aortic stenosis.[6,18,19] Likewise, as indicated in Table 7–1, the group means for patients with mild, moderate, and severe aortic stenosis differ significantly. Unfortunately, because of the large overlap between groups, the MACS shows little direct correlation with aortic valve area or peak systolic aortic valve gradient in patients with calcified

TABLE 7–1

RELATIONSHIP OF MAXIMAL AORTIC
LEAFLET SEPARATION TO SEVERITY OF
AORTIC STENOSIS IN ADULTS

Aortic Valve Area	MACS	
	Mean (mm)	Range (mm)
Normal persons	19.4[18] 20.5[6]	15–26
Mild (AVA > 1 cm²)	14.9	9–20
Moderate (AVA 1–0.75 cm²)	9.9	4–15
Noncritical (AVA > 0.75 cm²)	10.0	3–15
Severe (AVA < 0.75 cm²)	4.5[18] 6.4[19]	0–11

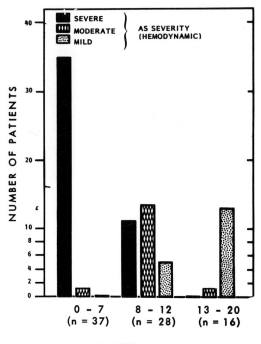

Fig. 7–5. Relationship of the maximum aortic cusp separation (in millimeters) to severity of aortic stenosis in a group of 81 patients. (From Godley, RW, et al.: Reliability of two-dimensional echocardiography in assessing the severity of valvular aortic stenosis. Chest, 79:657, 1981.)

valves.[18] The measurement does, however, identify certain subgroups at increased risk of having a critical lesion and permits exclusion of a critical lesion in others. Thus, in combined series, all patients with critical aortic stenosis (aortic valve area [AVA] of 0.75 cm² or less) have had an MACS of 11 mm or less.[6,18,19] An MACS of greater than 11 mm, therefore, would appear to exclude a critical lesion. Slightly larger leaflet separations (≥ 13 mm) have, with one exception, been associated with mild lesions (AVA of 1.0 cm² or greater), and this value, therefore, has a greater than 96% predictive accuracy for mild stenosis.[19]

In contrast, all patients with an MACS of 2 mm or less have had critical lesions, as have the large majority of those with an MACS of less than 8 mm.[6,18,19] In one series, an MACS of less than 8 mm was found to be predictive of critical aortic stenosis in 97%[19] of cases, whereas in another, an MACS of 8 mm or less was predictive of a critical lesion in 82%.[18] Importantly, 84 of 87 reported cases with an MACS of 8 mm or less have had an aortic valve area of 1 cm² or less. Likewise, 60 of 61 cases with an MACS of 12 mm or less have had an aortic valve area of 1.25 cm² or less. Figure 7–5 illustrates the relationship of

MACS to severity in a group of 81 patients with aortic stenosis.

Unfortunately, as Figure 7–5 demonstrates, the MACS value falls between 8 and 12 mm in a large number of patients. This group represents between 26 and 44% of study patients, and in these instances, discrimination between mild, moderate, and severe or critical and noncritical lesions is extremely difficult.[6,18] When the MACS is in this range, the use of some of the principles for qualitative short-axis evaluation of leaflet excursion discussed later may prove helpful. In many instances, however, quantitation beyond the fact that the lesion is hemodynamically significant may not be possible.

When evaluating these data, remember that the hemodynamic separation between a severe and mild lesion may be as little as 0.25 cm². These correlations further presume that the hemodynamic estimates are accurate at this level of discrimination. Because the MACS measurement is fundamentally limited in that it must assume that leaflet separation in one plane is representative of valve area (which, in the case of the deformed calcified valve, may be irregular), any better correlation within this narrow range is unlikely. The echocardiographic assessment of severity of aortic stenosis based on the MACS measurement, therefore, cannot be considered a substitute for cardiac catheterization. This measurement does, however, appear to represent a noninvasive method for identifying patients with anatomic evidence of valvular aortic stenosis whose leaflet separation places them at high risk of having a critical lesion. Further, it should exclude from catheterization patients whose leaflet separation indicates only a mild lesion.

This measurement is further limited because it must presume that the leaflets separate maximally during systole. When the forward cardiac output is low, the leaflets may not separate maximally, and the MACS may be inappropriately reduced.

Direct aortic valve area measurement. The direct determination of mitral valve orifice size has proved to be one of the most accurate and reliable quantitative measurements in clinical cross-sectional echocardiography (see Chap. 5). Visualization and measurement of the aortic valve orifice, in contrast, have proved far more difficult for a variety of reasons.[6,18,19] First, in the adult with calcific aortic stenosis, the valve orifice tends to be smaller, more irregular, and more densely calcified than that of the stenotic mitral valve. Second, the aortic valve moves more rapidly through the scan plane than does the mitral valve, thereby making localization of the true orifice more difficult. Finally, the range in valve areas from a mild to a severely stenotic aortic valve is small, and as a result, variations between the echocardiographic and hemodynamic measurements that are acceptable in mitral ste-

nosis have proved unacceptable with aortic lesions.

Reported success rates for direct recording of the aortic valve orifice have varied from 13%[19] to greater than 85%,[21] with the majority of clinical experience favoring the lower figure.[18,19] In patients in whom a well-defined orifice can be recorded, however, there does appear to be a reasonable correlation between the echocardiographic and hemodynamic estimate of orifice area. Figure 7–6 illustrates this relationship for a group of eight patients. Unfortunately, these 8 patients represent the only instances from a total group of 81 consecutive patients referred for cardiac catheterization for suspected aortic stenosis in whom a measurable aortic orifice could be recorded. Thus, although the clinical value of direct aortic valve area measurement would be enormous, visualization of the aortic valve orifice cannot, at present, be achieved in a large enough percentage of patients to play a major clinical role.

Qualitative assessment of short-axis leaflet motion. Two qualitative patterns of aortic leaflet motion are sufficiently distinctive to permit rapid, visual assessment of severity without the need for measure-

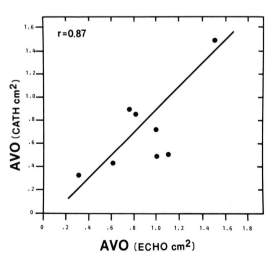

Fig. 7–6. Relationship of directly measured echocardiographic aortic valve orifice to the aortic valve orifice determined at cardiac catheterization.

ment of MACS or aortic orifice area. First, it can be presumed that if any leaflet in either short or long axis opens completely to the margin of the aortic wall, there can be no more than mild stenosis. This presumption applies because full opening of one leaflet of a three-leaflet valve means that the orifice can be reduced by no more than 66%, which is less than the degree of stenosis required for the development of a significant gradient. Secondly, if the valve is severely deformed and there is no observable leaflet motion, the lesion can be considered severe.

In other instances, although not directly reflecting severity, qualitative assessment of the pattern of leaflet motion in short axis can improve the accuracy of the MACS measurement. This is based on the observation that, although the MACS tends to overestimate severity, it rarely underestimates severity. Thus, although an MACS of 11 mm or less correctly identifies the vast majority of patients with critical aortic stenosis, it also includes a significant number of patients (between 21 and 27% of the total group) with mild or moderate lesions.[18,19]

Qualitative evaluation of aortic leaflet motion helps to identify those patients in whom the MACS alone would overestimate severity by identifying the orifice configurations most frequently associated with this overestimation. The most common of these are the *elliptic and the eccentric orifices*, which are illustrated in Figure 7–7. In the instance of the elliptic or fish-mouthed orifice (2), the longest dimension is oriented perpendicular to the path of the scan plane, and the MACS, taken from anterior to the posterior margins of this orifice, would obviously underestimate the true valve area. In the instance of the eccentric orifice (3 and 4), the degree of leaflet separation varies with the commissure between the right and noncoronary leaflets being more completely fused than are those between the right and left and the left and noncoronary

cusps. When viewed in long axis, the more deformed commissure tends to be more highly reflective and is generally predominant. An MACS measurement taken from this commissure, however, would greatly overestimate the true severity of the lesion.

Recognition of these patterns, even when the orifice is not adequately recorded to make a direct area measurement, permits these potential sources of inaccuracy to be identified and the severity to be more appropriately categorized. This is of particular value in patients with an MACS between 8 and 12 mm. In this range, approximately 40% of patients have severe lesions, 40% have moderate lesions, and 20% have mild obstruction. The combination of the short-axis assessment of leaflet motion with long-axis MACS measurement in this group, however, has been demonstrated to improve the predictive accuracy for overall patient separation from 46 to 86%.[19]

Table 7–2 presents an approach to the evaluation of the patient with calcific aortic stenosis. This approach combines both the short- and long-axis assessment of valve orifice size and permits the correct classification of more than 90% of patients with aortic stenosis. One must recognize, however, that this noninvasive assessment still fails to predict accurately the hemodynamic valve area in individual patients.

Indirect estimation of severity based on the constant wall stress hypothesis. The final echocardiographic method for estimating the severity of aortic stenosis is based on the observation that the normal left ventricle hypertrophies in response to a chronic pressure load in a manner that maintains wall stress within a constant narrow range. Using Laplace's relationship, it can be shown that wall stress is directly related to left ventricular systolic pressure and cavity size and inversely related to wall thickness. Peak left ventricular wall stress, therefore, can be approximated by the expression:

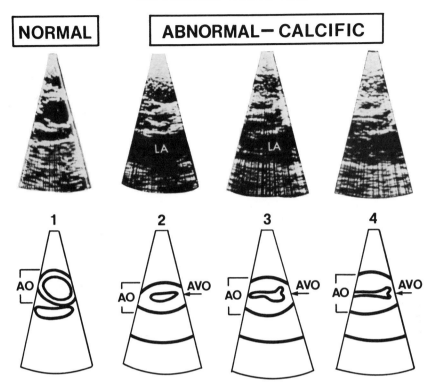

Fig. 7–7. Parasternal short-axis recordings of the aortic valve illustrate the characteristic valve orifice configurations that result in an MACS measurement that overestimates the severity of stenosis. (1) The normal circular valve orifice. Any linear dimension passing through the center of the orifice should show a direct correlation with the valve area. 2, 3, and 4, The orifice either appears elliptic (2) or leaflet separation is uneven with the maximum separation eccentrically positioned (3 and 4). In these cases, an anteroposterior dimension characteristically underestimates the valve area and thereby overestimates the severity of an obstructive lesion. LA = left atrium; AO = aorta; AVO = aortic valve orifice. (From Godley, RW, et al.: Reliability of two-dimensional echocardiography in assessing the severity of valvular aortic stenosis. Chest, 79: 657, 1981.)

$$\text{Wall stress} = \frac{\text{LVIDs} \times \text{LVPs}}{\text{LVWTs}}$$

LVIDs is the left ventricular internal dimension at end-systole, LVPs is the peak systolic intracavitary pressure, and LVWTs is the maximal end-systolic wall thickness. Because, in the absence of left ventricular failure, left ventricular hypertrophy maintains stress at a constant level, a wall stress constant can be calculated and the equation rearranged to:

Left ventricular systolic pressure

$$= \frac{\text{Constant} \times \text{LVWTs}}{\text{LVIDs}}$$

The stress constant has varied in differ-

ent studies. In the majority of studies, however, a numeric value of 225 has been derived. Using this constant:

Left ventricular systolic pressure

$$= \frac{225 \times \text{LVWTs}}{\text{LVIDs}}$$

Once the left ventricular peak systolic pressure is known, the peak pressure gradient across the aortic valve can then be estimated as the difference between the left ventricular systolic pressure and the systolic blood pressure. The systolic blood pressure is determined by a cuff sphygmomanometer. Using this method, a strong correlation has been demonstrated between the echocardiographically determined and the hemodynamically determined aortic valve gradient,[22–27] and the

TABLE 7–2

A SUGGESTED APPROACH TO THE
CROSS-SECTIONAL EXAMINATION OF
THE STENOTIC AORTIC VALVE

1. Long-axis recording to:
   — locate valve
   — detect stenosis
2. If stenotic—determine maximal cusp
   separation
   — < 8 mm   (85% severe aortic ste-
                nosis)
   — 8–12 mm   (40% severe, 40% mod-
                erate, 20% mild)
   — > 12 mm   (95% mild aortic steno-
                sis)
3. Evaluate short-axis aortic valve orifice
   — Measure aortic valve area (AVA)
     when possible
   — If AVA cannot be measured, at-
     tempt to qualitatively assess ori-
     fice geometry
4. Add qualitative orifice evaluation to
   MACS as follows:
   — MACS ≤ 11 mm, 75% will be crit-
     ical ∴
   — Presumed critical unless
     (a) one leaflet opens fully (SAX)—
         lesion mild
     (b) MACS between 8–12 mm and
         orifice elliptic or eccentric;
         MACS overestimates severity
         and lesion likely to be moder-
         ate or less
   — > 90% of remaining cases should
     be severe, and discrimination be-
     yond this point is probably not
     possible.

technique has been reported to be useful
for both the initial and the sequential assessment of aortic stenosis.[25]

This method is inaccurate in patients
with left ventricular failure and chamber
dilatation because, as the ventricle dilates,
wall stress increases, and the assumptions
of the formula are no longer valid. The
validity of the method has also been questioned following valvotomy.[27]

Use of the wall stress hypothesis to predict aortic valve gradient presumes that a
diagnosis of aortic stenosis is already established and that the aortic valve lesion
is the only cause of the increased afterload.
Left ventricular hypertrophy is also presumed to develop as a secondary phenomenon and the method is, therefore, invalid
in patients with hypertrophic or infiltrative myopathies.

From a technical standpoint, the left
ventricular posterior wall must be clearly
recorded because small variations in the
wall thickness measurement cause significant changes in the calculated left ventricular pressure.

Because of the many assumptions and
variables inherent in this method, it is primarily applicable in children in whom
changes in wall thickness are more clearly
related to a single lesion.[23–26] Despite the
positive correlations that have been reported, the frequency of left ventricular
failure, systemic hypertension, and ischemic heart disease in adults makes reliance on this type of indirect predictive
measurement less sound.

Congenital Aortic Stenosis

Congenital valvular aortic stenosis (Fig.
7–8) is characterized by an increase in echo
production from the thickened aortic
cusps, systolic doming of the stenotic
valve, and a decrease in cusp separation
at the valve orifice.[28] The increased reflectivity tends to involve the leaflets symmetrically, but is less intense than that
noted in the calcified valve of the adult.
Reflectivity typically permits the full expanse of the valve cusps to be recorded
during both diastole and systole, whereas
diastolic visualization of the valve cusps
may be difficult in the normal valve. More
importantly, tipping or doming motion of
the leaflets occurs during systolic opening
with loss of their normal parallel orientation as they swing to a fully open position. At peak systolic opening (Fig. 7–8,

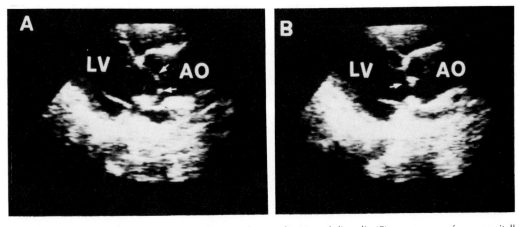

Fig. 7–8. Parasternal long-axis recordings illustrate the systolic (*A*) and diastolic (*B*) appearance of a congenitally stenotic aortic valve. Systolic doming of the valve is indicated by the arrowheads in *A*. During diastole, reflectivity from the coaptation line increases, but the leaflets themselves appear thin and are not highly reflective.

A), one or both leaflets curve inward toward the center of the aortic lumen, producing the characteristic systolic domed pattern of the congenitally stenotic valve.

The diastolic configuration of the congenitally stenotic valve is variable. Leaflet coaptation may be normal or eccentric, or multiple linear echoes may arise from the region of coaptation. On occasion, the leaflets may prolapse into the left ventricular outflow tract (see Fig. 7–13, *D*). Although, as discussed later in this chapter, eccentric coaptation is commonly associated with a bicuspid valve and valvular insufficiency is frequently noted with aortic valve prolapse, there does not appear to be any precise correlation between the long-axis diastolic coaptation pattern and leaflet structure or valvular insufficiency.

Quantitation of severity in congenital valvular stenosis rests primarily on the measurement of maximal aortic cusp separation. In congenitally stenotic valves, the MACS measurement shows a more consistent relationship with valve orifice area (Fig. 7–9) than is noted with the calcified valve of the adult.[28] This improved correlation apparently occurs because the pliable valve orifice naturally assumes a more symmetric or circular shape when fully distended, and the linear measurement of cusp separation, therefore, more closely

approximates a diameter of the circular orifice.

Although the MACS appears to correlate with valve area, some correction is necessary in the child to relate both of these measurements to individual size. In early studies, attempts were made to correct cusp separation for patient size, using body surface area.[28] Such attempts resulted in a consistent underestimation of severity, and the degree of underestimation increased as patient size decreased. Consequently, maximum aortic cusp separation was related to individual size using a constant internal reference. The base of the aorta was chosen as this reference because this region had been previously used as a reference for patient size in both anatomic[29] and echocardiographic studies[30] and could be recorded in the same scan plane as the aortic valve. Because maximal aortic cusp separation appeared to be a reflection of actual valve orifice size, whereas the aortic annulus seemed to represent a potential orifice when the valve was excised, it was possible to express the diameter of the actual orifice (AO-D) as a percentage of the potential orifice or MACS/AO-D.

Figure 7–10 depicts the method of measurement of MACS and AO-D, whereas Figure 7–11 illustrates the relationship of MACS expressed as a percentage of AO-D

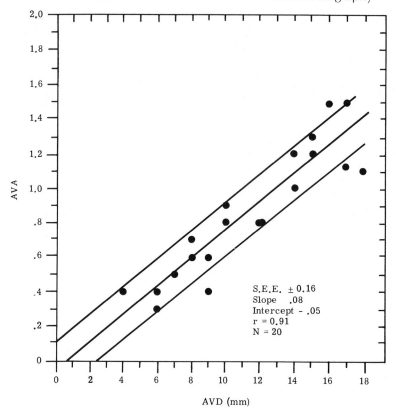

Fig. 7–9. Relationship of the maximum aortic cusp separation (MACS) to aortic valve area for a group of 20 children with congenital valvular aortic stenosis. (From Weyman, AE, et al.: Cross-sectional echocardiographic assessment of the severity of aortic stenosis in children. Circulation, 55:773, 1977. Reproduced by permission of the American Heart Association.)

to severity of stenosis in normal persons and in a group of children with congenital aortic stenosis. In normal persons, MACS represents a high percentage of aortic root diameter (mean 73%). In children with mild stenosis, this percentage decreases to a mean of 53%, whereas in those with more severely stenotic lesions, MACS represents only 30% of AO-D. A direct correlation can also be shown between MACS, expressed as a percentage of AO-D, and both peak systolic aortic valve gradient and calculated aortic valve area.[28] In these correlations, however, there is wide variability between individual points, and it is not possible to predict directly either valve area or peak systolic gradient from the echocardiographic measurement. The cross-sectional method, however, does provide a simple and rapid method for de-

tecting congenital aortic stenosis and for separating patients with mild stenosis from those with more critical lesions.

Bicuspid Aortic Valve

The bicuspid aortic valve is the most common congenital cardiac anomaly and is found in 0.9 to 1.3% of patients in autopsy series.[17,31] Bicuspid valves are clinically important because they may be associated with hemodynamically significant aortic stenosis in the child or may undergo progressive thickening, fibrosis, and, eventually, calcification leading to critical obstruction in later life. In addition, bicuspid valves are frequently insufficient, are a common site of infection in

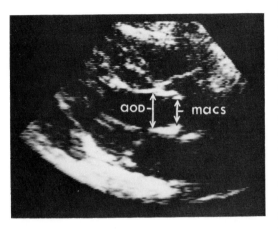

Fig. 7–10. Parasternal long-axis recording of a congenitally stenotic aortic valve illustrates the method of measurement of the maximum aortic cusp separation (MACS) and aortic diameter (AO-D). The MACS is taken from the inner margins of the echoes of the anterior and posterior borders of the aortic orifice, whereas the AO-D is taken at the level of the aortic annulus.

bacterial endocarditis, and may be associated with a variety of other congenital disorders of the heart.[17]

Anatomically, bicuspid valves have two primary orientations. In approximately 50% of cases, one cusp is positioned anteriorly and the second is positioned posteriorly. The commissures are to the right and left, respectively. In this configuration, both coronary arteries arise in front of the anterior cusp. A raphe, present in roughly one half of these cases, is always located in the anterior cusp. Alternatively, the cusps may be positioned to the right and left, and the two commissures may have an anteroposterior orientation. In this configuration, the right coronary artery arises from behind the right cusp and the left coronary artery from behind the left. A raphe is also present in approximately 50% of valves with this orientation and is always situated in the right cusp.[17]

The percentage of bicuspid valves that becomes stenotic or insufficient and the mechanism by which this occurs are unknown.[17] Theoretically, in the absence of leaflet redundancy, the straight line distance between the points of lateral attachment of a bicuspid valve would be the same as the length of the free edges of the leaflets, and the valve should be inherently stenotic. It has been suggested pathologically, however, that, although bicuspid valves are frequently stenotic, sufficient redundancy exists in many instances to permit the normal opening of the bicuspid valve.[17,32]

Insufficiency of a bicuspid valve may develop for several reasons. The redundancy of the valve leaflets required to permit systolic opening may result in diastolic leaflet prolapse. Although the exact incidence of prolapse of one or both leaflets of a bicuspid valve is not known, it is clearly not uncommon. Another cause of valvular insufficiency is leaflet damage due to bacterial endocarditis. The incidence of bicuspid valves in patients dying of acute aortic endocarditis ranges from 9 to 31%,[33–36] whereas in patients with bicuspid valves and pure aortic regurgitation, the valvular incompetence in as many as 73% of the patients may be due to infective endocarditis.[17] In addition, valvular insufficiency may develop as a result of degeneration of the leaflets caused by the effects of aging and the continued stress of improper closure or superimposed rheumatic disease.[17]

The echocardiographic diagnosis of a bicuspid aortic valve is based on the demonstration of two cusps and two commissures during direct short-axis recording. Additional short-axis features that support this diagnosis include leaflet redundancy and infolding and eccentric valve closure. In long axis, an abnormal or eccentric coaptation line may also be apparent with systolic leaflet doming and an abnormal pattern of systolic opening.[37,38]

The characteristic two-leaflet, two-commissure pattern of the bicuspid aortic valve is illustrated in Figures 7–12 and 7–13. In Figure 7–12, the two commissures are positioned to the right and left. The leaflets, therefore, have an anterior and posterior

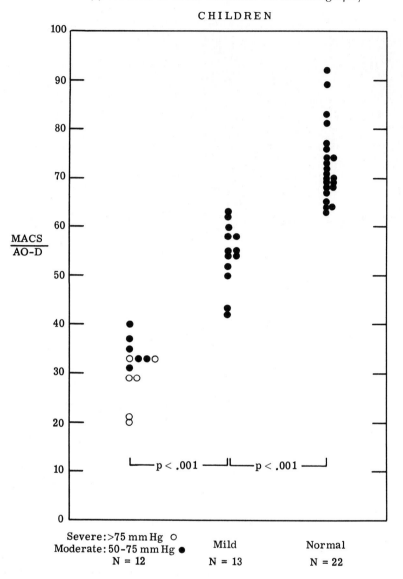

Fig. 7–11. Relationship of the maximum aortic cusp separation (MACS), expressed as a percentage of the aortic root diameter (AO-D), to severity of aortic stenosis in children. (From Weyman, AE, et al.: Cross-sectional echocardiographic assessment of the severity of aortic stenosis in children. Circulation, *55:*773, 1977. Reproduced by permission of the American Heart Association.)

orientation. During diastole (*A*), a single linear echo arises from the coaptation line between the two leaflets, which divides the aortic root horizontally. The anterior leaflet in this example is larger than the posterior leaflet, and both the left and the right coronary arteries arise from behind this anterior cusp. Figure 7–13, *A*, illustrates a bicuspid valve with a vertically

oriented line of coaptation and a prominent raphe in the right-sided cusp. As the leaflets begin to separate, marked redundancy is evident (Fig. 7–13, *B*), and the fully open systolic leaflet configuration is demonstrated in panel *C*. During diastole (*D*), the redundant leaflets prolapse into the left ventricular outflow tract. The appearance of these bicuspid valves can be

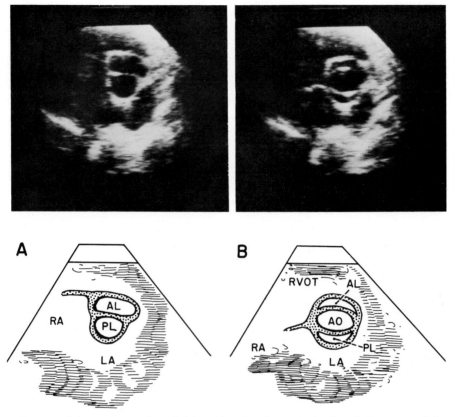

Fig. 7–12. Parasternal short-axis recording of a bicuspid aortic valve. *A,* In the diastolic frame, a single horizontal coaptation line separates the anterior (AL) and posterior (PL) leaflets. The anterior leaflet in this example is the larger of the two leaflets, and both coronary arteries arise from behind this cusp. *B,* During systole, the open leaflets produce a circular orifice, which is apparent within the margins of the aortic root. AO = aorta; RVOT = right ventricular outflow tract; LA = left atrium; RA = right atrium.

contrasted with the tricuspid valves illustrated in Figures 7–2, 7–3, and 7–15.

The sensitivity of the cross-sectional technique in detecting the bicuspid aortic valve is unknown. In studies in which angiographic and surgical confirmation have been available, sensitivity has been excellent; however, these patients represent only a small percentage of the total population with bicuspid valves.[37] Both false-positives and false-negatives may be encountered. A false-negative diagnosis is most likely when a prominent raphe is evident, giving the appearance of a third coaptation line. This is compounded when leaflet redundancy obscures the typical opening pattern of a bicuspid valve. False-positives occur when one leaflet and coaptation line are poorly visualized. In the adult, when a bicuspid valve becomes fibrotic or calcified, the underlying disorder is frequently no longer apparent.

Figure 7–14 depicts a bicuspid valve in long axis. During systole (A), the full open aortic leaflets are parallel to the aortic root, suggesting that, in this example, leaflet redundancy was sufficient to permit full opening of the valve. Although normal leaflet opening may be observed, systolic doming is common and is reported in approximately 50% of patients.[37] The degree of doming becomes more prominent as the degree of stenosis increases. During diastole (B), the coaptation line between the two leaflets of the bicuspid aortic valve is positioned eccentrically within the aortic

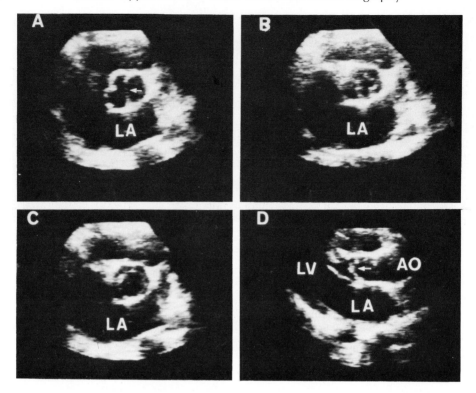

Fig. 7–13.   Series of recordings of a bicuspid aortic valve. *A,* A vertically oriented coaptation line (arrow) and a prominent raphe in the right cusp are noted during diastole. *B,* During initial systolic opening, redundancy and infolding of the valve leaflets are obvious. *C,* At full systolic opening, the leaflets parallel the concentric margins of the aorta, producing a circular orifice. *D,* In the parasternal long-axis view, diastolic prolapse of the bicuspid valve is evident (horizontal arrow). LA = left atrium; LV = left ventricle; AO = aorta.

root.[38] The degree of eccentricity can be expressed quantitatively by calculating an eccentricity index using the formula:

$$EI = {}^1/_2 \frac{A}{a}$$

where "A" is the aortic root diameter at the onset of diastole and "a" is the distance from the line of aortic cusp coaptation to the nearest aortic wall at the same point in the cardiac cycle. It was originally suggested that all bicuspid valves had an eccentricity index of greater than 1.5, whereas all tricuspid valves had a degree of eccentricity of 1.25 or less. This index, therefore, would permit discrimination of a tricuspid valve from a bicuspid valve.[39] Subsequently, approximately 25% of patients with bicuspid valves were shown to have normal eccentricity indexes, whereas

on occasion, tricuspid valves appeared eccentric.[37,40] Despite these difficulties, eccentric valve closure in the long axis should always suggest the possibility of a bicuspid valve and should prompt a more detailed short-axis examination in an attempt to demonstrate the leaflet structure.

Aortic Leaflet Thickening Without Stenosis

Focal thickening of the free edges of one or more of the aortic leaflets without associated valvular stenosis is not uncommon, particularly in older patients. The cause of these focal areas of increased reflection is unclear because they are usually incidental findings. Their more common appearance in elderly patients suggests that they represent some form of valvular degeneration with or without associated calcium deposition.

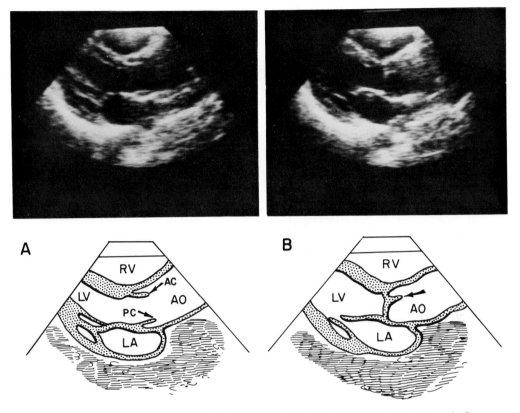

Fig. 7–14. Parasternal long-axis recording of a bicuspid aortic valve. *A,* During systole, the aortic leaflets separate widely and lie parallel to the margins of the aortic root. *B,* During diastole, the coaptation line of the aortic leaflets is markedly eccentric and is displaced closer to the anterior margin of the aortic root. RV = right ventricle; LV = left ventricle; AO = aorta; LA = left atrium; AC = anterior cusp; PC = posterior cusp.

Diffuse thickening of the aortic leaflets may be seen with cardiac amyloidosis and appears to be useful in differentiating this disorder from other infiltrative myopathies. Figure 7–15 is an aortic valve recording from a patient with amyloidosis that illustrates this diffuse aortic leaflet thickening.

AORTIC INSUFFICIENCY

Aortic insufficiency may result from a primary disorder of either the aortic valve, the aortic root, or a combination of both. Aortic insufficiency on a valvular basis may be either acquired (occurring most often as a result of rheumatic fever or bacterial endocarditis) or congenital (in association with congenital valvular aortic stenosis, bicuspid aortic valve, or aortic

valve prolapse).[17,41–43] Disorders of the aortic root associated with valvular insufficiency are characterized by either focal or generalized dilatation of the ascending aorta with loss of the normal annular support for the aortic cusps.[44]

Echocardiographically, the diagnosis of aortic insufficiency is based on indirect findings, including a left ventricular volume overload pattern[45–47] and a high-frequency diastolic fluttering of the anterior mitral leaflet,[48–50] and, on occasion, of the interventricular septum.[51,52] Additional features include an abnormal short-axis diastolic configuration of the anterior mitral leaflet (see Chap. 5) and a characteristic pattern of diastolic septal motion (see Chap. 12). Once the diagnosis of aortic insufficiency is established on either clinical or echocardiographic grounds, how-

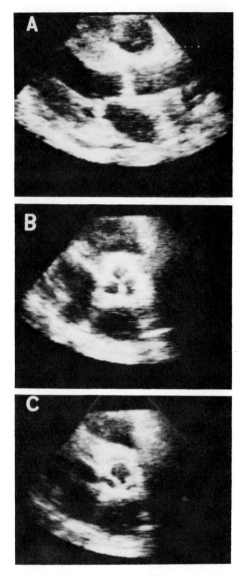

Fig. 7–15. Illustration of the marked aortic leaflet thickening, which may be noted in patients with amyloidosis. *A*, Parasternal long-axis recording. *B*, Parasternal short-axis recording during diastole. *C*, Parasternal short-axis systolic recording.

ever, direct recording of the aortic valve and root usually permits the cause of the valvular insufficiency to be determined.

Rheumatic Aortic Insufficiency

Rheumatic involvement of the aortic cusps is characterized by leaflet thickening, scarring, and retraction with failure of the cusps to coapt completely during diastole. Some degree of aortic stenosis is common.[53] The echocardiographic features of rheumatic aortic insufficiency are similar to those of rheumatic valvular stenosis and include increased reflectivity from the thickened deformed leaflets, leaflet fixation beginning at the bases of one or more of the aortic cusps, impaired systolic leaflet motion, and occasional systolic leaflet doming. During diastole, the valve cusps are more highly reflective than normal, and multiple linear echoes may be found along the coaptation line. Unfortunately, although the various patterns of leaflet coaptation have been studied extensively, a consistent pattern of diastolic leaflet closure that can uniformly be associated with aortic insufficiency has not been defined.

Aortic Valve Vegetations

The aortic valve is a common site of involvement in patients with bacterial endocarditis. Although mitral valve endocarditis has been noted more frequently in postmortem studies,[54] the predominance of aortic valve involvement in surgical series suggest that operative intervention is more common when the aortic valve is affected.[54-58] Combined infections of both the aortic and mitral valves are also frequently observed.[54,55] Predisposing factors for endocarditis include rheumatic deformity of the valve leaflets,[59,60] bicuspid aortic valve,[17] and, in the elderly, atheromatous deposits, degeneration, and calcification of the aortic cusps.[61] Echocardiographically, aortic vegetations appear as masses or clumps of echoes attached to the ventricular surface of the aortic leaflet(s). These echo-producing masses may be small or large, fixed or mobile, and have been described as fuzzy or shaggy in appearance. When mobile and large, the vegetations may prolapse into the left ventricular outflow tract during diastole and swing forward with the stream of blood into the aorta during systolic ejection.[62-66]

Figure 7–16 illustrates a vegetation on the ventricular surface of a congenitally stenotic valve.

The identification of aortic vegetations depends on their location, size, relationship to underlying valvular deformities, and association with valvular destruction. Valvular vegetations characteristically involve the bodies or free edges of the aortic leaflets. They are commonly focal, involving only a single or two adjacent leaflets. Although visualization of vegetations as small as 2 mm has been reported,[62] larger lesions are obviously more easily detected. Prominent underlying valvular deformities may make the identification of vegetations more difficult, and when a vegetation is superimposed on a severely deformed calcified valve, recognition of the vegetation as a distinct lesion may be difficult. Although vegetations generally move in unison with the leaflets to which they are attached, exaggerated motion of a pedunculated vegetation or a friable portion of a fixed vegetation may aid in their recognition. Figure 7–17 is an apical five-chamber view of a freely moving aortic vegetation. In this diastolic frame, the vegetation is hanging into the left ventricular outflow tract, beneath the aortic valve.

Fenestrated and Flail Aortic Leaflets

Some degree of valvular destruction is commonly seen in patients with aortic vegetations and may vary from a small fenestration to a completely torn, flail leaflet. Leaflet fenestration is characterized by high-frequency, diastolic fluttering within or at the margins of the echo-producing,

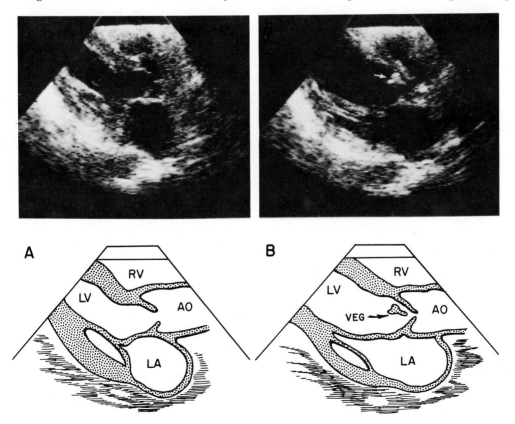

Fig. 7–16. The parasternal long-axis recording of an aortic valve vegetation (VEG). *A,* During systole, leaflet doming occurs, but vegetation is not apparent. *B,* In diastole, however, a large vegetation is visualized hanging beneath the anterior leaflet. RV = right ventricle; LV = left ventricle; AO = aorta; LA = left atrium.

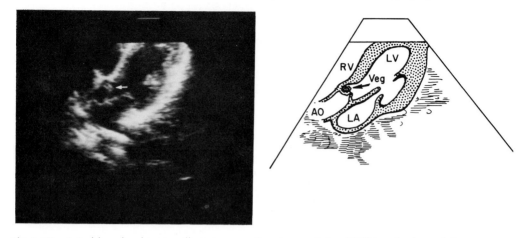

Fig. 7–17. Apical five-chamber view illustrates an aortic valve vegetation (VEG) hanging beneath the noncoronary aortic cusp. RV = right ventricle; LV = left ventricle; AO = aorta; LA = left atrium.

vegetative mass.[67,68] This high-frequency fluttering is caused by the regurgitant stream of blood flowing past the freely mobile piece of leaflet tissue. Diastolic fluttering of the aortic valve has been noted to date only in cases of fenestrated or partially flail aortic leaflets and may be considered pathognomonic for this type of disorder. Flail leaflets exhibit a more dramatic motion pattern, swinging freely into the left ventricular outflow tract during diastole such that their normal convex orientation toward the left ventricle is reversed and they become concave inferiorly.[67] During systole, the partially detached leaflet reverses its orientation, swinging in a 180-degree arch through the aortic annulus into the ascending aorta. When a flail leaflet is present, lack of diastolic coaptation with the remaining normally attached leaflets is usually evident. Figure 7–18 illustrates a flail right coronary aortic leaflet.

Septal Abscess

Extension of the infectious process into the interventricular septum with septal abscess formation characteristically results in swelling or thickening at the base of the interventricular septum in the area where the septum normally tapers to join

the aortic root. Thickening in this area is unusual and is generally noted only with a septal abscess or with a surgical patch covering a repaired ventricular septal defect. The area of the abscess is usually more highly reflective than is the surrounding tissue, and may appear linear or speckled internally. Paravalvular abscesses extending into the aortic root produce similar thickening or widening of the aortic wall. The infected portion of the wall is typically more reflective than surrounding normal tissue.

Hemodynamic Sequelae of Aortic Endocarditis

When the bacterial process causes valvular destruction and severe aortic insufficiency, the echogram may be of value in assessing the sequelae of this increased hemodynamic burden on the left ventricle. Thus, in addition to the left ventricular volume overload and mitral leaflet fluttering, which are characteristic of aortic insufficiency, abnormalities in the pattern of mitral leaflet closure may provide important hemodynamic information.[69–71] As discussed in Chapter 5, mitral valve closure is normally initiated by atrial relaxation and completed by ventricular systole. With acute severe aortic insuffi-

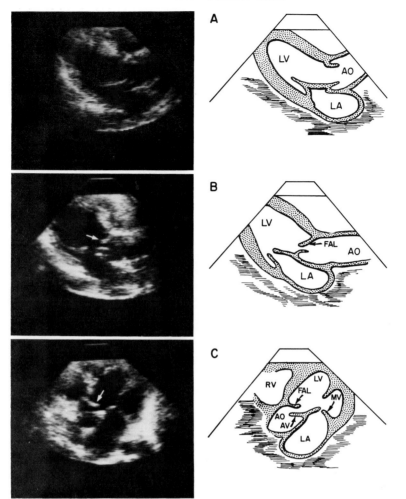

Fig. 7–18. Flail right coronary aortic leaflet. *A,* Parasternal long-axis recording indicates the relatively normal systolic appearance of the flail valve. *B,* Diastolic recording demonstrates the reversal in direction of the freely moving leaflet. The leaflet tip (FAL) points down toward the left ventricle (LV). *C,* An obliquely recorded apical five-chamber view that again illustrates lack of coaptation of the flail leaflet and reversal of the normal diastolic orientation. RV = right ventricle; AO = aorta; AV = aortic valve; LA = left atrium; MV = mitral valve; LV = left ventricle; FAL = flail aortic leaflet.

ciency, diastolic pressure in the left ventricle may rise rapidly, thereby causing the mitral valve to close prematurely. Premature mitral valve closure has been associated with severe left ventricular failure suggesting the need for urgent surgical intervention.[70–72] One caution must be noted in this regard. Patients with extensive bacterial destruction of the aortic valve often develop septal abscesses with resulting conduction delay and prolongation of the PR interval. When first-de-

gree heart block is present, the mitral valve normally closes completely in response to atrial relaxation, and closure prior to ventricular systole is therefore neither unexpected nor abnormal. Truly premature mitral valve closure must occur earlier than would be expected as a result of atrial relaxation or ventricular systole.

When aortic valve vegetations are large and freely mobile, it is frequently questioned whether surgical removal is warranted on the basis of their appearance alone. Although little data are available to resolve this question, no association has been observed to date between the size or mobility of vegetations and the development of subsequent complications.[73]

Aortic Insufficiency Associated with Congenitally Stenotic and/or Bicuspid Valves

Aortic insufficiency may frequently be associated with congenitally stenotic and/or bicuspid aortic valves. In the former situation, the valvular deformity is evidenced by the characteristic systolic leaflet doming, whereas in the latter, the two-leaflet, two-commissure pattern evident on short-axis diastolic recording confirms that the valve is bicuspid. Although no specific features of either the congenitally stenotic or the bicuspid valve indicate incompetency, aortic valve prolapse appears to be noted more commonly when the valve is insufficient.

Aortic Valve Prolapse

Aortic valve prolapse can be defined as an inferior or apical diastolic displacement of one or more aortic cusps below the plane of the aortic annulus. Aortic valve prolapse has been reported in as many as 20% of patients with mitral valve prolapse[74] and may be noted with bicuspid and/or congenitally stenotic aortic valves, complex congenital disorders of the great vessels, such connective tissue disorders as Marfan's syndrome, sinus of Valsalva aneurysms, following aortic valvulotomy and, on occasion, with ventricular septal defect located immediately beneath the valve. Figure 7–19 is an example of aortic valve prolapse involving the right and noncoronary aortic leaflets.

The natural history and hemodynamic consequences of aortic valve prolapse remain to be defined, as does its association with aortic insufficiency. In one study, aortic insufficiency was clinically evident in only 20% of patients with aortic valve prolapse.[74] When prolapse is associated with congenital aortic stenosis or bicuspid aortic valve, however, valvular insufficiency appears more common.

THE AORTA

The aorta is the major arterial trunk connecting the left ventricle with the systemic arterial system. The aorta has a thick, tough musculoelastic wall that normally is able to withstand pressures in the thousands of millimeters of mercury without bursting.[75] The aortic wall is composed of three primary layers: a thin, inner, tunica intima; a thick tunica media; and a thin, outer tunica adventitia. Structurally, the tunica media is the most important of these layers, comprising more than 80% of the arterial wall. This layer is composed of multiple, concentric, elastic sheets made of broad, interwoven, fenestrated bands. These sheets are connected by interposed smooth muscle, collagen, and ground substance. The inner portion of the medial layer is nourished by diffusion from the vascular lumen, whereas its outer portion is supplied by small, diffusely branching intramural arteries, the vasa vasorum.[76,77]

In addition to its role as a conduit, the aortic wall, because of its elastic properties, also serves as a compression chamber, damping the surge of aortic pressure during systole and, when inflow ceases, using the stored tension within the vascular wall to continue to drive blood through the peripheral capillaries. This dual function prevents wide swings in systemic arterial pressure and maintains a relatively constant perfusion pressure throughout the peripheral vascular system.[75]

The aorta can be divided anatomically into three primary regions: the ascending aorta, the aortic arch, and the descending aorta. The descending aorta can be further divided at the diaphragm into thoracic and abdominal segments.[1]

From an echocardiographic viewpoint, disorders involving the tubular aorta can

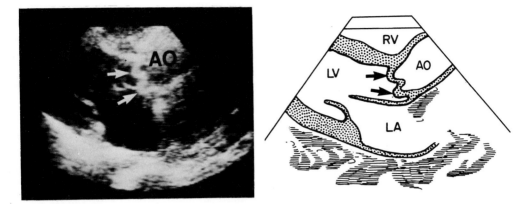

Fig. 7–19. Parasternal long-axis recording of the aortic valve illustrates prolapse of both the right and noncoronary aortic leaflets (horizontal arrows). LV = left ventricle; RV = right ventricle; LA = left atrium; AO = aorta.

be grouped into those that produce luminal narrowing or stenosis and those that are characterized by dilatation of the vessel walls.

The Ascending Aorta

The ascending aorta begins at the aortic valve and extends roughly 5 cm to its junction with the aortic arch. Its origin typically lies beneath the third costal cartilage along the left sternal margin.[1] From this point, it courses anteriorly, superiorly, and rightward, joining the arch beneath the superior border of the second right costal cartilage. Three outpouchings (the sinuses of Valsalva) appear at the origin of the ascending aorta and are discussed earlier in this chapter in conjunction with the aortic valve.

Figure 7–20 diagrammatically illustrates the normal appearance of the ascending aorta from its origin at the aortic annulus to its disappearance beneath the sternum. The diameter of the vessel normally varies in this region, increasing from the aortic annulus (level 1) to the sinuses of Valsalva (level 2) by a mean of 5.4 mm (range, 2 to 10 mm).[78] At the sinotubular junction (level 3), the diameter decreases to equal or slightly exceed (mean, 3.1 mm) that recorded at the aortic annulus. The normal decrease in diameter from the sinuses (level 2) to the beginning of the tubular portion of the aorta (level 3) averages 10% (range, 0 to 26%). Importantly, the diameter of the tubular portion of the ascending aorta in normal persons is never less than that recorded at the aortic annulus.[78]

Supravalvular Aortic Stenosis

Supravalvular aortic stenosis is an obstructive, congenital deformity of the ascending aorta that originates just distal to the coronary arteries and produces either localized or diffuse narrowing of the vessel.[79] Although the designation, "supravalvular aortic stenosis," encompasses a heterogeneous group of lesions, three specific anatomic types have been characterized. First is the so-called membranous type, which consists of a simple fibrous diaphragm containing a single perforation. At the opposite extreme is a uniform hypoplasia of the entire ascending aorta, designated the hypoplastic type. Between these two is the hourglass lesion. This type of obstruction is characterized by extreme thickening of the media of the ascending aorta with an hourglass-like narrowing of the external aspect of the affected segment and corresponding narrowing of the aortic lumen. Intimal fibrous thickening may appear over the narrowed segment, further accentuating the degree of obstruction.[79]

The hourglass deformity is clearly the

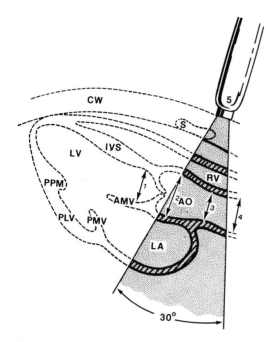

Fig. 7–20. Diagram illustrates the relationship of a 30-degree cross-sectional scan to the supravalvular portion of the ascending aorta. The aortic diameter is generally measured at the levels indicated by the vertical arrows: (1) the aortic annulus, (2) the sinuses of Valsalva, (3) the junction of the superior margin of the sinuses of Valsalva and the tubular ascending aorta (the sinotubular junction), (4) the ascending aorta at the most distal margin of the scan plane or at its junction with the aortic arch. CW = chest wall; S = sternum; IVS = interventricular septum; LV = left ventricle; PPM = posterior papillary muscle; PLV = posterior left ventricular wall; PMV = posterior mitral valve leaflet; AMV = anterior mitral valve leaflet; LA = left atrium; AO = aorta; RV = right ventricle. (From Weyman, AE, et al.: Cross-sectional echocardiographic characterization of aortic obstruction. 1. Supravalvular aortic stenosis and aortic hypoplasia. Circulation, 57:491, 1978. Reproduced by permission of the American Heart Association.)

most common, representing roughly 66% of cases, whereas diffuse narrowing of the vessel accounts for more than 20%. Membranous lesions are the least common, occurring in no more than 10% of patients with supravalvular obstruction.[80–82] Although supravalvular stenosis is not common (it accounts for only 0.6 to 6% of obstructive lesions[79,83,84] occurring in the region of the aortic valve), it does occur with sufficient frequency to warrant continued diagnostic consideration.

In addition to the different anatomic types of supravalvular aortic stenosis, three separate clinical presentations have also been described. The most common of these is the sporadic form in which the lesion occurs in otherwise normal individuals. In approximately a third of cases, the supravalvular stenosis is found in association with an extended syndrome, which includes an abnormal elfin facies, mental retardation, and idiopathic hypercalcemia.[85–88] Finally, there have been reports of familial aggregates of patients in which the disorder appears to be transmitted as an autosomal dominant disorder with variable expression.[89,90]

Echocardiographically, supravalvular aortic stenosis is characterized by an obvious decrease in aortic diameter originating at the superior border of the sinuses of Valsalva.[78] The area of obstruction may vary in both severity and extent, but the point of peak aortic narrowing usually is found just anterior to the junction of the superior border of the left atrium and the aortic root.[78]

The membranous lesion generally appears as a discrete, thin, linear echo extending inward from the walls of the aorta and encroaching on the vascular lumen. The membrane is usually located at the sinotubular junction just above the insertion of the superior left atrial wall into the posterior aortic root. The lesion is considered obstructive when the separation between the inner margins of the membrane is less than the diameter of the outflow tract at the annulus. Figure 7–21 is a long-axis, cross-sectional scan of the ascending aorta and illustrates such a supravalvular membrane.

Figure 7–22 is an example of an hourglass-like lesion. In this example there is more marked luminal narrowing as well as a more extensive area of involvement of the ascending aorta. Figure 7–23 is an aortic angiogram from the same patient and illustrates a similar degree of obstruction and extent of aortic involvement.

Figure 7–24 illustrates aortic hypo-

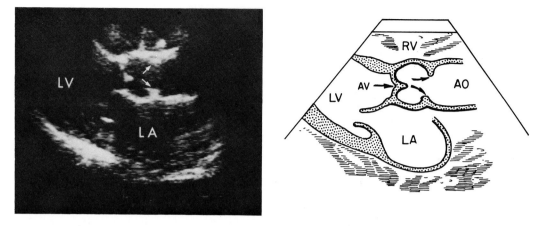

Fig. 7–21. Parasternal long-axis recording of the ascending aorta illustrates a discrete supravalvular membrane. The membrane, indicated by the oblique arrows, appears as two discrete linear bands of echoes arising from the anterior and posterior margins of the aortic root encroaching on the lumen of the vessel. RV = right ventricle; AV = aortic valve; LV = left ventricle; AO = aorta; LA = left atrium.

plasia. In this example, the aorta appears small, thin, and strand-like. The area of hypoplasia involves the entire ascending aorta and aortic arch. The diminutive vessel is evident throughout the scan plane and, as indicated in the accompanying diagram, was associated with hypoplasia of the left ventricle and mitral valve. In the left-hand portion of the scan, a small area of dilatation reflects the rudimentary sinuses of Valsalva. Figure 7–25 is an angiogram from the same patient and confirms the extent and severity of the aortic hypoplasia.

Comparisons between cross-sectional echocardiographic and angiographic studies of the aortic root have revealed a good correlation in both morphologic appearance and estimates of severity.[78] Likewise, in the small group of patients examined to date, the echocardiographic diameter of the aorta at the point of maximal narrowing has been within 3 mm of the corresponding angiographic measurement. The echogram has tended toward slight underestimation of the angiographic value.[78] When the full extent of the lesion can be encompassed, the extent of involvement can also be measured accurately. Using the diameter of the aorta at the annulus as a reference, a mean decrease in diameter of 47%

was noted in four patients with hourglass lesions.[78] This finding is in contrast to the normal mean increase of 12.5%. In addition, a rough correlation existed in this small patient group between the percent decrease in diameter and the severity of obstruction. Thus, in one patient with an 18-mmHg gradient, a 25% decrease in diameter was noted, whereas in 3 patients with gradients of 74 mmHg or larger, a mean decrease of 55% was observed. When the aorta is diffusely hypoplastic, the annulus is frequently also involved and can no longer be used as a reference for estimating severity. In such instances, correlation of absolute measurements with published normal values may be necessary.

Aneurysms of the Ascending Aorta

Aneurysms are abnormal, localized areas of dilatation of the wall of a blood vessel, usually an artery.[91,92] Aneurysms may be saccular (involving only a portion of the vascular wall) or fusiform (encompassing all or almost all of the circumference of the vessel). True aneurysms involve all the layers of the vascular wall. False aneurysms, in contrast, result from destruction of the vessel wall, usually by trauma. The

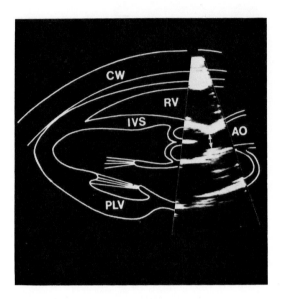

Fig. 7–22. Parasternal long-axis recording of the ascending aorta illustrates the hourglass type of supravalvular obstruction. The area of peak obstruction is indicated by the vertical arrowheads. CW = chest wall; RV = right ventricle; IVS = interventricular septum; AO = aorta; PLV = posterior left ventricle. (From Weyman, AE, et al.: Cross-sectional echocardiographic characterization of aortic obstruction. 1. Supravalvular aortic stenosis and aortic hypoplasia. Circulation, 57:491, 1978. Reproduced by permission of the American Heart Association.)

external border of the false aneurysm is composed of perivascular clot and connective tissue. Dissecting aneurysms are characterized by separation of the layers of the aortic wall. The process of dissection is commonly initiated by rupture of a vasa vasorum with subsequent formation of an intramural hematoma. This intramural hematoma separates the medial layers and produces an intimal tear, which allows the hematoma to communicate with the vascular lumen. Once this connection is established, the force of aortic pressure continues the process of dissection.[91]

Aortic aneurysms may be congenital or acquired. The most common congenital aneurysms include those arising from a

sinus of Valsalva and those associated with Marfan's syndrome. Acquired aneurysms may result from atherosclerosis, idiopathic cystic medial necrosis, syphilis, trauma, or infection (mycotic aneurysms).[91]

Regardless of their cause or location, aneurysms of the aorta result from disease of the musculoelastic media, which is the major barrier against aortic pressure. Deterioration of the media progressively weakens the aortic wall, resulting in dilatation at the site of involvement. Dilatation increases wall stress in the affected region, which may lead to continued local expansion and, finally, to rupture.

Congenital Aneurysms of the Aorta

Sinus of Valsalva aneurysm. Congenital aneurysms of the sinuses of Valsalva appear to result from a lack of continuity between the media of the aortic root and the annulus of the aortic valve.[93] These aneurysms are reported to involve the right coronary sinus in approximately 69% of the cases, the noncoronary sinus in 26%, and the left coronary sinus in 5%.[94] Because the sinuses are largely intracardiac, their relationship to adjacent structures determines the direction of aneurysmal expansion and the site of rupture. Aneurysms of the right coronary sinus tend to project into the right ventricle and, occasionally, the right atrium, whereas those of the noncoronary sinus almost invariably project into the right atrium.[95] More rarely, sinus of Valsalva aneurysms may protrude into the right ventricular outflow tract, causing outflow obstruction;[96] dissect into the interventricular septum and then rupture into the right or left ventricles;[97] or communicate directly with the left atrium, ventricle, or pericardial space. Occasionally, dilatation of a sinus may cause prolapse of the associated aortic leaflet with resulting valvular insufficiency.[98–101]

Echocardiographically, sinus of Val-

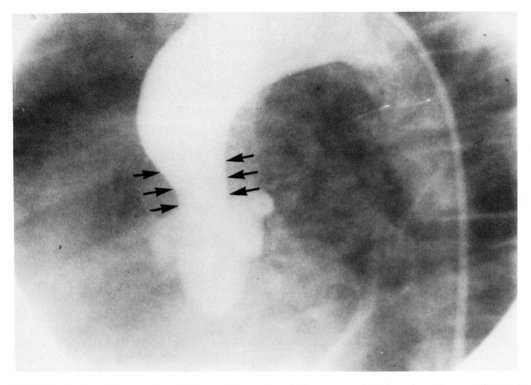

Fig. 7–23. Angiographic recording of the ascending aorta, which corresponds to the echocardiogram illustrated in Figure 7–22. The area of obstruction is indicated by the horizontal arrows and corresponds in both severity and extent to the cross-sectional appearance of the lesion. (From Weyman, AE, et al.: Cross-sectional echocardiographic characterization of aortic obstruction. 1. Supravalvular aortic stenosis and aortic hypoplasia. Circulation, 57:491, 1978. Reproduced by permission of the American Heart Association.)

salva aneurysms are best visualized in a parasternal short-axis view of the aortic root. The aneurysmal sinus is typically larger and has a thinner wall than do the nonaffected sinuses. Figure 7–26 is a short axis recording of a right coronary sinus aneurysm that illustrates these features.

When a sinus ruptures (Fig. 7–27), the resulting echocardiographic pattern is determined largely by the size of the leak, the rapidity with which the leak develops, and the chamber that receives the aortic blood. When the shunt is into the right side of the heart, the increased flow must pass through the pulmonary artery, the left atrium, and the left ventricle before reaching the aorta again. Therefore, a left ventricular volume overload pattern can always be expected. When the aneurysm ruptures into the right ventricle, volume overload of this chamber is also present,

whereas rupture into the right atrium causes volume overload of both the right atrium and the ventricle. Despite the right ventricular volume overload, paradoxic septal motion should not be expected because the right and left ventricular volume loads should balance each other.

Rupture into the right side of the heart has also been associated with premature opening of the pulmonary valve caused by the rapid rise in right ventricular diastolic pressure.[102]

Marfan's syndrome. Marfan's syndrome is a generalized disorder of connective tissue inherited as an autosomal dominant trait. Marfan's syndrome is characterized by abnormalities of the eye (myopia and ectopia lentis); the skeletal system (excessive limb length, loose joints, kyphoscoliosis, arachnodactyly, pectus excavatum, and pectus carinatum); and the

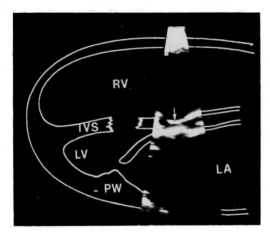

Fig. 7–24. Cross-sectional echogram of the supravalvular aorta from a patient with severe hypoplasia of the aortic annulus and ascending vessel. The area of greatest narrowing is indicated by the vertical arrow. Proximal to the obstruction, rudimentary sinuses of Valsalva are visible. Distally, hypoplasia of the entire ascending aorta continues. As indicated in the accompanying diagram, there was also hypoplasia of the left ventricle (LV) and mitral valve, a ventricular septal defect, and a dilated right ventricle (RV) and pulmonary artery. IVS = interventricular septum; PW = posterior wall; LA = left atrium. (From Weyman, AE, et al.: Cross-sectional echocardiographic characterization of aortic obstruction. 1. Supravalvular aortic stenosis and aortic hypoplasia. Circulation, 57:491, 1978. Reproduced by permission of the American Heart Association.)

cardiovascular system.[103] Cardiovascular abnormalities include aortic aneurysm, which may be complicated by dissection; aortic insufficiency due to dilatation of the aortic root and annulus; and myxomatous degeneration of the aortic leaflets.[103–105] Myxomatous degeneration of the mitral valve and chordal apparatus is also frequently noted. Although not evident in all cases of Marfan's syndrome, cardiovascular abnormalities are present in at least 60% of affected adults.[103–105] Cardiac abnormalities tend to be progressive and are believed to represent the response of the defective connective tissue to prolonged hemodynamic stress.[103,106] This hypothesis is supported by the fact that such abnormalities are less pronounced and rarely involve the aortic root in children, whereas in adults, the abnormalities center about

the areas of greatest hemodynamic stress—the left-sided cardiac valves and the proximal aorta.[104] Aortic dissection is the most serious complication, and dissection, together with the other aortic valve abnormalities, is the leading cause of death.[107]

The primary defect underlying the aortic root abnormality of Marfan's syndrome is unknown. Histologically, there is striking loss of medial elastic tissue in the affected segment, disorganization of smooth-muscle bundles, and an increase in collagen. In addition, there is evidence of cystic medial necrosis with focal accumulation of mucopolysaccharide.[103–106] Echocardiographically, the aortic root is typically dilated (often massively), and the aortic walls appear thin. The pattern of dilatation is unique because it involves the annulus, sinuses of Valsalva, and the distal ascending aorta, symmetrically.[108] The aortic leaflets are elongated, and the orifice that the leaflets must occlude is enlarged. When aortic insufficiency is present, the left ventricle dilates, and the left ventricular stroke volume increases. The mitral valve is also typically redundant, and prolapse of both mitral leaflets may be noted. Figures 7–28, A and B, are long- and short-axis recordings of the aortic root, which illustrate the characteristic changes noted in Marfan's syndrome. In long axis, the aortic root is markedly dilated, and the aortic leaflets are elongated. The pronounced dilatation at the level of the sinuses of Valsalva compresses the left atrium from above, thereby reducing its anteroposterior expanse. In short axis, the marked dilatation of the aortic root is again evident, as is the symmetric dilatation of the three sinuses of Valsalva. The extended commissure of the coapted aortic leaflets can also be appreciated.

Acquired Aneurysms

Two types of acquired aneurysms of the ascending aorta have been characterized echocardiographically: the dissecting aneurysm and the mycotic aneurysm.[108]

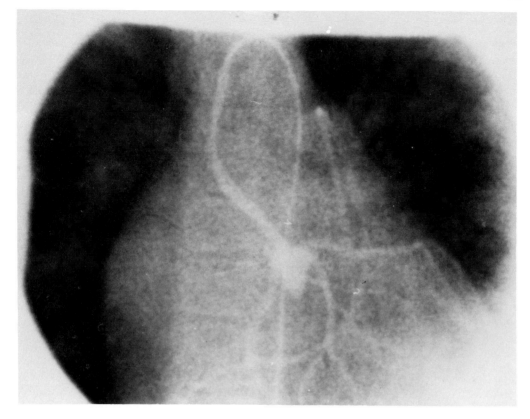

Fig. 7–25. Angiographic recording of the ascending aorta corresponds to the cross-sectional echogram in Figure 7–24. This recording again demonstrates severe hypoplasia of the entire ascending aortic arch. Diminutive sinuses of Valsalva, from which the coronary arterial system arises, are also evident. (From Weyman, AE, et al.: Cross-sectional echocardiographic characterization of aortic obstruction. 1. Supravalvular aortic stenosis and aortic hypoplasia. Circulation, 57:491, 1978. Reproduced by permission of the American Heart Association.)

Dissecting aneurysms. Dissecting aneurysms develop as a result of degenerative or destructive disease of the aortic media, usually in association with systemic hypertension.[109,110] The most common underlying cause is idiopathic cystic medial necrosis. Dissection may also occur in other conditions that are associated with weakening of the aortic media or that place an increased stress on the aortic wall, such as Marfan's syndrome, Ehlers-Danlos syndrome, idiopathic kyphoscoliosis, Turner's syndrome, and coarctation of the aorta. Dissection may also be seen in younger women in the third trimester of pregnancy and following cardiac surgery.

Echocardiographically, dissecting aneurysms of the ascending aorta are characterized by dilatation of the aortic root and by separation of the normal single dominant echo from the aortic wall in the region of the dissection into two discrete echoes that move in unison with one another.[108] The inner echo arises from the tunica intima, whereas the outer echo is produced by medial and adventitial structures external to the tear. When the dissection follows a spiral course, the region of echo separation likewise appears to curve around the vessel as its course is followed with superior-inferior short-axis scans.

Figure 7–29 is an example of a dissection involving both the anterior and posterior aorta. The intimal margins of the dissection are indicated by the vertical

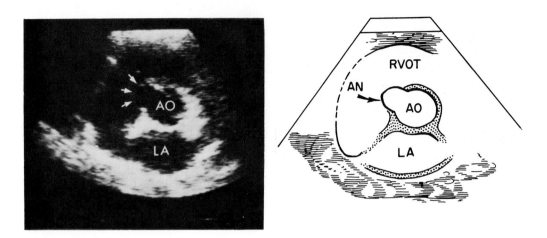

Fig. 7–26. Parasternal short-axis recording illustrates aneurysmal dilatation (AN) of the right coronary sinus of Valsalva. The aneurysm is thin-walled and, in this instance, projected into the right atrium. RVOT = right ventricular outflow tract; AO = aorta; LA = left atrium.

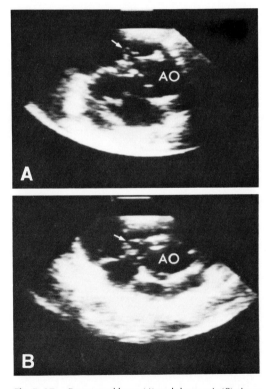

Fig. 7–27. Parasternal long- (A) and short-axis (B) views of a ruptured right sinus of Valsalva aneurysm. The aneurysm is thin-walled, and the area of rupture is indicated by the oblique arrow at its tip.

arrows. This dissection occurred several years after aortic valve replacement, and a Starr-Edwards valve can be seen in the aortic position. Figure 7–30 is an example of a second dissection. In this example, the aortic root is dilated, and the dissection is confined to the posterior aortic wall. The importance of repeated short-axis scan has been emphasized in these lesions because their focal nature and variable position may result in failure to visualize the dissection in any single imaging plane.[108]

Mycotic aneurysms. Mycotic aneurysms are produced by growth of microorganisms within the aortic wall, which results in focal destruction of the media. The microorganisms may reach the aortic wall by embolization from bacterial vegetations, by direct extension from infected aortic valves, or by internal or external invasion. Mycotic aneurysms may also arise at the site of surgical aortotomy. In the only instance of mycotic aneurysm I have observed to date, the aneurysm developed following aortic valvotomy. In this patient, a massive false aneurysm with a large mass of echoes in the shape of a fir tree extended anteriorly into the false aneurysm from the anterior border of the aorta in the region of the aortotomy.

The Aortic Arch

The aortic arch begins beneath the su-

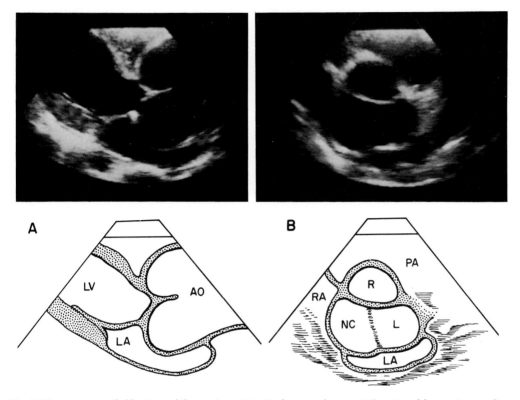

Fig. 7–28. Aneurysmal dilatation of the aortic root in Marfan's syndrome. *A,* Parasternal long-axis recording of the aortic root illustrates the dilatation of the aortic root and the thinning of the vascular wall, which are characteristic of Marfan's syndrome. The prominent posterior sinus of Valsalva compresses the left atrium (LA) from above. The aortic leaflets appear thin and elongated. *B,* Short-axis recording illustrates the symmetric dilatation of the three sinuses of Valsalva. Although only one coaptation line is apparent in this recording, the valve was tricuspid. PA = pulmonary artery; R = right coronary aortic cusp; NC = noncoronary aortic cusp; L = left coronary aortic cusp; RA = right atrium; AO = aorta; LV = left ventricle.

perior border of the second right costal cartilage and curves superiorly, posteriorly, and to the left, passing in front of the trachea and then curving inferiorly along its left-hand border. It joins the descending aorta at the inferior border of the fourth thoracic vertebra, posteriorly. At its most superior point, it is roughly 2.5 cm below the upper border of the sternum. The aortic arch gives off three major arterial branches: the innominate, the left common carotid, and the left subclavian arteries.[1]

The aortic arch is recorded with the transducer placed directly in the suprasternal notch and the scan plane directed posteriorly, inferiorly, and leftward to align it parallel to the long axis of the aorta.[111,112] In this position, the transducer is between the innominate and left common carotid branches of the aortic arch. When displayed, the left common carotid is positioned to the right of the apex of the sector, and the innominate artery is to the left. The ascending aorta courses superiorly along the left margin of the scan, whereas the descending aorta sweeps posteriorly along the right-hand margin. Figure 7–31 illustrates the probe position and scan plane orientation used to record the aortic arch. In this example, the sector is only 30 degrees wide, and a limited area of the arch and descending aorta is visualized. Using a wider scan angle, as illustrated in Chapter 4, both the ascending and

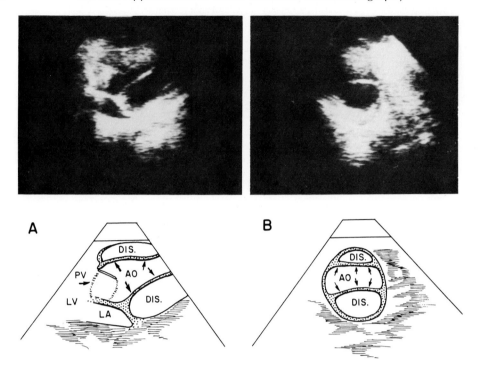

Fig. 7–29. Parasternal long- and short-axis recordings of the ascending aorta illustrate aortic dissection (DIS). In the long-axis recording (A), large echo-free space posterior to the aortic root and a smaller, anterior, echo-free space are produced by the dissection. The aortic intima is indicated by the vertical arrowheads. A Starr-Edwards valve is present in the aortic position. In the short-axis view (B), the posterior dissection elevates the intima from below. This pattern suggests that the pressure in the false channel is high enough to deform the aorta (AO) and thus excludes the left atrium as a possible cause of this echo-free area. PV = prosthetic valve; LV = left ventricle; LA = left atrium.

descending aorta and the full sweep of the arch can be visualized simultaneously.

The normal aortic arch appears as an arcuate echo-free structure. Its walls are parallel and roughly equidistant throughout the scan area. Figure 7–32 is a long-axis, cross-sectional recording of a normal aortic arch and proximal descending aorta. In this example, the inital sweep of the vessel from left to right reflects the distal aortic arch, whereas the continuation of the arc from right to left represents the proximal descending aorta. The origin of the left carotid artery is indicated in the accompanying diagram. The right pulmonary artery is commonly recorded beneath the aortic arch with the left atrium behind the pulmonary artery. Although not apparent in Figure 7–32, these structures can be easily visualized in Figure 4–16, C.

In addition to its characteristic appearance, the systolic pulsations of this arterial vessel also aid in its recognition.[111]

The close proximity of the aortic arch to the suprasternal notch makes this portion of the aorta relatively easy to record. In earlier M-mode studies, it was noted that the arch, right pulmonary artery, and left atrium could be visualized in as many as 94% of cases,[113–115] whereas in cross-sectional studies, the arch has been recorded uniformly in normal subjects.[111,112] The branches of the arch are slightly more difficult to record with visualization of the carotid and subclavian being reported in 92% of cases and the innominate in 60%.[112]

Coarctation of the Aorta

Coarctation of the aorta is characterized

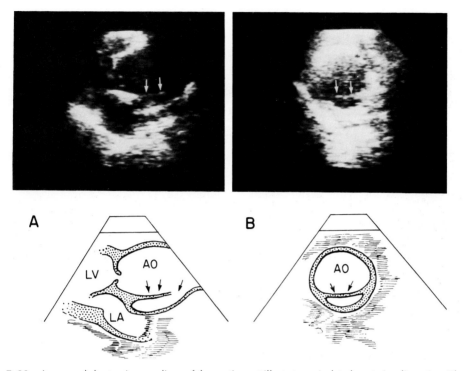

Fig. 7–30. Long- and short-axis recordings of the aortic root illustrate an isolated posterior dissection. The intimal flap is indicated by the vertical arrowheads. The aortic root is markedly dilated. LV = left ventricle; LA = left atrium; AO = aorta.

anatomically by a localized deformity of the media of the aortic wall that produces a curtain-like infolding that eccentrically narrows the vascular lumen. Externally, the aorta exhibits an indentation or localized concavity.[116] Although coarctation may occur at any level of the thoracic or abdominal aorta,[117] it is most commonly located just beyond the origin of the left subclavian artery or distal to the insertion of the ligamentum arteriosum.[118] The area of coarctation may be well defined and localized, or the aortic segment may be diffusely narrowed.

Coarctation is commonly divided at the ductus arteriosus into the postductal, or adult, type and the preductal, or infantile, type. Postductal coarctation is usually localized and appears almost as a diaphragm with the aorta widening immediately below the area of constriction to a diameter greater than that above the obstruction.[119]

In the preductal or infantile type, the constriction is proximal to the entrance of the ductus arteriosus. Preductal coarctation can be further subdivided into three general categories: (1) localized constriction just above the entrance to the ductus, (2) diffuse isthmic narrowing extending from the entrance of the ductus superiorly to the left subclavian artery, and (3) constriction involving not only the isthmus, but extending to include a variable portion of the aortic arch.[119] Isolated coarctations are usually postductal, whereas coarctation occurring in association with other congenital cardiac anomalies is more frequently preductal. In preductal lesions, there is a further association between the location and extent of narrowing and the presence of other major defects. Thus, studies have shown that focal preductal constriction is associated in 16% of patients with other major abnormalities; isthmic hypoplasia in 28% and more diffuse obstruction involving the isthmus and aortic arch in 80%.[119]

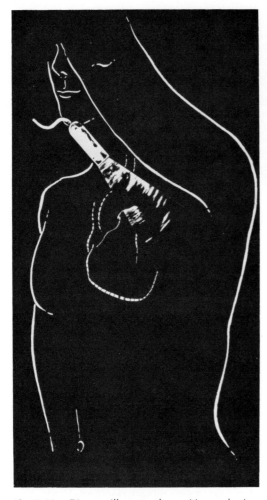

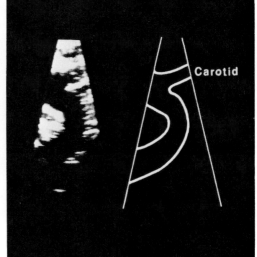

Fig. 7–32. Suprasternal long-axis recording of a normal aortic arch and descending aorta. In the upper left-hand portion of the scan, the distal portion of the aortic arch is initially visualized sweeping from left to right. The left carotid artery arises from the arch and courses to the right and superiorly. Distal to the left carotid artery, the vessel continues its sweep away from the transducer, arching initially from left to right and then back across the plane of the scan from right to left as the proximal descending aorta. The diameter of the aortic lumen is consistent throughout the plane of the scan. (From Weyman, AE, et al.: Cross-sectional echocardiographic detection of aortic obstruction. 2. Coarctation of the aorta. Circulation, 57:498, 1978. Reproduced by permission of the American Heart Association.)

Fig. 7–31. Diagram illustrates the position and orientation of the cross-sectional probe in the suprasternal notch. This orientation is utilized to record the aortic arch and proximal descending aorta. The probe is normally directed inferiorly, posteriorly, and slightly to the left when recording this region. The scan plane is oriented approximately 45 degrees to both the sagittal and coronal planes of the body. (From Weyman, AE, et al.: Cross-sectional echocardiographic detection of aortic obstruction. 2. Coarctation of the aorta. Circulation, 57:498, 1978. Reproduced by permission of the American Heart Association.)

Direct echocardiographic visualization of the area of coarctation has been reported by several groups with success rates varying from 89[111] to 100%.[112] Differentiation of lesion structure has also been achieved.[112] Coarctation appears echocardiographically as a localized decrease in the diameter of the aortic lumen, with the area of maximal narrowing distal to the origin of the left subclavian artery. The area of coarctation is characteristically more reflective than is the surrounding vascular wall because of the focal thickening in the affected region and the tendency for the obstructing shelf to be more perpendicular than the curvilinear wall of the normal descending aorta to the path of the scan plane.[111,112] Proximal to the area of obstruction, the left carotid and left subclavian arteries may be enlarged, and the aortic pulsations are increased. Distal to the lesion, the aorta again dilates, but in this region, the normal arterial pulsations are damped.[111] This striking disparity between the markedly pulsatile proximal vessel and the quiescent distal vessel highlights the presence of the obstructing lesion. In many cases, it is this discrepancy in pulsation that initially alerts the examiner to the possible presence of a coarctation.[111]

Figure 7–33 illustrates an area of discrete coarctation. In this example, a localized area of luminal narrowing is distal to the left subclavian artery. The area of coarctation is small and well demarcated and produces almost complete obliteration of the aortic lumen. Figure 7–34 is an angiogram from the same patient and illustrates the similarity in the appearance of the lesion in these two imaging formats. Figure 7–35 is a recording from a child with a more diffuse area of luminal narrowing. In this example, the area of coarctation begins proximal to the origin of the left carotid artery and extends distally beyond the origin of the left subclavian. The

corresponding angiogram illustrates a relatively diffuse area of coarctation similar to that seen on the cross-sectional scan (Fig. 7–36).

Aortic Arch Aneurysms

Aneurysms of the aortic arch and proximal descending aorta are not uncommon.[120] Traumatic aneurysms arise most commonly in the isthmic region between the left subclavian artery and ligamentum arteriosum.[121] Congenital aneurysms may also occur in this area.[120] The entire arch may likewise be involved in aortic dissection,[122,123] with fusiform atherosclerotic aneurysms,[120] and in such connective tissue disorders as Marfan's syndrome and Ehlers-Danlos syndrome.[3] Figure 7–37 is a long-axis recording of the ascending aorta

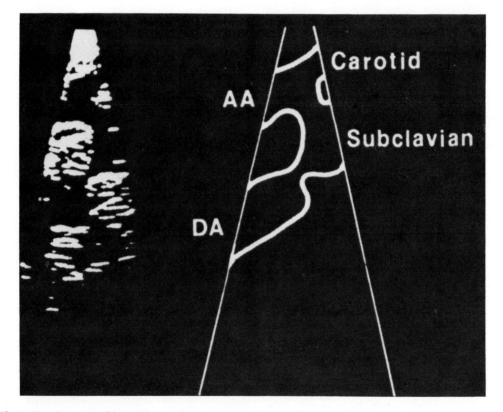

Fig. 7–33. Suprasternal long-axis scan from a patient with a localized area of aortic narrowing distal to the origin of the left subclavian artery. AA = ascending aorta; DA = descending aorta. (From Weyman, AE, et al.: Cross-sectional echocardiographic detection of aortic obstruction. 2. Coarctation of the aorta. Circulation, 57:498, 1978. Reproduced by permission of the American Heart Association.)

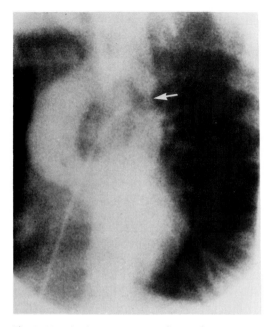

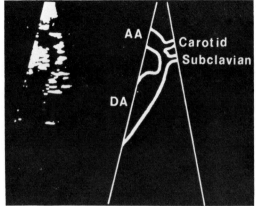

Fig. 7–35. Suprasternal long-axis scan from a patient with a more diffuse area of aortic obstruction that begins in the region of the aortic arch and extends to a point of maximal narrowing, which is distal to the left subclavian artery. Beyond the area of maximal obstruction, the aortic diameter returns toward normal. AA = aortic arch; DA = descending aorta. (From Weyman, AE, et al.: Cross-sectional echocardiographic detection of aortic obstruction. 2. Coarctation of the aorta. Circulation, 57:498, 1978. Reproduced by permission of the American Heart Association.)

Fig. 7–34. Angiogram corresponding to the cross-sectional study in Figure 7–33. In this recording, a localized area of narrowing of the aortic lumen is distal to the origin of the left subclavian artery (horizontal arrow), which corresponds in both location and appearance to the obstruction seen on the cross-sectional scan. (From Weyman, AE, et al.: Cross-sectional echocardiographic detection of aortic obstruction. 2. Coarctation of the aorta. Circulation, 57:498, 1978. Reproduced by permission of the American Heart Assocation.)

and aortic arch and illustrates aneurysmal dilatation in a patient with Ehlers-Danlos syndrome.

Unfortunately, despite the relative ease of recording diffuse aneurysmal dilatation of this region, the echocardiographic diagnosis of dissecting aneurysms of the aortic arch has proved difficult. This difficulty occurs because of the multiple linear echoes normally encountered in this area that not only complicate the diagnosis of actual dissections, but also result in frequent false-positive results. At present, the echocardiographic detection of dissecting aneurysms of the aortic arch is a poorly defined area that will require more study before such lesions can be clearly characterized.

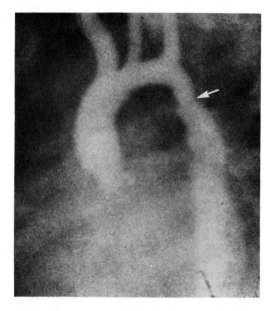

Fig. 7–36. Angiographic recording corresponding to the cross-sectional scan in Figure 7–35. Again, a fairly extensive area of aortic narrowing is noted. The maximal decrease in luminal diameter occurs distal to the origin of the left subclavian artery (horizontal arrow). (From Weyman, AE, et al.: Cross-sectional echocardiographic detection of aortic obstruction. 2. Coarctation of the aorta. Circulation, 57:498, 1978. Reproduced by permission of the American Heart Association.)

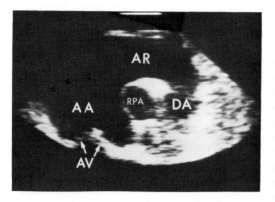

Fig. 7–37. Diffuse dilatation of the ascending aorta (AA) and aortic arch (AR) in a patient with Ehlers-Danlos syndrome. AV = aortic valve; DA = descending aorta; RPA = right pulmonary artery.

The Descending Aorta

The descending aorta originates at the lower border of the fourth thoracic vertebra and extends inferiorly to its bifurcation into the common iliac arteries in front of the fourth lumbar vertebra. It can be divided at the diaphragm into the thoracic and abdominal segments. At its origin, the descending thoracic aorta lies to the left of the vertebral column. As it descends, it curves toward the midline and is positioned directly in front of the vertebral column at its termination.[1]

The Thoracic Aorta

The descending thoracic aorta is best visualized from a parasternal transducer location as it passes behind the left side of the heart.[124–126] In the typical long-axis view of the left ventricle, the descending thoracic aorta appears as a pulsatile, circular or oval, echo-free space located beneath the posterior atrioventricular groove. During short-axis scans from the apex to the base of the left heart, the position of the descending aorta appears to shift relative to the center of the left ventricle because of the acute angle at which the long axes of these two structures intersect (Fig. 7–38). At the papillary muscle level, the descending aorta is generally medial to the

center of the left ventricle; at the mitral valve level, it is more directly behind the left ventricle; at the left atrial level, it is slightly lateral or leftward in position; and at the pulmonary artery level, it lies beneath the arterial bifurcation.[125] The long-axis position of the descending aorta is also reported to vary when there is left atrial or left ventricular dilatation.[125] When the left atrium is enlarged, the descending aorta is typically displaced superiorly from its normal position behind the atrioventricular groove, whereas with left ventricular hypertrophy, the descending aorta is displaced inferiorly. These variations in relative positions do not represent movement of the aorta, but rather a shift in cardiac position relative to the aorta produced by the variation in chamber size. The normal descending thoracic aorta is smaller than the aortic root or ascending aorta. It has a reported mean diastolic diameter of 17 ± 3.3 mm in contrast to a mean diastolic diameter of 22 ± 4.0 mm for the ascending aorta. The descending aorta is reported to be larger than normal in patients with hypertension, aortic valve disease, and coronary atherosclerosis.[125] It is also enlarged in patients with thoracic aortic aneurysms.

An additional cause of dilatation of the descending thoracic aorta in the newborn is cerebral or hepatic arteriovenous malformations.[126] These arteriovenous connections increase venous return to the right side of the heart during intrauterine life. This increased flow is transmitted to the descending aorta via the ductus arteriosus, thereby causing the aortic dilatation. This aortic dilatation is commonly associated with four-chamber cardiac enlargement and congestive failure. The combination of features suggests the appropriate diagnosis. Figure 7–39 compares a normal descending thoracic aorta to a markedly dilated vessel.

An abnormally small descending thoracic aorta may be noted with aortic hypoplasia.[125]

The position of the descending thoracic aorta may also be useful in differentiating pleural from pericardial effusion because

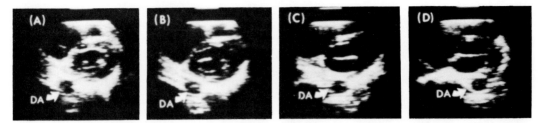

Fig. 7–38. Short-axis scans recorded as the transducer is swept from the left ventricle (A) to the aortic root (D). Because the aorta crosses obliquely beneath the left ventricle, its position shifts from left to right as the scan plane is moved superiorly. DA = descending aorta.

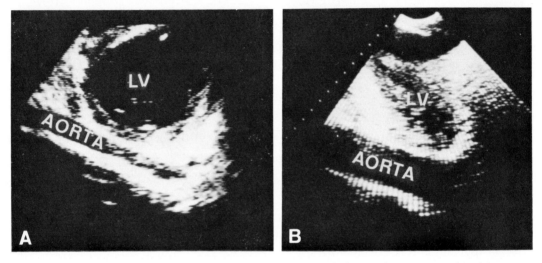

Fig. 7–39. Cross-scans of the descending thoracic aorta obtained with the transducer positioned on the anterior chest wall and the scan plane aligned parallel to the long axis of the thoracic vessel. A, A normal aorta. B, The thoracic vessel is dilated. In each case, the left ventricle (LV) is positioned anteriorly to the descending aorta.

pericardial effusion displaces the extra pericardial thoracic aorta posteriorly; whereas a pleural effusion should not change the position of the aorta relative to the left side of the heart.

The Abdominal Aorta

The abdominal aorta is readily examined throughout its course. Areas of aneurysmal dilatation, external compression, and abdominal coarctation can likewise be appreciated. This structure, however, is usually evaluated as part of an abdominal ultrasound examination rather than in conjunction with the echocardiographic examination and, therefore, is not considered further in this discussion.

THE SUBVALVULAR LEFT VENTRICULAR OUTFLOW TRACT

The subvalvular portion of the left ventricular outflow tract is a funnel-shaped area extending from the free edges of the mitral leaflets to the aortic annulus. It is bounded anteriorly by the interventricular septum and posteriorly by the anterior mitral leaflet. Disorders of primary interest in this region are those that obstruct left ventricular outflow. Such disorders can be divided both anatomically and functionally into the fixed anatomic obstructive lesions located immediately beneath the aortic valve, the discrete subaortic stenoses, and obstructive lesions occurring deeper in the left ventricle that typically have both an anatomic and functional component.

Discrete Subaortic Stenosis

Discrete subvalvular aortic stenosis is a relatively frequent cause of left ventricular outflow obstruction and accounts for approximately 10% of all cases of aortic stenosis in childhood.[127,128] This obstruction is generally produced by either a thin, discrete fibrous membrane located immediately beneath the aortic valve and obstructing an otherwise normal outflow tract (type 1) or a thick, fibrous ring associated with muscular hypertrophy and located approximately 1 cm below the valve and extending downward 1 to 2 cm (type 2).[129] The type 2 lesions not only produce a more diffuse area of left ventricular outflow obstruction, but also frequently encroach on the anterior mitral leaflet. A third variety, the fibromuscular tunnel, may narrow the outflow tract for several centimeters.[130,131] Subvalvular tunnels are relatively uncommon, representing only 6[120] to 20%[130] of fixed subvalvular obstructive lesions. The subvalvular tunnels, however, produce the greatest deformity of the outflow region.

Separation of the various types of subvalvular obstruction is important because, as a rule, simple surgical resection of the thin membrane relieves the obstruction in type 1 lesions, whereas fibromuscular rings and subvalvular tunnels require more extensive surgical revision of the outflow tract with frequent, residual obstruction.[129] Associated defects are common in the discrete subvalvular stenoses and are present in from 10[131] to 57% of reported cases.[130] The most common associated lesions are ventricular septal defects and associated areas of obstruction at other levels of the left ventricular outflow tract.[130]

Echocardiographically, discrete areas of subvalvular obstruction are optimally visualized in a parasternal long-axis view. When visualization of the lesion is difficult (particularly when a discrete membrane is suspected), the apical five-chamber view may be a useful adjunct because it places the membrane perpendicular to the path of the scan plane, thereby enhancing visualization. Short-axis scanning of the outflow tract in an attempt to directly record the decrease in outflow area has proved less useful because precise alignment of the short-axis scan plane across the area of maximal obstruction is difficult.

Discrete Membranous Subaortic Stenosis

Discrete subvalvular membranes appear echocardiographically as thin, linear bands of echoes protruding from both the anterior and posterior margins of the outflow tract immediately beneath the aortic valve.[7,132,133] The inner margins of the membrane are characteristically more highly reflective than the membrane itself. In the original cross-sectional description of discrete subvalvular membranes, only the linear echoes from these inner margins were noted and were felt to represent the characteristic feature of the subvalvular membrane.[132] With improvements in instrumentation, however, it has become possible to record the full extent of the membrane and to visualize its pattern of movement.

Figure 7–40 illustrates a thin, subvalvular membrane lying immediately beneath the aortic valve. The membrane extends downward into the outflow tract from the interventricular septum, partially obstructing the outflow area. In this systolic recording, the membrane domes or curves slightly toward the aortic valve. These membranes are generally mobile and move toward the aortic valve during systole and shift back into the left ventricle during diastole. When a membrane is present, the rest of the outflow tract is usually normal, and the subvalvular fibrous curtain, or separation between the insertion of the left and the noncoronary aortic leaflets and the anterior mitral leaflet, is not elongated.

Diffuse Fibromuscular Subvalvular Obstruction

Subvalvular fibromuscular collars or

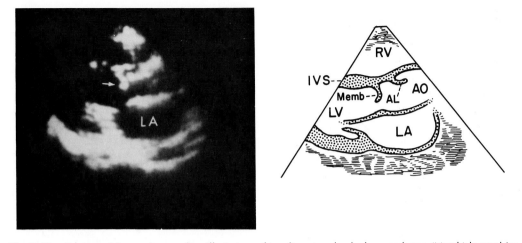

Fig. 7–40. Parasternal long-axis recording illustrates a thin, discrete subvalvular membrane (Memb) located immediately beneath the aortic valve. The membrane protrudes from the anterior margin of the outflow tract in the region of the membranous septum and partially obstructs an otherwise normal outflow space. In this systolic recording, the membrane appears to bow toward the aorta (AO). RV = right ventricle; IVS = interventricular septum; LV = left ventricle; AL = anterior leaflet; LA = left atrium.

tunnels produce a more extensive area of obstruction, which is characterized by an inward bowing of the echoes from the anterior and posterior margins of the outflow tract immediately beneath the aortic valve.[131] Both the anterior and posterior borders of the outflow tract must be deformed before this diagnosis can be considered. Focal areas of upper septal hypertrophy, which encroach on the anterior margin of the outflow tract, are common but are not, as a rule, obstructive. Obstructive lesions almost invariably involve the base of the anterior mitral leaflet as well as the upper septum. They elongate the subvalvular fibrous curtain and thereby increase the separation between the noncoronary and the left coronary aortic leaflets and the anterior mitral leaflet. The area of obstruction may extend for several centimeters, with increased narrowing of the outflow space being commonly noted as systole progresses. Figure 7–41 is an example of diffuse subvalvular obstruction. In this example, the area of obstruction is located approximately 1 cm below the aortic valve and extends downward roughly 1.5 cm. Other examples of sub-

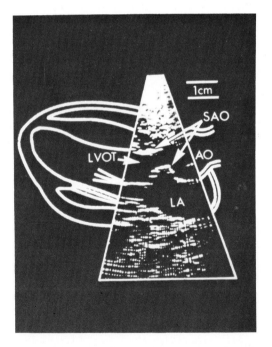

Fig. 7–41. Parasternal long-axis recording of the left ventricular outflow tract (LVOT) illustrates diffuse subvalvular aortic obstruction (SAO). In this example, the echoes from the interventricular septum and anterior mitral leaflet bow inward from the anterior and posterior margins of the outflow tract, producing an elongated area of outflow obstruction. AO = aorta; LA = left atrium.

valvular obstruction can be found in Chapter 13.

An additional type of outflow obstruction has been noted echocardiographically in one patient. In this example, illustrated in Figure 7–42, a narrow, shelf-like protrusion of the basal end of the muscular interventricular septum encroached on the outflow tract from above. A corresponding shelf-like bulge protruded anteriorly from the midportion of the anterior mitral leaflet. Although there was systolic anterior motion of this abnormal anterior mitral leaflet echo, the leaflet abnormality was also present during diastole, suggesting a fixed deformity of the valve associated with an additional functional obstructive component.

Postoperative Studies

After surgical intervention, the subvalvular left ventricular outflow tract generally remains abnormal.[134] Following membrane resection, residual fragments of the base of the membrane are often visible both anteriorly and posteriorly. These fragments may be isolated or superimposed on more diffuse areas of subvalvular narrowing and are commonly associated with a residual gradient. Figure 7–43 is a recording obtained following surgical resection of a subvalvular membrane. Both basal

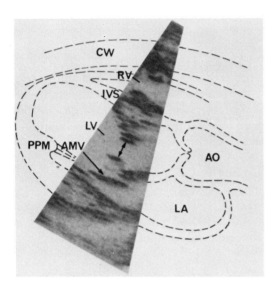

Fig. 7–42. Parasternal long-axis scan of the subvalvular left ventricular outflow tract illustrates a third type of fixed subvalvular obstruction. In this example, a prominent muscular shelf arises from the base of the interventricular septum (IVS) and is associated with a fixed deformity in the midportion of the anterior mitral leaflet. This type of obstruction can be distinguished from idiopathic hypertrophic subaortic stenosis (IHSS) because the anterior protrusion from the mitral valve (AMV) is present during both systole and diastole, whereas the functional obstruction of IHSS is noted only during the systolic phase of the cardiac cycle. CW = chest wall; RV = right ventricle; LV = left ventricle; PPM = posterior papillary muscle; AO = aorta; LA = left atrium. (From Weyman, AE, et al.: Cross-sectional echocardiography in evaluating patients with discrete subaortic stenosis. Am J Cardiol, 37:358, 1976.)

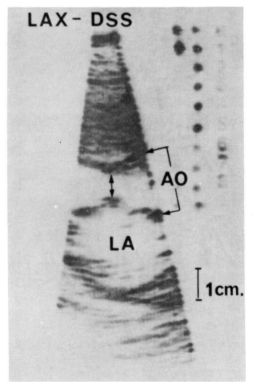

Fig. 7–43. Parasternal long-axis recording of the left ventricular outflow tract obtained following surgical resection of a subvalvular membrane. The basal remnants of the resected membrane and a more diffuse generalized narrowing of the outflow space are apparent. The area of peak narrowing is indicated by the vertical arrows. AO = aorta; LA = left atrium. (From Weyman, AE, et al.: Cross-sectional echocardiography in evaluating patients with discrete subaortic stenosis. Am J Cardiol, 37:358, 1976.)

remnants of the resected membrane and an associated area of more diffuse outflow tract narrowing are present.

With more extensive outflow obstruction, the residual postoperative deformity of the outflow tract is usually greater than that noted following simple membrane resection and, in some patients, little change may be seen from the preoperative study. Although experience with these lesions is not great, we have not observed any cases to date in which the outflow tract appeared totally normal following resection of a subvalvular lesion.

Functional Subvalvular Aortic Stenosis

The term, functional subvalvular aortic stenosis, encompasses a heterogeneous group of disorders with common features, including (1) anatomic narrowing of the left ventricular outflow tract in the region between the interventricular septum and the anterior mitral leaflet and (2) variable anterior systolic displacement of the mitral valve into this narrowed outflow space, producing outflow obstruction. Narrowing of the outflow tract is most commonly due to septal hypertrophy. The septal hypertrophy may be asymmetric (ASH), as in idiopathic hypertrophic subaortic stenosis (IHSS), or may be associated with hypertrophy of the remainder of the ventricle (concentric hypertrophy).

The functional component of this type of obstruction, systolic anterior motion of the mitral valve (SAM), has been postulated to occur through one of several mechanisms: (1) the anterior mitral leaflet might be drawn upward against the protruding interventricular septum by systolic contraction of the papillary muscles;[135–139] (2) the mitral valve leaflets could be pushed forward into the narrowed outflow tract from behind by hyperdynamic contraction of the left ventricular posterior wall;[140–143] or (3) the anterior mitral leaflet might be sucked into the outflow tract by the high-velocity stream of blood that is passing through the narrowed outflow space (the Venturi effect).[143,144]

Cross-sectional studies of the mitral valve in IHSS have excluded the first two mechanisms.[144,145] Thus, the systolic anterior motion of the mitral valve has been shown to develop at a right angle to a line drawn from the free edges of the mitral leaflets to the tips of the papillary muscles. This pattern indicates that the systolic anterior motion cannot be caused by abnormal papillary muscle contraction pulling the valve against the septum. In addition, the systolic anterior motion of the mitral valve has been shown to exceed the systolic excursion of the posterior left ventricular wall and, therefore, occurs independently of posterior wall motion. Consequently, the mitral valve cannot be pushed into the outflow tract by the contracting posterior wall.

Exclusion of these two possibilities has reinforced the hypothesis that the mitral valve is drawn into the outflow tract by Venturi forces acting on the anterior mitral leaflet which increase as flow velocity increases, and the space through which ejected blood must pass (the left ventricular outflow tract) becomes increasingly narrow.[144]

Given the high intracavitary pressures that may occur with this type of obstruction, one might question how the mitral leaflet can be drawn into the left ventricular cavity because, normally, the force of left ventricular pressure acts to hold the mitral leaflet in a posterior or closed position. Consideration of the effects of papillary muscle position and chordal tension on mitral leaflet closure (see Chap. 5, Papillary Muscle Dysfunction) may offer some insight into how this might occur. Specifically, in IHSS, the papillary muscles are displaced anteriorly and toward the center of the left ventricular cavity.[144,145] The mitral valve apparatus at the onset of systole has likewise been shown to be relatively anteriorly positioned in the ventricle, and the degree of anterior displacement has been related to the severity of obstruction.[144] Anterior displacement of the papillary muscles should decrease the relative tension on the chordae to the body of the anterior mitral leaflet. (This situation is the converse of that in papillary muscle dysfunction in which posterior displacement of the papillary muscles increases tension in this area.) This decrease in tension should be even more prominent when the distance from the papillary muscle tips to the leaflet is decreased by hypertrophy of the left ventricular myocardium at the base of the papillary muscles or by reduced cavity size.

Displacement of the papillary muscles toward the center of the left ventricular cavity should also increase tension at the margins of the leaflets in comparison to that exerted at their midportion. (This situation, again, is the exact opposite of that in papillary muscle dysfunction.) This combination of forces should produce redundancy or buckling in the midportion of the anterior mitral leaflet, thereby predisposing the leaflet to be drawn into the left ventricular outflow tract by a negative or sucking Venturi force acting on its ventricular surface or to be pushed anteriorly and superiorly by the stream of blood rushing through the outflow tract. If this combination of factors could result in anterior leaflet redundancy, it might also explain the frequently noted association between systolic anterior motion of the mitral valve and mitral valve prolapse.

Figure 7–44 is an example of SAM in a patient without ASH or outflow tract narrowing. In this and other examples of this type of SAM without ASH, the systolic anterior motion is confined to the midportion of the leaflet as might be anticipated from the preceding discussion.

Idiopathic Hypertrophic Subaortic Stenosis

Idiopathic hypertrophic subaortic stenosis is the classic and, by far, the most widely studied example of functional subvalvular aortic obstruction.[146–153] This familial disorder, transmitted in an autosomal dominant pattern,[154] is characterized by focal or asymmetric myocardial hypertrophy of unknown cause that preferentially involves the interventricular septum.[146,155–158,159] Histologically, the area of hypertrophy is composed of large numbers of bizarrely shaped, disorganized, cardiac muscle cells.[159–162] The hypertrophied segment typically encroaches on the left ventricular cavity and, when the septum is involved,[144] on the left ventricular outflow tract.[144] Obstruction, when present, is associated with systolic anterior motion of the mitral valve into the narrow outflow space.[163–166]

The two primary echocardiographic features of idiopathic hypertrophic subaortic stenosis (IHSS), asymmetric hypertrophy of the interventricular septum (ASH),[155,156,167,168] and systolic anterior motion of the mitral valve (SAM) are illustrated in Figure 7–45.[163–166] In addition, a variety of nonspecific abnormalities are frequently noted with IHSS, including anterior displacement of the mitral valve apparatus within the left ventricle,[144] a decrease in left ventricular cavity size,[144] an unusual reflective pattern from the area of hypertrophied myocardium,[169] left atrial enlargement, abnormal systolic motion of the aortic valve,[13,14] and a surprisingly high incidence of pericardial effusion.

Asymmetric septal hypertrophy (ASH), defined as an interventricular septal/free-wall ratio of 1.3 to 1 or greater, was initially felt to be so characteristic of IHSS that it could be used to identify not only affected patients but also asymptomatic carriers.[154–156] Subsequently, it has been shown that concentric left ventricular hypertrophy with symmetric thickening of the septum and free left ventricular wall may, on occasion, be seen in patients with IHSS, whereas disproportionate septal hypertrophy (DSH) may be found in a variety of congenital and acquired lesions in the

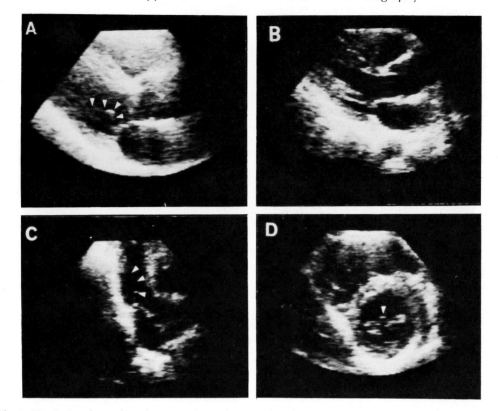

Fig. 7–44. Series of recordings from a patient with systolic anterior motion of the mitral valve without evidence of asymmetric septal hypertrophy or outflow obstruction. *A,* A parasternal long-axis recording obtained from the midportion of the left ventricle illustrates the systolic anterior motion (arrowheads). *B,* A recording from the same patient but with the transducer angled medially through the posterior-medial papillary muscle. With the scan plane shifted from the midportion of the mitral valve, systolic anterior motion is not noted. *C,* An apical long-axis view again illustrates the systolic anterior motion in the midportion of the valve. *D,* A parasternal short-axis recording that demonstrates how this abnormal motion pattern is clearly confined to the center of the mitral leaflet.

absence of hypertrophic cardiomyopathy.[153] Disproportionate septal hypertrophy appears to be a normal finding in the fetus and disappears by the age of 1 to 2 years. In the older child and adult, DSH may be seen with lesions producing long-standing right ventricular hypertension, such as valvular pulmonary stenosis and primary pulmonary hypertension. It may also be seen, albeit less frequently, in patients with combined aortic and mitral valve disease, Eisenmenger's syndrome, coronary artery disease, systemic hypertension, and a variety of other lesions.[153,170] Thus, although the reported specificity of ASH as an echocardiographic marker of IHSS remains high, in individual cases, one may not be able to discriminate reli-

ably between secondary disproportionate septal thickening (DSH) and a primary hypertrophic cardiomyopathy on the basis of simple echocardiographic measurement alone.[153] The distribution and extent of hypertrophy, however, may provide additional diagnostic information. Focal areas of marked hypertrophy within the septum and/or free wall are clearly more specific for a hypertrophic myopathy than is generalized septal thickening.

To date, studies indicate that the distribution of septal and ventricular hypertrophy may vary considerably in individual cases of hypertrophic myopathy. The focal hypertrophy is noted most frequently in the upper and middle portions of the septum. Hypertrophy of the lower third of the

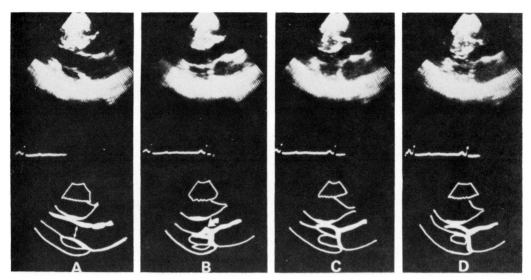

Fig. 7–45. Series of parasternal long-axis recordings illustrates the septal hypertrophy and systolic anterior motion of the mitral valve, which are characteristic of IHSS. *A,* An end-diastolic recording demonstrates the open mitral leaflets (arrowheads in the accompanying diagram). *B,* Recorded during early systole, this view illustrates the initial motion of the anterior mitral leaflet toward the septum. *C,* A midsystolic frame that illustrates more extensive motion of the mitral leaflet and chordal apparatus toward the septum. *D,* A late systolic image in which the systolic anterior motion (SAM) is fully developed. The mitral valve appears to press against the septum. (From Martin, RP, Rakowski, H, French, J, and Popp, RL: Idiopathic hypertrophic subaortic stenosis viewed by wide-angle phase array echocardiography. Circulation, 59:1206, 1979. Reproduced by permission of the American Heart Association.)

septum is less common.[169,171] Involvement of the anterolateral free wall of the ventricle is frequent.[171] Atypical patterns, such as concentric midventricular constricting rings and medial-lateral dumbell-like areas of hypertrophy, may also be noted, but the significance of individual patterns remains uncertain. In general, the more extensive the ventricular involvement, the more severe the functional impact and more marked the outflow obstruction. Upper septal hypertrophy, when combined with extensive hypertrophy elsewhere in the ventricle, for example, is associated with high gradients (greater than 60 mmHg), whereas isolated hypertrophy of the upper septum is of less clear significance and is usually associated with latent or no obstruction.

The area of focal hypertrophy frequently has a speckled or ground-glass-like reflective pattern that is distinct from that seen in uninvolved areas of the ventricle. A similar, but more diffuse, pattern is also encountered in infiltrative disorders, such as cardiac amyloid. This unusual reflection pattern may represent an echocardiographic expression of the abnormal cellular architecture.

The actual functional outflow obstruction of IHSS is produced by independent anterior displacement of the mitral valve (with the chordae tendinae) into the outflow tract. The severity of obstruction has been related to both the absolute reduction in outflow tract size and the degree and duration of systolic anterior mitral valve motion. An outflow tract diameter of less than 20 mm has been reported in as many as 66% of patients with obstructive IHSS, whereas such a reduction in outflow tract size was not observed in normal persons and occurred rarely in patients with non-obstructive hypertrophic myopathy.[144] The magnitude and duration of the systolic anterior motion has been demonstrated to correlate with the severity of the intraventricular gradient under both basal conditions and with provocative maneuvers.[166] The SAM also decreases or disappears following surgical intervention when the outflow gradient is abolished.[172,173] Figure 7–46 is an example of this abnormal systolic motion as it appears in the apical four-chamber view. In this patient with severe IHSS, the mitral leaflets swing medially against the septum during systolic contraction, totally filling the inferior portion of the outflow space.

In any consideration of the systolic motion of the mitral valve, one must remember that the coapted mitral leaflets are fixed at the papillary muscle level and at the mitral valve ring. During systole, therefore, the mitral apparatus normally moves anteriorly in unison with the anterior motion of the posterior left ventricular wall, annulus, and papillary muscles. Any phenomenon that exaggerates the normal systolic anterior motion of these points of mitral valve attachment, of necessity, increases the anterior motion of the coapted leaflets. It is not surprising, therefore, that increased systolic motion of the mitral apparatus has been described in conditions associated with exaggerated left ventricular posterior wall motion, such as left ventricular aneurysm, anterior wall myocardial infarction, and left ventricular volume overload.[153,174] This mitral valve motion is not, by itself, abnormal, but merely represents the obligatory anterior motion of the mitral apparatus in unison with the exaggerated movement of its points of attachment. Pericardial effusion

of at least moderate size may be seen in as many as one third of patients with IHSS. The reason for this high incidence of effusion is unclear, and it does not appear to have functional significance.

Other Causes of Functional Outflow Obstruction

Although, in the past, narrowing of the left ventricular outflow tract and systolic anterior motion of the mitral valve have been associated almost exclusively with IHSS, there is growing evidence that functional outflow obstruction may occur in a variety of less well-defined circumstances.[175–177] In a recent study, less than 28% of patients with echocardiographic evidence of ASH and SAM had true hypertrophic myopathy at autopsy. If the mechanism of outflow obstruction discussed earlier is correct, it might be anticipated that for any given ejection velocity, functional subvalvular obstruction would occur anytime the distance between the interventricular septum and the anterior mitral leaflet reached a critical point. This further assumes that there is sufficient flexibility of the mitral valve apparatus to permit the anterior leaflet to be drawn into the outflow tract. Given these relationships, any factor that increased ejection velocity, decreased the space between the anterior mitral leaflet and septum, or increased leaflet redundancy should increase the tendency for obstruction.

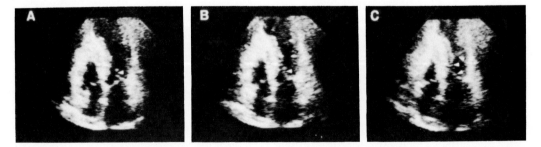

Fig. 7–46. Apical four-chamber view illustrates the evolution of the systolic anterior motion of IHSS in this projection. *A,* The initial coaptation of the mitral leaflets in the midportion of the annular plane. *B,* Recorded slightly later in the systolic period, the coapted leaflets have drifted toward the hypertrophied interventricular septum. *C,* The coapted leaflets fully abut the interventricular septum (horizontal arrows), completely filling the inferior portion of the outflow space.

Two clinical settings in which functional subvalvular obstruction often develops illustrate these points. The first is the elderly patient, usually a female with long-standing hypertension, who is admitted to the hospital with hypovolemia due to gastrointestinal bleeding or excessive diuresis. A harsh systolic murmur noted early in the hospital stay prompts an echocardiographic examination that typically reveals concentric left ventricular hypertrophy, a small left ventricular cavity, and systolic anterior motion of the mitral valve. With volume replacement and/or correction of anemia, the murmur disappears as does the echocardiographic SAM. The combination of anemia and hypovolemia in such persons presumably increases ejection velocity and decreases the outflow space, thereby producing obstruction.[176]

The second group of patients has fixed outflow obstruction at the subvalvular, valvular, or supravalvular level with secondary left ventricular hypertrophy. Following surgical relief of the outflow obstruction, these patients develop functional obstruction at the ventricular level, which is commonly transient. Relief of the fixed obstruction may allow ejection velocity to increase and, given the narrowed outflow space, functional subvalvular obstruction may result.

Functional subvalvular aortic stenosis, therefore, appears to develop in response to a series of geometric and hemodynamic alterations within the left ventricle and, as such, seems to be a functional derangement with multiple causes.

REFERENCES

1. Gray, H: Gray's Anatomy. Edited by CM Goss. Philadelphia, Lea & Febiger, 1959.
2. Seward, JB, and Tajik, AJ: Non-invasive visualization of the entire thoracic aorta: a new application of wide-angle two dimensional sector echocardiographic technique. Am J Cardiol, 43:387, 1979.
3. Bansal, RC, Tajik, AJ, Seward, JB, and Offord, RP: Feasibility of detailed two-dimensional echocardiographic examination in adults: prospective study of 200 patients. Mayo Clin Proc, 55:291, 1980.
4. Rushmer, RF: Cardiovascular Dynamics. Philadelphia, Saunders, 1970, p. 45.
5. Tajik, AJ, et al.: Two-dimensional real-time ultrasonic imaging of the heart and great vessels, technique, image orientation, structures identification and validation. Mayo Clin Proc, 53:271, 1978.
6. Weyman, AE, Feigenbaum, H, Dillon, JC, and Chang, S: Cross-sectional echocardiography in assessing the severity of valvular aortic stenosis. Circulation, 52:828, 1975.
7. Weyman, AE, et al.: Localization of left ventricular outflow obstruction by cross-sectional echocardiography. Am J Med, 60:33, 1976.
8. Lange, LW, Sahn, DJ, Allen, HD, and Goldberg, SJ: Subxyphoid cross-sectional echocardiography in infants and children with congenital heart disease. Circulation, 59:513, 1979.
9. Yeh, HC, Winsberg, F, and Mercer, EM: Echocardiographic aortic valve orifice dimension: its use in evaluating aortic stenosis and cardiac output. J Clin Ultrasound, 1:182, 1973.
10. Rasmussen, S, et al.: Forward stroke volume derived from aortic valve echograms. Clin Res, 27:672, 1979. (Abstract)
11. Davis, RA, et al.: Echocardiographic manifestations of discrete subaortic stenosis. Am J Cardiol, 33:277, 1974.
12. Laurenceau, JL, Guay, JM, and Gagne, S: Echocardiography in the diagnosis of subaortic membranous stenosis. Circulation (Suppl IV), 48:46, 1976. (Abstract)
13. Gramiak, R, Shah, PM, and Kramer, DH: Ultrasound cardiography: contrast studies in anatomy and function. Radiology, 92:939, 1969.
14. Feigenbaum, H: Clinical applications of echocardiography. Prog Cardiovasc Dis, 14:531, 1972.
15. Roberts, WC: Valvular, subvalvular and supravalvular aortic stenosis: morphologic features. Cardiovasc Clin, 5:97, 1973.
16. Friedberg, CW: Diseases of the Heart. Philadelphia, Saunders, 1966, p. 1129.
17. Roberts, WC: The congenitally bicuspid aortic valve. Am J Cardiol, 26:72, 1970.
18. DeMaria, AN, et al.: Value and limitations of cross-sectional echocardiography of the aortic valve in the diagnosis and quantification of valvular aortic stenosis. Circulation, 62:304, 1980.
19. Godley, RW, et al.: Reliability of two-dimensional echocardiography in assessing the severity of valvular aortic stenosis. Chest, 79:657, 1981.
20. Grossman, W (Ed): Cardiac Catheterization and Angiography. Philadelphia, Lea & Febiger, 1980.
21. Leo, LP, et al.: Determination of aortic valve area by cross-sectional echocardiography. Circulation, 60:203, 1979.
22. Bennett, DH, Evans, DW, and Raj, MVJ: Echocardiographic left ventricular dimensions in pressure and volume overload. Their use in assessing aortic stenosis. Br Heart J, 37:971, 1975.
23. Glanz, S, Hellenbrand, WE, Berman, MA, and

Talner, NS: Echocardiographic assessment of the severity of aortic stenosis in children and adolescents. Am J Cardiol, 38:620, 1976.

24. Johnson, GL, et al.: Echocardiographic evaluation of fixed left ventricular outlet obstruction in children. Pre- and postoperative assessment of ventricular systolic pressures. Circulation, 56:299, 1977.

25. Blackwood, AR, Bloom, KR, and Williams, CM: Aortic stenosis in children; experience with echocardiographic prediction of severity. Circulation, 57:263, 1978.

26. Azia, KU, Van Grondelle, A, Paul, MH, and Muster, AJ: Echocardiographic assessment of the relation between left ventricular wall and cavity dimensions and peak systolic pressure in children with aortic stenosis. Am J Cardiol, 40:775, 1977.

27. Schwartz, A, et al.: Echocardiographic estimation of aortic valve gradient in aortic stenosis. Ann Intern Med, 89:329, 1978.

28. Weyman, AE, et al.: Cross-sectional echocardiographic assessment of the severity of aortic stenosis in children. Circulation, 55:773, 1977.

29. Becu, LM, et al.: Anatomic and pathologic studies in ventricular septal defect. Circulation, 14:349, 1956.

30. Brown, OR, Harrison, DC, and Popp, RL: An improved method for echographic detection of left atrial enlargement. Circulation, 50:58, 1974.

31. Osler, W: The bicuspid condition of the aortic valve. Trans Assoc Am Physicians, 2:185, 1886.

32. Edwards, JE: The congenital bicuspid aortic valve. Circulation, 23:485, 1961.

33. Lewis, T, and Grant, RT: Observations relating to subacute infective endocarditis. Heart, 10:21, 1923.

34. Grant, RT, Wood, JE, and Jones, TD: Heart valve irregularities in relation to subacute bacterial endocarditis. Heart, 14:247, 1928.

35. Fulton, MN, and Levine, SA: Subacute bacterial endocarditis with special reference to the valvular lesions and previous history. Am J Med Sci, 183:60, 1932.

36. Bayles, TB, and Lewis, WH: Subacute bacterial endocarditis in older people. Ann Intern Med, 13:2154, 1940.

37. Fowles, RE, et al.: Two-dimensional echocardiographic features of bicuspid aortic valve. Chest, 75:434, 1979.

38. Nanda, NC, and Gramiak, R: Evaluation of bicuspid valves by two-dimenstional echocardiography. Am J Cardiol, 11:372, 1978.

39. Nanda, NC, et al.: Echocardiographic recognition of the congenital bicuspid aortic valve. Circulation, 49:870, 1974.

40. Radford, DJ, et al.: Echocardiographic assessment of bicuspid aortic valves. Angiographic and pathological correlates. Circulation, 53:80, 1976.

41. Stapleton, JF, and Harvey, WP: A clinical analysis of aortic incompetence. Postgrad Med, 46:156, 1969.

42. Carter, JB, Sethi, S, Lee, GB, and Edwards, JE:

Prolapse of semilunar cusps as causes of aortic insufficiency. Circulation, 43:922, 1971.

43. Frahm, CJ, Braunwald, E, and Morrow, AG: Congenital aortic regurgitation, clinical and hemodynamic findings in four patients. Am J Med, 31:63, 1961.

44. Braunwald, E: Heart Disease: A Textbook of Cardiovascular Medicine. Philadelphia, Saunders, 1980.

45. McDonald, IF: Echocardiographic assessment of left ventricular function in aortic valve disease. Circulation, 53:860, 1976.

46. Gaasch, WH, Andrias, WC, and Levine, HJ: Chronic aortic regurgitation. The effect of aortic valve replacement on left ventricular mass and function. Circulation, 58:825, 1978.

47. Henry, WL, et al.: Observations on the optimum time for operative intervention for aortic regurgitation. I: Evaluation of the results of aortic valve replacement in symptomatic patients. Circulation, 61:471, 1980.

48. Dillon, JC, et al.: Significance of mitral fluttering in patients with aortic insufficiency. Clin Res, 18:304, 1970. (Abstract)

49. Joyner, CR, Dyrda, I, and Reid, JM: Behavior of the anterior leaflet of the mitral valve in patients with the Austin-Flint murmur. Clin Res, 14:251, 1966. (Abstract)

50. Winsberg, F, Gabor, GE, and Hernberg, JG: Fluttering of the mitral valve in aortic insufficiency. Circulation, 41:225, 1970. (Abstract)

51. Cope, GD, Kisslo, JA, Johnson, ML, and Myers, S: Diastolic vibration of the interventricular septum in aortic insufficiency. Circulation, 51:589, 1975.

52. Friedewald, VE, Futral, JE, Kinard, SA, and Phillips, B: Oscillations of the interventricular septum in aortic insufficiency. J Clin Ultrasound, 2:229, 1974. (Abstract)

53. Friedberg, CW: Diseases of the Heart. Philadelphia, Saunders, 1966, p. 1103.

54. Lepeschkin, E: On the relation between the site of valvular involvement in endocarditis and the blood pressure resting on the valve. Am J Med Sci, 224:318, 1952.

55. Watanakunakorn, C: Changing epidemiology and newer aspects of infective endocarditis. Adv Intern Med, 22:21, 1977.

56. Pelletier, LLJ, and Petersdorf, RG: Infective endocarditis: a review of 125 cases from the University of Washington hospitals, 1963–72. Medicine, 56:287, 1977.

57. Richardson, JV, Karp, RB, Kirklin, JW, and Dismulses, WE: Treatment of infective endocarditis: A 10-year comparative analysis. Circulation, 58:589, 1978.

58. Boyd, AD, et al.: Infective endocarditis, an analysis of 54 surgically treated patients. J Thorac Cardiovasc Surg, 73:23, 1977.

59. Lerner, PJ, and Weinstein, L: Infective endocarditis in the antibiotic era. N Engl J Med, 274:199, 259, 323, 387, 1966.

60. Kelson, SR, and White, PD: Notes on 250 cases of subacute bacterial (streptococcal) endocar-

ditis studied and treated between 1927 and 1939. Ann Intern Med, 22:40, 1940.

61. Braunwald, E: Heart Disease: A Textbook of Cardiovascular Medicine. Philadelphia, Saunders, 1980.
62. Dillon, JC, et al.: Echocardiographic manifestations of valvular vegetations. Am Heart J, 86:698, 1973.
63. Wann, LS, Dillon, JC, Weyman, AE, and Feigenbaum, H: Echocardiography in bacterial endocarditis. N Engl J Med, 295:135, 1976.
64. Gilbert, BW, et al.: Two-dimensional echocardiographic assessment of vegetative endocarditis. Circulation, 55:346, 1977.
65. Gregoratos, G, and Karliner, JS: Infective endocarditis diagnosis and management. Med Clin North Am, 63:173, 1979.
66. Stafford, A, et al.: Serial echocardiographic appearance of healing bacterial vegetations. Am J Cardiol, 44:754, 1979.
67. Mintz, GS, Kotler, MN, Segal, BL, and Parry, WR: Comparison of two-dimensional and M-mode echocardiography in the evaluation of patients with infective endocarditis. J Cardiol, 43:738, 1979.
68. Wray, TM: Echocardiographic manifestations of flail aortic valve leaflets in bacterial endocarditis. Circulation, 51:832, 1975.
69. Winsberg, F: Aortic valve. In Cardiac Ultrasound. Edited by R Gramiak, and RC Waag. St. Louis, CV Mosby, 1975.
70. Pridie, RB, Beham, R, and Oakley, CM: Echocardiography of the mitral valve in aortic valve disease. Br Heart J, 33:296, 1971.
71. Botvinick, EH, et al.: Echocardiographic demonstration of early mitral valve closure in severe aortic insufficiency. Its clinical implications. Circulation, 51:836, 1975.
72. Mann, T, McLaurin, L, Grossman, W, and Craige, E: Assessing the hemodynamic severity of acute aortic regurgitation due to infective endocarditis. N Engl J Med, 293:108, 1975.
73. Wann, LS, et al.: Comparison of M-mode and cross-sectional echocardiography in infective endocarditis. Circulation, 60:728, 1979.
74. Mardelli, TJ, et al.: Cross-sectional echocardiographic identification of aortic valve prolapse. Circulation (Suppl II), 60:204, 1979. (Abstract).
75. Rushmer, RF: Cardiovascular Diagnosis. Philadelphia, Saunders, 1970, p. 13.
76. Weiss, L, and Greep, R: Histology. New York, McGraw-Hill, 1977.
77. Quinquera, L, Carneiro, J, and Contopoulos, A: Basic Histology. Los Altos, Lange Medical Publications, 1977.
78. Weyman, AE, et al.: Cross-sectional echocardiographic characterization of aortic obstruction. I. Supravalvular aortic stenosis and aortic hypoplasia. Circulation, 57:491, 1978.
79. Peterson, TA, Todd, B, and Edwards, JE: Supravalvular aortic stenosis. J Thorac Cardiovasc Surg, 50:734, 1968.
80. Denie, JJ, and Verleugt, AP: Supravalvular aortic stenosis. Circulation, 18:902, 1958.

81. Morrow, AG, et al.: Supravalvular aortic stenosis. Circulation, 20:1003, 1959.
82. Keith, JD, Rowe, RD, and Vlad, P: Heart Disease in Infancy and Childhood. New York, Macmillan, 1978.
83. Beureu, AJ, Apitz, J, and Ronceg, J: Die Diagnose und Beurteilung der Verschiedenen Formen der Supravalvularen Aortenstenose. Zeitschrift fuer Kreislaufforschung, 51:829, 1962.
84. Hancock, EW: Differentiation of valvar, subvalvar and supravalvar aortic stenosis. Guys Hosp Rep, 110:1, 1961.
85. Williams, JC, Barratt-Boyes, BG, and Lowe, JB: Supravalvular aortic stenosis. Circulation, 24:1311, 1961.
86. Beuren, AH, et al.: The syndrome of supravalvular aortic stenosis, peripheral pulmonary stenosis, mental retardation, and similar facial appearance. Am J Cardiol, 13:471, 1964.
87. Black, JA, and Bonham-Carter, RE: Association between aortic stenosis and facies of severe infantile hypercalcemia. Lancet, 2:745, 1963.
88. Garcia, RE, Friedman, WF, Kaback, MM, and Rowe, RD: Idiopathic hypercalcemia in supravalvular aortic stenosis: documentation of a new syndrome. N Engl J Med, 271:117, 1964.
89. McCue, CM, Spicuzza, TT, Robinson, LW, and Mauck, HP: Familial supravalvular aortic stenosis. J Pediatr, 73:889, 1968.
90. Wooley, CF, et al.: Supravalvular aortic stenosis. Clinical experience with four patients including familial occurrence. Am J Med, 31:717, 1961.
91. Friedberg, CW: Diseases of the Heart. Philadelphia, Saunders, 1966, p. 1434.
92. Hopps, HC: Principles of Pathology. New York, Appleton-Century Crofts, 1959.
93. Edwards, JE, and Burchell, HB: The pathologic anatomy of deficiencies between the aortic root and the heart including aortic sinus aneurysms. Thorax, 12:125, 1957.
94. Sawyers, JL, Adams, JE, and Scott, HW: Surgical treatment for aneurysms of the aortic sinuses with aorticoatrial fistula. Surgery, 41:26, 1957.
95. Sakakibara, S, and Konno, S: Congenital aneurysms of the sinus of Valsalva: anatomy and classification. Am Heart J, 63:405, 1962.
96. Kerber, RE, et al.: Unruptured aneurysm of the sinus of Valsalva producing right ventricular outflow obstruction. Am J Med, 53:775, 1972.
97. Onat, A, Ersanli, O, Kanuni, A, and Aykan, TB: Congenital aortic sinus aneurysms with particular reference to dissection of the interventricular septum. Am Heart J, 72:158, 1966.
98. Davidson, HG, Tabricium, J, and Husfeldt, E: Five cases of congenital aneurysm of the aortic sinuses of Valsalva and notes of the prognosis. Acta Med Scand, 160:455, 1968.
99. Falholt, W, and Thomson, G: Congenital aneurysm of the right sinus of Valsalva diagnosed by aortography. Circulation, 8:549, 1953.
100. London, SB, and London, RE: Production of aortic regurgitation by unperforated aneurysm

of the sinus of Valsalva. Circulation, *24*:1403, 1961.

101. Rothbaum, DA, Dillon, JC, Chang, S, and Feigenbaum, H: Echocardiographic manifestation of right sinus of Valsalva aneurysm. Circulation, *49*:768, 1974.

102. Weyman, AE, Dillon, JC, Feigenbaum, H, and Chang, S: Premature pulmonic valve opening following sinus of Valsalva aneurysm rupture into the right atrium. Circulation, *51*:556, 1975.

103. McKusick, VA: Heritable Disorders of Connective Tissue. 4th Ed. St. Louis, CV Mosby, 1972.

104. Hirst, AE, and Gore, I: Marfan's syndrome: a review. Prog Cardiovasc Dis, 16:187, 1973.

105. Phorphutkul, C, Rosenthal, A, and Nadas, AS: Cardiac manifestations of Marfan's syndrome in infancy and childhood. Circulation, 47:587, 1973.

106. Bowers, D: Pathogenesis of primary abnormalities of the mitral valve in the Marfan's syndrome. Br Heart J, *31*:679, 1969.

107. Murdoch, JL, et al.: Life expectancy and causes of death in the Marfan's syndrome. N Engl J Med, 286:804, 1972.

108. DeMaria, AN, et al.: Identification and localization of aneurysms of the ascending aorta by cross-sectional echocardiography. Circulation, 59:755, 1979.

109. Hirst, AE, Johns, VJ, and Kime, SE: Dissecting aneurysm of the aorta: a review of 505 cases. Medicine, 37:217, 1958.

110. Braunstein, H: Pathogenesis of dissecting aneurysm. Circulation, 28:1071, 1963.

111. Weyman, AE, et al.: Cross-sectional echocardiographic detection of aortic obstruction II. Circulation, *57*:498, 1978.

112. Shan, DJ, Allen, HD, McDonald, G, and Goldberg, SJ: Real-time cross-sectional echocardiographic diagnosis of coarctation of the aorta: a prospective study of echocardiographic angiographic correlations. Circulation, 56:762, 1977.

113. Goldberg, BB: Suprasternal ultrasonography. JAMA, *215*:245, 1971.

114. Goldberg, BB: Ultrasonic measurement of the aortic arch, right pulmonary artery and left atrium. Radiology, *1*:383, 1971.

115. Allen, HD, and Goldberg, SJ: Usefulness of left atrial dimension measurement by echocardiography. Ultrasound, *2*:222, 1974.

116. Edwards, JE, Casey, IS, Neufeld, HN, and Lester, RG: Congenital Heart Disease. Philadelphia, Saunders, 1965.

117. Bahnson, HT, Cooley, RN, and Sloan, RD: Coarctation of the aorta at unusual sites. Am Heart J, *38*:905, 1949.

118. Elliot, LP, and Schiebler, GL: X-ray Diagnosis of Congenital Cardiac Diseases. Springfield, Charles C Thomas, 1968.

119. Keith, JD, Rowe, RD, and Vlad, P: Heart disease in infancy and childhood. New York, Macmillan, 1978.

120. Friedberg, CW: Diseases of the Heart. Philadelphia, Saunders, 1966.

121. Parmley, LF, Mattingly, TW, Manrun, WC, and Jahnke, EJ: Non-penetrating traumatic injury of the aorta. Circulation, *17*:1086, 1958.

122. DeBakey, ME, et al.: Surgical management of dissecting aneurysms of the aorta. J Thorac Cardiovasc Surg, 49:130, 1965.

123. Sethi, GF, Hughes, RK, and Takaro, T: Dissecting aortic aneurysms. Am J Thoracic Surgery, 18:201, 1974.

124. Seward, JB, and Tajik, AJ: Non-invasive visualization of the entire thoracic aorta: a new application of wide-angle two-dimensional sector echocardiographic technique. Am J Cardiol, 43:387, 1979.

125. Mintz, GS, Kotler, MN, Segal, BL, and Parry, WR: Two-dimensional echocardiographic recognition of the descending thoracic aorta. Am J Cardiol, 44:232, 1979.

126. Sapire, PW, et al.: Dilatation of the descending aorta: a radiologic and echocardiographic diagnostic sign in arteriovenous malformations in neonates and young infants. Am J Cardiol, 44:493, 1979.

127. Braunwald, E, et al.: Congenital aortic stenosis. I. Clinical and hemodynamic findings in 100 patients. Circulation, *27*:426, 1963.

128. Campbell, M: The natural history of congenital aortic stenosis. Br Heart J, *30*:514, 1968.

129. Kelly, DT, Wulfsberg, E, and Rowe, RD: Discrete subaortic stenosis. Circulation, 46:309, 1972.

130. Newfeld, EA, et al.: Discrete subvalvular aortic stenosis in childhood. Study of 51 patients. Am J Cardiol, 38:53, 1976.

131. Reis, RL, et al.: Congenital fixed subvalvular aortic stenosis: an anatomic classification and correlations with operative results. Circulation, (Suppl I), 43:1, 1971.

132. Weyman, AE, et al.: Cross-sectional echocardiography in evaluating patients with discrete subaortic stenosis. Am J Cardiol, 37:358, 1976.

133. Williams, DE, Sahn, DJ, and Friedman, WF: Cross-sectional echocardiographic localization of sites of left ventricular outflow obstruction. Am J Cardiol, 37:250, 1976.

134. Shariatzadel, AN, King, H, Girod, D, and Shumacker, HB: Discrete subaortic stenosis. A report of 20 cases. J Thorac Cardiovasc Surg, 63:258, 1972.

135. Dinsmore, RE, Sanders, CA, and Harthorne, JW: Mitral regurgitation in idiopathic hypertrophic subaortic stenosis. N Engl J Med, *275*:1225, 1966.

136. Simon, AL, Ross, J, and Gault, JH: Angiographic anatomy of the left ventricle and mitral valve in idiopathic hypertrophic subaortic stenosis. Circulation, 36:852, 1967.

137. Roberts, WC: Valvular, subvalvular, and supravalvular aortic stenosis: morphologic features. Cardiovasc Clin, 5:98, 1973.

138. King, JF, et al.: Superior-to-inferior septal hypertrophy in IHSS: the fundamental determinant of obstruction. Circulation (Suppl IV), 48:6, 1973. (Abstract)

139. Reis, RL, et al.: Anterior-superior displacement of anterior papillary muscle (APM) producing obstruction and mitral regurgitation in IHSS:

operative relief by posterior-medial realignment of APM following ventricular septal myectomy. Circulation (Suppl II), 50:181, 1974.

140. Criley, JM, Lennon, PA, Basi, AS, and Blaufuss, AH: Hypertrophic cardiomyopathy. *In* Clinical Cardiovascular Physiology. Edited by HJ Levine. New York, Grune and Stratton, 1976.

141. Criley, JM, Lewis, KB, White, RI, and Ross, RS: Pressure gradients without obstruction. A new concept of "hypertrophic subaortic stenosis." Circulation, 32:881, 1965.

142. White, RI, Criley, JM, Lewis, KB, and Ross, RS: Experimental production of intracavitary pressure differences. Possible significance in the interpretation of human hemodynamic studies. Am J Cardiol, 19:806, 1967.

143. Wigle, ED, Adelman, AG, and Silver, MD: Pathophysiological considerations in muscular subaortic stenosis. *In* Hypertrophic Obstructive Cardiomyopathy. Edited by GEW Wolstenholme, M O'Connor. London, Churchill, 1971.

144. Henry, WL, Clark, CE, Griffith, JM, and Epstein, SE: Mechanism of left ventricular outflow obstruction in patients with obstructive asymmetric septal hypertrophy (idiopathic hypertrophic subaortic stenosis). Am J Cardiol, 35:337, 1975.

145. Martin, RP, Rakowski, H, French, J, and Popp, RL: Idiopathic hypertrophic subaortic stenosis viewed by wide-angle, phased array echocardiography. Circulation, 59:1206, 1979.

146. Teare, D: Asymmetrical hypertrophy of the heart in young patients. Br Heart J, 20:1, 1958.

147. Braunwald, E, et al.: Idiopathic hypertrophic subaortic stenosis. Clinical, hemodynamic and angiographic manifestations. Am J Med, 29:924, 1960.

148. Goodwin, JF, Hollman, A, Cleland, WP, and Teare, RD: Obstructive cardiomyopathy simulating aortic stenosis. Br Heart J, 22:403, 1960.

149. Braunwald, E, et al.: Idiopathic hypertrophic subaortic stenosis. I. A description of the disease based upon an analysis of 64 patients. Circulation (Suppl IV), 30:3, 1964.

150. Ross, J, et al.: The mechanism of the intraventricular pressure gradient in idiopathic hypertrophic subaortic stenosis. Circulation, 34:558, 1966.

151. Braunwald, E, Brockenbrough, EC, Morrow, AG: Hypertrophic subaortic stenosis—a broadened concept. Circulation, 26:161, 1962.

152. Cohen, J, et al.: Hypertrophic obstructive cardiomyopathy. Br Heart J, 26:16, 1964.

153. Mason, BJ, and Epstein, SE: Hypertrophic cardiomyopathy. Am J Cardiol, 45:141, 1980.

154. Clark, CE, Henry, WL, and Epstein, SE: Familial prevalence and genetic transmission of idiopathic hypertrophic subaortic stenosis. N Engl J Med, 289:709, 1973.

155. Henry, WL, Clark, CE, and Epstein, SE: Asymmetric septal hypertrophy (ASH): echocardiographic identification of the pathognomonic anatomic abnormality of IHSS. Circulation, 47:225, 1973.

156. Epstein, SE, et al.: Asymmetric septal hypertrophy. Ann Intern Med, 81:650, 1974.

157. Menges, H, Brandenburg, RO, and Brown, AL: The clinical, hemodynamic and pathologic diagnosis of muscular subvalvular aortic stenosis. Circulation, 24:1126, 1961.

158. Roberts, WC: Valvular, subvalvular and supravalvular aortic stenosis: morphologic features. Cardiovasc Clin, 5:104, 1973.

159. VanNoorden, S, Olsen, EG, and Pearse, AG: Hypertrophic obstructive cardiomyopathy. A histological, histochemical and ultrastructural study of biopsy material. Cardiovasc Res, 5:118, 1971.

160. Ferrans, VJ, Morrow, AG, and Roberts, WC: Myocardial ultrastructure in idiopathic hypertrophic subaortic stenosis. A study of operatively excised left ventricular outflow tract muscle in 14 patients. Circulation, 45:769, 1972.

161. Maron, BJ, and Roberts, WC: Quantitative analysis of cardiac muscle cell disorganization in the ventricular septum of patients with hypertrophic cardiomyopathy. Circulation, 59:689, 1979.

162. Maron, BJ, et al.: Quantitative analysis of cardiac muscle cell disorganization in the ventricular septum: comparison of fetuses and infants with and without congenital heart disease and patients with hypertrophic cardiomyopathy. Circulation, 60:685, 1979.

163. Shah, PM, Gramiak, R, and Kramer, DH: Ultrasound location of left ventricular outflow obstruction in hypertrophic obstructive cardiomyopathy. Circulation, 40:3, 1969.

164. Popp, RL, and Harrison, DC: Ultrasound in the diagnosis and evaluation of therapy in idiopathic hypertrophic subaortic stenosis. Circulation, 40:905, 1969.

165. Shah, PM, Gramiak, R, Adelman, AG, and Wigle, ED: Role of echocardiography in diagnostic and hemodynamic assessment of hypertrophic subaortic stenosis. Circulation, 44:891, 1971.

166. Henry, WL, Clark, CE, Glancy, DL, and Epstein, SE: Echocardiographic measurement of the left ventricular outflow gradient in idiopathic hypertrophic subaortic stenosis. N Engl J Med, 288:989, 1973.

167. Abbasi, AS, MacAlpin, RN, Eber, LM, and Pearce, ML: Echocardiographic diagnosis of idiopathic hypertrophic cardiomyopathy without outflow obstruction. Circulation, 46:897, 1972.

168. Abbasi, AS, MacAlpin, RN, Eber, LM, and Pearce, ML: Left ventricular hypertrophy diagnosed by echocardiography. N Engl J Med, 289:118, 1973.

169. Martin, RP, Rakowski, H, French, J, and Popp, RL: Idiopathic hypertrophic subaortic stenosis viewed by wide-angle, phased-array echocardiography. Circulation, 59:1206, 1979.

170. Maron, BJ, et al.: Prevalence and characteristics of disproportionate ventricular septal thickening in patients with acquired or congenital heart disease: echocardiographic and morphologic findings. Circulation, 55:489, 1977.

171. Tajik, AJ, Seward, JB, and Hagler, DJ: Detailed analysis of hypertrophic obstructive cardiomyopathy by wide-angle two dimensional sector echocardiography. Am J Cardiol, 43:348, 1979. (Abstract)

172. Shah, PM, Gramiak, R, Adelman, AG, and Wigle, ED: Echocardiographic assessment of the effects of surgery and propranolol on the dynamics of outflow obstruction in hypertrophic subaortic stenosis. Circulation, 45:516, 1972.

173. Bolton, MR, et al.: The effects of operation on the echocardiographic features of idiopathic hypertrophic subaortic stenosis. Circulation, 50:897, 1974.

174. Greenwald, J, Yap, JF, Franklin, M, and Lichtman, AM: Echocardiographic mitral systolic motion in left ventricular aneurysm. Br Heart J, 37:684, 1975.

175. Boughner, DR, Rakowski, HE, and Wigle, D: Mitral valve systolic anterior motion in the absence of hypertrophic cardiomyopathy. Circulation, 57, 58 (Suppl. II):235, 1978.

176. Levisman, JA: Systolic anterior motion of the mitral valve due to hypovolemia and anemia. Chest, 70:687, 1976.

177. Wei, JY, Weiss, JL, and Bulkley, BH: The heterogeneity of hypertrophic cardiomyoathy. An autopsy and one-dimensional echocardiographic study. Am J Cardiol, 45:24, 1980.

Chapter 8

Left Ventricle

Arthur E. Weyman and W. Daniel Doty

The primary function of the heart is to provide the energy necessary to propel blood through the vascular channels of the body to supply oxygen and metabolites to tissues and to remove the waste products of cellular metabolism.[1] Rhythmic contraction of the muscular left ventricle creates the force needed to overcome systemic vascular resistance and to initiate and maintain this circulation of blood.[2] An assessment of left ventricular function is, therefore, of primary importance in the overall evaluation of any patient with cardiac disease. This functional assessment further represents one of the major challenges of cross-sectional echocardiography because it requires greater quantitative accuracy than does any other application of this imaging format.

Anatomically, the left ventricle is a thick-walled, bullet-shaped chamber with a large, roughly cylindric base and a smaller, cone-shaped apical cap.[2,3] In cross section, the ventricle has a nearly circular configuration that increases in area from apex to base.[2,3]

The left ventricle is positioned obliquely in the chest such that its apex points to the left, inferiorly and anteriorly. It lies posterior and to the left of the right ventricle and inferior and anterior to the left atrium. The anteromedial portion of the left ventricle is formed by the triangular interventricular septum, which is shared with the right ventricle. The remainder of the ventricular wall is not in contact with any other cardiac chamber and is, therefore, termed the free wall.[3]

The left ventricle has a number of important internal and external anatomic features or landmarks that serve as references for locating the scan plane during cross-sectional imaging and permit the division of the chamber into specific regions of interest. The major internal landmarks include the mitral valve, the papillary muscles and the apical tip.

The mitral valve divides the ventricle at its base into an anterior outflow and a posterior inflow region. It also forms a reference for determining the position of the ventricular long axis and the anteroposterior minor dimension. In short axis, the plane of the mitral commissures can be

267

used to define the orientation of orthogonal minor diameters and to align radial coordinate systems.

The two large papillary muscles arise from the anterolateral and posteromedial left ventricular free walls inferior to the medial and lateral mitral commissures. They are positioned such that a line joining their tips parallels a similar line connecting the mitral commissures. The mitral valve and papillary muscles, therefore, combine to provide a constant spatial reference at two separate levels within the ventricle.

The left ventricular apex is a particularly important landmark because it represents the most clearly defined intercept of the left ventricular long axis and forms the reference for transducer placement in each apical view.

The primary external landmarks are the anterior and posterior junctions of the right and left ventricular free walls. These points define the boundaries of the interventricular septum and the paths of the left anterior descending and posterior descending coronary arteries.[3]

The muscular walls that surround the left ventricle are between 9 and 12 mm thick or approximately 3 times as thick as those of the right ventricle.[2,3] These walls are composed of sheets of muscle fibers, which encircle the ventricular cavity like the windings of a turban.[4-6] Contraction of these muscular sheets decreases both the radius of the cylindric portion of the ventricle and the ventricular long axis. The major power and volume of ejection, however, are produced by contraction of the circumferentially oriented muscle bundles because the volume of a cylinder decreases with the square of its radius. Long-axis shortening is less effective in ejecting blood because volume displacement is only in direct proportion to change in length.[2]

The inner surface of the ventricle is lined by multiple small muscular bands—the trabeculae carneae.[2,3] Although they do not contribute directly to tension development, the trabeculae represent preformed wrinkles in the ventricular wall that provide a template for further endocardial infolding during ventricular contraction. They also displace volume and permit more complete systolic emptying than would be possible if the inner walls of the ventricle were smooth.[2]

GENERAL PRINCIPLES OF ECHOCARDIOGRAPHIC IMAGING PERTINENT TO THE LEFT VENTRICULAR EXAMINATION

A number of basic principles of ultrasonic imaging should be considered when attempting to record, interpret, or quantitate cross-sectional images of the left ventricle. First, remember that, in any evaluation of the left ventricle, the structures of primary interest are the endocardial and epicardial interfaces. The endocardial interface is the most important of the two because the area encompassed within the boundaries of the endocardium corresponds to the left ventricular blood pool and, hence, the chamber volume. Endocardial motion, likewise, is the primary determinant of volume change and, hence, overall ventricular function. Neither the structure nor the function of the ventricle can be evaluated unless the endocardium is well visualized.

The epicardial interface, in contrast, encompasses both the intracardiac blood pool and the ventricular musculature. By itself, the epicardial interface provides little information about the relative magnitude or the functional integrity of the muscle contained within its boundaries. From an echocardiographic standpoint, the epicardial interface serves primarily as a reference in determining wall thickness, systolic thickening, and ventricular muscle mass.

Ideally, both the endocardium and epicardium should be visualized in their entirety throughout the cardiac cycle, and point targets along their surfaces should be recorded accurately and uniformly. Unfortunately, the closed-loop configuration of these interfaces results in only a small portion being aligned perpendicular to the path of the scan plane in the majority of the standard views. The ability to record individual segments of these interfaces, therefore, varies with the difference in the acoustic impedance of the tissues that form the interface, their orientation in the scan plane, and their surface characteristics.[7] When the interfaces are perpendicular to the path of the scan plane, as occurs in the parasternal and subcostal long-axis views, the primary determinant of reflectivity is the difference in acoustic density of the tissues that border the interface. Because the difference in acoustic impedance between lung and heart muscle is greater than that between heart muscle and intracavitary blood, the reflectivity of the posterior-wall epicardium is greater than that of any of the internal borders of the ventricle.[7] The anterior right ventricular epicardium, in contrast, abuts the soft tissue of the anterior chest wall, which differs little from the right ventricular epicardium in acoustic impedance. As a result, the right ventricular epicardium is the most difficult surface to visualize.

When the interfaces are oblique or parallel to the path of the scan plane, their spatial orientation and surface characteristics play a more important role in determining their reflectivity. Figure 8–1 illustrates the relationship of the endocardial and epicardial interfaces of the left ventricle to the scan plane in a representative short-axis view. If the chamber were smooth walled (Fig. 8–1, A), only a small portion of the anterior segment of each surface and a slightly larger portion of the posterior segment would be visualized. This problem is even more marked in the apical views, where only the apical tip is perpendicular to the ultrasonic beam. Fortunately, the endocardial surface is irregular, and such rough surfaces scatter a por-

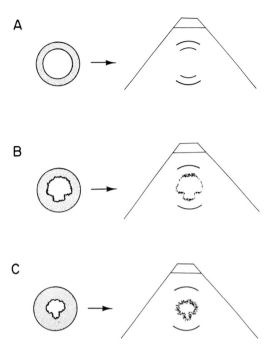

Fig. 8–1. Series of diagrams illustrates the relationship of the left ventricular endocardial and epicardial interfaces to the path of the ultrasonic scan plane in the short-axis projection. *A,* Reflections that would arise from a smooth-walled chamber. *B,* Change in the reflective pattern occurs when the interface is irregular. *C,* Increased reflectivity from the medial and lateral walls of the endocardium due to more marked systolic infolding. In each of these examples, the epicardial interface remains smooth; consequently, its medial and lateral borders are not clearly defined.

tion of the incident sound energy in all directions. This scatter decreases the reflected energy recorded from surfaces that are perpendicular to the sound beam but permits some reflections to originate from areas that are oblique or parallel to the incidence sound energy. Figure 8–1, *B,* illustrates the effect of this surface irregularity on a representative diastolic image. Endocardial infolding increases during systolic contraction, further increasing the reflective characteristics of the walls that are parallel or oblique to the path of the scan plane (Fig. 8–1, *C*). The epicardial interface, in contrast, remains smooth, and its reflective characteristics vary little from systole to diastole.

The resolution and display characteristics of individual targets along the endocardial and epicardial surfaces also vary depending on the position of the targets within the ultrasonic beam (Fig. 8–2). From a resolution standpoint, only targets that are perpendicular to the path of the scan plane are viewed with the axial resolution of the imaging system. Points that are oblique or parallel to the scan plane are resolved to varying degrees using the lateral resolution of the system and, hence, are widened by the point-spread function of the beam at any given depth. Again, using the short-axis view as an example, the greatest point spreading occurs along the medial and lateral walls of the ventricle, which are oriented parallel to the path of the ultrasonic beam (Fig. 8–2, B). Spreading of individual points along these interfaces causes the resulting echoes to

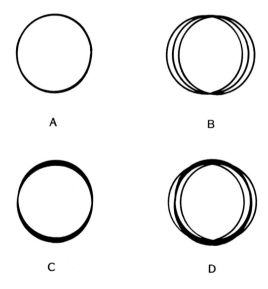

A   B

C   D

Fig. 8–2. Series of diagrams illustrating the effects of beam width and pulse width on the image recorded from a circular target in this example. *A,* It is assumed that the scan plane originates above the test object and that the beam is swept from left to right. *B,* The effect of beam width, which broadens the echoes from targets positioned around the medial and lateral surfaces of the circular test object. *C,* The effect of pulse width thickens the echoes arising from the anterior and posterior margins of the test object. *D,* The combined effects of beam width and pulse width thicken the echoes from targets that are anteriorly and posteriorly positioned and broaden those arising from targets that are oriented medially and laterally.

encroach on contiguous chamber or muscle areas. Because the degree of point spreading varies, depending on the gain level and on the position of individual targets within the beam (see Chap. 1), direct correction for these errors is difficult, and their recognition, therefore, becomes even more important. The length of the ultrasonic pulse also affects the perceived axial width of individual targets (Fig. 8–2, C), but to a much lesser degree than the lateral beam width distortion.[8,9] The combined effects of beam width and pulse duration on a circular target are illustrated in Figure 8–2, D.

Finally, accurate description of the motion of targets along any interface is affected by the position of the target within the scan plane and its direction of motion. Motion of targets perpendicular to the path of the ultrasonic beam (axial motion) can be precisely recorded to the millimeter or submillimeter range. Motion across the scan plane, however, is recorded as movement of the target echo from one data line to the next and is, therefore, measured in degrees. The accuracy with which lateral motion can be determined depends on the separation between data lines and, therefore, is inversely related to the line density and varies from the apex to the base of the sector. In addition, the ability to perceive motion is related to the amount of movement and to the size of the moving object. For example, a fly may move only 1 or 2 millimeters and, yet, this small movement will be apparent, whereas a suspension bridge or skyscraper may sway many feet in the wind but will appear motionless. The motion of interfaces that are oriented parallel to the path of the sound beam and move laterally is therefore more difficult to appreciate and can be less accurately measured than that of perpendicularly oriented and axially moving regions. For this reason, wall motion is recorded less accurately in the apical than in the long-axis views. Likewise, the excursion of the anterior and posterior walls of the ventricle is more easily defined in the short-axis views than is the excursion of the medial and lateral walls.

EXAMINING PLANES AND LINEAR DIMENSIONS

The primary imaging planes used to record the left ventricle are listed in Table 8–1. The orientation of these planes is based on the assumed geometric symmetry of the ventricle and is fixed by specific internal and/or external references. Because these planes are positioned with reference to the left ventricular major or minor axes (see Chaps. 3 and 4), the axes themselves, portions thereof, or dimensions that parallel these axes should be included in the recorded images. The short-axis planes, for example, use the circular configuration of the ventricle when viewed in cross section to align the individual planes parallel to the true ventricular short axes. As a result, when appropriately positioned, these planes should inherently include orthogonal minor ventricular dimensions. The use of geometric assumptions to define these planes makes the areas and dimensions contained by the planes naturally suited to the reconstruc-

TABLE 8–1
LEFT VENTRICULAR IMAGING PLANES

(A) Parasternal long axis
    1. Left ventricle
    2. Left ventricular apex
(B) Parasternal short axis
    1. Mitral valve level
    2. Papillary muscle level
    3. Apical level
(C) Apical
    1. Four chamber
    2. Two chamber
    3. Long axis
(D) Subcostal
    1. Long axis (four chamber)
    2. Short axis

tion of the geometric figures on which these assumptions are based.

Unfortunately, as the length of Table 8–1 suggests, no single view or simple combination of views provides all the data necessary for a complete evaluation of the left ventricle. This occurs primarily because access to the ventricular chamber is restricted by the available acoustic windows. As a result, with the exception of the short-axis planes, some compromise must uniformly be made in terms of completeness of the image or appropriate orientation to achieve optimal interface definition. Thus, although linear and/or area measurements can be derived from the majority of these views, data must frequently be combined from multiple planes to assemble a complete picture of ventricular structure and function.

The Parasternal Long-Axis Views

The parasternal long axis is the initial and most commonly used plane for recording the left ventricle. As illustrated in Figure 8–3, the parasternal long-axis view transects the ventricle along a line extending from the anterior portion of the interventricular septum to the posterolateral free wall. It includes the basal two thirds of the septum and the posterolateral free wall from the atrioventricular groove to the base of the papillary muscles. This orientation places both the right and left septal surfaces and the endocardial and epicardial borders of the posterior wall perpendicular to the path of the ultrasonic beam. As a result, visualization of these interfaces is optimal and motion is along the beam axis. This combination of factors makes the parasternal long-axis view ideal for defining the distances between contralateral points along the ventricular walls and for measuring endocardial excursion and myocardial thickness and thickening.

Because this plane fails to include the ventricular apex, no area measurement can be obtained. Likewise, only an anteropos-

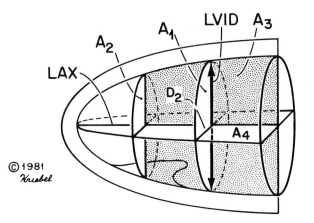

NORMAL LEFT VENTRICLE

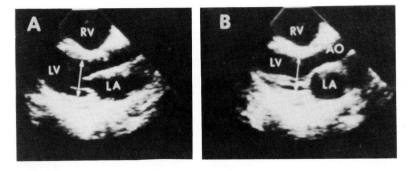

Fig. 8–3. Parasternal long-axis recording of the left ventricle (LV) during diastole (A) and systole (B) illustrates the method for obtaining the left ventricular internal dimension (LVID). The LVID is the distance between the tips of the vertically oriented arrowheads in each panel. RV = right ventricle; AO = aorta; LA = left atrium. The accompanying diagram illustrates the position of this dimension within an idealized left ventricular cavity and its relationship to areas and dimensions derived from the other ventricular views. The absence of shading at the apex is to emphasize that this plane does not include the apex and hence, does not provide an area measurement.

terior linear dimension is available. This dimension, also referred to as the left ventricular internal dimension (LVID), however, has formed the basis for most of the M-mode determinations of left ventricular function and,[10–15] as such, is probably the most important single echocardiographic measurement. In M-mode studies, the LVID has conventionally been taken at the chordal level between the free edges of the mitral leaflets and the tips of the papillary muscles.[16] This point was chosen because it could be readily defined, and, in the absence of spatial orientation, provided a means for standardization of data between patients, examinations, and laboratories. The inherent spatial orientation of the

cross-sectional image makes the chordal reference less critical. Because of the established historical precedent, however, its use has persisted.

In the cross-sectional format, the anteroposterior internal dimension (LVID) is taken as the length of a line that extends from the left septal surface to the posterior wall endocardium, passes through the tips of the mitral leaflets, and is perpendicular to the ventricular long axis (see Fig. 8–3). The ventricular long axis in this view is drawn such that it divides the chamber into roughly equal halves. Because the ventricle is cylindric at this level, the LVID should approximate a maximal dimension in this plane. Various methods have been used to define the end-diastolic and end-systolic LVID. The simplest method, however, is to take these measurements from the frames containing the maximum and minimum cavity areas, respectively.

The cross-sectional LVID may be the same as or smaller than the corresponding M-mode measurement. The reason for this variation is illustrated in Figure 8–4. Specifically, when the M-mode transducer is positioned on the chest below the chordal level or when the left ventricle slopes posteriorly from apex to base, the M-mode beam transects the ventricle obliquely and the LVID is artifactually elongated. The ability in the cross-sectional format to orient this dimension perpendicular to the long axis should overcome this problem and should result in a more accurate and reproducible measurement.

A similar anteroposterior dimension (D_1) can be obtained from a short-axis view at the free edge of the mitral valve. As with the left atrial anteroposterior dimension (see Chap. 6), this measurement is better taken from the long-axis plane because the true anteroposterior orientation and motion of the ventricle parallel to its long axis are more easily appreciated in long axis.

The parasternal long-axis view of the cardiac apex is illustrated in Figure 8–5. In this view, the imaging plane transects the apex in an anteroposterior direction, and the scan plane is oriented parallel to and passes through the ventricular long axis and the apical tip. Because the parasternal long-axis view of the cardiac apex contains no internal references but the apex itself, this view provides no standardizable linear dimensions. Likewise, because the basal side of the scan is not enclosed, area measurements cannot be recorded.

It has been suggested that the parasternal long-axis views at the base and apex might be superimposed by using the anterior mitral leaflet as a reference to enclose the entire ventricular cavity.[17] Once these views are combined, a long axis could then be drawn from the apical tip to either the mitral aortic junction, the mi-

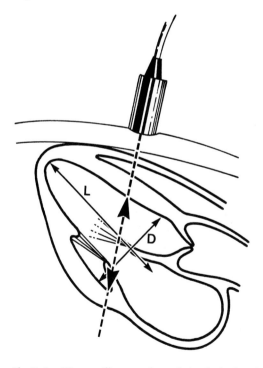

Fig. 8–4. Diagram illustrates the variation in the length of the M-mode left ventricular internal dimension that can arise as a result of apical displacement of the transducer or oblique orientation of the heart within the chest. L = length; D = diameter. (From Rodgers, EW, et al.: Echocardiography for quantitation of cardiac chambers. *In* Progress in Cardiology. Edited by PN Yu, and JF Goodwin. Philadelphia, Lea & Febiger, 1979.)

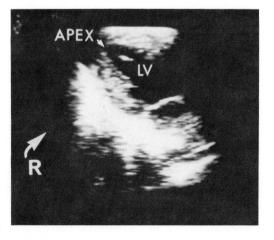

Fig. 8–5. Parasternal long-axis recording of the cardiac apex.

tral ring, or the insertion point of the posterior mitral leaflet into the left ventricular posterior wall. The greater ease of long-axis measurement in the apical views, lack of accuracy in image superimposition, and overall complexity of this method, however, have limited its application.

The long-axis view of the apex is primarily used for evaluating apical configuration and wall motion. Apical wall motion is optimally recorded because the long-axis view of the apex is the only view in which both the anterior and the posterior margins of the apex are perpendicular to the path of the scan, and thus, motion is along the beam axis.[18]

Short-Axis Planes

Theoretically, an almost limitless number of planes might be oriented parallel to the true short axes of the left ventricle. The lack of internal references by which these planes can be standardized, however, has limited reproducible sampling to three levels. These levels include the parasternal short-axis views through the mitral valve leaflets, through the bodies of the papillary muscles, and through the apex between the papillary muscles and the apical tip.

The parasternal short-axis view of the left ventricle at the mitral valve level is illustrated in Figure 8–6, A. This plane transects the ventricle from its anterior to its posterior surfaces, is parallel to the plane of its true short axes, and passes through the free edges of the mitral leaflets. The free edges of the mitral leaflets are normally defined as the point at which maximal leaflet excursion occurs. In low flow states or mitral stenosis, this may not pertain because maximal leaflet separation may be less than the annular diameter. In these instances, the free edges can be defined by sweeping the short-axis scan plane down the mitral valve to a point just prior to the disappearance of the leaflet echoes.

Because this plane passes through the ventricle at its cylindric base, the image should appear roughly circular. The circular short-axis configuration of the ventricle permits measurement of a chamber area and provides a number of options for obtaining ventricular diameters and chordal or radial measurements. The simplest method for drawing perpendicular short-axis diameters relates these dimensions to the scan plane, thereby defining an antero-posterior diameter and a perpendicular, medial-to-lateral ventricular diameter. Though attractive from the standpoint of simplicity, dimensions related to the transducer may vary considerably in their orientation relative to specific points around the ventricular circumference in different individuals, with examination from different transducer angles, or when ventricular rotation occurs from systole to diastole. This variance may affect the reproducibility of data, particularly when the radial excursions of individual points around the ventricular circumference are compared.[19] These differences are not trivial because the position of the papillary muscles and, hence, the orientation of the mitral commissures may vary considerably.[20] The ventricle may also rotate about its long axis by as much as 29 degrees.[19]

A second method relates the orientation of the minor axes to a fixed internal reference(s). Different references have been used for this purpose. In one approach, an axis was constructed from the midpoint of the interventricular septum to the posterolateral wall such that it divided the diastolic ventricular cavity in half.[21] Once this orientation was established, a second perpendicular diameter or a number of diameters at varying angles could then be defined relative to the first. Unfortunately, this method is limited because the anterior and posterior borders of the interventricular septum are frequently difficult to define. An alternative method for orienting the short-axis diameters of the ventricle uses the mitral valve commissures as the

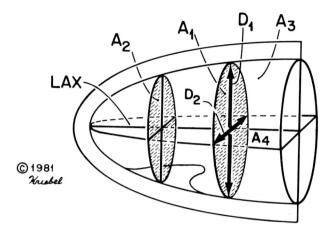

NORMAL LEFT VENTRICLE

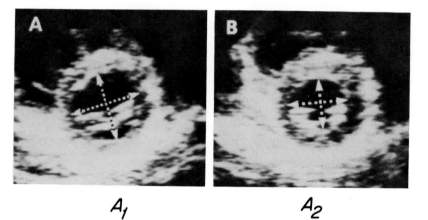

Fig. 8–6. Parasternal short-axis view of the left ventricle at the mitral valve and papillary muscle levels (*B*). The method we prefer for aligning ventricular diameters is illustrated. Because these views encompass the circumference of the ventricular cavity, an area can be measured at both the mitral valve (A_1) and the papillary muscle levels (A_2). The accompanying diagram again illustrates the relative positions of these areas and dimensions to those obtained from the other standard ventricular views.

internal references. The initial diameter is then drawn through the midpoint of the ventricular cavity such that it parallels a line connecting these commissures. A second diameter can be constructed perpendicular to and can bisect the first diameter, which should pass through the midpoint of the mitral valve orifice. This method is illustrated in Figure 8–6, *A* and discussed in detail in Appendix A.

The parasternal short-axis view of the left ventricle at the papillary muscle level is depicted in Figure 8–6, *B*. This view, like the short axis at the mitral valve level, provides a left ventricular area and orthogonal minor dimensions. In addition, multiple radial measurements can be obtained once the center of the cavity is defined. The minor ventricular dimensions obtained in the view can be aligned with reference to the scan plane, the interventricular septum, or the papillary muscles. Again, we prefer to relate these dimensions to the papillary muscles and to draw the initial diameter through the center of the left ventricular cavity from the medial to the lateral walls such that it parallels a line connecting the tips of the papillary muscles. A second dimension can then be obtained that is perpendicular to and bisects the first dimension and, thus, should pass vertically between the two papillary muscles. The left ventricular area obtained from this view is an integral part of several of the volume formulas discussed later in this chapter. Likewise, the radial excursion of individual points on the ventricular circumference is of major importance in the evaluation of patients with ischemic heart disease.

In symmetric or circular ventricles, almost any method for measuring minor ventricular diameters suffices as long as the linear dimensions are obtained from consistent points along the ventricular circumference.

When the ventricle is asymmetric, however, the lengths of individual minor dimensions may differ significantly. It has been suggested, in these instances, that the noncircular shape of the ventricle itself be used as a means of orientation.[22] In one format, which highlights the discrepancy between the major and minor ventricular short axes, an ellipse is constructed with the posterior wall of the left ventricular endocardium comprising the posterior arc of its circumference (Fig. 8–7).[22,23] The major axis (B) of the ellipse is taken as the longer of the two minor axes of the left ventricle. The minor axis (A) is then defined as the length of a line that bisects and is perpendicular to the major axis. An eccentricity index can then be defined as the ratio of B to A. For circular ventricles, this ratio equals unity, but increases as the degree of ventricular deformity becomes greater.[22]

The parasternal short-axis view of the left ventricular apex is illustrated in Figure 4–9, C. Although this plane encompasses a ventricular area, this measurement cannot be precisely fixed and, therefore, has little quantitative value. Likewise, any linear dimension that might

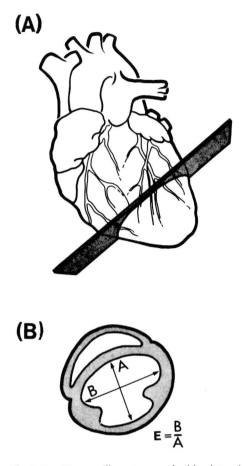

(A)

(B)

$$E = \frac{B}{A}$$

Fig. 8–7. Diagram illustrates a method for determining the degree of left ventricular eccentricity. The scan plane in this example is aligned to transect an eccentric ventricle parallel to its short axis at the papillary muscle level. To determine the degree of eccentricity, one must view the chamber as an ellipse with the posterior wall comprising the posterior arc of its circumference. The major axis of the ellipse (*B*) is taken as the longer of the two minor axes of the ventricle. A second minor axis (*A*), which bisects and is perpendicular to the major axis, is then constructed. The eccentricity index (E) can then be defined as a ratio of B to A.

be obtained from this plane could not be considered reproducible. This view is used primarily to determine the degree of apical involvement in patients with ischemic heart disease, to visualize the circumferential extent of apical thrombus, and to define the position of the apical tip and ventricular long axis for the orientation of subsequent long-axis and apical views.

Effects of Ventricular Motion on Short-Axis Measurements

Because the short-axis planes are fixed in space, whereas the ventricle moves about all its axes as it contracts, one must appreciate the effects of the various components of ventricular motion on any derived data. Three types of motion are important: (1) rotation of the ventricle about its long axis, (2) motion of the ventricle in space, and (3) motion of the ventricle parallel to its long axis or through the scan plane. The left ventricle normally rotates by as much as 7 degrees in a counterclockwise direction about its long axis as it contracts.[19] This rotation may increase to 29 degrees in patients with ostium secundum atrial septal defects[19] and may occur in a reverse or clockwise direction in patients with ostium primum defects and AV canals.[23]

Rotation must be considered in any system that measures radially directed endocardial excursion or wall thickening. When rotation is not considered and excursion is sampled, for example, at 10-degree intervals around the circumference of a ventricle that rotates 20 degrees as it contracts, a given target on the endocardial surface will be 2 radii away from its starting point by the end of the contraction sequence. Orientation of the coordinate system around fixed internal references that move with the ventricle corrects for rotation and permits constant sampling of similar points along the ventricular circumference.

Motion of the ventricle along its minor axes causes the center of ventricular mass or area to shift as the heart contracts. Because this centroid forms the point of origin of all radial systems, failure to appreciate or to correct for this type of motion results in an underestimation of the radial excursion of points toward which the centroid moves and in a corresponding artifactual augmentation of the excursion of points on the opposite surface of the ventricle.[24] Figure 8–8 illustrates the effects of movement of the ventricle in space on the perceived excursion of individual points along the ventricular wall. It also illustrates how realignment of each frame about the centroid for that frame can correct for this type of motion in the symmetrically contracting ventricle.

Motion of the ventricle parallel to its long axis is caused by long-axis shortening, which draws the base of the ventricle inferiorly toward the apex and the apex superiorly toward the base. Consequently, a more basal portion of the ventricle is transected by the scan plane at end-systole than at end-diastole. Because the base of the ventricle is larger than the apex, this type of motion artifactually increases both the end-systolic cavity area and decreases the apparent endocardial excursion. The effects of this type of motion are illustrated diagrammatically in Figure 8–9. Long-axis shortening also increases the muscle mass contained within the fixed area of the scan plane at end-systole when compared to the end-diastolic mass.

Ventricular rotation and spatial motion of the ventricle along any of its minor axes can be appreciated from the short-axis image and, therefore, direct correction can be achieved. Motion of the ventricle parallel to its long axis cannot be appreciated from the short-axis image alone, and direct correction for this type of motion is not possible. Although the motion of the ventricle from systole to diastole could be tracked by varying the angle of the scan plane to hold it on a fixed point within the chamber, this is clearly not practical. As a result, when excessive motion of the left ventricle along its long axis is noted, linear dimensions may preferably be obtained from one of the long-axis or apical views.

The Apical Views

The apical views are recorded with the transducer positioned directly over the tip of the left ventricular apex and, therefore,

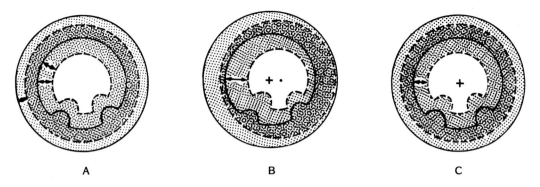

Fig. 8–8. Series of diagrams illustrates the effects of spatial motion of the left ventricle during contraction on the perceived amplitude of wall motion. (*A*), There is no spatial motion of the ventricle, and contraction around the circumference of the chamber is symmetric. (*B*), The ventricular chamber shifts to the right as it contracts. This motion augments the perceived contraction of the left-sided endocardial surface (horizontal arrow) and diminishes the perceived contraction of the right-hand margin of the chamber. The diastolic center of the ventricle is indicated by the cross and the systolic center by the point. The distance between the two centers is the motion of the centroid during contraction. (*C*), Both the systolic and diastolic frames have been realigned about the centroid for each frame. Appropriate correction has been made for motion of the ventricle in space, and contraction again is correctly perceived.

at the distal extreme of the ventricular long axis. The scan plane is then angled until the maximal minor dimension at the ventricular base is recorded. The apical views are thus aligned by definition such that they include the full extent of the left ventricular long axis. Once positioned to include the long axis, a plane originating at the left ventricular apex theoretically could be rotated a full 360 degrees about this axis. The lack of internal and external references available to fix such a plane in space, however, has limited apical sampling to three primary views. These views include the apical four-chamber, long-axis, and two-chamber views.

The *apical four-chamber view,* illustrated in Figure 8–10, *A*, is the most commonly utilized apical imaging plane. In this view, the plane is rotated such that it transects the midportion of the interventricular septum and the lateral left ventricular free wall in the region of the anterolateral papillary muscle. It includes a ventricular long axis that extends from the left ventricular apex to the midportion of the mitral annular plane as illustrated in the diagram accompanying Figure 8–10, *A.* Minor dimensions can be drawn per-

pendicular to this long axis at any desired point(s) along the major axis. The area of the left ventricle within this plane can also be determined.

Unfortunately, targets along the septum and the left ventricular free wall are positioned such that they are parallel to the path of the scan plane. As a result, the echoes arising from point targets along these interfaces are widened by the point-spread function of the beam and encroach on the ventricular cavity. This artifactually reduces the measured cavity area and the length of linear distances between points along these walls.

The motion of the ventricular walls in this and the other apical views is also laterally rather than axially directed and, thus, is not optimally appreciated. As with the short-axis views, point spreading may be corrected by using the leading edge method for measurement or by realigning the images about the center of these echoes.[9] This phenomenon probably explains, in part, why volumes calculated from the areas and dimensions obtained in this and other apical views tend to underestimate true ventricular volume.

Assessment of apical wall motion using

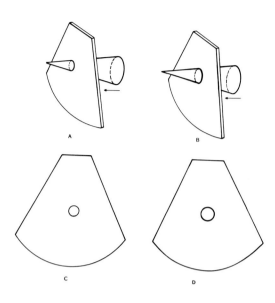

Fig. 8–9. Diagram illustrates the effects of apical motion of the ventricle during systolic contraction on the recorded short-axis area. (A), A representative imaging plane passes through the apical segment of a cone. (C), The cross-sectional area that appears on the display. When the cone advances through the plane, as indicated in B, the cross-sectional area on the display increases correspondingly (D). These variations in the cross-sectional area of the cone are analogous to the changes in the area of the ventricle, that can be produced by apical motion relative to a fixed imaging plane.

the apical four-chamber view may be misleading. A normal apex frequently appears hypokinetic because of the combined effects of poor near-field endocardial definition, motion of the apex into the scan plane, and positioning of the transducer above or below the true apical tip.

The major role of the apical four-chamber view is to provide a ventricular long axis and to permit the total extent of the ventricular borders that surround this long axis to be defined (albeit not optimally). This view is particularly useful for identifying ventricular thrombi, apical aneurysms, and in certain instances, pseudoaneurysms. It is also useful when assessing relative right and left ventricular chamber areas.

*The apical long-axis view of the left ven-*tricle is illustrated in Figure 8–10, *B*. In this view, the scan plane is rotated approximately 45-degrees clockwise from the four-chamber view and is positioned such that it includes the aortic and mitral orifices. As illustrated in the diagram accompanying Figure 8–10, *B*, a ventricular long axis can theoretically be drawn from the apical tip to the junction of the mitral and aortic valves, the midportion of the mitral annulus, or the insertion point of the posterior mitral leaflet. The midpoint of the ventricular base appears to be the most consistent basal intercept of this axis because it corresponds to the method used for defining this dimension in the parasternal long axis and other apical views. Once this long axis is defined, any number of orthogonal minor dimensions can be drawn perpendicular to the major axis at selected points within the ventricle. As with all other apical views, targets along the ventricular walls are resolved with the lateral resolution of the scan plane, and their motion is laterally directed.

The apical two-chamber view is illustrated in Figure 8–10, *C*. In this view, the scan plane transects the anterolateral and posteromedial left ventricular free walls and is oriented by definition such that it fails to intersect any part of the right ventricle. This view, like the other apical views, contains a ventricular long axis extending from the tip of the left ventricle to a point that bisects the plane of the mitral annulus, multiple minor dimensions, and a ventricular area. Importantly, this plane is rotated approximately 90 degrees to the apical four-chamber view. The apical two- and four-chamber views are the only two imaging planes that are orthogonally positioned about the ventricular long axis and include all the points around the circumference of the ventricle. They are, therefore, the ideal combination of planes for calculating ventricular volumes using either the ellipsoid area-length or the Simpson's rule method. Figure 8–11 illustrates how, in the idealized ventricular

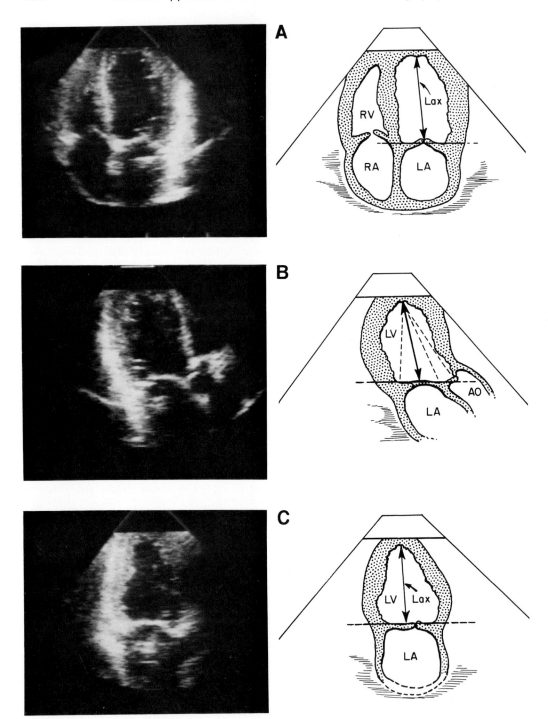

Fig. 8–10. Apical four-chamber (*A*), long-axis (*B*), and two-chamber (*C*) views of the left ventricle (LV) and accompanying diagrams illustrate the ventricular long axis (Lax). The interrupted lines in the apical long-axis view (*B*) indicate alternative basal intercepts of the long axis (i.e., the aortic annulus, insertion point of the noncoronary aortic leaflet, or insertion point of the posterior mitral leaflet). For consistency, the basal intercept of the ventricular long axis in this view should be defined as the midpoint of the ventricular base. LA = left atrium. AO = aorta.

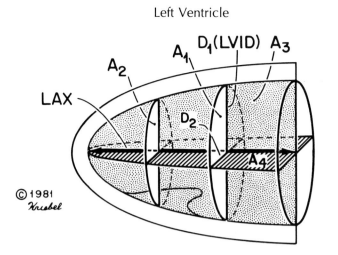

NORMAL LEFT VENTRICLE

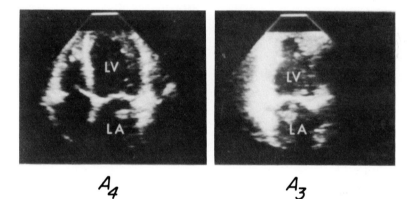

A_4 A_3

Fig. 8–11. Diagram illustrating how the orthogonal areas derived from the apical four chamber (A_4) and two chamber (A_3) views and the left ventricular long axis relate to the areas and dimensions obtainable from the other left ventricular imaging planes. The position of these apical planes in space obviously varies with that of the internal landmarks about which they are fixed, and their positions in the diagram are intended to illustrate geometric and not necessarily anatomic relationships.

model, these orthogonal apical areas and the apically derived long axis relate to the areas and dimensions derived from the other standard views of the left ventricle.

The Subcostal Views

The left ventricle can be visualized from the subcostal transducer location in either the long-axis or the multiple short-axis projections.

The subcostal long-axis (four-chamber) view of the left ventricle is illustrated in Figure 8–12, A. In this projection, the im-

aging plane passes through the posterior third of the right ventricle, the posterior segment of the interventricular septum, the left ventricular long axis, and the antero-lateral left ventricular free wall at or just above the anterolateral papillary muscle. This orientation places both the septum and the lateral left ventricular free wall perpendicular to the path of the scan plane and is theoretically optimal for recording targets along their surfaces. Left ventricular wall motion is also axially directed in this view and should be accurately recorded. In children, this view is extremely

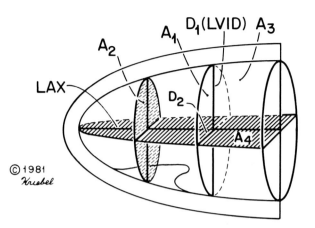

NORMAL LEFT VENTRICLE

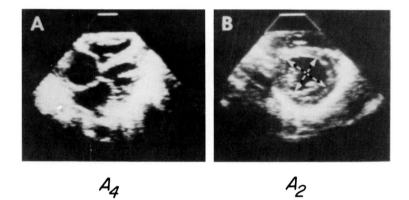

Fig. 8–12.   A, Subcostal long-axis view of the left ventricle. B, Subcostal short-axis view with the minor dimension aligned relative to the papillary muscles. The diagram illustrates how the planes fit into the idealized model of the left ventricle.

valuable for recording left ventricular structure and function. In the adult, the left ventricle is so deep to the transducer face that clear structure visualization is frequently difficult to obtain. When the ventricle can be clearly recorded, however, a major and multiple minor dimension can be obtained. A cavity area can also be outlined, and the excursion of points along the ventricular walls can be recorded.

Multiple *short-axis views* of the left ventricle can theoretically be obtained from the subcostal transducer location. The landmarks available to orient these planes, however, are similar to those in the para-

sternal short-axis views and limit sampling to the levels of the mitral valve, papillary muscles, and cardiac apex. In the subcostal position, the transducer and hence the origin of the scan plane are rotated counterclockwise between 60 and 90 degrees from the parasternal transducer location. This rotation causes the images to appear rotated in the opposite or clockwise direction. Figure 8–12, B, is a subcostal short-axis view of the left ventricle taken at the papillary muscle level. This view contains the same dimensions and area that are available in the corresponding parasternal short-axis view. Furthermore, when these dimensions are aligned relative to an internal reference, such as the papillary muscle tips, they should, as indicated, be identical to comparable parasternal measurements. The same relationships apply at the mitral valve and apical levels, and when available, the subcostal views should offer an alternative to the parasternal views. In addition, because of the shift in transducer orientation, the subcostal views may permit the recording of some areas of the ventricle that are less well visualized from the precordium.

LEFT VENTRICULAR VOLUME

The collection of imaging planes described in the preceding section contains a variety of dimensions and areas that can be used to calculate left ventricular volume. Before the volume of any chamber can be determined from a planar image or group of images, however, the chamber must first be represented by a mathematical model with dimensions that are directly available or can be calculated from the image(s). A variety of geometric figures or combinations of figures have been used to represent the left ventricle. The most common of these are illustrated in Figure 8–13. They represent three basic approaches to ventricular volume calculation: (1) representation of ventricular volume as the volume of a single figure, e.g., the prolate ellipsoid; (2) the sum of the volumes of multiple smaller figures of like configuration (the Simpson's rule method); or (3) the volumes of a combination of different figures, e.g., a cylinder and a cone. The first two methods have been extensively studied and validated angiographically.[25–32] The third uses the short-axis area measurements that are unique to cross-sectional echocardiography, but that greatly increase the number and variety of geometric models that can be conveniently used to represent the ventricular chamber.

Ventricular Volume Calculations Using the Prolate Ellipsoid Model

The single figure that has been used most extensively to represent the left ventricle is the prolate ellipsoid. This figure forms the basis for most angiographic calculations of left ventricular volume, and its validity as a model of the left ventricle has been well documented.[25–30] The prolate ellipsoid is illustrated in Figures 8–14, A and B. This figure has two minor axes, (D_1) and (D_2), and a major axis, (L). It can also be sectioned through its long axis to provide orthogonal areas, (A_1) and (A_2), or through its short axes to yield a third area, (A_3). The volume of the ellipsoid can be calculated by using the formula:

$$\text{Volume} = \frac{4}{3}\,\pi\left(\frac{L}{2}\right)\left(\frac{D_1}{2}\right)\left(\frac{D_2}{2}\right) \quad (1)$$

The ellipsoid model can be applied to echocardiographic images by (1) extension of the M-mode D^3 method; (2) adaptation of angiographic ellipsoid volume formulas; or (3) use of the short-axis area to derive a unique echocardiographic ellipsoid area-length formula.

D^3 Method

The D^3 method is the simplest approach to left ventricular volume calculation because it permits volume to be estimated from a single linear dimension.[11] This method was originally developed specifically for M-mode echocardiographic studies where only one ventricular dimension was available. It is based on the following observations.

1. Left ventricular dilatation occurs primarily along the minor axis. Consequently, a linear relationship can be demonstrated between minor-axis length[33] and chamber volume over a wide range of ventricular sizes.

2. A good correlation can be demonstrated between the M-mode left ventric-

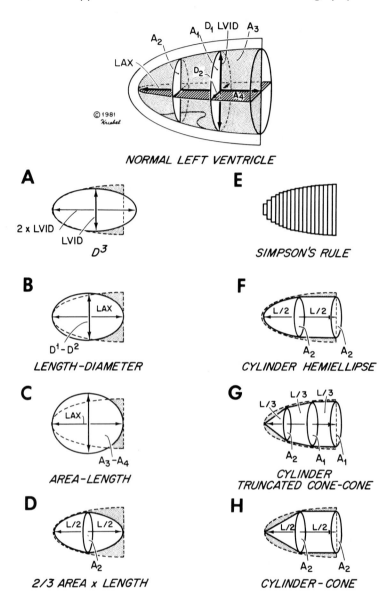

Fig. 8–13. Series of diagrams illustrates the primary geometric figures that have been used to represent the left ventricle, and the echocardiographic dimensions and areas used to construct these figures. (A) The prolate ellipsoid—D³ method; (B) the prolate ellipsoid-length diameter method; (C) the prolate ellipsoid using the biapical areas and the ventricular length. (D) the prolate ellipsoid using the short-axis area and length; (E) Simpson's rule; (F) the cylinder-hemiellipse; (G) the cylinder truncated cone-cone; (H) the cylinder cone.

ular internal dimension (LVID) and the angiographic minor axis.

3. The LVID is directly related to left ventricular volume,[33–35] and this relationship improves when the linear dimension is cubed.[10,11]

The same method for approximating left ventricular volume can be derived from the ellipsoid volume formula if it is assumed that the LVID is equal to one of the minor axes of the ellipse (D_1), that both minor dimensions are equal ($D_1 = D_2$), and

PROLATE ELLIPSOID

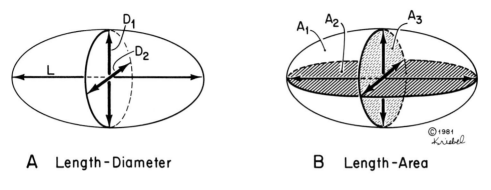

A   Length-Diameter   **B   Length-Area**

Fig. 8–14. Diagram illustrating the prolate ellipsoid figures. (A) The minor diameters (D_1 and D_2) and long-axis length (L); and (B) the three areas that can be obtained either by projecting the figure or by sectioning it through its long or short axes. For reasons of convention, planer labelling in this figure does not correspond to the normal left ventricular illustration in Figure 8–13, and these should not be confused.

that the major axis (L) is equal to twice the minor axis ($L = 2D_1$). After substitution, the formula for the volume of the ellipsoid becomes:

$$\text{Volume} = \frac{4}{3}\,\pi\left(\frac{2D_1}{2}\right)\left(\frac{D_1}{2}\right)\left(\frac{D_1}{2}\right)$$

or $\qquad V = \dfrac{\pi}{3} \times D^3 \qquad\qquad$ (2)

or $\qquad V = 1.047 \times D^3$

  or $\simeq D^3$

Because the ventricle becomes more spherical as it dilates, the ratio of (L) to (D) decreases. As a result, the D^3 method may seriously overestimate the volume of larger ventricles.[13,36–44] Several regression formulas have been developed to correct for the effect of ventricle size on the relationship of L to D. The most widely used formula is that derived by Teichholz, et al.,[45] in which:

$$\text{Volume} = \left(\frac{7.0}{2.4 + D}\right) \times D^3 \qquad (3)$$

This correction permits more direct correlation between echocardiographic and angiographic volumes over a wide range of ventricular sizes[45] and has recently been determined the most accurate M-mode method for calculating stroke volume.[46]

The D^3 method is easily adapted to the cross-sectional format.[21,47] As illustrated in Figure 8–3, the LVID can be directly obtained from the parasternal long-axis view or an orthogonal short-axis projection. Measurements taken from the cross-sectional image should be more reliable and, thereby, should increase the accuracy of the method. Unfortunately, although the simplicity of this method is attractive, it has major limitations. The most important limitation is that the method seeks to define left ventricular size and function from a single arbitrary dimension and, consequently, must assume that the recorded measurement actually corresponds to one of the minor axes of the ellipsoid model and that the function of the ventricle in the region in which the dimension is taken is representative of global ventricular function.

TABLE 8–2
LEFT VENTRICULAR VOLUME MEASUREMENTS AND CORRELATIONS

Geometric Model	Volume Formula	Reference	Subjects of Study	Segmental Disease	Dilated Ventricle	Standard of Comparison	Cross-sectional Views	Ejection Fraction r	Ejection Fraction SEE	End-systolic Volume r	End-systolic Volume SEEml	End-diastolic Volume r	End-diastolic Volume SEEml	In vitro Volume r	In vitro Volume % error	In vitro Volume SEEml
Prolate Ellipsoid (Length-Diameter)	$\left(\dfrac{7.0}{2.4+D}\right)D^3$	Folland, et al.[21]	35 patients	20	8	Single-plane cineangiogram	4 Ch SAX-MV Pap	.55	.130	.81	37	.72	46			
	$\dfrac{4}{3}\pi\left(\dfrac{L}{2}\right)\left(\dfrac{D_1}{2}\right)\left(\dfrac{D_2}{2}\right)$	Chaudry, et al.[54]	30 patients	20	Unspecified number	Single-plane cineangiogram	2 Ch SAX-MV	.73		.91		.86				
	D^3	Wyatt, et al.[47]	21 dogs in vitro			Direct volume measurements	SAX-LAX							.84	40.4	
	D^3	Wyatt, et al.[56]	10 dogs in vitro	Symmetric ventricles		Direct volume measurements	Not specified							.967	29.8	
			8 dogs in vitro	Asymmetric ventricles										.840	46.0	
	$\dfrac{\pi}{6}D_1D_2L$	Wyatt, et al.[47]	21 dogs in vitro			Direct volume measurements	SAX-LAX							.956	8.7	
Prolate Ellipsoid (Length-Area)	$\dfrac{\pi}{6}L\left(\dfrac{4A_1}{\pi D}\right)\left(\dfrac{4A_1}{\pi L}\right)$	Folland, et al.[21]	35 patients	20	8	Single-plane cineangiograms	4 Ch SAX-MV LAX-apex	.78	.098	.72	44	.67	49			
	$\dfrac{8(A_1)^2}{3\pi L}$						4 Ch LAX-apex	.76	.101	.64	48	.61	52			
	$\dfrac{\pi}{6}L\left(\dfrac{4A_3}{\pi D}\right)\left(\dfrac{4A_1}{\pi L}\right)$	Carr, et al.[17]	22 patients	6		Single plane (8 patients) Biplane (14 patients)	SAX-MV Pap 2 Ch, 4Ch LAX-apex Parasternal	.93		.93		.93 (.46)				
	$\dfrac{8(A_1)^2}{3\pi L}$	Roelandt, et al.[57]	50 patients			Single-plane cineangiogram	LAX			.74		.61				
	$\dfrac{8(A_1)^2}{3\pi L}$	DiSessa, et al.[55]	24 normal adults	No	No	Single-plane cineangiogram	2 Ch 4 Ch	.70		.96		.96				
			22 children	No	Unspecified number			.76		.97		.94				
	$\dfrac{8(A_1)^2}{3\pi L}$	Wyatt, et al.[56]	10 dogs in vitro	Symmetric ventricles		Direct volume measurements	LAX							.972	21.6	
			8 dogs in vitro	Asymmetric ventricles										.837	47.0	
	$\dfrac{8(A_1)^2}{3\pi L}$	Wyatt, et al.[47]	21 dogs in vitro			Direct volume measurements	LAX							.903	9.5	
Simpson's Rule	$\dfrac{\pi}{4}H\sum_{0}^{20}D_1\times D_2$	Schiller, et al.[63]	30 patients	18		Biplane cineangiograms	Sax-Pap 2 Ch	.87	.076	.90	8.5	.80	15			
		Silverman, et al.[64]	10 children			Biplane cineangiograms	4 Ch 2 Ch			.91		.94				
	Computer biplane formula															

Formula	Reference	Sample	Control	n	Method	View	Detail	.84	.80	.80	.80	r	SEE
	Bommer, et al.[60]	20 patients			Biplane cineangiograms	"Biplane"							
	Gueret, et al.[65]	11 dogs in vitro	Control		Single-plane cineangiograms	SAX-5 levels		.89–.92	.89–.92				
			LAD occlusions			Length unspecified		.89–.92	.89–.92				
	Wyatt, et al.[56]	10 dogs in vitro	Symmetric ventricles		Direct volume measurements	Multiple SAX views						.996	5.6
		8 dogs in vitro	Asymmetric ventricles									.980	9.9
$\dfrac{N}{3\,mm}\displaystyle\sum_{o} area$	Eaton, et al.[62]		No		Volumetric chamber measurements	SAX-15–19 views						.962	2.51
						8–10 views						.956	2.84
						5–6 views						.960	2.83
						4 views						.926	3.96
						3 views						.918	4.28
						2 views						.833	5.51
						1 view						.827	7.24
	Eaton, et al.[61]	6 dogs (67 volumes) in vitro			Volumetric chamber measurements	SAX-3 mm intervals						.972	2.93
	Bommer, et al.[60]	18 human casts				"Biplane apical"						.97	
Cylinder-Cone $\tfrac{2}{3}$ AL		2 contracting heart models			Cineangiography			.98	.97	.97			
$(A_1 + A_2 + A_3)h + \dfrac{A_4 h}{2} + \dfrac{\pi}{6}h^3$	Wyatt, et al.[47]	21 dogs in vitro			Direct volume measurements	LAX / 4-SAX		.99	.97	.97		.98	6.6
	Wyatt, et al.[47]	21 dogs in vitro			Direct volume measurements	SAX / LAX						.97	8.6
Cylinder-Truncated Cone-Cone $(A_1)\dfrac{L}{3} + \left(\dfrac{A_1 + A_2}{2}\right)\dfrac{L}{3} + \dfrac{1}{3}(A_2)\dfrac{L}{3}$	Folland, et al.[21]	35 patients	20	8	Single-plane cineangiograms	SAX-MV, Pap / 4 Ch		.78 / .097	.86	32 / .76		43	
Cylinder-Hemiellipsoid $\tfrac{5}{6}$ AL	Folland, et al.[21]	35 patients	20	8	Single-plane cineangiograms	SAX-MV / 4 Ch		.66 / .116	.75	42 / .68		49	
	Wyatt, et al.[47]	21 dogs in vitro			Direct volume determinations	SAX / LAX						.97	10.9
	Gueret, et al.[65]	11 dogs in vivo	Control		Single-plane cineangiogram	SAX-MV		.81	.95	.97			
						SAX-Pap		.84	.89	.81			
			LAD occlusion			SAX-MV		.60	.56	.90			
						SAX-Pap		.92	.87	.82			
	Wyatt, et al.[56]	10 dogs in vitro	Symmetric ventricles		Direct measurement	"LAX"						.993	10.1
		8 dogs in vitro	Asymmetric ventricles			SAX						.971	21.7

There are important exceptions to both of these assumptions. In ischemic heart disease, for example, major local abnormalities in left ventricular structures and function may be present in areas of the ventricle that are removed from the region sampled by the LVID. Not surprisingly, a number of studies have demonstrated the inaccuracy of M-mode volume determinations in patients with regional dyssynergy.[38,42,46,48,49] In right ventricular volume overload, the LVID may also fail to reflect accurately left ventricular volume. This occurs because the interventricular septum is frequently displaced toward the left ventricle. Such displacement alters the relationship of the two minor dimensions, and because the LVID more closely approximates the smaller dimension, chamber volume is underestimated. Even within in vitro studies of symmetric formalin-fixed ventricles, the D^3 method correlated less well with measured ventricular volumes than did methods based on more extensive substitution into the ellipsoid formula or on combined geometric figures (Table 8–2).[47] Likewise, in clinical studies, the corrected D^3 method correlated less well with angiographic stroke volume than did the single or biplane angiographic formula or a modified Simpson's rule approach.[21] Thus, despite its historical import and the large body of data that has been generated by the use of this method, the D^3 formula, with or without correction, appears to be the least accurate echocardiographic approach to volume calculation.

Angiographic Ellipsoid Volume Formulas—The Length-Diameter and Area-Length Methods

Many of the echocardiographic sections of the left ventricle contain dimensions and areas that appear similar to those found in angiographic projections of the ventricular chamber. As a result, a number of the angiographic ellipsoid volume formulas have been applied to echocardiographic volume calculations. There are two basic angiographic approaches to volume calculation that use the ellipsoid model: the length-diameter method, in which the minor ventricular dimension is measured directly from the image,[26–28] and the area-length method, in which the minor dimension is calculated rather than directly measured.[25,29,30] The rationale for and the method by which each of these angiographic approaches can be applied to cross-sectional echocardiography are more easily understood if the angiographic derivations of the formulas are first considered.

Angiographic Derivations

Figure 8–15 illustrates how the ellipsoid model is applied angiographically. This figure contains two orthogonal angiographic images of the left ventricle recorded in the anteroposterior and left lateral projections. As indicated in the accompanying diagrams, each of these images contains a long axis drawn from the aortic valve to the ventricular apex, a minor axis that is perpendicular to the major dimension, and an elliptic area that is contained within the ventricular silhouette. Together, the two planar images provide the orthogonal minor dimensions and ventricular length required by the prolate ellipsoid formula. Application of this formula, however, requires two assumptions: (1) the ventricle must be oriented parallel to at least one of the angiographic planes so that a true long axis is projected, and (2) the ventricle must be a true ellipse. In practice, the true left ventricular long axis generally cannot be determined angiographically, and since (L) is not usually equal in the two projections, the larger length must be assumed to approximate more nearly the ventricular long axis.[25,29] Likewise, the ventricle is rarely a true ellipse, and as a result, correction for shape becomes necessary. This can be done by

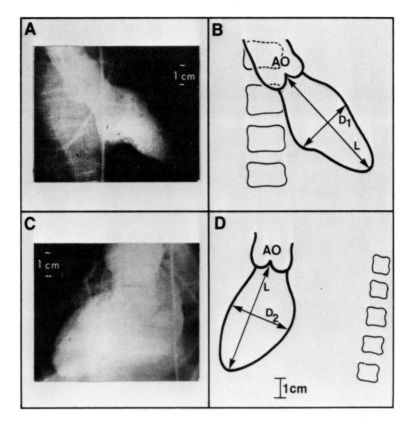

Fig. 8–15. Anterior-posterior (*A* and *B*) and lateral angiographic (*C* and *D*) projections of the left ventricle and accompanying diagrams illustrate how the ellipsoid figure can be used to represent the angiographic silhouette of the ventricular chamber. AO = aorta; L = length; D_1, D_2 = diameter. (From Rogers, EW, et al.: Echocardiography for quantitation of cardiac chambers. *In* Progress in Cardiology. Vol. 8. Edited by PN Yu, and JF Goodwin. Philadelphia, Lea & Febiger, 1979.)

assuming that the projected area of the ventricle (A) represents a true ellipse. By knowing the ventricular length (L), the minor axis for that projection (D) can be calculated from the relationship:

$$\text{Area} = \pi \times \frac{L}{2} \times \frac{D}{2} \text{ or } D = \frac{4A}{\pi L} \quad (4)$$

This correction permits the irregular silhouette of the left ventricle in each projection to be represented by a true ellipse, and the volume formula then becomes:

$$\text{Volume} = \frac{4}{3}\pi \left(\frac{L\max}{2}\right)\left(\frac{4\,A_1}{2\pi L_1}\right)\left(\frac{4\,A_2}{2\pi L_2}\right)$$

$$(5)$$

Ventricular volume can also be calculated from a single planar image (generally the RAO angiographic image) using the length-diameter method if the two minor diameters are assumed equal. If $D_1 = D_2$, then:

$$\text{Volume} = \frac{4}{3}\pi \left(\frac{L}{2}\right)\left(\frac{D_1}{2}\right)\left(\frac{D_1}{2}\right) \quad (6)$$

$$\text{or} \qquad V = \frac{\pi}{6}L \times D^2$$

The area-length method can also be used, by assuming the ventricular area and long axis in the two projections are the same with the result that:

$$\text{Volume} = \frac{4}{3}\pi \left(\frac{L_1}{2}\right)\left(\frac{4A_1}{2\pi L_1}\right)\left(\frac{4A_1}{2\pi L_1}\right)$$

$$(7)$$

or $V = \dfrac{8A^2}{3\pi L}$

Either the single plane or the biplane ellipsoid formulas can be applied to any appropriately derived planar image of the ventricle.

For angiographic use, two additional corrections are required. The first correction is necessary to allow for the image magnification that occurs as a result of divergence of the x-ray beam as it passes from the tube, through the ventricular chamber, and to the recording film.[25,50] The appropriate correction factor must be derived independently for each projection because the distance from the tube to the heart and from the heart to the recording film varies depending on the projection used. Each correction factor must then be included in the volume calculation.

The second correction is necessary to compensate for the slight overestimation of ventricular volume that is observed when the angiogram is compared to postmortem ventricular injection.[25,30] This overestimation has been attributed to the failure of the angiographic method to allow for the volume displaced by the trabeculae papillary muscles and mitral valve apparatus. A regression equation, $V_t = 0.928 V_c - 3.8$, has been derived to correct for this inaccuracy,[25] and the final biplane angiographic volume formula including both of these corrections can be expressed[51] as

$$V_t = \frac{0.788 \, Aa \times A_L}{Lmin}$$

$$\times \, (CFm)^2 \, (CFs) - 3.8 \quad (8)$$

where CFm is the correction factor for the image with the larger major axis, CFs is the correction factor for the second image, Aa is the area in the anteroposterior projection, A_L is the area in the lateral projection, and Lmin is the smaller of the two uncorrected major axes.

In clinical practice, this method has a standard error of approximately 5%.[30] To arrive at this formula, however, it has been necessary to (1) assume that the ventricle can be represented by a prolate ellipse, (2) assume that the maximal angiographic long axis is representative of the true long axis, (3) derive the minor axis to correct for deviation from a true ellipse, (4) correct for magnification, and (5) allow for the volume displaced by the trabeculae, papillary muscles and mitral valve apparatus.

In the single-plane format, other elements of the formula may also be less accurately derived because (1) only a single projection of the long axis is available and, thus, must be assumed to be the true long axis and (2) only one correction factor for image magnification can be determined and must be cubed. This magnification correction factor is also less accurate because the true center of the ventricle cannot be determined from a single plane. Despite these additional assumptions, the single plane method has an error of only approximately 9%.[30]

Echocardiographic Applications of the Length-Diameter and Area-Length Ellipsoid Volume Formulas

The role of the angiographic length-diameter and area-length methods in echocardiographic left ventricular volume calculation has been examined in a variety of clinical and experimental studies.[17,21,46,50,52,53]

The echocardiographic application of these formulas is slightly more complicated because most angiographic studies are limited to two orthogonal planes that include the ventricular long axis, whereas the echocardiogram provides a number of additional short-axis planes. These additional planes increase both the available points for data sampling and the methods of substitution into the ellipsoid formula.[47] Despite these differences, the basic assumptions of the formulas are similar, and the data required for their use appear to be readily available. These similarities can be appreciated by comparing the echocardiographic areas and dimensions illustrated in the idealized ventricular model in Figure 8–13 with those of the ellipsoid figures illustrated in Figure 8–14.

The length-diameter method. The length-diameter method is easily adapted to the echocardiographic format. The ventricular length (L) can be obtained from any of the apical views,[47,54] whereas the minor diameters (D_1 and D_2) can be taken from lines drawn perpendicular to the long axis in orthogonal apical views or, more commonly from a short-axis plane.[46,54] All the dimensions are taken from the inner margins of the endocardial echoes.

The echocardiographic length-diameter method has been compared in experimental studies to direct in vitro volume measurements[47] and clinically to angiographically derived volume.[54] The results of these correlations and their relationship to other methods of volume calculation are illustrated in Table 8–2. Although these data are preliminary, full substitution into the ellipsoid equation appears to result in better correlation with other methods of volume calculation than can be achieved using the cubed linear dimension with or without correction for ventricular shape.

Area-length method. It has been observed in angiographic studies that because of the irregular outline of the left ventricle, choice of the location and direction of the minor dimensions used in the length-diameter format may be somewhat arbitrary and inconsistent. Furthermore, these measurements can be more accurately derived from the ventricular area (A) and major axis length (L) (see formula 4).[25,30]

Although the fixed internal references that are available in the cross-sectional images should permit more reproducible orientation of the minor dimensions, the variable nature of their placement is again apparent in the different short-axis planes from which they have been obtained.[21,47] To avoid the inaccuracies that appear inherent in the arbitrary placement of ventricular dimensions and to better allow for irregularities in ventricular shape, it seems reasonable to make use of the angiographic experience and calculate the echocardiographic minor axis from the ventricular area and major dimension.

Both the biplane and single-plane area-length formulas have been employed echocardiographically.[17,21,47,55–57] In the biplane format, one left ventricular area (A_4) and length (L) are obtained from one of the apical planes, usually the four-chamber view. Two methods have been employed to obtain the second orthogonal plane. One format uses the short axis at the mitral valve level, where the area is equal to A_1 (see Fig. 8–13) and the length is equal to the larger of the minor dimensions (D_1) in this plane.[17,21] The ellipsoid volume formula then becomes:

$$\text{Volume} = \frac{\pi}{6}(L_1)\left(\frac{4A_4}{\pi L}\right)\left(\frac{4A_1}{\pi D_1}\right) \quad (9)$$

The second method uses an orthogonal apical plane, usually the two-chamber view, in which the area is equal to A_3 (see Fig. 8–13) and the length should be equal to the ventricular length in the orthogonal apical plane.

Volume is then calculated as:

$$\text{Volume} = \frac{\pi}{6}(L_1)\left(\frac{4A_3}{\pi L_1}\right)\left(\frac{4A_4}{\pi L_2}\right) \quad (10)$$

Use of any short-axis view appears inappropriate in this equation because, for a circular ventricle, the calculated dimension is the same as the measured dimension, D_1, and is prejudiced by the level at which the plane is taken. In addition, the calculated minor axes, in all likelihood, will not intersect the long axis at the same point and, therefore, will not be truly orthogonal. It would appear that the minor dimensions are more appropriately calculated from two orthogonal planes that include the ventricular long axis, such as the apical two- and four-chamber views.

Volume can also be determined using the area-length method from a single projection using the single-plane formula:[21,47,56–58]

$$\text{Volume} = \frac{8 \, (A_4)^2}{3 \pi L}$$

The single-plane formula is only valid for projections that include the true ventricular long axis (i.e., the apical view). The correlations that have been achieved using the area-length method are listed in Table 8–2. In general, the biplane area-length method has proved superior to the biplane length-diameter and the single-plane area-length methods.[21] Likewise, in comparative studies of formalin-fixed left ventricles, the biplane length-diameter method has proved more accurate than the single-plane area-length calculation. These data suggest that, in any application of the ellipsoid model, the greater the number of dimensions that are either directly measured or directly calculated, the greater the accuracy of the volume determinations.

Determining ventricular volume using the ellipsoid model from the short-axis area and ventricular length. A third method for determining ventricular volume from the ellipsoid figure utilizes the short-axis area (A_2) (Fig. 8–13) and the ventricular length (L).[47] Because the short-axis area is equal to

$$\pi \times \left(\frac{D_1}{2}\right) \times \left(\frac{D_2}{2}\right),$$

the ellipsoid volume equation then becomes:

$$\text{Volume} = \frac{4}{3} A \times \frac{L}{2} \qquad (11)$$

$$\text{or} \qquad \frac{2}{3} A \times L$$

In formalin-fixed hearts, volumes calculated using this derivation have correlated extremely well with directly measured volume.[47] Use of the constant $2/3$, however, results in a consistent, slight underestimation of true volume. The figures that are actually formed when the echocardiographic dimensions and areas are substituted into the ellipsoid volume formulas and their relationship to the idealized ventricle are illustrated in Figure 8–13, A to D.

Simpson's Rule Method

The second general method for calculating left ventricular volumes employs Simpson's rule. According to Simpson's rule, the volume of a large figure can be calculated from the sum of the volumes of a series of smaller, similar figures. The volume of an evenly sliced stick of butter, for example, might be determined from the sum of the volumes of each rectangular slice.

Figure 8–16 illustrates how this method can be applied to the left ventricle. In this example, the chamber is divided along its

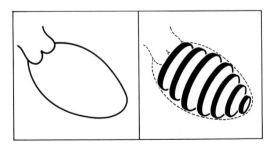

Fig. 8–16. Diagram illustrates the division of an ellipsoid ventricle into a series of cylinders using Simpson's rule. (From Rogers, EW, et al.: Echocardiography for quantitation of cardiac chambers. In Progress in Cardiology. Vol. 8. Edited by PN Yu, and JF Goodwin. Philadelphia, Lea & Febiger, 1979.)

long axis into a series of cylinders or ellipsoid cylinders. The volume of each cylinder is determined from the formula:

$$\text{Volume} = \pi \left(\frac{D_1}{2}\right)\left(\frac{D_2}{2}\right) \times H \quad (12)$$

Where H equals the height of the cylinder and D_1 and D_2 are the orthogonal diameters. This method can be applied echocardiographically in several ways. The first method, illustrated in Figure 8–17, records serial short-axis cross-sectional scans of the ventricle at known increments from apex to base. The height of each cylindric section is then determined directly as the distance between short-axis scans (in this example, 5 mm) and the area of the cylinder either planimetered from the short-axis section or calculated from two measured minor diameters. The volume of the ventricle can then be determined by summing the volumes of the individual sections,[59] or

$$\text{Volume} = (A_1 + A_2 + A_3 \ldots) \times H \quad (13)$$

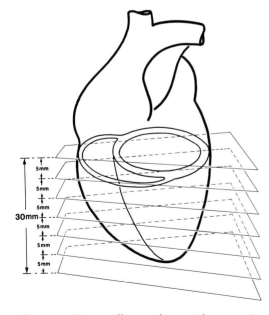

Fig. 8–17. Diagram illustrates how serial cross sections of the ventricle can be obtained at fixed increments and then summed to determine the volume of the entire ventricle.

In experimental studies, this method has yielded accurate volume measurements with correlation coefficients greater than .97 and low standard errors (Table 8–2).[60–62] The accuracy of this method is influenced by the sampling intervals, and a clear relationship is demonstrated between the number of sections recorded and both the correlation coefficient and standard error (Table 8–2).[62] Unfortunately, although accurate, this method is not applicable clinically because the limited acoustic windows do not permit the scan plane to be stepped down the ventricle in fixed increments from base to apex.

A second adaptation of Simpson's rule, which can be applied clinically, uses two cross-sectional views that are orthogonal about the long axis to define the margins of the left ventricle and divides the chamber along this common axis into a series of even slices.[63,64] Each of these slices is then represented by an ellipsoid cylinder, and the height of each cylinder (H) is determined by dividing the ventricular long axis by the number of slices. The orthogonal diameters of each cylinder are then derived from the two planes by taking the distances between the endocardial intercepts of lines drawn perpendicular to the long axis at each interval and ventricular volume calculated as:

$$\text{Volume} = \frac{\pi}{4} H \sum_{0}^{N} D_1 \times D_2 \quad (14)$$

The Simpson's rule method is attractive because it does not require that the ventricle correspond to any geometric figure and, as illustrated in Figure 8–18, readily adapts to gross distortions in ventricular shape.

The data accumulated using the Simpson's rule approach to ventricular volume calculation are listed in Table 8–2. In general, excellent correlations have been obtained with this method provided that the sampling intervals taken are sufficiently narrow. Its major limitation lies in the

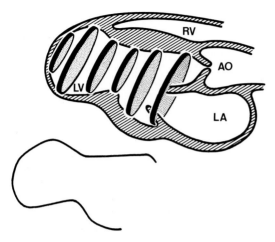

Fig. 8–18. Diagram illustrates how Simpson's rule readily adapts to gross distortions in ventricular shape. RV = right ventricle; AO = aorta; LV = left ventricle; LA = left atrium. (From Rogers, EW, et al.: Echocardiography for quantitation of cardiac chambers. *In* Progress in Cardiology. Vol. 8. Edited by PN Yu, and JF Goodwin. Philadelphia, Lea & Febiger, 1979.)

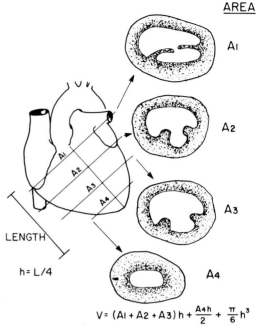

AREA

A_1

A_2

A_3

LENGTH

$h = L/4$

A_4

$$V = (A_1 + A_2 + A_3)h + \frac{A_4 h}{2} + \frac{\pi}{6}h^3$$

Fig. 8–19. Diagram illustrates a modified Simpson's rule approach to left ventricular volume calculation. The volume of the basal three quarters of the ventricle are determined using Simpson's rule, whereas the volume of the apex is determined as the volume of an ellipsoid volume segment. (From Wyatt, H, et al.: Cross-sectional echocardiography. 1. Analysis of mathematic models for quantifying mass of the left ventricle in dogs. Circulation, 60:1104, 1979. Reproduced by permission of the American Heart Association.)

complexity of the calculations, which are laborious by hand and generally require computer support.

A third method, illustrated in Figure 8–19, uses a modification of Simpson's rule.[47] In this model, the volume of the body of the ventricle is determined in the usual Simpson's rule format, whereas the apex is considered as a separate ellipsoid segment. The volume of the overall figure is calculated from the formula:

$$\text{Volume} = (A_1 + A_2 + A_3)\, h \qquad (15)$$
$$+ \frac{A_4 h}{2} + \frac{\pi}{6}\, h^3$$

A better correlation has been demonstrated with measured volume in vitro with use of this formula than with any of the ellipsoid formulas or the combined geometric figures. Although technically a combination of figures, this formula is included in this section because the majority of the data is derived using the Simpson's rule method.

Combined Geometric Figures

The final approach to left ventricular volume calculation uses the short-axis planes to divide the ventricle into two or more sections that can be represented individually by different geometric figures.[21,47,56,65] The figures most commonly used to represent these ventricular sections are the cylinder (volume = area of the base × height), the cone (volume = $1/3$ area of the base × height), the truncated cone

$$\text{Volume} = \frac{\pi \times H\, (r_1^2 + r_2^2 + r_1\, r_2)}{3}$$

$$(16)$$

where r_1 = the radius of the base and r_2

= the radius of the apex, and the ellipsoid segment (volume = $^2/_3$ area of the base × height). Once the volumes of each of these subfigures are known, they can be added to determine the volume of the whole ventricle. Three such combined figures, illustrated in Figure 8–13, F through H, are the cylinder-hemiellipse (F), the cylinder-truncated cone-cone (G), and the cylinder-cone (H).

In each of these combined figures, the overall length is equal to the ventricular length taken from one of the apical views. The areas are short-axis cavity areas recorded at the mitral valve level (A_1) or the papillary muscle level (A_2). In each instance, the short-axis sections presumably divide the long axis into segments of equal length. As a result, the height of each subfigure is the same and can be determined by dividing the ventricular length (L) by the total number of subfigures.

Each of these three models has been utilized in either clinical or experimental studies to estimate ventricular volume. A fourth combined figure, the truncated cone-hemiellipsoid has not been applied to volume calculation, but because of its favorable comparison to left ventricular shape is discussed in the section on methods for determining endocardial surface area.

The Cylinder-Cone

The simplest combined figure represents the base of the ventricle as a cylinder and the apex as a cone. The volume of this figure can be determined by using the formula:

$$V = A \frac{L}{2} + \frac{1}{3} A \frac{L}{2} \text{ or } \frac{2}{3} A \times L \quad (17)$$

where A is the short-axis ventricular area, and L is the ventricular length. An excellent correlation has been reported between volumes calculated using this model and directly measured volumes from formalin-fixed hearts.[47] It has not, to date, been evaluated in either the in vivo experimental setting or in clinical studies. Consequently, its true value remains unclear. It is interesting to note that this figure has the same formula as that of the ellipsoid figure, where volume is calculated from the short-axis area and ventricular length.[47] In the ellipsoid format, the formula has been more extensively tested in vitro[47] and again has been found to have an excellent correlation (r equals .97) with measured volume. The formula has a slight tendency to underestimate true ventricular volume. The underestimation appears related to the constant $^2/_3$ because volumes calculated using the same basic formula but with the constant $^5/_6$ show a similar correlation but more closely approximate true volume. It is assumed in this model that the short-axis plane divides the ventricle in half so that the height of each subfigure is equal to L/2.

The Cylinder-Truncated Cone-Cone

The volume of the second combined figure, the cylinder-truncated cone-cone (Fig. 8–13, G) can be calculated from the following formula:[21]

$$\text{Volume} = \frac{L}{3} (A_1)$$

$$+ \pi \frac{(r_1{}^2 + r_2{}^2 + r_1 r_2)}{3} \frac{L}{3} + \frac{1}{3} (A_2) \frac{L}{3}$$

$$(18)$$

where A_1 is the short-axis of the ventricle at the mitral valve level, and A_2 is the corresponding short-axis area at the papillary muscle level. In this model, it is assumed that the short-axis planes divide the ventricle into three equal parts such that the height of each figure is equal to one third of the overall ventricular length in the apical four-chamber view. Volumes calculated using this model have correlated well with single plane angiographic volumes in clinical studies.[21] The overall correlation has proved superior to that observed with either the single or the biplane ellipsoid volume method, the cylinder hemiellipsoid model (see the following), or the corrected D^3 method.[21]*

The Cylinder Hemiellipsoid

The final combined figure that has been applied clinically is the cylinder-hemiellipsoid (Fig. 8–13, F). The volume of this figure is calculated from the formula:

$$\text{Volume} = A\frac{L}{2} + \frac{2}{3}A \times \frac{L}{2} \quad (19)$$

$$\text{or} \quad V = \frac{5}{6}A \times L$$

This model has been evaluated in both experimental[47] and clinical studies.[21] In the experimental model, the area (A) was taken at the papillary muscle level and assumed to divide the ventricle in half such that the height of each subfigure was equal to L/2. During in vitro studies, volumes calculated using this model correlated well with ventricular volume with individual points aggregating closely about the line of identity.[47] On this basis, the formula was considered to represent the best of the combined geometric figure models for ventricular volume calculation. In clinical studies, however, these excellent correlations have not been observed (see Table 8–2).[21] Unfortunately, in the clinical series, the area (A) was taken at the mitral valve level, thereby preventing precise comparison of these data. In addition, because the area taken at the papillary muscle level has been shown experimentally to yield a better comparison with measured volume when abnormal segmental

---

*The clinical studies presented in Table 8–2 use the formula: volume = $\frac{1}{2}$ (area at the base + area at the apex) × height for the volume of the truncated cone. This approximation is acceptable when both areas are similar but become increasingly less accurate as the truncated cone more closely approaches a cone.

wall motion is present, the comparison becomes more difficult.[65]

Summary

Despite the large volume of data presented in Table 8–2, no optimal method for the clinical determination of ventricular volume is apparent. No study compares the accuracy of all the available formulas nor do studies using the same formulas employ similar methods. These data do, however, provide important insight into the accuracy and limitations of echocardiographic volume calculations.

First, they demonstrate that echocardiographic volumes consistently underestimate true ventricular cavity volume because of (1) the effects of pulse width and beam width, which broaden the echoes from the endocardial interface and thereby encroach on the ventricular chamber; (2) the use of the plane of the mitral valve annulus as the basal intercept of the ventricular long axis, which slightly foreshortens ventricular length measurements when compared with angiographic measurements taken from the aortic valve; (3) frequent failure to identify the true apical extreme of the ventricular cavity, resulting in an underestimation of ventricular length; (4) the exclusion of the portion of the cavity volume contained within the trabeculae; and (5) the systolic motion of the ventricle through the scan plane with artifactual reduction in either diastolic or systolic volume.[17,47,63,66]

These limitations of the echocardiographic method are in almost direct contrast to the angiographic silhouette image in which true volumes are consistently overestimated because of (1) inclusion of the papillary muscles and mitral valve apparatus in the calculated volume; (2) the effects of the silhouette format, which gives a maximal projected area, and (3) inclusion of the trabeculae in the ventricular volume because dye within the invaginations between the muscles extends to the edge of the projected silhouette.

Secondly, end-systolic echocardiographic volumes almost uniformly show a better correlation with angiographic volumes than do end-diastolic volumes. This difference apparently relates to the more reliable definition of the endocardial interface at end-systole than at end-diastole.

Finally, the overall accuracy of the various formulas appears to relate to the frequency of sampling and the ease with which the model adapts to changes in ventricular contour. Thus, the Simpson's rule method, with sections taken at 3-mm intervals, is clearly the most accurate, whereas the D^3 method, which utilizes the least amount of available data and requires the greatest number of assumptions, is the least precise.

A theoretic "worst case" comparison of these formulas can be used to point out individual strengths and weaknesses. Figure 8–20 illustrates a cross-sectional image of a large ventricular aneurysm originating below the papillary muscles. The accompanying diagram shows the points at which the standard measurements of ventricular length (L), mitral valve short-axis area (A_1), papillary muscle short-axis area (A_2), and LVID would be taken. The figures that would be calculated from each of these measurements are then superimposed on the outline of the actual echo. The only figures that truly approximate the "worst case" ventricle are the Simpson's rule method and the area-length ellipsoid model. The Simpson's rule method provides the most accurate representation. The area-length method converts the irregular figure to an ellipse by deriving the minor dimension and thereby gives a reasonable representation of the area and volume of the ventricle. The D^3 method fails completely to approximate the ventricle, whereas the figures that rely on short-axis areas significantly underestimate true ventricular volume. Data derived from symmetric ventricles may be misleading because any reproducible area or dimension should show a relationship to the volume of a symmetric figure. Methods that are valid in both the symmetric ventricle and the "worst case" model should have the greatest applicability to the general cardiac population.

LEFT VENTRICULAR MASS

One of the primary mechanisms by which the left ventricle adapts to an abnormal pressure or volume load is muscular hypertrophy. The degree of hypertrophy parallels the severity of the increased load,[67–70] and extreme hypertrophy may indicate a poor prognosis.[71–73] Anatomically, left ventricular hypertrophy is characterized by an increase in muscle mass or weight. Left ventricular mass is determined by two factors: (1) chamber volume and (2) wall thickness. In chronic pressure loads, mass generally increases as a result of wall thickening without a marked increase in chamber volume (Fig. 8–21, A and B), whereas with volume overloads, the increase in mass is predominantly due to chamber dilatation (Fig. 8–21, C and D). The common association of the term "left ventricular hypertrophy" with wall thickening may lead to confusion because mass may increase without an increase in wall thickness.

All echocardiographic calculations of left ventricular mass are based on the assumption that the volume of the myocardium is equal to the total volume contained within the epicardial borders of the ventricle less the chamber volume[74–76,79]

$$\text{or} \qquad V_m = V_t \, (ep) - V_c \, (en) \qquad (20)$$

where V_m is the muscle volume, V_t is the total left ventricular volume or the volume contained within the epicardial interface, and V_c is the chamber volume or volume contained within the endocardial interface. The muscle volume (V_m) can then be converted to mass (LVM) by multiplying by the specific gravity of the cardiac muscle (1.05) such that

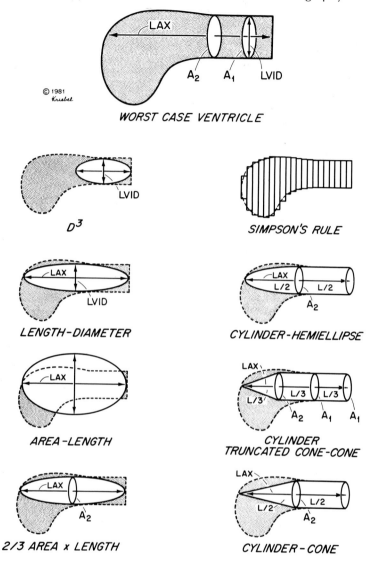

Fig. 8–20. Series of diagrams illustrates the adaptive ability of each of the ventricular volume formulas to a theoretic worst case ventricle. Only Simpson's rule and the area-length ellipsoid volume formulas accurately approximate the volume of this distorted figure. A_1 = short-axis area at the mitral valve level; A_2 = short-axis area at the papillary muscle level; LVID = left ventricular internal dimension; LAX = long axis.

$$LVM = [V_t (ep) - V_c (en)] \times 1.05 \quad [21]$$

In all left ventricular mass calculations, the interventricular septum is assumed to be a part of the left ventricle. As a result, the right septal surface is considered to form the external border of the left ventricle in the septal region.

A variety of echocardiographic methods have been described to calculate ventricular mass. These differ principally in (1)

the conventions used to measure wall thickness and chamber area and (2) the formula used to calculate volume.

The first major factor in any mass calculation is the definition of the endocardial and epicardial interfaces or, more specifically, whether the echoes from these interfaces are included in the wall thickness measurement, are considered part of the chamber volume, or, in the case of the

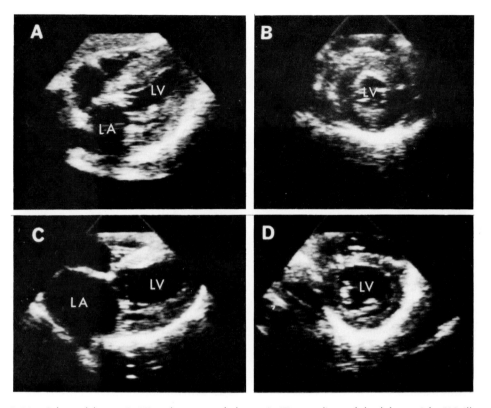

Fig. 8–21. Subcostal long-axis (*A*) and parasternal short-axis (*B*) recordings of the left ventricle (LV) illustrate concentric left ventricular hypertrophy. The ventricular walls are thickened, and the chamber size is decreased. (*C* and *D*), Corresponding subcostal long- and short-axis views that illustrate eccentric hypertrophy. In these examples, there is a predominant increase in the chamber volume and a corresponding, although lesser, increase in wall thickness. LA = left atrium.

epicardial echo, are excluded completely. At least four different conventions have been described for making these measurements: (1) standard,[74,77] (2) Penn,[76] (3) ASE,[78] and (4) Wyatt.[79] These measurement formats are illustrated in Figure 8–22.

The first three formats were developed specifically for M-mode echocardiography, whereas the fourth has been applied solely to cross-sectional studies. Both the standard and the ASE conventions appear inappropriate for use in the cross-sectional format because they require the line of measurement to cross at least one interface at some point around the circumference of the ventricle. In the Penn and Wyatt conventions, the line of measurement follows the same border of the interface around the ventricular circumfer-

ence, and they appear better suited to the cross-sectional method. We prefer to use the Wyatt method because the internal margins of both the endocardial and epicardial interfaces are usually more easily defined than are the external margins and because this method is consistent with the other dimensional and area measurements described in this text. Although seemingly a trivial point, the inclusion of these echoes is important because a 1-mm variation represents approximately a 10% difference in wall thickness.[76] These differences become even more significant when determining mass because the calculated volumes vary with the cube of the linear measurement.

The volume component of the mass formula can be derived using any of the

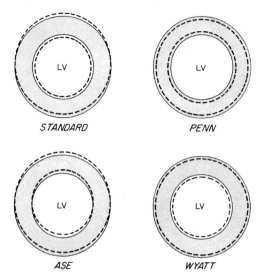

Fig. 8–22. Series of diagrams illustrates the adaptation of the four major conventions for defining the endocardial and epicardial interfaces to the short-axis, cross-sectional image of the left ventricle. The shaded areas correspond to the myocardium, while the interrupted lines follow the path of the line of measurement using each convention.

methods described in the preceding section for ventricular volume calculation: (1) Simpson's rule, (2) the combined geometric figure, or (3) the single figure.

Simpson's Rule Method

The most accurate method for calculating ventricular mass appears to be the Simpson's rule method or a modification thereof. In the Simpson's rule mass calculation, the myocardium is represented as a series of thick-walled, hollow cylinders. The volume of each cylinder is determined from the planimetered muscle area and the section height.[79,80] The myocardial area of each cylinder is derived from serial echocardiographic short-axis cross sections, and the height is determined (1) by direct measurement of the interval between sections,[79] or (2) by assuming that the sections are evenly spaced and dividing the ventricular long axis by the total number of sections.[80]

In pathologic studies, the echocardiographically derived area of individual sections has correlated extremely well with

the photographic section area (r = .95) and the section volume (r = .97) as have the calculated mass and section weight.[80]

In the experimental model, a modification of this method has been applied (see Fig. 8–19) in which the ventricular long axis (L) is divided into four presumably equal segments (h) by short-axis planes taken at the mitral valve, at the high and low papillary muscle levels, and at the apex.[79] The first three sections are then represented as thick-walled, hollow cylinders, and the apex is viewed as an ellipsoid volume segment. The volume of the whole figure is expressed as:

$$V = (A_1 + A_2 + A_3) h$$
$$+ \frac{A_4 L}{2} + \frac{\pi}{6} h^3 \quad (22)$$

This method has yielded a good correlation with actual mass (r = .95) and should be applicable clinically.

Combined Geometric Figures

Only one combined figure has been tested to date for determining the volume component of the mass formula.[79] This figure is the cylinder-hemiellipsoid (Fig. 8–14, F) where

$$V = \frac{5}{6} A \times L \quad (23)$$

The same formula is used to determine the volumes contained within both the endocardial and epicardial interfaces, and mass is calculated as

$$LVM = (LVV \text{ of epicardium}$$
$$- LVV \text{ endocardium}) \quad (24)$$
$$\times \text{ muscle density}$$

The areas within each interface are measured directly from a short-axis scan of the ventricle at the high papillary muscle level, and the length (L) for each figure is taken from the base to the respective epicardial and endocardial interfaces at the apex.

In experimental studies, this method has yielded an excellent correlation with ventricular weight with a small standard error and even scatter of individual points about the line of identity.[79] This model further allows for the absence of myocardium at the base of the ventricle because the length measurement is derived such that the bases of the concentric shells are parallel. It also makes allowance for the contribution of the papillary muscles to overall mass. Although this model does not readily adapt to gross changes in ventricular shape (as noted in the "worst case" example in Figure 8–20), clinically important changes in mass are most commonly sought when the ventricle is symmetric. This model, therefore, appears to represent a simple and reliable method for volume calculation for which the necessary data should be available in most patients.

Single-Figure Method

The single-figure method for calculating the volume component of the mass equation has been tested using both the prolate ellipsoid model and the simple cylinder.[79,80] Although valuable in volume calculation, the ellipsoid model appears to fail in this setting because, when constructing concentric ellipsoid figures, it is necessary to assume that the ventricle is surrounded by a uniform shell of even thickness (D^3) or by a shell that tapers at both extremes of the long axis (area-length or length-diameter). In either case, the ellipsoid fails to allow for the absence of myocardium over the mitral and aortic orifices. This limitation has been previously demonstrated in postmortem measurements which indicate that, for mass calculation, the ventricle is better represented by a truncated ellipsoid.[81] Not surprisingly, therefore, comparative studies show that mass calculations using the

ellipsoid figure have correlated less well with measured mass than have those using either the Simpson's rule or the combined figure methods. The D^3 derivation of the ellipsoid model is least accurate.[81]

The simple cylinder has also been used for mass calculation in several studies.[79,80] This figure consistently overestimates true mass but, again, yields a reasonable correlation when an appropriate correction is introduced.

There is no general agreement about the optimal method for mass calculation. The Simpson's rule method appears to be the most accurate but also the most complex approach to mass calculation. In the symmetric ventricle of the experimental model, the ellipsoid figure has been less accurate than the combined cylinder-hemiellipsoid or the cylinder alone.[79] In more irregular ventricles, such as the "worst case" example presented in Figure 8–20, the accuracy of the area-length ellipsoid model might prove superior; however, mass is rarely determined in this setting. Thus, because of its simplicity and accuracy, the combined cylinder-hemiellipsoid appears, at this point, to be the best clinical alternative.

Relationship of Mass to Volume

As the ventricle enlarges, wall thickness must also increase proportionately to prevent an increase in wall stress. In volume overloads, therefore, the degree of compensatory or eccentric hypertrophy should maintain a constant relationship with chamber volume. In pressure loads, in contrast, the degree of hypertrophy should be disproportionate to the chamber volume. To determine the "appropriateness" of hypertrophy to chamber volume and, by inference, to define whether the ventricle is pumping against increased pressure (increased wall thickness relative to chamber volume) or is working at increased stress because of failure of the myocardium to hypertrophy appropriately (decreased wall thickness relative to chamber volume), an index that relates wall thickness to chamber volume has been proposed.[82] This index, the relative wall thickness (RWT), is without units and can be calculated using the formula:

$$RWT = \frac{1.612\ w}{\sqrt[3]{V}} \qquad (25)$$

where w represents the left ventricular free wall thickness at end-diastole, and V is the left ventricular chamber volume. In a series of normal postmortem hearts, the relative wall thickness was calculated as 53 ± .11 (SD).[81] The concept of relative wall thickness has been used echocardiographically in estimating left ventricular peak systolic pressure (see Chap. 7) and may play an additional role in other areas.

Dynamic or Ejection Phase Indices of Left Ventricular Performance

The principal dynamic- or ejection-phase indices that can be calculated echocardiographically[10–15, 17, 21, 47, 55,56, 60, 63, 65, 83–87] are the stroke volume (SV), ejection fraction (EF), shortening fraction (%ΔD),[84,86–88] and velocity of circumferential fiber shortening (Vcf).[12,39,89–93] Stroke volume can be determined directly as:

Stroke volume = end diastolic
                volume − end systolic volume

or indirectly from the M-mode echogram of the mitral valve.[94] In the direct approach, the end-diastolic and end-systolic volumes are calculated using one of the methods described earlier. As might be expected, the most accurate clinical correlations have been obtained using a modification of Simpson's rule (see Table 8–2). The echocardiographic stroke volume generally shows a better correlation with the comparable angiographic measurement than does the end-diastolic volume. How-

ever, the end-systolic volume correlates best with the comparable angiographic measurement. In absolute terms, the echocardiographic stroke volume appears to be a more accurate estimate of the comparable angiographic volume than are either the end-diastolic or the end-systolic volumes taken by themselves. This increased accuracy occurs because the consistent errors in both volume calculations cancel out when the values are subtracted. Angiographically, the normal stroke volume has been reported to average 45 ml/m² ± 13 ml.[95]

Indirect calculation of stroke volume from the M-mode mitral valve echogram is possible using the formula:[94]

$$MVSV = \left(\frac{EE(mm)}{HR\ [beats/min\ +\ PR(sec)]} \right)$$
$$\times\ 100\ +\ \frac{2\ \times\ DE\ (mm/sec)}{HR\ (beats/min)} \qquad (26)$$

where EE is the maximum vertical separation of the mitral leaflets, HR is the heart rate, PR is the PR interval derived from the electrocardiogram, and DE is the most rapid slope of the anterior mitral leaflet echo between the point of initial leaflet separation (D) and the point of maximal leaflet excursion (E). This method of stroke volume calculation is based on the assumption that the volume of blood entering the left ventricle through the mitral valve during diastole is equal to the amount ejected during the preceding systole. It is also based on the experimental observations that the pattern of mitral valve motion recorded echocardiographically closely resembles the directly measured flow pattern across the mitral valve.[96,97] The formula itself was derived from correlations of specific parameters of mitral valve motion with stroke volume and has been validated using an appropriate mathematical model.[94] It has the advantage of being independent of ventricular geometry, but its accuracy is based on the assumption that the mitral valve is anatomically intact and that flow through the valve is unimpeded. The formula, therefore, is invalid in patients with aortic insufficiency, mitral stenosis, and other abnormalities that distort the flow field through the mitral valve orifice.

Stroke volumes calculated using this formula have correlated well with those obtained by thermodilution and the Fick method. In clinical correlations, stroke volume is frequently determined by dividing the cardiac output by the heart rate. Remember that many techniques that measure cardiac output, such as the Fick method, reflect only the forward component of the stroke volume. In the presence of valvular regurgitation or ventricular septal defect, they may significantly underestimate the total volume ejected by the left ventricle and measured by the direct echocardiographic method.

The ejection fraction is the ratio of the stroke volume to the end-diastolic volume,

$$EF = \frac{EDV - ESV}{EDV} \times 100 \qquad (27)$$

The ejection fraction is a global index of left ventricular fiber shortening and is generally considered as one of the most meaningful measures of left ventricular pump function. Angiographic studies have shown that the normal ejection fraction averages 67% ± 8% (SD). Values below 50% in the resting supine individual are generally considered abnormal.[37,95]

The ejection fraction can also be estimated indirectly from the mitral valve echogram based on the minimum separation between the anterior mitral leaflet at its E point (see Chap. 5) and the most posterior excursion of the interventricular septum.[98] Patients with normal left ventricular function have little (less than 5 mm) or no E-point septal separation, whereas patients with reduced ejection fractions (less than 50%) have increased separation. This index, like the stroke volume calculation from the mitral valve echogram, has the advantage of being independent of ventricular geometry, and the E-point septal separation has been shown to have a reasonable correlation (r = − .86) with angiographic ejection fraction.[98] The index is limited, however, because it must assume normal mitral valve motion and unimpeded left ventricular inflow. Thus, it is inaccurate in such settings as aortic insufficiency.

The final two ejection phase indices, the shortening fraction and the Vcf, are primarily applicable to the M-mode method and rely on minor-axis shortening as a representation of overall ventricular systolic function. They are based on the angiographic observation that the systolic decrease in ventricular volume is primarily due to minor-axis shortening and that the percent change in the minor axis during systole shows a linear correlation with ejection fraction.[33,99] These assumptions are similar to those underlying the D^3 method of volume calculation, and their limitations have already been discussed. Fractional shortening represents a simple method for estimating ventricular function in the symmetrically contracting ventricle and can be calculated from the LVID using the following formula:

FS (% Δ D)

$$= \frac{LVID_d - LVID_s}{LVID_d} \times 100 \qquad (28)$$

In patients with normal left ventricular function, Δ D is usually greater than 25%.

The velocity of circumferential fiber shortening may be a more meaningful estimate of left ventricular function than the more familiar ejection fraction because it reflects not only the normalized amplitude but also the rate of fiber shortening.[12,87,90,91,93] The Vcf, expressed in circumferences per second, is normally calculated by assuming that the LVID is the diameter of the ventricular annulus and is expressed as

$$Vcf = \frac{LVID_d - LVID_s}{LVID_d \times E.T.} \quad (29)$$

where ET is the ejection time derived from the carotid pulse tracing, from the duration of aortic valve opening, or from the onset to the peak of posterior left ventricular wall movement. The lower limit of normal for Vcf is 1.1 circumferences per second.

The ejection-phase indices, although generally considered to reflect myocardial contractility, are also subject to changes of preload and afterload. When either end-diastolic volume (preload) is reduced or aortic pressure (afterload) is elevated, the ejection phase indices decline. Conversely, the ejection phase indices may appear normal when afterload is reduced, as in acute mitral insufficiency or ventricular septal defect, even though contractility may be depressed.

Left Ventricular Response to Exercise

Various forms of controlled stress are frequently employed in conjunction with the echocardiographic examination to assess the ability of the left ventricle to respond to increased demand.[100–105] These challenges are directed primarily toward identifying early global abnormalities of left ventricular function that are not apparent at rest or toward inducing wall motion abnormalities in patients with ischemic heart disease. Exercise is the most convenient and commonly used form of stress. Both dynamic (supine bicycle)[100–103,105] and isometric (handgrip) exercises are employed.[100,104]

The left ventricular response to pharmacologic variation in afterload and preload, to cold exposure, and to a variety of physiologic maneuvers, such as the Valsalva and Müller maneuvers, can also be assessed echocardiographically. The general cardiac response to all forms of exercise is an increase in heart rate, blood pressure, and cardiac output.[100] Dynamic exercise produces a greater increase in heart rate for a given change in blood pressure than does isometric exercise. Isometric exercise, in contrast, causes a predominant increase in blood pressure.

The changes in left ventricular size and function that are noted during various forms of exercise are listed in Table 8–3. Dynamic exercise normally causes a progressive decrease in the left ventricular end-systolic dimension and end-systolic volume, and an increase in stroke volume.[100] Controversy exists concerning the response of the end-diastolic dimension and volume to dynamic exercise. In general, end-diastolic volume changes little during mild or moderate dynamic exercise. An increase in diastolic volume is noted during severe exercise.[106–109] In supine studies, diastolic volume changes little following the initiation of exercise. This is in contrast to upright exercise, where an initial increase in diastolic volume is noted and attributed to increased venous return following initial contraction of the leg muscles.[100]

The normal response to handgrip exercise is complex and appears, in part, to depend on the severity of the handgrip stress. At 50% or greater maximum voluntary contraction, an increase in left ventricular systolic diameter has been reported with a decrease in the shortening fraction.[100] The diastolic volume is typically unchanged. At lower levels of handgrip, the results have been more variable with little, if any, change noted at 33% of maximal voluntary contraction in one study.[104] Changes similar to those produced by handgrip stress can be observed following pharmacologically induced increases in systolic blood pressure.[100]

REGIONAL WALL MOTION ABNORMALITIES

Acute coronary occlusion results in almost immediate cessation of myocardial

TABLE 8–3
CHARACTERISTIC RESPONSES TO DYNAMIC AND ISOMETRIC EXERCISE

	HR	SBP	D_D	D_S	%ΔD	V_D
Handgrip 15% max	↑	↑	—	↑	↓	↓
50%	↑	↑	—	↑ ↑	↓ ↓	
Pharm —	↑	↑	—	↑	↓ ↓	↓
Supine Bicycle Exercise	↑	↑	—	↓	↑	↑
Upright Bicycle Exercise	↑	↑	—	↓	↑	↑

HR = Heart rate
SBP = Systolic blood pressure
D_D = Diastolic left ventricular dimension
D_S = Systolic left ventricular dimension
%ΔD = Percent left ventricular minor dimension shortening
V_D = Normalized mean rate of left ventricular dimension shortening

contraction in the region supplied by the obstructed vessel.[110] Once established, the area of abnormal function tends to persist, and repeated injury generally causes progressive deterioration of ventricular function. The characteristic association between regional myocardial blood flow and muscular function permits segmental contraction abnormalities to be used as early and sensitive markers of underlying ischemia and/or infarction.[111] These wall motion abnormalities are particularly significant because they appear within seconds after the onset of ischemia (prior to any important change in the electrocardiogram)[112] and because their extent can be related to overall pump function[113] and, as a result, to subsequent morbidity and mortality.[114] Echocardiographically, segmental contraction abnormalities are encountered in three general settings: (1) following acute myocardial infarction; (2) in patients with chronic ischemic heart disease, and (3) as a result of transient ischemia induced by exercise or some other controlled stress.

Acute Myocardial Infarction

A number of experimental studies have demonstrated that regional wall motion abnormalities can be visualized echocardiographically within five to ten beats after acute coronary ligation.[111,115,116] Clinically, abnormal wall motion can be observed almost coincidentally with the onset of pain in patients with unstable angina, and following acute infarction, abnormal wall motion is usually established by the time an examination can be initiated.

These regional contraction abnormalities are characterized by a decreased amplitude and rate of endocardial excursion and an associated decrease in subjacent wall thickening.[111,117–121] When present, they are usually of sufficient magnitude to permit identification by simple visual comparison with adjacent, more normally moving segments.[115,122–126] In addition to offering a convenient, noninvasive method for identifying the abnormal wall motion that occurs following acute infarction, echocardiography also permits evaluation of the severity, extent, anatomic location, and natural history of these abnormally contracted segments.

Sensitivity and Specificity of Abnormal Wall Motion as an Echocardiographic Marker of Acute Infarction

Several studies, to date, have suggested that some abnormality of left ventricular wall motion can be detected echocardiographically in almost all patients with acute transmural myocardial infarction and in every patient in which the ventricle is completely recorded.[122,123,125,127] Although, on occasion, individual ventricular segments that do not show evidence of infarction pathologically may move abnormally and areas containing limited or old infarction may appear to move normally,[122,125] no cases of adequately studied, documented transmural infarction have been reported in which no wall motion abnormalities were noted. Quantitation of the extent of abnormal wall motion, however, is only possible when the ventricle is completely visualized, or in roughly 85% of the cases.

When myocardial infarction is *nontransmural* or *subendocardial*, abnormal wall motion is noted less consistently. In one study, the echocardiogram detected only one of two subendocardial infarcts involving less than 5% of the myocardium,[128] whereas in a second, wall motion was considered normal in each of two patients with clinical evidence of subendocardial infarction.[125]

Myocardial infarction is not the only cause of abnormal segmental wall motion. Abnormal motion of the anteroapical segments may be seen in aortic regurgitation, and as discussed in Chapter 12, there are a variety of causes of abnormal septal motion. Wall thickening, in these instances, is usually normal and permits identification of these abnormalities as nonischemic. Focal myocarditis decreases both wall motion and thickening and is usually indistinguishable echocardiographically from myocardial infarction or ischemia.

Degree of Abnormal Motion Within Infarcted Segments

The severity of abnormal motion within infarcted segments can be described in qualitative terms or the endocardial excursion and wall thickening at specific points measured directly. Qualitatively, motion within abnormal segments is usually described as hypokinetic (normally directed but reduced), akinetic (absent), or dyskinetic (paradoxic). Following acute transmural myocardial infarction, the majority of affected segments (more than 72%) are either akinetic or dyskinetic.[122] Hypokinesis, when present, is usually profound, with a mean decrease from normal of 50 to 75% reported.[118,119,129]

Direct measurement of the radial excursion and thickening at individual points within the abnormal region is also possible. These measurements can be related to control normal values or to comparable measurements from adjacent normal areas. Description of wall motion in absolute terms is of somewhat limited value, however, because of the many factors other than myocardial infarction that can affect endocardial excursion and because of the wide normal variation in the absolute excursion of individual points around the ventricular circumference.[130,131]

Wall thickening appears to be a more specific quantitative indicator of ischemic dysfunction because it is not affected by the spatial motion of the ventricle or by alterations in ventricular shape. In clinical studies, normal systolic wall thickening has averaged 36% (range 14 to 57%),[132] and experimentally, mean thickening has ranged from 5 to 100%.[133] Wall thickening characteristically decreases in areas of scar or acute ischemia, whereas wall thinning is noted only with acute ischemia and infarction.[119,133,134] Direct correlations between wall thickening and extent of transmural pathologic infarct suggest that when less than 20% of the transmural myocardium is infarcted, mean thickening decreases by roughly 50%, whereas infarction of more than 20% of the transmural myocardium is uniformly associated with wall thinning.[135]

The ability of two-dimensional echocardiography to visualize myocardial thickness of the entire left ventricle is unique among currently available techniques for evaluating left ventricular function. Improvement in quantitation of regional thickening is thus an important and exciting challenge to allow more sensitive and specific evaluation of segmental left ventricular dysfunction.

Methods of Quantitation

There are three general methods for quantitating the extent of abnormal wall motion in patients with acute myocardial infarction: (1) the segmental approach in which the ventricle is divided into a number of segments, and the function within each segment is added to derive an index representing overall ventricular performance,[120,122–124,136–138] (2) representation of the endocardial surface area as the area of a geometric figure or combination of figures and the area of abnormal wall motion as a segment of the area of a subfigure to derive a "functional infarct size,"[126,139] or (3) measurement of the extent of abnormal wall motion within serial short-axis sections that can be related individually to histology, blood flow, or tracer kinetics within comparable anatomic sections or can be summed using Simpson's rule.[115,128,140,141]

The Segmental Approach

The segmental approach is the easiest but quantitatively the least precise method for describing infarct location and area. This approach divides the ventricle into a number of segments of roughly equal size whose margins are defined relative to fixed anatomic landmarks. Segmental systems have been described that differ both in the number of segments used and in their orientation within the ventricle. Figure 8–23 illustrates one such system. In this format, the ventricle is divided into nine segments—four at the base, four at the papillary muscle level, and one representing the cardiac apex. The individual segments are positioned such that they bracket the

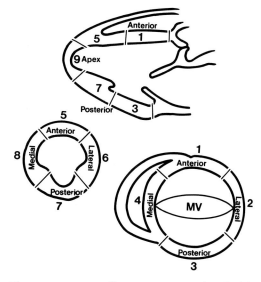

Fig. 8–23. Diagram illustrates a segmental method for defining specific anatomic areas of the left ventricle. (Adapted from Heger, J, et al.: Cross-sectional echocardiography in acute myocardial infarction: detection and localization of regional left ventricular asynergy. Circulation, 60:531, 1979. Reproduced by permission of the American Heart Association.)

orthogonal short-axis minor dimensions that are aligned relative to the mitral commissures and papillary muscles. The wall motion within each segment can then be determined, usually on a visual basis, and assigned a numeric score. By adding the performance values for each segment, a "wall motion index" that reflects the overall function of the ventricle can be derived and related to other indices of ventricular performance.

The Geometric Figure Method

A more quantitative method for determining the extent of abnormal wall motion uses the surface area of a single or combined geometric figure to represent the ventricular endocardial surface area.[126,139] The figure that has been used most commonly to represent the left ventricle in endocardial surface area calculations is the truncated cone. This figure has been used either alone, with an arbitrary area assigned to the apical cap,[126] or in combination with an ellipsoid segment, which is used to represent the cardiac apex.[139] Figure 8–24 illustrates the former method. In this format, the area of the truncated cone is calculated from the radii of short-axis segments at the mitral valve level and at the base of the papillary muscles. The height is taken as the long-axis length of the ventricle, and the apical cap is assigned an arbitrary area of 10%. Once the endocardial surface area of the whole ventricle (A_{Lv}) is known, the percent that functions abnormally or the functional infarct size (FIS) can be calculated as illustrated in Figure 8–25. In this example, a small area of abnormal wall motion is located posteriorly at the base of the ventricle. The extent of this "infarct area" (A_I) can be calculated by constructing a second truncated cone with a height that corresponds to the long-axis length of the asynergic segment. The radii of the base and apex of this cone are derived from short-axis scans at the basal and apical margins of the asynergic area. Because the asynergic area is

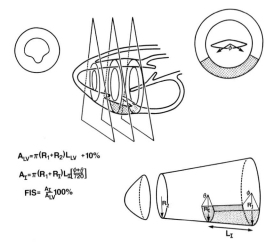

$$A_{LV} = \pi(R_1+R_2)L_{LV} + 10\%$$

$$A_I = \pi(R_1+R_I)L_I[\tfrac{\phi+\theta}{720}]$$

$$FIS = \tfrac{A_I}{A_{LV}} \cdot 100\%$$

Fig. 8–25. Diagram illustrates a method for calculating functional infarct size (FIS). In this format, the endocardial surface area of the left ventricle is initially calculated as in Figure 8–24. The area of a second figure that encompasses the infarct is then calculated separately. L_I is the length of the asynergic segment; R_1 is the radius of a short-axis scan taken at the base of the area of asynergy; and R_I is the radius of a scan at the apical margin of the asynergic segment. The functionally abnormal area within this subfigure can then be calculated from the percentage of the circumference of the short-axis scan at the base and apex of the infarct area which demonstrates asynergy. The area of abnormal function can then be expressed as a percentage of the total left ventricular endocardial surface area.

only a small percentage of the total area of this subfigure, the area of the whole subfigure is multiplied by the percent of the circumference that moves abnormally at each margin (see Fig. 8–25). The functional infarct size (FIS) is then expressed as a percentage of the total ventricular endocardial surface area by the relationship:

$$\text{FIS} = \text{asynergic area } (A_I) \div \text{total endocardial area } (A_{Lv}) \times 100 \quad (30)$$

Although the truncated cone has been the primary figure used in endocardial surface area calculations to date, any of the geometric models described in the section on volume calculation might be employed for this purpose.

Individual or Summed Short-Axis Sections

The final and most precise method for quantitating the extent of abnormal wall

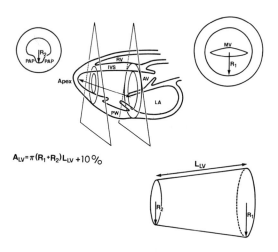

$$A_{LV} = \pi(R_1+R_2)L_{LV} + 10\%$$

Fig. 8–24. Diagram illustrates a method for determining the endocardial surface area of the left ventricle. With this approach, the area of the left ventricle is represented by the area of a truncated cone. The apex is assigned an arbitrary value of 10%. R_1 = the radius of the ventricle at the mitral valve level; R_2 = radius obtained from a short-axis scan at the low papillary muscle level. The long-axis length of the left ventricle (L_{LV}) is obtained in one of the apical views. PAP = papillary muscle; RV = right ventricle; IVS = interventricular septum; AV = aortic valve; LA = left atrium; PW = posterior wall; MV = mitral valve.

motion utilizes individual short-axis ventricular sections. In clinical studies, these sections are recorded at specific levels of the ventricle as identified by internal references. In experimental studies, short-axis sections can be recorded serially from apex to base as indicated in Figure 8–17. The regional wall motion within each section can then be analyzed in detail and, when serial sections are available, can be summed using Simpson's rule to describe the overall function of the ventricle.

Figure 8–26, A through C, illustrates the normal appearance and contraction pattern of a typical short-axis cross section from an experimental study. In panel A, recorded at end-diastole, the ventricular walls are relatively thin, and the cavity area is large. As systole progresses (B and C), there is inward excursion of the endocardium toward the center of the ventricle, a decrease in cavity area, and a thickening of the myocardium. Figure 8–27, in contrast, is a comparable section recorded following an experimentally induced infarction. In this example, there is loss of normal wall motion and thickening in the area of the infarct.

Short-axis sections are ideally suited to more detailed manual or computer analyses. Because short-axis motion is directed radially toward or away from the center of the ventricle, analysis is generally based on some form of radial coordinate system. Figure 8–28 illustrates such a system. In this example, 8 radii are constructed such that ventricular motion and thickening can be sampled at 45-degree intervals around the ventricular circumference. The end-diastolic position of the ventricular endocardium is indicated by the solid line, and the end-systolic position is indicated by the interrupted line. An area of dyskinesis involving roughly 25% of the ventricular circumference between the 90- and 180-degree radii is indicated.

Using this type of system, a number of parameters can be examined, including (1)

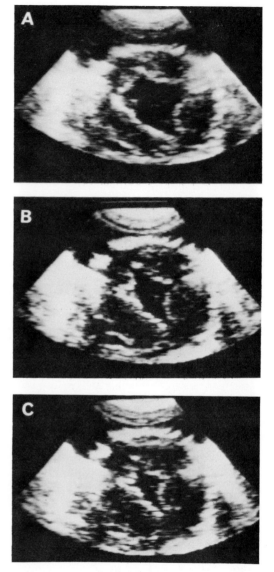

Fig. 8–26. Serial short-axis scans of the left ventricle from end-diastole (A) to end-systole (C). As the ventricle contracts, there is symmetric inward motion of the endocardium and an increase in wall thickness.

radial endocardial excursion, (2) radial wall thickening, (3) circumferential extent of abnormal wall motion (in this example 90 degrees/360 degrees or 25%), (4) expansion or contraction of an infarct area, and (5) changes in cavity and cavity section areas. Obviously, each of these measurements must be related to some central point within the ventricle that defines the

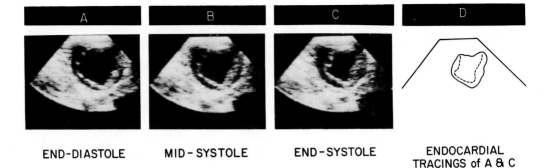

END-DIASTOLE   MID-SYSTOLE   END-SYSTOLE   ENDOCARDIAL
                                                       TRACINGS of A & C

Fig. 8–27. Parasternal short-axis scans of the left ventricle illustrate the loss of normal contraction that characterizes an area of infarction. (A) = end-diastole, (B) = mid-systole, (C) = end-systole. During this contraction sequence, there is symmetric inward motion of the endocardium in all areas except the anterior quadrant (from approximately the 11:00 to the 1:30 positions). The accompanying diagram (D) indicates this area of asynergy.

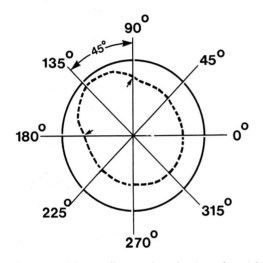

Fig. 8–28. Diagram illustrates how the circumferential extent of an area of asynergy can be quantitated using a radial coordinate system.

origin of the coordinate system. To date, fixed, floating, and mean centroids have been used for this purpose. Although a floating centroid appears to correct most appropriately for the spatial motion of the normal ventricle, a fixed reference is necessary to detect the abnormal motion of ischemic segments. Once the center of the ventricle is established, detailed analyses of individual sections are possible as illustrated in Figures 8–29 and 8–30. In Figure 8–29, serial tracings of the endocardial and epicardial interface positions from end-diastole to end-systole have been digitized and overlaid. The endocardial cen-

troid for each frame has also been determined, and the pattern of centroid motion has been plotted in the center of the ventricular cavity. It has been our preference to use the mean of the centroids for each frame as the initial reference for our radial coordinate system. This point forms a fixed reference in space, while still allowing for transitional motion of the ventricle.[24] Wall motion is then radially sampled at 10-degree intervals around the circumference of the ventricle, and a three-dimensional plot is constructed describing the amplitude and timing of excursion at each point from end-diastole to end-systole (Fig. 8–30). This type of plot condenses a large volume of data and illustrates the significant normal variation in the excursion of individual points around the ventricular circumference as well as the variation in the timing of peak excursion at each point.[130,131,133] This type of analysis is useful for detailed comparisons of wall motion with other parameters, such as regional myocardial flow or tracer kinetics.

Relationship of the Location and Extent of Abnormal Wall Motion to Pathologic Infarction

The relationship of the area of abnormal wall motion to underlying pathologic infarct distribution has been examined both clinically and experimentally. Infarction

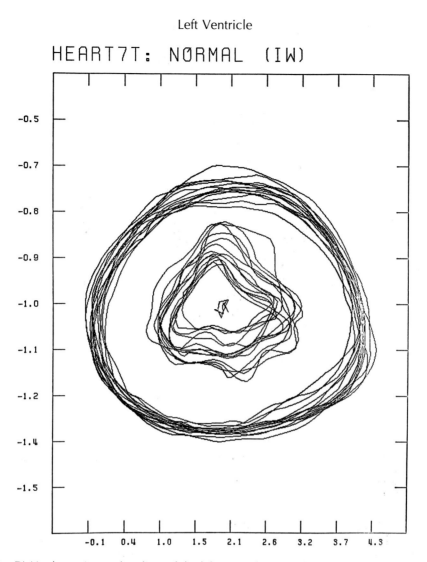

Fig. 8–29. Digitized superimposed outlines of the left ventricular epicardium and endocardium illustrate the contraction sequence from end-diastole to end-systole. The endocardial centroid for each frame is calculated and plotted within the center of the ventricular cavity.

was evident at pathologic examination in more than 95% of segments exhibiting abnormal wall motion in one study[122] and in all abnormally contracting segments with greater than 5% transmural infarction in another.[115] Experimentally, the circumferential extent of abnormal wall motion within individual short-axis sections has been shown to correlate well with both the pathologic infarct area[115] and the linear extent of the infarction in comparable anatomic sections.[140] The area of abnormal wall motion, however, consistently over-estimates both the area and the marginal extremes of the underlying infarct.[115,140] Figure 8–31 illustrates the relationship of the extent of abnormal wall motion, expressed as a percentage of the end-diastolic circumference of the ventricle, to the percent of the myocardial area that shows evidence of infarction in 47 ventricular sections.

Relationship of Abnormal Wall Motion to Electrocardiographic Infarct Location

Traditionally, the location of acute myocardial infarction has been determined

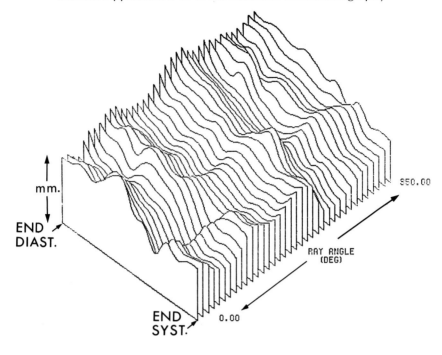

HEART7N: NORMAL (IW)

Fig. 8–30. Three-dimensional display of the endocardial excursion of individual points at 10-degree intervals around the circumference of the ventricle obtained from the digitized data in Figure 8–29. This plot depicts the distance from end-diastole (left) to end-systole (right) of points along radii that are separated by 10-degrees from the center of the left ventricle.

clinically by the Q-wave distribution on the standard 12-wave electrocardiogram.[142–144] The relationship of the electrocardiographically predicted location and extent of infarction to the echocardiographically recorded area of abnormal wall motion has been examined in several studies.[122,125] These relationships can be described best by using one of the segmental systems. This approach permits direct correlation between events occurring at specific anatomic locations within the ventricle.

Figure 8–32 illustrates a method that has been derived to display graphically these data. This format incorporates the segmental system illustrated in Figure 8–23 and depicts the heart as a series of three concentric rings.[122] The cardiac apex forms the central ring, and the four segments at the base of the heart form the outer ring. The ventricle is thereby displayed as if viewed from the apex. The interventricular septum is to the viewer's left, the lateral wall is to the right, the anterior wall is positioned superiorly, and the posterior wall is positioned inferiorly.

Inferior Infarction

The patterns of abnormal wall motion observed in patients with electrocardiographic evidence of isolated inferior, inferoposterior, and inferolateral infarction are illustrated in Figure 8–33. In this series, 95% of patients with electrocardiographic evidence of infarction involving the inferior wall (Q waves and leads 2,3, AVF) had dyssynergy involving at least one of the two posterior segments. When iso-

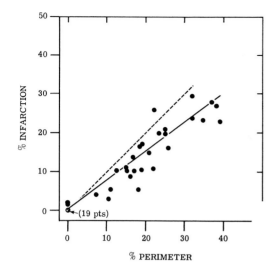

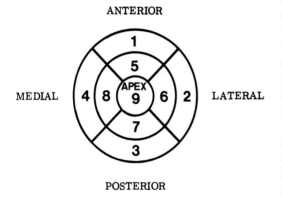

lated inferior infarction was present electrocardiographically (Fig. 8–33, *A*), asynergy was typically confined to the posterior quadrant and limited to one or, at most, two segments. The specific area of posterior involvement was evenly distributed between the base of the ventricle and the papillary muscle region. When inferior wall infarction was complicated by acute ventricular septal defect (Fig. 8–33, *B*), the region of asynergy uniformly involved the two medial segments, which correspond anatomically to the posterior portion of the interventricular septum. In each instance, septal aneurysm formation was noted.[122] None of these patients had electrocardiographic evidence of septal involvement, and the wall motion abnormality, therefore, was a better predictor of the extent and location of infarction. Patients in the electrocardiographic subgroups of inferoposterior infarction (Fig. 8–33, *C*) had asynergy extending to the lateral segments in addition to their posterior involvement. Those in the electrocardiographic inferolateral group (Fig. 8–33, *D*) had the most extensive involvement, which included the whole posterior quadrant, the lateral wall at the base, and variable involvement of the lateral wall in the midventricle. In this group, abnormal wall motion was also frequently noted in the cardiac apex, the midanterior wall, and the septum.

Unfortunately, this segmental system is not ideally aligned to depict the anatomic location of inferior infarction. The location of the abnormal inferior wall motion in this system is rotated roughly 30-degrees counterclockwise from its true anatomic location, and most inferior infarctions actually involve a portion of the medial and posterior segments.

Anterior Infarction

Figure 8–34, *A* through *C*, illustrates the patterns of abnormal wall motion observed in patients in the electrocardiographic subgroups of anterior infarction.[122]

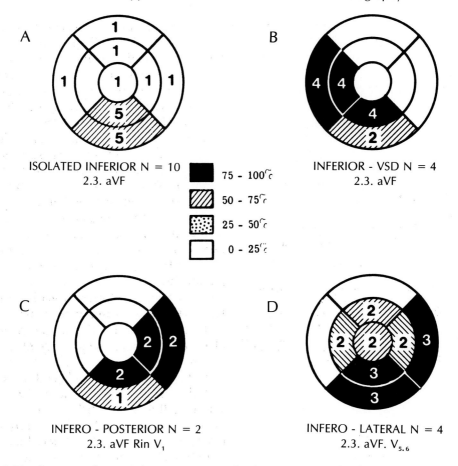

Fig. 8–33. Frequency of segmental asynergy associated with ECG subgroups of patients with inferior infarction. The shading indicates the percentage of patients within each group who show asynergy in a particular segment. VSD = ventricular septal defect. (From Heger, J, et al.: Cross-sectional echocardiography in acute myocardial infarction: detection and localization of regional left ventricular asynergy. Circulation, 60:531, 1979. Reproduced by permission of the American Heart Association.)

In all instances of anterior infarction, one of the anterior segments, either at the base or midventricular level, was abnormal.[122] In patients with anteroseptal infarction, abnormal motion occurred most frequently in the anterior segment at the midventricular level with associated involvement of the cardiac apex and the interventricular septum at the midventricle. The anterobasal and medial-basal segments were also frequently involved, but less so than were the more distal portions of the ventricle. Involvement of the base of the ventricle in anteroseptal infarction appears to depend on the level of obstruc-

tion of the left anterior descending coronary artery.

When the obstruction occurs proximal to the first septal perforator, the full extent of the anterior wall is abnormal, whereas obstruction below the first septal perforator characteristically spares the basal portions of the anterior wall.[145] In the subgroup of patients with anterolateral infarction, asynergy was observed to involve uniformly the cardiac apex and the anterior segment of the ventricle at the midventricular level. In the majority of these patients, the lateral segment at the midventricular level was also abnormal with an extensive but heterogeneous pattern of involvement

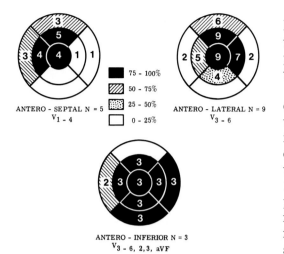

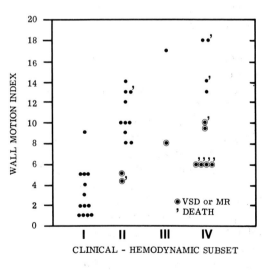

Fig. 8–34. Frequency of segmental asynergy associated with the ECG subgroups of patients with anterior wall infarction. (Adapted from Heger, J, et al.: Cross-sectional echocardiography in acute myocardial infarction: detection and localization of regional left ventricular asynergy. Circulation, 60:531, 1979. Reproduced by permission of the American Heart Association.)

lationship could be established between the degree of abnormal wall motion, expressed as a "wall motion index," and patient status.

Figure 8–35 illustrates the results of one of these studies. In this series, the ventricle was divided into 9 segments, as illustrated in Figure 8–23, and wall motion within each segment was assigned a numerical value (normal motion = 0, hypokinesis = 1, akinesis = 2, dyskinesis = 3, and hyperkinesis = −1) to derive an index reflecting both the extent and degree of dysfunction. In this format, when all nine segments functioned normally, the overall wall motion index equaled zero. When all segments were dyskinetic, the index was 3 (the numerical value for dyskinesis) × 9 (the number of segments), or 27. With this approach, the indices noted in pa-

of the remainder of the ventricle. Finally, patients with combined anterior and inferior infarction had extensive ventricular motion abnormalities. Only the anterobasal segment was completely spared.

These observations are consistent with older pathologic data and suggest that, in general, inferior infarction tends to be oriented more toward the base of the ventricle, whereas anterior infarctions tend to involve the cardiac apex. They also suggest that apical dysfunction is poorly reflected electrocardiographically and that inferior wall infarction may extend into the interventricular septum and may be associated with severe septal damage without electrocardiographic evidence of septal involvement.

Relationship of Abnormal Wall Motion to Ventricular Performance

The extent and severity of the abnormal wall motion that is recorded echocardiographically have been compared to both clinical and hemodynamic evidence of ventricular performance in several clinical studies.[123,136,137] In each study, a clear re-

Fig. 8–35. Relationship of extent and severity of abnormal wall motion (expressed as a wall motion index) to the clinical-hemodynamic performance of individual patients. Group I = uncomplicated myocardial infarction; group II = pulmonary congestion without peripheral hypoperfusion; group III = peripheral hypoperfusion without pulmonary congestion; and group IV = cardiogenic shock (Swan-Forrester classification). (From Heger, J, et al.: Cross-sectional echocardiographic analysis of the extent of left ventricular asynergy in acute myocardial infarction. Circulation, 61:1113, 1980. Reproduced by permission of the American Heart Association.)

tients with uncomplicated infarctions were significantly lower than those in patients with evidence of pulmonary congestion or peripheral hypoperfusion. Further, in the absence of acute ventricular septal defect or mitral regurgitation, death was noted only in patients with the highest wall motion indices.

When ventricular septal rupture or acute mitral regurgitation complicated infarction, the mean wall motion index, although still significantly higher than that observed with uncomplicated infarction, was less than expected given the severity of the hemodynamic dysfunction and the high mortality within this group.[123] Apparently, allowance for hyperkinesis in the noninfarcted segments inappropriately weighted the index, and in this setting, areas of apparent compensatory hyperfunction do not favorably affect outcome.

Relationship of Abnormal Wall Motion to Survival

Survival following acute myocardial infarction has been related to two echocardiographic parameters, functional infarct size[126] and infarct expansion.[145] Figure 8–36 illustrates the relationship of survival to functional infarct size derived using the truncated cone formula illustrated in Figures 8–23, and 8–24 and expressed as a percentage of overall left ventricular endocardial surface area. In this group of 32 patients, the mean functional infarct area for survivors was significantly less than the mean for nonsurvivors. Importantly, all patients with functional infarct areas involving 35% or less of the ventricle survived. In the group with infarct areas of greater than 35%, approximately 60% were nonsurvivors. Thus, although patients with large functional infarct sizes (up to 68%) may survive, such patients are at high risk, and survival is associated with major pump dysfunction.[126] Because wall motion becomes abnormal immediately following an acute is-

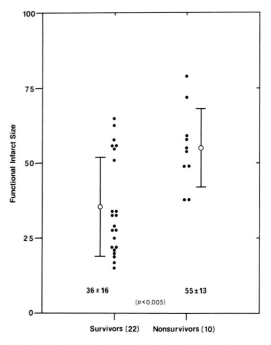

Fig. 8–36. Relationship of functional infarct size, expressed as a percentage of total left ventricular endocardial surface area, to patient survival.

chemic event, this method should identify patients at high risk early in their clinical course.

The second parameter that is associated with a significant mortality is infarct expansion.[146] The majority of evidence, to date, suggests that once the margins of an infarct are established, they remain fairly constant over time in the absence of reinfarction. Significant expansion within the infarct area, however, may occur in as many as 25% of patients. Infarct expansion can be observed as early as 3 days after acute infarction and, once initiated, appears to continue through the first several weeks. When present, expansion has been associated with significant risk of ventricular rupture and subsequent death (50%).[146]

A Simplified Visual Method for Estimating Functional Infarct Size During the Cross-Sectional Examination

Each of the methods described earlier in this chapter for infarct quantitation requires detailed analysis of wall motion or extensive calculation. Figure 8–37 illustrates a simplified method by which infarct size can be estimated visually during the course of a cross-sectional examination. With this approach, the maximal long-axis extent of the abnormally moving segment is first defined and expressed as a percentage of the total long-axis length of the ventricle. In this illustration, for example, the abnormally moving segment, indicated by the stippled region, involves 50% of the posterior wall.

The next step is to determine the maximal short-axis extent of the abnormally contracting area. This determination is made by looking at the ventricular short axis as the face of a clock and determining the extent of the infarct area in terms of hours (see Fig. 8–37). In this example, the abnormally moving segment (stippled area) extends from the 4 to the 8 o'clock position or encompasses a 4-hour segment of the 12-hour clock face. Thus, the abnormal segment involves 33% (12 divided by 4) of the ventricular circumference. The total percentage of infarction is then calculated by multiplying the long-axis percent involvement (in this example, 50% or .5) by the short-axis percentage (33% or 0.33). In this example, functional infarct

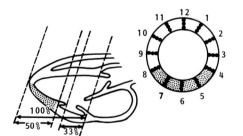

PERCENT INF. = PERCENT LAx x PERCENT SAx

Fig. 8–37. A simplified method for the visual calculation of the functional infarct area. In this format, the long-axis extent of the asynergic segment is expressed as a percentage of the total long axis (LAx) and is multiplied by the percentage of the circumference in short axis (SAx) that is asynergic to obtain the overall percentage of the ventricle that shows functional evidence of infarction.

size would equal roughly 17% of the ventricle.

This simplified method has been compared with the truncated cone method (see Fig. 8–24) for calculating functional infarct size with surprisingly good results. It is particularly useful in the emergency room or coronary care unit, where some numerical estimate of infarct size is frequently helpful and detailed immediate analysis is impractical.

Chronic Ischemic Heart Disease

Chronic ischemic changes in the left ventricle that can be appreciated echocardiographically include fixed segmental wall motion abnormalities,[138,147–150] myocardial scar,[151] and ventricular aneurysm.[152–154] Regional wall motion abnormalities may be the result of a single small area of infarction, a prior massive event, or may be the sum of the multiple small areas of ventricular damage. As such, they vary widely in severity, distribution, and extent. At present, the left ventricular cineangiogram is the standard clinical method for evaluating regional left ventricular wall motion, and a number of studies have compared the echocardiographic and angiographic assessment of regional ventricular function. When examining these comparative data, one must first appreciate the relationship of the areas of the ventricle imaged in the more commonly obtained angiographic views to the standard echocardiographic imaging planes.

Figure 8–38 illustrates the path along which the x-ray beam transects the left ventricle in the standard angiographic views and the relationship of the ventricular borders delineated in these angiographic projections to a standard echocardiographic short-axis cross section. In each of the angiographic projections, the margins of the ventricle that are imaged are orthogonal to the direction of the x-ray beam. The margins of the ventricular wall,

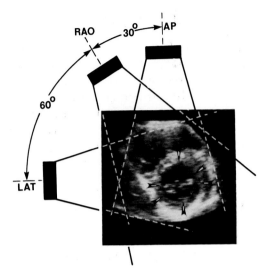

Fig. 8–38. Parasternal short-axis recording of the left ventricle indicates the points on the ventricular circumference that are imaged by using the standard cineangiographic anteroposterior (AP), right anterior oblique (RAO), and right lateral projections (LAT). Because the angiogram is a silhouette image, the margins of the ventricle that are projected in each of these standard planes are orthogonal to the direction of the x-ray beam.

which are imaged in the anteroposterior projection, roughly correspond to the 3 and 9 o'clock positions of the short-axis plane; the 30-degree right anterior oblique projection to the 1 and 7 o'clock positions; the 30-degree left anterior oblique projection to the 11 and 5 o'clock positions; and the left lateral projection to the ventricular borders at 12 and 6 o'clock. Given these relationships, the parasternal long-axis view of the left ventricle appears to correspond most closely to the 30-degree left anterior oblique angiographic projection. The apical four-chamber view images the ventricular walls at a point between the 30- and 60-degree left anterior oblique projections, and the apical two-chamber view roughly approximates an RAO projection.

When comparing angiographic and echocardiographic data, therefore, one must analyze the views that look at similar areas of the ventricle. In many older studies, comparisons were made between the M-mode assessment of ventricular wall motion and the RAO angiographic projec-

tions. These studies, unfortunately, look at different areas of the ventricle. In addition, comparisons between two-dimensional echocardiographic and angiographic analyses of wall motion cannot be precisely made because of the different physiologic stresses imposed by the examinations and because of basic differences in the data obtained. The echocardiographic image is tomographic in nature, whereas the angiogram is a silhouette image, which lies within a single plane only when ventricular geometry is symmetric. Even when comparable areas of the ventricle are examined, some differences in angiographic and echocardiographic wall motion can be expected because the angiogram is oriented relative to the axes of the body, whereas the echocardiogram is aligned relative to the heart.

A number of studies have compared echocardiographic and angiographic assessments of regional wall motion. These studies generally employ a segmental system and compare qualitative performance in individual regions. Available data suggest that echocardiographic visualization of at least a portion of the ventricle can be achieved in between 89 and 95% of the patients with chronic ischemic disease.[18,149] Complete visualization of the ventricle can be achieved in from 60 to 88% of patients.[138,149] The percentage of individual segments of the ventricle recorded varies with the segmental system employed; when general areas of interest are considered, 72 to 87% of segments are usually recordable.[138,149] Comparisons of wall motion in areas that are adequately visualized by both techniques have been excellent, and the major sources of discrepancy relate to differences in definition or visual grade.[18,149]

Many patients with coronary artery disease and normal left ventricular function develop wall motion abnormalities during exercise in areas that are marginally perfused.[102,105] Echocardiographic studies performed during exercise can identify these transient motion abnormalities. When present, the abnormalities appear to be highly specific for identifying ischemic disease, as evidenced by high-grade coronary obstruction of the vessels supplying the abnormal region and by transient thallium-201 perfusion defects.[104] The sensitivity of exercise-induced asynergy as a marker of coronary artery disease is low, however.[102,105] This is due to the imprecise correlation of regional ischemia with coronary arterial narrowing and to the technical limitations in performing an echocardiographic study during exercise.

Left Ventricular Scar

Scar formation is common following myocardial infarction. Scar tissue is typically more dense than surrounding muscle, and the ventricular wall in the scarred area is thinner than normal (Fig. 8–39). Echocardiographically, scar is characterized by an increase in echo production from the dense fibrous area and a decrease in diastolic wall thickness (less than 7 mm or 30% less than surrounding normal areas).[155] Systolic wall motion and thickening are usually decreased in the scarred area. On occasion, however, both motion and thickening may appear normal. Echocardiography appears to be a sensitive and specific method for detecting myocardial scar with surgical or pathologic confirmation being demonstrated in 95% of patients in one series.[155]

Left Ventricular Aneurysms

Left ventricular aneurysms may be acquired or congenital. Acquired aneurysms most commonly develop following acute myocardial infarction, although more rarely they may result from trauma or myocardial abscess. Pathologically, left ventricular aneurysms can be divided into true aneurysms, false or pseudoaneurysms, and congenital aneurysms or diverticula. These types of aneurysms differ in both their clinical significance and their echocardio-

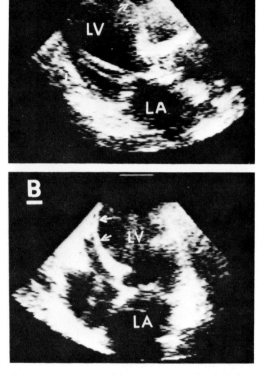

Fig. 8–39. Parasternal long-axis (A) and apical four-chamber views (B) illustrate an area of anteroapical scar (arrowheads). The area of scar is thinner than the normal muscle and, in real time, was dyskinetic. LV = left ventricle; LA = left atrium.

graphic appearance, and therefore, they are discussed separately.

True Aneurysms

By far, the most common type of aneurysm is the true aneurysm. True aneurysms usually develop following acute myocardial infarction and have been noted in as many as 15% of reported cases.[156–158] True aneurysms form through gradual expansion and thinning of the myocardium in the infarcted area and characteristically contain all the layers of the ventricular wall.[158] Initially, the wall of the aneurysm is composed predominantly of necrotic muscle and fibrous tissue.[158] With time, fibrosis and, occasionally, calcification increase.[159] Though early rupture of these aneurysms may be noted on rare occasions, late rupture almost never occurs.[151,160] Once formed, ventricular aneurysms may contribute to the development of cardiac decompensation and may underlie such serious secondary complications as refractory congestive heart failure, recurrent ventricular arrhythmias, and systemic emboli.[158]

Echocardiographically true aneurysms distort the shape of the left ventricle during both diastole and systole.[152] This definition distinguishes aneurysms from dyskinetic segments (where the distortion in shape is only present during systole). The wall of the aneurysm is typically thin in comparison to the normal myocardium, and motion of the aneurysmal segment is paradoxic. True aneurysms characteristically have a wide neck, and the diameter of the neck is comparable to the maximal diameter of the aneurysm.

The presence of the aneurysm is frequently highlighted by a prominent junction or hinge point between the more normally moving areas of the ventricle and the paradoxic motion of the aneurysmal segment.[152] The sensitivity of the echocardiographic diagnosis of ventricular aneurysms has ranged from 93 to 100%.[152,154] Occasional false-negatives have also been reported.[153,154] These occur most commonly when the aneurysms are small and extend from the tip of the cardiac apex or involve the high anterolateral wall. Between 85 and 95% of true aneurysms involve the cardiac apex, and extension into the anterior wall is common.[152,153,161] Thrombus is frequently present within left ventricular aneurysms and is reported pathologically in 15 to 77% of cases[162,163] and echocardiographically in as many as 34% of patients.[153]

Figure 8–40 is an example of a large anteroapical aneurysm. The aneurysm, indicated by the arrowheads, creates a distortion in the apical segment of the left ventricle. The neck of the aneurysm is wide, and when viewed in real-time, the aneurysmal segment moved paradoxically. Figure 8–41 illustrates a second large anteroapical aneurysm. In this example, the aneurysm is larger than the remaining normally functioning ventricle. Despite their predominant apical location, true aneurysms may develop anywhere in the ventricular wall. Figure 8–42, for example, illustrates a large aneurysm arising from the posterolateral surface of the ventricle.

False or Pseudoaneurysms

A rare type of left ventricular aneurysm is the false or pseudoaneurysm.[151,160,164] Pseudoaneurysms result from myocardial rupture, with the extravasated blood being contained by adherent parietal pericardium.[164] The rupture most commonly follows acute myocardial infarction, though it may also result from trauma, laceration, or abscess.[162–164] Pathologically, pseudoaneurysms are characterized by a small, narrow-necked channel that connects the ventricle with a larger aneurysmal sac containing blood and thrombus and lined by fibrous pericardial tissue without any myocardial elements. Pseudoaneurysms may be associated with the same complications noted with true aneurysms, but are particularly important because of their greater overall incidence of rupture and particularly because of their tendency for late rupture.[163,164]

Echocardiographically, the pseudoaneurysms appear as large, saccular or globular, echo-free chambers that are external to the left ventricular cavity.[165–168] They are connected to the ventricular cavity by a narrow neck the diameter of which is generally less than 40% of the maximal diameter of the aneurysm.[168] The neck typically produces an abrupt interruption in the ventricular wall in contrast to the gradual tapering of the myocardium into the aneurysm (which is characteristic of a true aneurysm). Figure 8–43 illustrates a large pseudoaneurysm that appears as an echo-free space external to the lateral wall of

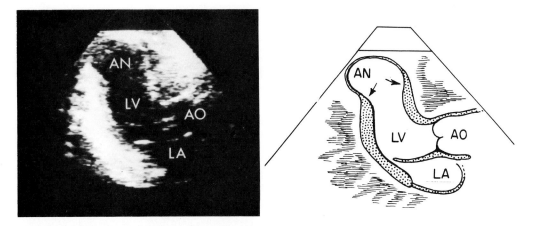

Fig. 8–40. Parasternal long-axis recording illustrates a large anteroapical aneurysm (AN). LA = left atrium; LV = left ventricle; AO = aorta.

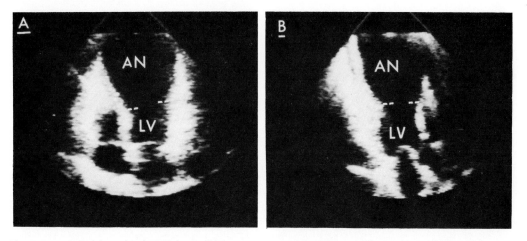

Fig. 8–41. Apical four-chamber and apical long-axis views of the left ventricle (LV) from a patient with a large anteroapical aneurysm (AN). In this example, the aneurysm is twice the size of the residual left ventricular cavity.

the ventricle. This aneurysm was produced by laceration of the ventricle, and the aneurysmal neck is small in comparison to the diameter of the aneurysm.

Left Ventricular Diverticula

Left ventricular diverticula are uncommon but well-recognized congenital cardiac malformations.[169–174] These diverticula are classified as either muscular or fibrous.[171] The muscular type is typically associated with midline thoracoabdominal defects and other cardiac malformations, whereas the fibrous variety usually occur as isolated ventricular lesions located in the subvalvular or apical regions. These diverticula, often referred to as aneurysms, may be associated with a number of complications, including mitral incompetence, angina pectoris, cardiac arrhythmias, systemic emboli, and cardiac rupture.[171,173,174] Figure 8–44 illustrates both the angiographic and cross-sectional echocardiographic appearance of a small diverticulum arising from the posterior surface of the left ventricle and communicating with the ventricular cavity. Echocardiographically, the diverticulum appeared as a small, circular, echo-free space

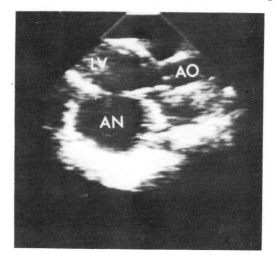

Fig. 8–42.   Parasternal long-axis recording of a large posterior aneurysm (AN). LV = left ventricle; AO = aorta.

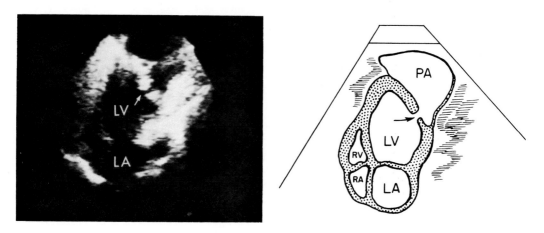

Fig. 8–43.   Apical four-chamber recording of a left ventricular pseudoaneurysm (PA). The pseudoaneurysm appears as a large echo-free space anterior and lateral to the apex and lateral wall of the left ventricle (LV). The narrow neck of the aneurysm is indicated by the horizontal arrow. RV = right ventricle; RA = right atrium; LA = left atrium.

behind and apparently communicating with the left ventricular cavity.[175]

Ventricular Septal Rupture

Ventricular septal rupture is a rare complication of acute myocardial infarction occurring in 0.5 to 1.0% of patients.[176] Ventricular septal rupture is associated with a grave prognosis, and death occurs in 54% of the patients within the first week following perforation and in as many as 87% within the first 2 months.[176] Most septal perforations are located in the postero-apical region and are characteristically associated with extensive myocardial infarction. The size of the perforation may vary considerably, but is usually less than 4 cm in diameter.[176] Although in the majority of cases a single perforation is noted, multiple perforations have been reported. Roughly 75% of septal perforations occur following left coronary artery occlusion and anterior wall infarction. The interval from the onset of pain to perforation av-

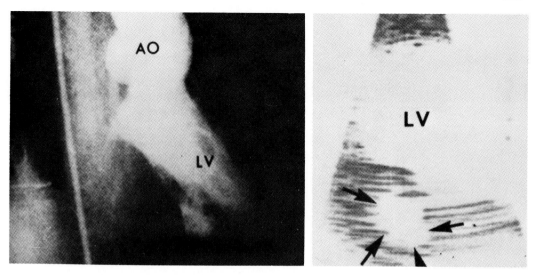

Fig. 8–44. Angiogram and cross-sectional echogram from a patient with a congenital left ventricular diverticulum. The diverticulum echocardiographically appears as a well-circumscribed, echo-free space posterior to the left ventricular cavity, which communicates to the left ventricular chamber through a narrow neck. LV = left ventricle; AO = aorta.

erages 3.5 days; intervals of from several hours to 9 days have been reported.[176,177]

Clinically, septal perforation is heralded by the sudden appearance of a new systolic murmur and by rapid hemodynamic deterioration. The differential diagnosis in these instances is generally between septal rupture and acute mitral regurgitation due to papillary muscle dysfunction or chordal rupture.[176–178]

Echocardiographically, septal perforation is detected primarily through direct visualization of the septal defect.[179–181] These defects appear as abrupt interruptions in the septal musculature and are usually surrounded by an extensive area of asynergy. They are typically located posteriorly in close proximity to the cardiac apex, and associated septal aneurysm formation is common.[181] Their method of formation and echocardiographic appearance are similar to those of a pseudoaneurysm. When septal perforation complicates anterior infarction, anteroapical dyskinesis is characteristically present. When septal rupture complicates inferior infarction, the apex is generally spared,

and there is an extensive area of posterior wall dyskinesis.

Variation in the size of the perforation is frequently noted. During systole, the perforation typically expands and may increase by as much as three times its diastolic diameter.[179,181]

Because of the higher left ventricular systolic pressure, shunt flow through these septal perforations is predominantly from left to right.[179] Peripherally injected contrast may be helpful in confirming the diagnosis of ventricular septal perforation. In general, this is based on a negative contrast effect at the right ventricular margin of the defect where the contrast containing blood in the right ventricular cavity is displaced by the blood flowing from the left ventricle that does not contain contrast.[179]

Additional findings that can be noted with acute ventricular septal rupture are right ventricular dilatation, left atrial dilatation, and exaggerated contraction of noninfarcted areas of the left ventricle.[177] Paradoxic septal motion, when present, is usually the result of septal dyskinesis.

Figure 8–45 is an example of ventricular septal rupture complicating acute myo-

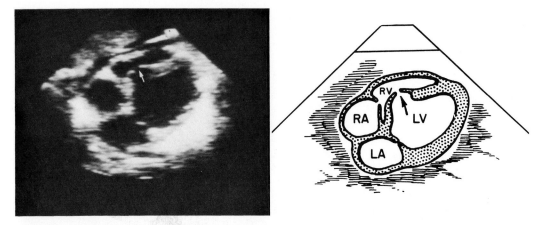

Fig. 8–45. Subcostal long-axis recording illustrates ventricular septal rupture complicating acute myocardial infarction. The defect (vertical arrow) is at the tip of a septal aneurysm. RV = right ventricle; RA = right atrium; LA = left atrium; LV = left ventricle.

cardial infarction. In this instance, the ventricular septal defect lies at the posterior margin of the interventricular septum, just superior to the posteromedial papillary muscle.

LEFT VENTRICULAR THROMBI

Left ventricular mural thrombi are a relatively common complication of acute myocardial infarction being noted in from 20 to 60% of cases in postmortem series.[157,162,163,182–184] Thrombus formation appears more often with larger infarcts, and the incidence of mural thrombus increases when there is left ventricular aneurysm formation. Detection of these thrombi may be of major clinical importance because they presumably underlie the arterial embolic events noted in as many as 5% of patients following acute infarction.[185–187]

Echocardiographically, mural thrombi appear as focal, echo-producing masses superimposed on and interrupting the normal endocardial contour of the ventricle in regions of akinesis or dyskinesis.[188–196] They may be fixed, pedunculated and freely mobile or may have a fixed base with mobile filaments extending from the surface. Thrombi characteristically have a speckled appearance and, when organized, may contain areas that are brighter

than surrounding myocardium. Thrombi that occur in the absence of aneurysm formation almost invariably involve the cardiac apex. However, on a rare occasion, a thrombus may be noted arising from the anterior or anterolateral free wall when no aneurysm is present. Apical thrombi are best visualized in one of the apical views. When thrombus is suspected in an apical view, however, confirmation usually requires its visualization in at least one other projection.

Thrombi generally become visible echocardiographically between the sixth and tenth day following an acute infarction.[194] The natural history of these thrombi is unclear. In small series, however, little change has been noted within the first few months after formation, but regression and ultimate disappearance during long-term observation is possible.[189] To date, thrombi have only been observed following anterior wall infarction. This association is not surprising because anterior infarctions tend to be larger than and tend to involve the cardiac apex more frequently than do inferior wall infarcts. The critical underlying factors appear to be size and associated apical involvement rather than infarct location. Inferior wall infarction with apical dyskinesis is also expected to underlie apical thrombus formation.

Figure 8–46, *A*, illustrates the appearance of a globular thrombus within the cardiac apex of a patient with an established anterior wall myocardial infarction. This thrombus is well defined and has a speckled internal appearance. Figure 8–46, *B* and *C*, are two examples of laminar thrombus within an apical aneurysm. In panel *B*, the thrombus appears confined to the anterior margin of the aneurysm; however, as the scan is continued inferiorly, a second area of laminar thrombus along the posterior wall of the aneurysm is apparent. The posterior thrombus is more dense and appears better organized than the thrombus that is recorded anteriorly.

LEFT VENTRICULAR TUMORS

Tumors involving the left ventricle are rare, and limited data are available concerning their echocardiographic manifestations.[193] In general, left ventricular tumors, like those of the other cardiac chambers, may be intracavitary, intramural, or extramural. Most tumors that involve the left ventricle are extramural, arising within the posterior mediastinum and deforming the left ventricular chamber by external compression. Figure 8–47 is an example of a large sarcoma (located behind the left ventricle) that pushes against the posterior border of this chamber, thereby producing a posterior concavity. Intramural tumors produce focal thickening of the ventricular wall and may extend into the ventricular chamber.[193]

Figure 6–11 is an example of an intramural left ventricular fibroma. This example is included in the section on the left atrium because the tumor extended into the atrial cavity. Its site of origin, however, was the left ventricular myocardium. Figure 15–11 is an example of a metastatic adenocarcinoma involving the myocardium. In this example, the primary manifestation is pericardial effusion; however, the echocardiographic pattern suggests myocardial involvement. Intracavitary

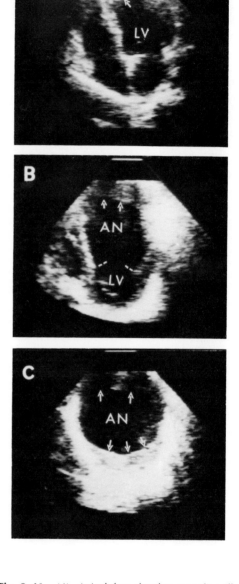

Fig. 8–46. (*A*), Apical four-chamber recording illustrates a circumscribed thrombus within the apex of the left ventricle (LV). The thrombus is clearly demarcated and has a speckled internal pattern. (*B*), A recording from a second patient with an anteroapical aneurysm (AN) containing a large laminar thrombus (vertical arrowheads). The origin of the aneurysm from the left ventricle (LV) is indicated by the interrupted lines. (*C*), Short-axis recording through the aneurysm (AN). Anteriorly, the faint laminar thrombus is apparent, whereas posteriorly, an equally large area of thrombus is more highly reflective, suggesting that it is better organized.

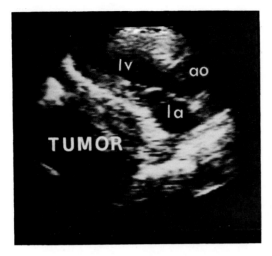

Fig. 8–47. A posterior mediastinal sarcoma that compresses the left ventricle (lv) from behind, creating a posterior concavity in the ventricular wall. ao = aorta; la = left atrium.

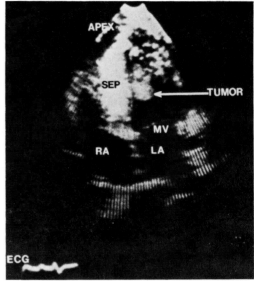

Fig. 8–48. Metastatic malignant melanoma within the left ventricular cavity. The tumor appears as an intracavitary mass of echoes that is similar in appearance to the left ventricular thrombus (illustrated in Figure 8–44). SEP = septum; RA = right atrium; LA = left atrium; MV = mitral valve. (From Ports, TA, Cogan, J, Schiller, NB, and Rapaport, E: Echocardiography of left ventricular masses. Circulation, 58:528, 1978.)

tumors are encountered even less frequently. When present, however, they generally appear as fixed or mobile masses of echoes with the ventricle.[193] Figure 8–48 is an example of an intracavitary melanoma. The appearance of this tumor mass does not differ greatly from that of the thrombi discussed earlier, and echocardiographic differentiation may be difficult.

CARDIOMYOPATHIES

The cardiomyopathies are a large heterogeneous group of disorders that primarily affect the heart muscle. The cardiomyopathies are unique in that the muscular derangement does not result from ischemic, hypertensive, valvular, or pericardial disease.[197] The cardiomyopathies are usually subdivided on a functional basis into the congestive, restrictive or infiltrative, and hypertrophic forms.[197] Hypertrophic cardiomyopathy or idiopathic hypertrophic subaortic stenosis is classically associated with left ventricular outflow obstruction and is discussed in Chapter 7.

Congestive Cardiomyopathies

The congestive cardiomyopathies are characterized primarily by a generalized decrease in systolic pump function.[198,199] The reduced contractile function typically involves both the right and left ventricles and is associated with an increase in both diastolic and systolic chamber volumes. Wall motion is symmetrically reduced, and this symmetric dysfunction permits differentiation from ischemic disease in which wall motion abnormalities are typically segmental.[200] Wall thickness is usually normal, and hypertrophy, when present, is not proportionate to the increase in chamber volume. Wall thickening may also decrease. Diastolic mitral valve excursion is reduced, and the E-point septal separation is usually increased. Left ventricular dilatation may result in incomplete mitral valve closure (see Chap. 5), and both the anterior and posterior mitral leaflets may fail to reach the plane of the mitral annulus.[201] Left and right atrial dilatation are also common. When right ventricular dilatation is marked, incomplete closure of the tricuspid valve may also be noted. Figure 8–49 is an example of a patient with congestive cardiomyopathy and biventricular failure.

The echocardiographic features of congestive cardiomyopathy provide little insight into the underlying cause and support the general observation that the congestive pattern may represent a final common pathway for a variety of disorders.[202]

Restrictive Myopathies

Endocardial Fibroelastosis

Endocardial fibroelastosis is a disorder of infants and young children characterized by diffuse hyperplasia of the endocardium caused by proliferation of collagenous and elastic tissue.[203,204] This disorder may be primary or secondary. The primary form is unassociated with other congenital cardiac defects and involves the left ventricle almost exclusively.[205–208] The endocardium is thicker, and the area of involvement is greater than that noted in the secondary variety. Primary endocardial fibroelastosis can be subdivided on the basis of left ventricular size into the dilated and contracted forms.[203,204] The dilated form, in which the ventricular chamber is enlarged and the walls hypertrophied, is the more common. Fibrosis and thickening of the aortic and mitral leaflets with chordal shortening and fibrosis are also common and may lead to mitral regurgitation.[204]

Secondary endocardial fibroelastosis is pathologically indistinguishable from the primary form. In general, however, the secondary variety is more focal in nature,

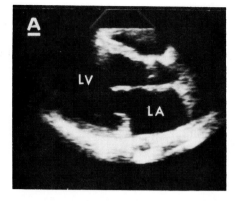

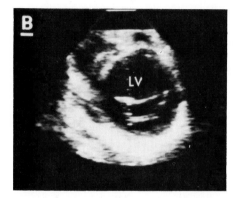

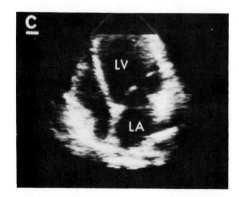

Fig. 8–49. Parasternal long-axis (A), short-axis (B), and apical four-chamber views (C) of a patient with congestive cardiomyopathy. The left ventricle (LV) is dilated and the ventricular walls appear thin. Each frame is recorded at peak diastolic mitral valve opening and indicates the reduction in mitral leaflet excursion that results from the reduced flow through the mitral valve orifice. LA = left atrium.

and the endocardial proliferation is less marked. Mural thrombi commonly complicate both varieties.[209] The secondary form is most commonly associated with obstruction to left ventricular outflow, particularly aortic stenosis[210] and coarctation of the aorta,[211] but may be observed in a variety of other anomalies, including anomalous origin of the left coronary artery from the pulmonary artery and hypoplastic left heart syndrome. Echocardiographically, subendocardial fibroelastosis appears as a focal or diffuse area of increased echo production arising from the endocardial interface. This dense band of echoes is usually homogeneous and may be several millimeters thick.[212] It stands out in sharp contrast to the normal epicardial echoes. Figure 8–50 is a parasternal long-axis recording from a patient with subendocardial fibroelastosis and illustrates the endocardial predominance.

Löffler's Endocarditis

Löffler's endocarditis (eosinophilic endomyocardial disease) is a rare form of endocardial fibrosis that is characteristically associated with a chronic persistent elevation in circulating eosinophils.[213–217] The endocardial fibrosis usually involves the subvalvular areas and cardiac apex and, when pronounced, may cause valvular insufficiency due to thickening of the chordae tendineae and interference with their normal function.[213–222] Mitral and tricuspid stenosis may also occur and appear to result from entrapment of the subvalvular apparatus in the fibrous material.[223–225]

Superimposed thrombus formation is frequent.[213,217–219] Echocardiographically, the subendocardial fibrous accumulation results in a generalized increase in ventricular wall thickness, a local increase in reflectivity, and layering of the endocardial echoes particularly in the subvalvular regions.[225,226] Nonspecific features, including atrial and ventricular enlargement and pericardial effusion, have also been reported.[226] Figure 9–8 is an example of Löffler's endocarditis that presented as mitral and tricuspid stenosis. In this example, there is a focal accumulation of echogenic material along the endocardial surface of the right ventricular free wall and reduced tricuspid valve opening.

Infiltrative Cardiomyopathies

Amyloidosis

Amyloidosis is a disease of unknown cause characterized by the deposition of an abnormal eosinophilic fibrous protein in various tissues and organs of the body.[227] Cardiac involvement is common, and amyloidosis is reported to account for between 5 and 10% of noncoronary cardiomyopathies.[228] In patients with amyloidosis, heart failure is the most common cause of death and is noted in as many as 20% of patients.[229]

In amyloidosis, the abnormal protein is deposited between the myocardial fibers, which it may surround, compress, and finally replace.[228,230] It may also be found in the papillary muscles, conduction system,

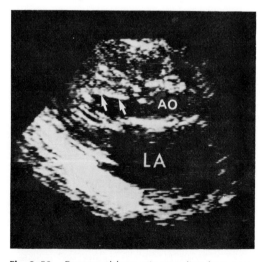

Fig. 8–50. Parasternal long-axis recording from a patient with subendocardial fiber elastosis. In this case, the ventricular cavity is small, and a dense rim of echo-producing material surrounds the endocardial surface of the ventricle (arrowheads). AO = aorta; LA = left atrium.

and pericardium. Amyloid deposition in the left atrium has been reported, and atrial involvement may be useful echocardiographically in differentiating amyloidosis from other infiltrative myopathies. Endocardial involvement of both the atrium and ventricles is not uncommon and may be associated with overlying thrombus. Amyloidosis also frequently causes focal or diffuse thickening of the cardiac valves (see Fig. 7–15), but valvular dysfunction is not characteristic.

There are four principal forms of amyloidosis:

1. Primary amyloidosis, which occurs independent of other systemic diseases and in which the tissue involvement is localized primarily to the heart, tongue, skin, gastrointestinal tract, and carpal ligaments.[229]

2. Secondary amyloidosis, which usually occurs in association with chronic disorders, such as rheumatoid arthritis or tuberculosis, and in which tissue involvement is primarily localized to the spleen, kidney, liver, and adrenals.

3. Familial amyloidosis of which multiple varieties have been described that differ in either clinical presentation or primary organ involvement.[231] Primary involvement of the heart is rare in familial amyloidosis,[231,232] but may be more common than previously suspected.

4. Senile amyloidosis, which appears to be a clinically distinct form of primary amyloidosis and is characterized by the advanced age of the affected person and the almost entirely cardiac location of the amyloid deposits.[230,233] Available data suggest that senile amyloidosis may be the most common form of amyloid, and its incidence can be expected to increase as the average age of the population increases. Senile amyloidosis has been reported at autopsy in 2 to 15% of the population over the age of 80, and its incidence is 3 to 4 times greater in patients dying of heart failure than in those without overt cardiac disease.[230,233]

The echocardiographic features in amyloid are illustrated in Figure 8–51. Amyloidosis typically produces an increase in right and left ventricular wall thickness. The thickened myocardium frequently has a speckled or ground glass sparkling appearance, chamber sizes may be normal or reduced, and wall motion is frequently decreased.[234–236] Pericardial effusion is not uncommon.[236] The interatrial septum and free atrial wall may also show an increase in thickness, and this picture may aid in differentiation of amyloid from other cardiac disorders.[236]

Hemochromatosis

Hemochromatosis is a systemic disorder characterized by increased deposition of iron in tissue and is usually associated with hepatic cirrhosis.[237] Hemochromatosis may occur as an idiopathic or hereditary disease, in association with chronic liver disease, as a result of congenital or acquired defects of erythrocytes or erythrocyte production, from anemia, or may be the result of excess oral or parenteral iron intake.[237] Cardiac iron deposition is common in hemochromatosis but is never noted in the absence of iron accumulation in other tissues. Iron deposits in myocardial cells are typically perinuclear but may extend to occupy much of the muscle fiber.[237] They are most common in the working tissues of the heart, particularly the left ventricular myocardium in which they are greatest in the subepicardial region, intermediate in the subendocardium and the papillary muscles, and least prominent in the middle third of the myocardium. The atrial myocardium may also be involved, but this involvement typically occurs later in the course of the disease and is less marked than the ventricular involvement.

Cardiac iron deposits appear to cause fiber degeneration, and fibrosis can result in congestive heart failure. Both phenomena appear related to the severity of the iron deposition. M-mode studies have

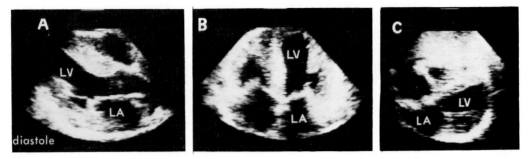

Fig. 8–51. Parasternal long-axis (A), apical four-chamber (B), and subcostal long-axis (C) views of the left ventricle (LV) from a patient with familial amyloidosis. The walls of the left and right ventricles and the interatrial septum are thickened. The valves are also thickened, and the myocardium has a diffusely speckled appearance.

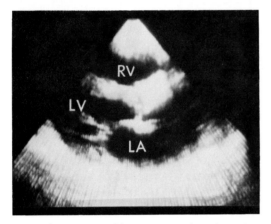

Fig. 8–52. Parasternal long-axis recording of a patient with hemochromatosis. The ventricular walls are slightly thicker than normal. Left ventricular systolic function was normal; however, the right ventricle (RV) and right atrium were dilated.

demonstrated that patients with hemochromatosis characteristically have an increase in left ventricular wall thickness. The wall thickening, however, is not as marked as that seen in amyloidosis.[234] Left ventricular mass is increased, and left ventricular chamber size may be normal or increased.[234] The left atrium may also be dilated. Figure 8–52 is a cross-sectional scan from a patient with hemochromatosis.

REFERENCES

1. Schlant, RC: Normal physiology of the cardiovascular system. *In* The Heart. Edited by JW Hurst. New York, McGraw-Hill, 1974.
2. Rushmer, RF: Cardiovascular Dynamics. Philadelphia, Saunders, 1970.
3. Gray, H: Gray's Anatomy. Edited by CM Goss. Philadelphia, Lea & Febiger, 1962.
4. Mall, FP: On the muscular architecture of the ventricles of the human heart. Am J Anat, 11:211, 1911.
5. Robb, JS, and Robb, RC: The normal heart. Am Heart J, 23:455, 1942.
6. Streeter, DD: Gross morphology and fiber geometry of the heart. *In* Handbook of Physiology. Vol. 1. Edited by P. Dow. Baltimore, Williams & Wilkins, 1962.
7. Wells, PNT: Biomedical Ultrasonics. New York, Academic Press, 1977.
8. Roelandt, J, et al.: Resolution problems in echocardiography: a source of interpretation errors. Am J Cardiol, 37:256, 1976.
9. Garrison, JB, et al.: Quantifying regional wall motion and thickening in two-dimensional echocardiography with a computer-aided contouring system. *In* Proceedings of Computers in Cardiology 1977. Edited by H Ostrow, and K Ripley. Long Beach, CA, Institute of Electrical and Electronics Engineers, 1977.
10. Feigenbaum, H, et al.: Correlation of ultrasound with angiocardiography in measuring left ventricular diastolic volume. Am J Cardiol, 23:111, 1969.
11. Feigenbaum, H, Popp, RL, and Wolfe, SB: Ultrasound measurements of the left ventricle: a correlative study with angiocardiography. Arch Intern Med, 129:461, 1972.
12. Fortuin, NH, Hood, WP, and Craige, E: Evaluation of left ventricular function by echocardiography. Circulation, 46:26, 1972.
13. Gibson, DG: Estimation of left ventricular size by echocardiography. Br Heart J, 35:128, 1973.
14. Pombo, JF, Troy, BL, and Russell, RO: Left ventricular volumes and ejection fraction by echocardiography. Circulation, 43:480, 1971.
15. Popp, RL, and Harrison, DC: Ultrasonic cardiac echocardiography for determining stroke volume and valvular regurgitation. Circulation, 41:493, 1970.
16. Feigenbaum, H: Echocardiography. Philadelphia, Lea & Febiger, 1976.
17. Carr, K, et al.: Measurement of left ventricular ejection fraction by mechanical cross-sectional echocardiography. Circulation, 59:1196, 1979.

18. Hickman, H, et al.: Cross-sectional echocardiography of the cardiac apex. Circulation (Suppl III), 56:589, 1977.

19. Mirro, MJ, Rogers, EW, Weyman, AE, and Feigenbaum, H: Angular displacement of the papillary muscles during the cardiac cycle. Circulation, 60:327, 1979.

20. Bansal, RC, Tajik, AJ, Seward, JB, and Offord, KP: Feasibility of detailed two-dimensional echocardiographic examination in adults: prospective study of 200 patients. Mayo Clin Proc, 55:291, 1980.

21. Folland, E, et al.: Assessment of left ventricular ejection fraction and volumes by real-time two-dimensional echocardiography. Circulation, 60:760, 1979.

22. Schreiber, FL, Weyman, AE, Feigenbaum, H, and Stewart, J: Effects of atrial septal defect repair on left ventricular geometry and degree of mitral valve prolapse. Circulation, 61:888, 1980.

23. Rogers, EW, et al.: Abnormalities of left ventricular geometry and rotation in endocardial cushion defect. Circulation, 60 (Suppl II): 145, 1979.

24. Franklin, TD, et al.: Variation in cross-sectional echocardiographic radial target motion relative to a calculated mean centroid of the left ventricle. Circulation, 62:III, 132, 1980.

25. Dodge, HT, Sandler, H, Ballen, DW, and Lord, JDJ: The use of biplane angiocardiography for the measurement of left ventricular volume in man. Am Heart J, 60:762, 1960.

26. Arvidsson, H: Angiocardiographic determinations of left ventricular volume. Acta Radiol, 56:321, 1961.

27. Bunnell, IL, Grant, C, and Greene, DG: Left ventricular function derived from the pressure volume diagram. Am J Med, 39:881, 1965.

28. Herman, HJ, and Bartle, SH: Left ventricular volumes by angiocardiography: comparison of models and simplification of techniques. Cardiovasc Res, 4:404, 1968.

29. Sandler, H, and Dodge, HT: The use of single plane angiocardiograms for the calculation of left ventricular volume in man. Am Heart J, 75:325, 1968.

30. Dodge, HT, Sandler, H, Bailey, WA, and Henley, RR: Usefulness and limitations of radiographic methods for determining left ventricular volume. Am J Cardiol, 18:10, 1966.

31. Davila, JC, and SanMarco, ME: An analysis of the fit of mathematical models applicable to the measurement of the left ventricle. Am J Cardiol, 18:31, 1966.

32. Chapman, CB, Baker, O, Reynolds, J, and Bonte, FJ: Use of biplane cinefluorigraphy for measurement of ventricular volume. Circulation, 18:1105, 1958.

33. Lewis, RP, and Sandler, H: Relationship between changes in left ventricular dimension and the ejection fraction in man. Circulation, 44:548, 1971.

34. Murray, JA, Johnston, W, and Reid, JM: Echocardiographic determination of left ventricular dimensions, volumes and performance. Am J Cardiol, 30:252, 1972.

35. Belenkie, I, Nutter, DO, and Clark, DW: Assessment of left ventricular dimensions and function by echocardiography. Am J Cardiol, 31:755, 1973.

36. Ratshin, RA, Rackley, CE, and Russell, RO: Determination of left ventricular preload and afterload by quantitative echocardiography in man. Circ Res, 34:711, 1974.

37. Rackley, CE, and Hood, WP: Quantitative angiographic evaluation and pathophysiologic mechanisms in valvular heart disease. Prog Cardiovasc Dis, 15:427, 1973.

38. Fortuin, NJ, Wood, WP, Sherman, ME, and Craige, E: Determination of left ventricular volume by ultrasound. Circulation, 44:575, 1971.

39. Johnston, ML: Echocardiographic evaluation of left ventricular size and function and its application to coronary artery disease. Adv Cardiol, 17:105, 1976.

40. Ludbrook, P, et al.: Comparison of ultrasound and cineangiographic measurements in patients with and without wall motion abnormalities. Br Heart J, 35:1026, 1973.

41. Machii, K, et al.: Echocardiographic left ventricular volume determination by direct measurement of the major and minor axes. Jpn Circ J, 41:501, 1977.

42. Mashiro, I, et al.: Comparison of measurements of left ventricle by echocardiography and cineangiography. Jpn Circ J, 39:23, 1975.

43. Ratshin, RA, Rackley, CE, and Russell, RO: Quantitative echocardiography: accuracy of ventricular volume analysis by area length linear regression and quadratic regression formulae. Am J Cardiol, 35:165, 1975.

44. Redwood, DR, Henry, WL, and Epstein, SE: Evaluation of the ability of echocardiography to measure acute alterations in left ventricular volume. Circulation, 50:901, 1974.

45. Teichholz, LE, Kreulen, T, Herman, MV, and Gorlin, R: Problems in echocardiographic volume determinations: Echocardiographic-angiographic correlations in the presence or absence of asynergy. Am J Cardiol, 37:7, 1976.

46. Kronik, G, Slany, J, and Mosslacher, H: Comparative value of eight M-mode echocardiographic formulas for determining left ventricular stroke volume. Circulation, 60:1308, 1979.

47. Wyatt, H, et al.: Cross-sectional echocardiography: II. Analysis of mathematic models for quantifying volume of formalin fixed left ventricle. Circulation, 61:1119, 1980.

48. Feigenbaum, H: New aspects of echocardiography. Circulation, 47:833, 1973.

49. Popp, RL, Alderman, EL, Brown, OR, and Harrison, DC: Sources of error in calculation of left ventricular volume by echocardiography. Am J Cardiol, 31:152, 1973.

50. Rackley, CE, and Hood, WP: Quantitative angiographic evaluation and pathophysiologic mechanisms in valvular heart disease. Prog Cardiovasc Dis, 15:427, 1969.

51. Yang, SS, Bentivoglio, LG, Maranhao, V, and

Goldberg, H: Cardiac volumes. *In* From Cardiac Catheterization to Hemodynamic Parameters. Philadelphia, F.A. Davis, 1978.

52. King, DL, et al.: Left ventricular volume determination by cross-sectional cardiac ultrasonography. Radiology, 104:201, 1972.

53. Teichholz, LE, Cohen, MV, Sonnenblick, BM, and Gorlin, R: Study of left ventricular geometry and function by B-scan ultrasonography in patients with and without asynergy. N Engl J Med, 291:1220, 1964.

54. Chaudry, K, et al.: Biplane measurements of left and right ventricular volumes using wide angle cross-sectional echocardiography. Am J Cardiol, 41:391, 1978.

55. DiSessa, T, et al.: Evaluation of cardiac chamber size and left ventricular function in children using two-dimensional apex echocardiography. Am J Cardiol, 45:468, 1980.

56. Wyatt, H, et al.: Quantification of volumes in asymmetric left ventricles by 2-D echocardiography. Circulation (Suppl II), 58:730, 1978.

57. Roelandt, J, et al.: Limitations of quantitative determination of left ventricular volume by multiscan echocardiography. Circulation, 49 & 50 (Suppl III):111–28, 1974.

58. Greene, DG, Carlisle, R, Grant, C, and Bunnell, IL: Estimation of left ventricular volume by one-plane cineangiography. Circulation, 35:61, 1967.

59. Georke, RJ, and Carlsson, E: Calculation of right and left ventricular volumes: methods using standard computer equipment and biplane angiograms. Invest Radiol, 2:360, 1967.

60. Bommer, W, et al.: Biplane apex echocardiography versus biplane cineangiography in the assessment of left ventricular volume and function: validation by direct measurements. Am J Cardiol, 45:471, 1980.

61. Eaton, LW, Maughan, WL, Shoukas, AA, and Weiss, JL: Accurate volume determination in the isolated ejecting canine left ventricle by two-dimensional echocardiography. Circulation, 60:320, 1979.

62. Eaton, LW, Maughan, WL, and Weiss, JL: Accurate volume determination in the isolated ejecting canine heart from a limited number of two-dimensional echocardiographic cross sections. Am J Cardiol, 45:470, 1980.

63. Schiller, N, et al.: Left ventricular volume from paired biplane two-dimensional echocardiography. Circulation, 60:547, 1979.

64. Silverman, N, Schiller, NB, Yaeger, R, and Ports, T: Left ventricular volume analysis by two-dimensional echocardiography in children. Circulation (Suppl II), 58:781, 1978.

65. Gueret, P, Wyatt, J, Meerbaum, S, and Corday, E: A practical two-dimensional echocardiographic model to assess volume in the ischemic left ventricle. Am J Cardiol, 45:471, 1980.

66. Rakowski, H, Martin, RD, and Popp, RL: Left ventricular function: assessment by wide angle two-dimensional ultrasonic sector scanning. Acta Med Scand (Suppl), 627:104, 1978.

67. Badeer, HS: Biologic significance of cardiac hypertrophy. Am J Cardiol, 14:133, 1964.

68. Hood, WB: Dynamics of hypertrophy of the left ventricular wall of man. *In* Cardiac Hypertrophy. Edited by N Alpert. New York, Grune and Stratton, 1971.

69. Sasayama, S, et al.: Adaptations of the left ventricle to chronic pressure overload. Circ Res, 38:172, 1971.

70. Ross, J: Afterload mismatch and preload reserve: a conceptual framework for the analysis of ventricular function. Prog Cardiovasc Dis, 18:255, 1976.

71. Sokolow, M, and Perloff, D: The prognosis of essential hypertension treated conservatively. Circulation, 23:697, 1961.

72. Spagnuolo, M, et al.: Natural history of rheumatic aortic regurgitation. Circulation, 34:368, 1971.

73. Tremouth, RS, Phelps, NC, and Neill, WA: Determinants of left ventricular hypertrophy and oxygen supply in chronic aortic valve disease. Circulation, 53:644, 1976.

74. Troy, BL, Pombo, J, and Rackley, CE: Measurement of left ventricular wall thickness and mass by echocardiography. Circulation, 40:602, 1972.

75. Murray, JA, Johnston, W, and Reid, JM: Echocardiographic determination of left ventricular dimension volumes and performance. Am J Cardiol, 30:252, 1972.

76. Devereux, R, and Reichek, N: Echocardiographic determination of left ventricular mass in man. Circulation, 55:613, 1977.

77. Feigenbaum, H, Popp, RL, Chip, JN, and Haine, CL: Left ventricular wall thickness measured by ultrasound. Arch Int Med, 121:391, 1968.

78. Sahn, DJ, DeMaria, A, Kisslo, J, and Weyman, AE: Recommendations regarding quantitation in M-mode echocardiography: results of a survey of echocardiographic measurements. Circulation, 58:1072, 1978.

79. Wyatt, H, et al.: Cross-sectional echocardiography. I. Analysis of mathematic models for quantifying mass of the left ventricle in dogs. Circulation, 60:1104, 1979.

80. Helak, J, et al.: Quantitation of human left ventricular (LV) mass and volume by cross-sectional echocardiography: In vitro anatomic validation. Am J Cardiol, 45:470, 1980.

81. Geiser, E, and Bove, K: Calculation of left ventricular mass and relative wall thickness. Arch Pathol, 97:13, 1974.

82. Grant, C, Green, DG, and Brunnell, IL: Left ventricular enlargement and hypertrophy. Am J Med, 39:895, 1965.

83. Gehrke, J, Leeman, S, Raphael, M, and Pridie, RB: Noninvasive left ventricular volume determination by two-dimensional echocardiography. Br Heart J, 37:911, 1975.

84. Fortuin, NH, Hood, WP, Sherman, E, and Craige, E: Determinations of left ventricular volumes by ultrasound. Circulation, 44:575, 1971.

85. Gibson, DG: Measurement of left ventricular volumes in man by echocardiography—comparison with biplane angiographs. Br Heart J, 33:614, 1971.

86. TenCate, FJ, et al.: Dimensions and volumes of

left atrium and ventricle determined by single-beam echocardiography. Br Heart J, 36:737, 1974.

87. Mason, S, and Fortuin, N: The use of echocardiography for quantitative evaluation of left ventricular function. Prog Cardiovasc Dis, 21:119, 1978.

88. Quinones, MA, Gaasch, WH, and Alexander, JK: Echocardiographic assessment of left ventricular function: with special reference to normalized velocities. Circulation, 50:42, 1974.

89. Cooper, RH, et al.: Comparison of ultrasound and cineangiographic measurements of the mean rate of circumferential shortening in man. Circulation, 46:914, 1972.

90. Cooper, RH, et al.: Ultrasound determinations of mean fiber shortening rate in man. Am J Cardiol, 29:257, 1972.

91. Quinones, MA, Gaasch, WH, and Alexander, JK: Influences of acute changes in preload, afterload, contractile state, and heart rate on ejection and isovolumic indices of myocardial contractility in man. Circulation, 53:293, 1976.

92. Ludbrook, P, et al.: Comparison of ultrasound and cineangiographic measurements of left ventricular performance in patients with and without wall motion abnormalities. Br Heart J, 35:1026, 1973.

93. Rosenblatt, A, Clark, R, Burgess, JE, and Cohn, K: Echocardiographic assessment of the level of cardiac compensation in valvular heart disease. Circulation, 54:509, 1976.

94. Rasmussen, S, et al.: Stroke volume calculated from the mitral valve echogram in patients with and without ventricular dyssynergy. Circulation, 58:125, 1978.

95. Dodge, H, Kennedy, J, and Peterson, J: Quantitative angiocardiographic methods in the evaluation of valvular heart disease. Prog Cardiovasc Dis, 16:1, 1973.

96. Nolan, ST, Dixon, SN, Fisher, RD, and Morrow, AG: The influence of atrial contraction and mitral valve mechanics on ventricular filling. Am Heart J, 77:784, 1969.

97. Laniado, S, et al.: A study of the dynamic relations between the mitral valve echogram and phasic mitral flow. Circulation, 51:104, 1975.

98. Massie, BM, Schiller, NB, Ratshin, RD, and Parmley, WW: Mitral-septal separation: new echocardiographic index of left ventricular function. Am J Cardiol, 39:1008, 1977.

99. Hood, WP, and Rolett, EL: Patterns of contraction in the human ventricle. Circulation (Suppl III), 40:109, 1969.

100. Crawford, MH, White, DH, and Amon, KW: Echocardiographic evaluation of left ventricular size and performance during handgrip and supine upright bicycle exercise. Circulation, 59:1188, 1979.

101. Sugishita, Y, and Kosekt, S: Dynamic exercise echocardiography. Circulation, 60:743, 1979.

102. Wann, LS, et al.: Exercise cross-sectional echocardiography in ischemic heart disease. Circulation, 60:1300, 1979.

103. Mason, SJ, et al.: Exercise echocardiography: detection of wall motion abnormalities during ischemia. Circulation (Suppl III), 56:III, 6, 1977.

104. DeMaria, AN, et al.: Evaluation of left ventricular responses to isometric exertion by two-dimensional echocardiography. Circulation, (Suppl), 59 & 60:II–152, 1979.

105. Morganroth, J, et al.: Exercise cross-sectional echocardiographic diagnosis of coronary artery disease. Am J Cardiol, 45:404, 1980.

106. Erickson, HH, Bishop, VS, Kardon, MB, and Horwitz, LD: Left ventricular internal diameter and cardiac function during exercise. J Appl Physiol, 30:473, 1971.

107. Braunwald, E, Goldblatt, A, Harrison, DC, and Mason, DT: Studies on cardiac dimensions in intact unanesthetized man. III. Studies of muscular exercise. Circ Res, 13:460, 1963.

108. Vatner, SF, et al.: Left ventricular response to severe exertion in untethered dogs. J Clin Invest, 51:3052, 1972.

109. Resych, SK, et al.: Cardiac function at rest and during exercise in normals and in patients with coronary heart disease: evaluation by radionuclide angiocardiography. Ann Surg, 187:449, 1978.

110. Tennant, R, and Wiggers, CJ: The effect of coronary occlusion on myocardial contraction. Am J Physiol, 112:351, 1935.

111. Theroux, P, et al.: Regional myocardial function in the conscious dog during acute coronary occlusion and responses to morphine, propranolol, nitroglycerin and lidocaine. Circulation, 53:302, 1976.

112. Pichler, M: Non-invasive assessment of segmental left ventricular wall motion: its clinical relevance in detection of ischemia. Clin Cardiol, 1:173, 1978.

113. Herman, MV, Heinle, RA, Klein, MD, and Gorlin, R: Localized disorders in myocardial contraction: asynergy and its role in congestive heart failure. N Engl J Med, 277:22, 1967.

114. Burggraf, GW, and Parker, JO: Prognosis in coronary disease, angiographic, hemodynamic and clinical factors. Circulation, 51:146, 1975.

115. Weyman, AE, Franklin, TD, Egenes, KM, and Green, D: Correlation between extent of abnormal regional wall motion and myocardial infarct size in chronically infarcted dogs. Circulation (Suppl II), 56:72, 1977.

116. Franklin, T, et al.: Differentiation of A-mode ultrasound signals from normal and ischemic myocardium by multivariate discriminant analysis of waveform parameters. Am J Cardiol, 45:403, 1980.

117. Kerber, R, and Abboud, F: Echocardiographic detection of regional myocardial infarction. Circulation, 47:997, 1973.

118. Kerber, R, et al.: Effects of acute coronary occlusion on the motion and perfusion of the normal and ischemic interventricular septum. Circulation, 54:928, 1976.

119. Corya, B, et al.: Echocardiography in acute myocardial infarction. Am J Cardiol, 36:1, 1975.

120. Heikkila, J, and Nieminen, M: Echoventriculographic detection, localization, and quantifi-

cation of left ventricular asynergy in acute my-ocardial infarction. Br Heart J, 37:46, 1975.

121. Heikkila, J, and Nieminen, M: Echoventricu-lography in acute myocardial infarction. IV. In-farct size and reliability by pathologic anatomic correlations. Clin Cardiol, 3:26, 1980.

122. Heger, J, et al.: Cross-sectional echocardiog-raphy in acute myocardial infarction: detection and localization of regional left ventricular asynergy. Circulation, 60:531, 1979.

123. Heger, J, et al.: Cross-sectional echocardio-graphic analysis of the extent of left ventricular asynergy in acute myocardial infarction. Cir-culation, 61:1113, 1980.

124. Visser, C, et al.: Quantification and localization of uncomplicated acute myocardial infarction by cross-sectional echocardiography. Circula-tion, 59 & 60:II, 152, 1979.

125. Bloch, A, Morard, J, Mayor, C, and Perrenoud, J: Cross-sectional echocardiography in acute myocardial infarction. Am J Cardiol, 43:387, 1979.

126. Rogers, EW, et al.: Predicting survival after my-ocardial infarction by cross-sectional echo. Cir-culation (Suppl), 58:II, 233, 1978.

127. Drobac, M, et al.: Complicated acute myocardial infarction: the importance of two-dimensional echocardiography. Am J Cardiol, 43:387, 1979.

128. Weiss, J, Bulkley, B, Hutchins, G, and Mason, S: Correlation of real-time 2-dimensional echo-cardiography with postmortem studies. Am J Cardiol, 41:369, 1978.

129. Kerber, RE, Martins, JB, and Marcus, ML: Effect of acute ischemia, nitroglycerin and nitroprus-side on regional myocardial thickening stress and perfusion: experimental echocardiographic studies. Circulation, 60:121, 1979.

129a. Moynihan, DE, Parisi, AE, and Feldman, CM: Quantitative detection of regional left ventric-ular contraction abnormalities by two-dimen-sional echocardiography. Circulation (Suppl I), 63:752, 1981.

130. Franklin, TD, et al.: Variation in cross-sectional echocardiographic radial target motion relative to a calculated mean centroid of the left ven-tricle. Circulation, 62:III, 132, 1980.

131. Franklin, TD, et al.: Three-dimensional graphic representation of left ventricular endocardial wall motion from two-dimensional echocardi-ography. Circulation, 62:III, 185, 1980.

132. Corya, BC, et al.: Systolic thickening and thin-ning of the septum and posterior wall in pa-tients with coronary artery disease, congestive cardiomyopathy and atrial septal defect. Cir-culation, 56:109, 1977.

133. Pandian, N, and Kerber, R: Ultrasonic sono-micrometers vs 2-D echocardiography in the detection of transient myocardial dyskinesis. Circulation, 62:III, 329, 1980.

134. Laurenceau, J, Turcot, J, and Dumesnit, J: Echo-cardiographic evaluation of ventricular wall thickness during acute coronary occlusions in dogs. Circulation (Suppl), 59 & 60:II, 1979.

135. Weiss, JL, et al.: Relationship of systolic thick-ening to transmural extent of myocardial in-

farction in the dog. Circulation (Suppl), 62:III, 328, 1980.

136. Charuzi, U, et al.: A quantitative comparison of cross-sectional echocardiography and radio-nuclide angiography in acute myocardial in-farction. Circulation (Suppl II), 58:196, 1978.

137. Wynne, J, Birnholz, J, Finberg, H, and Alpert, J: Regional left ventricular wall motion in acute myocardial infarction as assessed by two-di-mensional echocardiography. Circulation, 55 & 56:III, 152, 1977.

138. Lengyel, M, Tajik, A, Seward, J, and Smith, H: Correlation of two-dimensional echocardio-graphic and angiographic segmental wall mo-tion abnormalities in patients with prior trans-mural myocardial infarction: a prospective double-blind study. Circulation (Suppl), 59 & 60:II, 153, 1979.

139. Meltzer, R, et al.: Two-dimensional echocar-diographic quantification of infarct size alter-ation by pharmacologic agents. Am J Cardiol, 43:387, 1979.

140. Weiss, J, Bulkley, B, and Mason, S: Two-di-mensional echocardiographic quantification of myocardial injury in man: comparison with post mortem studies. Circulation (Suppl II), 58:595, 1978.

141. Arnett, E, Weiss, J, Garrison, J, and Fortuin, N: Quantitative evaluation of regional left ventric-ular thickening in man by two-dimensional echocardiography. Am J Cardiol, 43:377, 1979.

142. Wilson, RN, et al.: The electrocardiogram in myocardial infarction with particular reference to the mitral deflections of the ventricular com-plex. Heart, 16:155, 1933.

143. Pardee, HEB: An electrocardiographic sign of coronary artery obstruction. Arch Int Med, 26:244, 1920.

144. Fenichel, NM, and Kugell, VH: The large Q-wave of the electrocardiogram: correlation with pathologic observations. Am Heart J, 7:235, 1931.

145. Kan, G, Visser, CA, Lie, KI, and Durrer, D: Cor-relation of 2-dimensional echocardiography with coronary arteriography and electrocardi-ogram in anterior wall infarction. Circulation, 62:III, 186, 1980.

146. Eaton, L, et al.: Regional cardiac dilatation after acute myocardial infarction. N Engl J Med, 300:57, 1979.

147. Kisslo, J: Evaluation of the left ventricle by two-dimensional echocardiography. Acta Med Scand (Suppl), 627:112, 1979.

148. Ross, A, and Michaelson, S: Left ventricular contraction patterns by mechanical, two-di-mensional real-time echocardiography. Clin Res, 25:250A, 1977.

149. Kisslo, J, et al.: A comparison of real-time, two-dimensional echocardiography and cinean-giography in detecting left ventricular asyn-ergy. Circulation, 55:134, 1977.

150. Jacobs, JJ, Feigenbaum, H, Corya, BC, and Phil-lips, JF: Detection of left ventricular asynergy by echocardiography. Circulation, 68:263, 1973.

151. VanTassel, RA, and Edwards, JE: Rupture of the

heart complicating myocardial infarction; analysis of 40 cases including nine examples of left ventricular false aneurysms. Chest, 61:104, 1972.

152. Weyman, AE, et al.: Detection of left ventricular aneurysms by cross-sectional echocardiography. Circulation, 54:936, 1976.

153. Lengyel, M, et al.: Sensitivity and specificity of two-dimensional echocardiography in the detection of left ventricular aneurysms. Am J Cardiol, 45:436, 1980.

154. Rakowski, M, et al.: Left ventricular aneurysm: detection and determination of resectability by two-dimensional ultrasound. Circulation, 56:III, 153, 1977.

155. Rasmussen, S, Corya, B, Feigenbaum, H, and Knoebel, S: Detection of myocardial scar tissue by M-mode echocardiography. Circulation, 57:230, 1978.

156. Berman, B, and McGuire, J: Cardiac aneurysms. Am J Med, 8:480, 1950.

157. Abrams, DL, Edelist, A, Luria, MH, and Miller, AJ: Ventricular aneurysm: a reappraisal based on a study of 65 consecutive autopsied cases. Circulation, 27:164, 1963.

158. Schiehter, J, Hellerstein, HK, and Katz, LN: Aneurysm of the heart: correlative study of 102 proved cases. Medicine, 33:43, 1954.

159. Williams, TW, Peabody, CA, and Pruitt, RD: Calcified aneurysm of the left ventricular apex associated with intraventricular block of the left bundle branch type. Am Heart J, 63:557, 1962.

160. Vlodaver, Z, Coe, JJ, and Edwards, JE: True and false aneurysms: propensity for the latter to rupture. Circulation, 51:567, 1975.

161. Gorlin, R, Klein, MD, and Sullivan, JM: Prospective correlative study of ventricular aneurysm. Am J Med, 42:512, 1967.

162. Rad, G, et al.: Experience with sixty consecutive ventricular aneurysm resections. Circulation (Suppl II), 49 & 50:149, 1974.

163. Graber, JD, et al.: Ventricular aneurysm, an appraisal of diagnosis and surgical therapy. Br Heart J, 34:830, 1972.

164. Roberts, WC, and Morrown, AG: Pseudoaneurysm of the left ventricle: an unusual sequel of myocardial infarction and rupture of the heart. Am J Med, 43:639, 1967.

165. Katz, RJ, et al.: Non-invasive diagnosis of left ventricular pseudoaneurysm: role of two-dimensional echocardiography and radionuclide gated pool imaging. Am J Cardiol, 44:372, 1979.

166. Sears, TD, Ong, YS, Starke, H, and Forker, AD: Left ventricular pseudoaneurysm identified by cross-sectional echocardiography. Ann Int Med, 90:935, 1979.

167. Nanda, NC, and Gatewood, RD: Differentiation of left ventricular pseudoaneurysm from true aneurysms by two-dimensional echocardiography. Circulation (Suppl II), 60:144, 1979.

168. Catherwood, E, et al.: Two-dimensional echocardiographic recognition of left ventricular pseudoaneurysm. Circulation, 62:294, 1980.

169. Skapinker, S: Diverticulum of the left ventricle of the heart. Arch Surg, 63:629, 1951.

170. Potts, WJ, DeBoer, A, and Johnson, FR: Congenital diverticulum of the left ventricle. Surgery, 33:301, 1953.

171. Chesler, E, Tucker, RBK, and Barlow, JB: Subvalvular and apical left ventricular aneurysms in the Bantu as a source of systemic emboli. Circulation, 35:1156, 1967.

172. Edgett, JW, et al.: Diverticulum of the heart. Am J Cardiol, 24:580, 1969.

173. Treistman, B, et al.: Diverticulum or aneurysm of left ventricle. Am J Cardiol, 32:119, 1973.

174. Kanarek, KS, et al.: Clinical aspects of submitral left ventricular aneurysms. S Afr Med J, 47:1225, 1973.

175. Estevez, CM, Weyman, AE, and Feigenbaum, H: Detection of left ventricular diverticulum by cross-sectional echocardiography. Chest, 69:544, 1976.

176. Sanders, RJ, Kern, WH, and Blount, SG: Perforation of the interventricular septum complicating myocardial infarction. Am Heart J, 81:736, 1956.

177. Vlodaver, Z, and Edwards, JE: Rupture of ventricular septum or papillary muscle complicating myocardial infarction. Circulation, 55:815, 1977.

178. Pagall, JC, Pryor, R, and Blount, SG: Systolic murmur following myocardial infarction. Am Heart J, 87:577, 1974.

179. Farcot, JC, et al.: Two-dimensional echocardiographic visualization of ventricular septal rupture after acute myocardial infarction. Am J Cardiol, 45:370, 1980.

180. Scanlan, JG, Seward, J, and Tajik, A: Visualization of ventricular septal rupture utilizing wide-angle two-dimensional echocardiography. Mayo Clin Proc, 54:381, 1979.

181. Rogers, EW, et al.: Cross-sectional echocardiographic identification of aneurysms of the posterior interventricular septum with post-infarction ventricular septal defect. Chest: In Press.

182. Yates, WM, Welsh, PP, Stapleton, JF, and Clark, ML: Comparison of clinical and pathologic aspects of coronary artery disease in men of various age groups: a study of 950 autopsied cases from the Armed Forces Institute of Pathology. Ann Intern Med, 34:352, 1951.

183. Jordan, RA, Miller, RD, Edwards, JE, and Parker, RL: Thrombi embolism in acute and healed myocardial infarction. I. Intracardiac mural thrombus. Circulation, 6:1, 1952.

184. Phares, WS, Edwards, JE, and Burchell, HB: Cardiac aneurysm: clinicopathologic studies. Mayo Clin Proc, 28:264, 1953.

185. Helden, T, Iversen, K, Rapschou, F, and Schwartz, M: Anticoagulants in acute myocardial infarction. Lancet, 2:327, 1961.

186. Report of the working party on anticoagulant therapy in coronary thrombosis to the medical research council: assessment of short-term anticoagulant adminstration after cardiac infarction. Br Med J, 1:335, 1969.

187. Veterans Administration Hospital Investigators: Anticoagulants in acute myocardial in-

farction: results of a cooperative clinical trial. JAMA, 225:724, 1973.

188. DeMaria, AN, et al.: Left ventricular thrombi identified by cross-sectional echocardiography. Ann Int Med, 90:14, 1979.

189. Meltzer, RS, et al.: Diagnosis of left ventricular thrombi by two-dimensional echocardiography. Br Heart J, 42:261, 1979.

190. Suzuki, S, et al.: Cross-sectional echocardiographic findings of left ventricular thrombi in a ten-year-old patient with cardiomyopathy. Jpn Heart J, 20:675, 1979.

191. Seward, JB, Gura, GM, Hagler, DJ, and Tajik, AJ: Evaluation of M-mode echocardiography and wide angle two-dimensional echocardiography in the diagnosis of intracardiac masses. Circulation (Suppl), 57 & 58:II–234, 1978.

192. Probae, M, et al.: Two-dimensional echocardiographic recognition of mural thrombi: in vivo and in vitro studies. Am J Cardiol, 45:435, 1980.

193. Ports, FA, Cogan, J, Schiller, NB, and Rapaport, E: Echocardiography of left ventricular masses. Circulation, 58:528, 1978.

194. Asinger, RW, et al.: Serial evaluation for left ventricular thrombus during acute transmural myocardial infarction using two-dimensional echocardiography. Am J Cardiol, 45:483, 1980.

195. Asinger, R, et al.: Serial evaluation for left ventricular thrombus during the first episode of acute myocardial infarction using two-dimensional echocardiography. Circulation, 62:III, 277, 1980.

196. Mikell, F, et al.: Experimental left ventricular thrombi: early detection by two-dimensional echocardiography. Circulation, 62:III, 330, 1980.

197. Baumwald, E: Heart Disease: A Textbook of Cardiovascular Medicine. Philadelphia, Saunders, 1980.

198. Goodwin, JF: Congestive and hypertrophic cardiomyopathies: a decade of study. Lancet, 1:731, 1970.

199. Goodwin, JF, and Oakley, CM: The cardiomyopathies. Br Heart J, 34:545, 1972.

200. Corya, BC, Feigenbaum, H, Rasmussen, S, and Black, MJ: Echocardiographic features of congestive cardiomyopathy compared with normal subjects and patients with coronary artery disease. Circulation, 49:1153, 1974.

201. Godley, RW, et al.: Relation of incomplete mitral leaflet closure to the site of dyssynergy in patients with papillary muscle dysfunction. Circulation (Suppl II), 60:204, 1979.

202. Adelman, AG, et al.: Current concepts of primary cardiomyopathy. Cardiovasc Med, 2:495, 1977.

203. Edwards, JE, Carey, LS, Neufeld, HN, and Lester, RG: Congenital Heart Disease. Philadelphia, Saunders, 1965.

204. Moller, JH, et al.: Endocardial fibroelastosis. Circulation, 30:759, 1964.

205. Fisher, JH: Primary endocardial fibroelastosis: a review of 15 cases. Can Med Assoc J, 87:105, 1962.

206. Kelly, J, and Andersen, DH: Congenital endocardial fibroelastosis: clinical and pathologic investigation of those cases without associated cardiac malformations including report of 2 familial instances. Pediatrics, 18:539, 1956.

207. Manning, JA, and Keith, JD: Fibroelastosis in children. Prog Cardiovasc Dis, 7:172, 1964.

208. Still, WJS: Endocardial fibroelastosis. Am Heart J, 61:579, 1961.

209. Branch, CL, and Castle, RF: Thromboembolic complications in primary endocardial fibroelastosis. J Pediatr, 69:250, 1966.

210. DuShane, JW, and Edwards, JE: Congenital aortic stenosis in association with endocardial sclerosis of the left ventricle. Mayo Clin Proc, 29:102, 1954.

211. Hallidie-Smith, KA, and Olsen, EGJ: Endocardial fibroelastosis, mitral incompetence, and coarctation of the abdominal aorta. Br Heart J, 30:850, 1968.

212. Yoshida, Y, et al.: Ultrasonic studies on endocardial fibroelastosis. Tohoku J Exp Med, 123:329, 1977.

213. Löffler, W: Endocarditis parietalis fibroplastica mit Bluteosinophilie. Ein cigenartiges Krankheitsbild. Schweiz Med Wochenschr, 66:817, 1936.

214. Benvenisti, DS, and Ultmann, JE: Eosinophilic leukemia. Report of five cases and review of literature. Ann Intern Med, 71:731, 1961.

215. Odeberg, B: Eosinophilic leukemia and disseminated eosinophilic collagen disease—a disease entity. Acta Med Scand, 177:129, 1965.

216. Hardy, WR, and Anderson, RE: The hypereosinophilic syndromes. Ann Intern Med, 68:1220, 1968.

217. Chusid, MJ, et al.: The hypereosinophilic syndrome: analysis of fourteen cases with review of the literature. Medicine, 54:1, 1975.

218. Brink, AJ, and Weber, HW: Fibroplastic parietal endocarditis with eosinophilia. Am J Med, 34:52, 1963.

219. Blair, HT, et al.: Unusual hemodynamics in Löffler's endomyocarditis. Am J Cardiol, 34:606, 1974.

220. Brockington, IF, and Olsen, EGJ: Löffler's endocarditis and Davis endomyocardial fibrosis. Am Heart J, 85:308, 1973.

221. Roberts, WC, Liegler, DG, and Carbone, PP: Endomyocardial disease and eosinophilia. A clinical and pathologic spectrum. Am J Med, 46:28, 1969.

222. Bell, JA, Jenkins, BS, and Webb-Peploe, MM: Clinical, hemodynamic and angiographic findings in Löffler's eosinophilic endocarditis. Br Heart J, 38:541, 1976.

223. Mumme, C: Zur Klinik und Pathologie der Endokarditis und Aortitis fibroplastica sowie Thromboendarteriitis obliterans mit hochgradiger Eosinophilie im Blut, Knochenmark und in den Organen. Klin Med, 138:22, 1940.

224. Hoffman, FG, Rosenbaum, D, and Genovese, PD: Fibroplastic endocarditis with eosinophilia (Löffler's endocarditis parietalis fibroplastica): case report and review of literature. Ann Intern Med, 42:668, 1955.

225. Weyman, AE, Rankin, R, and King, H: Löffler's

endocarditis presenting as mitral and tricuspid stenosis. Am J Cardiol, 40:438, 1977.

226. Parrillo, JE, et al.: The cardiovascular manifestations of the hypereosinophilic syndrome. Prospective study of 26 patients with review of the literature. Am J Med, 67:573, 1979.

227. Briggs, GW: Amyloidosis. Ann Int Med, 55:943, 1961.

228. Buja, LM, Khoi, NB, and Roberts, WC: Clinically significant cardiac amyloidosis. Am J Cardiol, 76:394, 1970.

229. Kyle, RA, and Baynd, ED: Amyloidosis: review of 236 cases. Medicine, 54:271, 1975.

230. Pomerance, A: Senile cardiac amyloidosis. Br Heart J, 27:717, 1965.

231. Mahloudi, M, et al.: The genetic amyloidoses. Medicine, 48:1, 1969.

232. Frederiksen, T, Gotzeche, H, Harbe, N, and Kiaer, W: Familial primary amyloidosis with severe amyloid heart disease. Am J Med, 33:328, 1962.

233. Pomerance, A: Pathology of the heart with and without cardiac failure in the aged. Br Heart J, 27:711, 1965.

234. Borer, JS, Henry, WL, and Epstein, SE: Echocardiographic observation in patients with systemic infiltrative disease involving the heart. Am J Cardiol, 39:184, 1977.

235. Child, JS, Krivokapich, J, and Abbasi, AS: Increased right ventricular wall thickness on echocardiography in amyloid infiltrative cardiomyopathy. Am J Cardiol, 44:1391, 1979.

236. Cunha, CLP, et al.: Characteristic two-dimensional echocardiographic appearance of amyloid heart disease. Circulation, 60:II, 18, 1979.

237. Buja, LM, and Robert, WC: Iron in the heart: etiology and clinical significance. Am J Med, 51:209, 1971.

Chapter 9

Right Ventricular Inflow Tract

The right ventricular inflow tract includes (1) the tricuspid valve and supporting apparatus, (2) the right atrium, and (3) the great systemic veins (the inferior and superior venae cavae). This region of the heart collects the returning venous blood from the systemic capillary beds and transports it to the right ventricle for subsequent ejection into the pulmonary vessels. The tricuspid valve, in addition to permitting unimpeded flow from the right atrium to the right ventricle during diastole, prevents systolic regurgitation and helps to direct ejected blood toward the right ventricular outflow tract. The coronary sinus, which is also a tributary of the right atrium, might functionally be considered a part of the right ventricular inflow tract. Because the coronary sinus is anatomically incorporated into the posterior wall of the left atrium and is uniformly recorded with this structure, it is included in the discussion of the left, rather than the right, ventricular inflow tract.

THE TRICUSPID VALVE

Historically, the tricuspid valve was one of the most difficult structures to record

using the M-mode echocardiographic technique.[1] This difficulty occurred because of its location immediately beneath the sternum and its plane of motion relative to the anterior chest wall. The improved visualization of the right side of the heart provided by the cross-sectional method, however, has facilitated tricuspid valve recording, and an evaluation of this structure along with the other areas of the right ventricular inflow tract should now be a routine part of the echocardiographic examination.[2-4]

Anatomy

The tricuspid valve is a complex anatomic structure composed of leaflet tissue, chordae tendineae, papillary muscles, and the supporting annular ring and right ventricular myocardium.[5,6] The tricuspid valve is larger and structurally more complicated than the mitral valve. The orifice it must occlude is likewise larger and more irregular than the mitral orifice.[6] The tricuspid leaflets are actually a continuous veil of thin fibrous tissue with a basal portion that is attached around the entire circumference of the tricuspid annulus. This

338

fibrous tissue veil can be separated into three distinct leaflets by indentations along its free edge; however, these areas of separation are less distinct than those that characterize the mitral valve.[6] The three major tricuspid leaflets, the anterior, septal, and posterior, are of unequal size. The anterior leaflet is the largest and stretches from the infundibular region anteriorly to the inferolateral wall posteriorly. The septal leaflet stretches posteriorly along the interventricular septum from the infundibulum to the posterior ventricular border, attaching to both the membranous and muscular portions of the septum. The insertion of the septal leaflet of the tricuspid valve is characteristically inferior or apical relative to the septal insertion of the anterior mitral leaflet. The posterior leaflet attaches along the posterior margin of the annulus from the septum to the inferolateral wall. These relationships can be seen in the short axis of the tricuspid valve.

Three papillary muscles or muscle groups typically support the tricuspid leaflets and lie beneath each of the three commissures.[5,6] The anterior papillary muscle is the largest and lies beneath the commissure between the anterior and posterior leaflets. It arises from both the moderator band and the free anterolateral wall of the right ventricle. The posterior papillary muscle lies inferior to the junction of the posterior and septal leaflets, whereas a small, septal papillary muscle, originating from the septal border of the infundibulum, tethers the anterior and septal leaflets high against the infundibular wall. At times, this papillary muscle may be virtually absent, and the chordae tendineae may arise from small tendinous connections to the infundibulum.[6] The chordae arising from each of these papillary muscles attach to the free edges and the proximal ventricular surfaces of both of the leaflets supported by the papillary muscle.

The tricuspid valve has several unique morphologic features that distinguish it from the mitral valve and frequently aid in identifying the anatomic right ventricle with which it is characteristically associated. These features include (1) the trileaflet configuration; (2) the presence of three separate papillary muscles; (3) the partial origin of the anterior papillary muscle from the moderator band; and (4) the inferior or apical insertion point of the septal leaflet of the tricuspid valve relative to the anterior leaflet of the mitral valve. These points of distinction are particularly valuable when ventricular structure is in question and are discussed further in Chapter 13.

Methods of Cross-Sectional Examination

The tricuspid valve is examined using three primary cross-sectional imaging planes. These include (1) *the parasternal long axis of the right ventricular inflow tract*,[2] (2) *the parasternal short axis of the right ventricular inflow tract at the tricuspid valve level*, and (3) *the apical four-chamber view*.[3] The tricuspid valve can also be recorded in both the subcostal long-axis view of the right ventricle and the subcostal long axis of the right ventricular outflow tract.[4] In addition, multiple short-axis views of the tricuspid valve can be obtained independently from the subcostal transducer location. The subcostal views, however, place the valve in the far field of the scan plane and, except in infants, do not provide the image quality available from the parasternal or apical transducer locations.

The parasternal long-axis view of the right ventricular inflow tract transects the anterior and posterior tricuspid leaflets from their points of annular insertion to their free edges. It also includes the proximal chordal attachments to these leaflets and the anterior and posterior extremes of the tricuspid annulus (Fig. 9–1). Although the right ventricular papillary muscles normally are not visualized, one or more of the papillary muscles may be visible when the ventricle is hypertrophic or di-

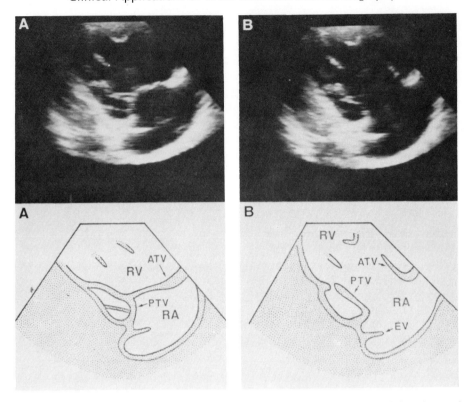

Fig. 9–1. Parasternal long-axis recording of a normal tricuspid valve during systole (*A*) and diastole (*B*). The right ventricular apex is displayed anteriorly and to the left, and the right atrium appears to the right and posteriorly. The tricuspid leaflets separate these two cavities. RV = right ventricle; RA = right atrium; ATV = anterior leaflet of tricuspid valve; PTV = posterior leaflet of tricuspid valve; EV = eustachian valve. Fragments of the anterior and posterior right ventricular papillary muscles are also evident in the apical segment of the right ventricular cavity.

lated. This imaging plane records the motion of the anterior and posterior tricuspid leaflets; their systolic and diastolic positions and spatial configurations; the anteroposterior tricuspid annular diameter; the motion pattern of the tricuspid annulus in both a superior-inferior and anteroposterior direction; and the temporal and spatial positions of the tricuspid leaflets in relation to the right ventricular cavity, annulus, and atrium. This view is difficult to standardize because there are not enough reference points to fix precisely the examining plane in space. As a rule, no left-sided structure should be recorded, and the tricuspid annulus should be visualized in a plane that passes through its maximal diameter. The maximal separation of the tricuspid leaflets at their free

edges should likewise be recorded (see Chap. 4).

The parasternal short axis of the right ventricle at the tricuspid level is recorded by angling the imaging plane rightward from the parasternal short axis of the left ventricle at the mitral valve level. Because the tricuspid annulus lies at a greater angle relative to the anterior chest wall than does the mitral annulus, the imaging plane must generally be angled toward the cardiac apex, and on occasion, the transducer must be moved up one interspace. Figure 9–2 illustrates the configuration of the tricuspid valve in the parasternal short-axis view. In normal persons, this type of image is difficult to obtain. Fortuitously, most diseases affecting the right side of the heart cause the right ventricle to dilate and/or to change shape, thereby making short-axis

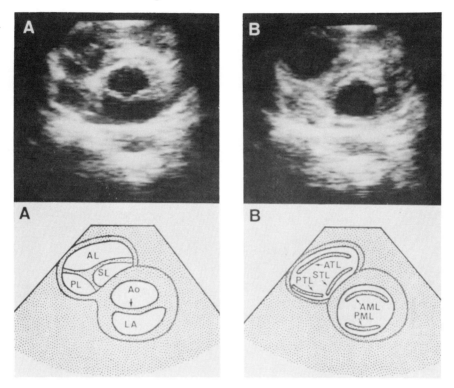

Fig. 9–2. Parasternal short-axis recording of a normal tricuspid valve during systole (*A*) and diastole (*B*). In the systolic frame (*A*), the commissures separating the three leaflets are recorded, and their relationships can be appreciated. AL = anterior tricuspid leaflet; SL = septal tricuspid leaflet; PL = posterior tricuspid leaflet; AO = aortic inlet; LA = left atrium. The vertical arrow in the accompanying diagram indicates the echo from the anterior mitral leaflet, which is transected just below the aortic valve. In the diastolic frame (*B*), the three tricuspid leaflets are recorded adjacent to the endocardial margins of the right ventricular cavity. The open mitral valve leaflets can also be visualized within the left ventricular cavity. AML = anterior mitral leaflet; PML = posterior mitral leaflet; ATL = anterior tricuspid leaflet; STL = septal tricuspid leaflet; PTL = posterior tricuspid leaflet.

tricuspid recording easier. This view is particularly useful because it permits direct visualization of the tricuspid orifice. It likewise permits the regions of circumferential involvement in focal disorders to be defined.

The apical four-chamber view passes through the tricuspid orifice along a line extending from roughly the 10 o'clock to the 4 o'clock positions relative to the corresponding short-axis plane transecting the anterior and septal tricuspid leaflets. The anterior leaflet is displayed laterally, and the septal leaflet is displayed medially (Fig. 9–3). This plane is ideal for determining the position of the right-sided atrioventricular ring and for defining the plane of leaflet closure relative to this an-

atomic landmark. It is also useful for defining the level of septal tricuspid leaflet insertion into the interventricular septum and for comparing this insertion point to that of the corresponding anterior mitral leaflet.

Normal Tricuspid Leaflet Motion— Long Axis

The normal tricuspid leaflets are thin, pliable structures that move passively in response to the forces acting on their surfaces. During diastole, overall leaflet movement represents the combination of the independent leaflet motion in response to phasic flow into the right ventricle and the motion of the tricuspid an-

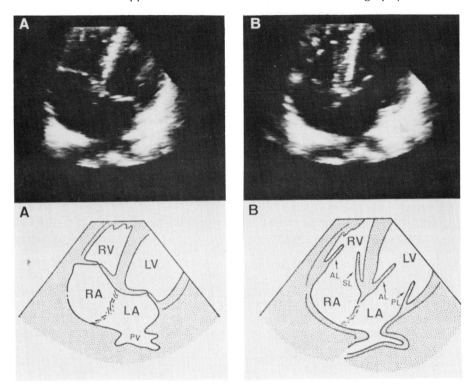

Fig. 9–3. Apical four-chamber view of a normal tricuspid valve during systole (A) and diastole (B). A, The slightly apical insertion of the septal tricuspid leaflet relative to the insertion of the anterior mitral leaflet is evident. In addition, the relationship of the coapted tricuspid leaflets to the tricuspid annulus can be appreciated. B, The leaflets are fully open and lie in close proximity to the endocardial surface of the right ventricle. AL = anterior leaflet of both the tricuspid and mitral valves; SL = septal leaflet of the tricuspid valve; PL = posterior leaflet of the mitral valve; RV = right ventricle; LV = left ventricle; RA = right atrium; LA = left atrium; PV = pulmonary veins.

nulus to which the leaflets are attached. During systole, no independent leaflet motion occurs, and the observed movement of the leaflets represents the motion of the tricuspid annulus and papillary muscles to which these leaflets are attached. Figure 9–4 depicts the normal patterns of tricuspid leaflet motion observed in the long-axis view.

Normal Tricuspid Leaflet Motion— Short Axis

The motion of the tricuspid leaflets in short axis is illustrated in Figure 9–5, A through F. In these examples, the imaging plane passes through the right ventricle just beneath the tricuspid annulus and the left ventricle at the mitral valve level. Because the plane is optimized to record the

right-sided structures, it is oblique to the left ventricle and mitral valve, and they appear distorted.

Normal Tricuspid Leaflet Motion— Apical Four-Chamber View

The normal motion of the tricuspid valve in the apical four-chamber view is depicted in Figure 9–6, A through E. In addition to permitting the recording of the pattern of tricuspid leaflet motion, this view also allows comparison of the timing of tricuspid leaflet movement with mitral leaflet movement because both valves are recorded in the same imaging plane. Tricuspid closure normally lags behind mitral closure, and as illustrated in Figure 9–6, E, the tricuspid leaflets may fail to close completely until the mitral valve has been closed for one or more frames.

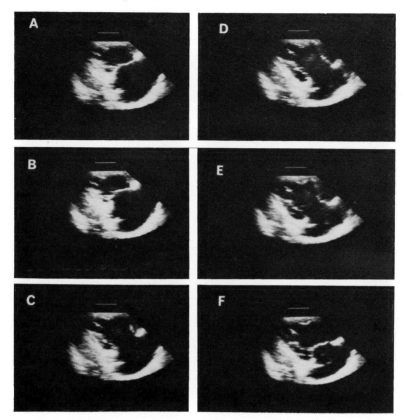

Fig. 9–4. Normal pattern of tricuspid leaflet motion in the parasternal long-axis view. *A,* Recorded at end-systole just prior to tricuspid leaflet opening. The right ventricular cavity is small, and the right atrium is maximally dilated. *B,* The initial downward motion of the tricuspid leaflets into the right ventricular cavity during isovolumic relaxation. *C,* The leaflets fly widely apart during rapid right ventricular filling, and at their maximal point of separation, the distance between the leaflet tips exceeds the diameter of the tricuspid annulus. *D,* The position of the valve during the slow-phase right ventricular filling. The leaflets lie parallel to one another and at right angles to the margins of the tricuspid annulus. *E,* Following atrial systole, the leaflet tips further separate. *F,* Atrial relaxation initiates leaflet closure, which is then completed by ventricular contraction. In the absence of an appropriately timed ventricular systole, however, leaflet closure is normally completed by atrial relaxation. Throughout the diastolic filling period, the tricuspid annulus moves posteriorly and superiorly and, at the onset of ventricular systole, is in its most posterior and superior position.

The diastolic motion of the tricuspid leaflets is more difficult to analyze in the apical four-chamber view than in either the long- or short-axis projections. This difficulty occurs because the leaflets are oriented parallel to the path of the ultrasonic beam during diastole and, hence, are poorly visualized. During systole, however, the leaflets lie perpendicular to the path of the beam and are well recorded. In addition, the plane of the tricuspid annulus is visualized more readily in this view than in any other imaging plane, and hence, this particular projection is optimal for recording systolic leaflet position relative to the plane of the annulus.

Factors Affecting the Timing, Amplitude, and Rate of Tricuspid Leaflet Motion

The factors that govern the timing, amplitude, and rate of tricuspid leaflet motion have been less well studied than those that determine the corresponding movement of the mitral valve. In general, these factors are presumably similar, and the discussion in Chapter 5 of the effects of pressure and flow on mitral leaflet motion,

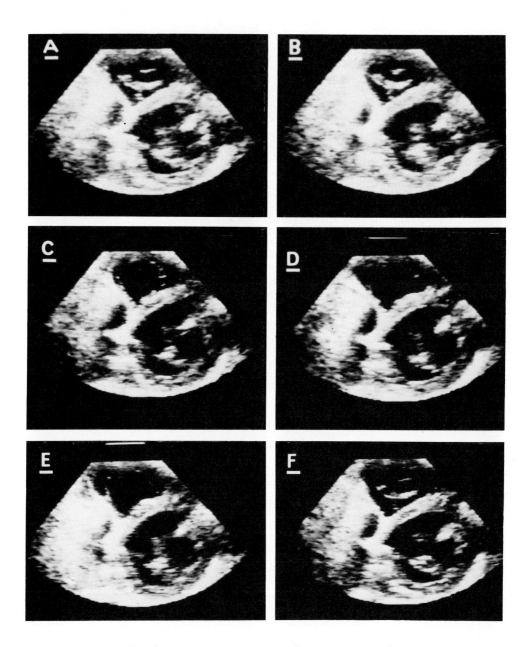

Fig. 9–5. Normal tricuspid leaflet motion in the parasternal short-axis view. *A,* The three commissures of the tricuspid valve within the right ventricular cavity recorded during systole. The anterior tricuspid leaflet is positioned anteriorly, the posterior leaflet is positioned to the left and posteriorly, and the septal leaflet is positioned to the right posteriorly. *B,* Recorded at end of ventricular systole. Right ventricular size decreases with continued appearance of the three leaflet commissures. *C,* At the onset of diastole, the leaflets separate widely and lie against the triangular margins of the right ventricular cavity. *D,* Recorded slightly later in diastole, this figure illustrates the leaflets against the margins of the right ventricle. *E,* Recorded at end-diastole just prior to the tricuspid leaflet closure. The apparent decrease in right ventricular cavity size reflects the motion of the right ventricular cavity superiorly through the imaging plane and the relatively lower level of the right ventricle recorded at this point in the cardiac cycle. *F,* Recorded following initial systolic closure of the valve. This panel is similar in configuration to *A,* although recorded slightly earlier in the cardiac cycle. AO = aorta.

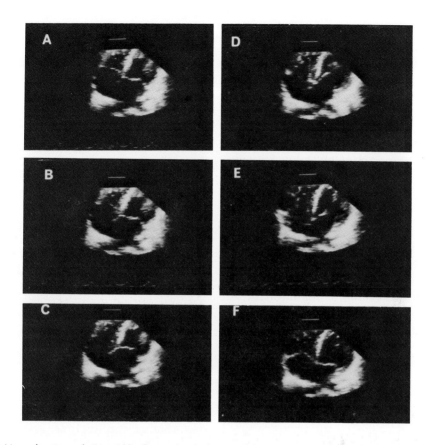

Fig. 9–6. Normal pattern of tricuspid leaflet motion in the apical four-chamber view. *A,* The position of the closed tricuspid leaflets at end of ventricular systole. *B,* Recorded during isovolumic relaxation, this panel demonstrates the initial downward displacement of the tricuspid valve leaflets into the right ventricle just prior to rapid leaflet opening. *C,* Recorded at the point of peak leaflet excursion. As demonstrated in this panel, tricuspid leaflet opening precedes mitral leaflet opening, and the tricuspid leaflets are in a fully opened position prior to the onset of mitral leaflet motion. *D,* Recorded during the diastasis phase. Both the mitral and tricuspid leaflets can be visualized in a neutral or resting position within the respective ventricular cavities. *E,* Recorded following atrial systole, this panel illustrates the reopening of the tricuspid leaflets in response to atrial contraction. *F,* The position of the tricuspid leaflets following atrial relaxation just prior to ventricular systole. At this point, the tricuspid leaflets have not reached their fully closed position, whereas the mitral valve is already closed. This view is particularly well suited for making comparisons between events on the right and left sides of the heart.

therefore, should also apply to the tricuspid valve.

Several differences in the timing of tricuspid and mitral motion, however, should be noted. First, tricuspid opening normally precedes mitral opening.[7] This earlier opening of the tricuspid valve occurs because the peak systolic pressure in the right ventricle is normally below that in the left ventricle, and the time required for right ventricular pressure to fall to the level of right atrial pressure, therefore, is much less than the corresponding time period on the left side of the heart. This leads to a shorter right ventricular isovolumic relaxation and an earlier tricuspid opening. Second, tricuspid closure occurs after mitral closure because electrical activation of the left ventricle precedes that of the right ventricle. This earlier contraction of the left ventricle results in earlier initial systolic pressure generation on the left side and, thus, earlier mitral valve closure. Finally, right atrial contraction and relaxation precede corresponding left atrial contraction and relaxation. The tricuspid valve A wave, therefore, should precede the mitral valve A wave, and because the tricuspid valve closes after the mitral valve, the AC interval (duration from the peak of the A wave [A] to the point of leaflet closure [C]) on the right side should normally be longer than the corresponding interval on the left side.

THE ABNORMAL TRICUSPID VALVE ECHOGRAM

Normal function of the tricuspid valve permits unimpeded flow of blood from the right atrium into the right ventricle during diastole and prevents regurgitation into the right atrium during systole. On the basis of these functional requirements, tricuspid valve lesions can be divided into (1) those that restrict diastolic inflow into the right ventricle and are characterized echocardiographically by decreased diastolic leaflet excursion and (2) those that primarily affect the systolic competence of the valve and are associated with abnormalities of leaflet closure on either a functional or a structural basis.

Right Ventricular Inflow Obstruction

Obstruction to right ventricular inflow may result from an acquired or congenital deformity of the tricuspid valve or may develop as a functional disorder associated with tumors, vegetations, or thrombi that occlude the tricuspid orifice.[8] Acquired tricuspid stenosis is seen most commonly in patients with rheumatic heart disease but may also develop in association with a malignant carcinoid, endocardial fibroelastosis,[9] and endomyocardial fibrosis. Congenital tricuspid stenosis associated with a normal right ventricle is rare and is characterized by leaflets that are fused at their commissures but are otherwise relatively normal.[11,12] A profound reduction in tricuspid valve size—tricuspid atresia—is commonly associated with hypoplasia of the right ventricle and pulmonary atresia.[13] This combination of disorders is discussed in Chapter 13. Likewise, the tumors and thrombi that produce functional right ventricular inflow obstruction usually arise within the right atrium and are discussed in that section.

Rheumatic Tricuspid Stenosis

Rheumatic fever is, by far, the most common cause of acquired valvular tricuspid stenosis. Rheumatic inflammation of the tricuspid valve produces scarring and fibrosis of the valve leaflets, fusion of the leaflet commissures, and associated fibrosis and thickening of the chordae tendineae.[14] These abnormalities combine to limit tricuspid leaflet mobility and to reduce the size of the tricuspid orifice. Rheumatic tricuspid stenosis occurs less frequently than, but is almost invariably associated with, mitral stenosis being reported in 2[15] to 15%[16] of patients with rheumatic mitral involvement. The mitral lesion, in addition to being more common, is typically more severe and clinically predominates.

Tricuspid stenosis is characterized echocardiographically by (1) an increase in echo production from the thickened deformed tricuspid leaflets; (2) an abnormal diastolic leaflet motion; and (3) a reduction in the tricuspid valve orifice size.

The increase in echo production from the deformed tricuspid leaflets occurs most commonly along their free edges, is typically less pronounced than that seen with mitral stenosis, and the chordae, likewise, are less severely involved. Calcification is rarely noted.

The abnormal diastolic leaflet motion in tricuspid stenosis is similar to that observed with mitral stenosis. It is characterized by restricted excursion of the leaflet tips, diastolic doming of both the

anterior and the posterior tricuspid leaflets, and decreased or absent initial diastolic closing motion of the anterior leaflet
(E–F slope).

The reduced opening excursion of the
leaflet tips results from the commissural
fusion, which prevents their normal separation. The bodies of the leaflets, in contrast, are more freely mobile and separate
widely. This dissociation of movement between the leaflet tips and bodies results in
a prominent doming of the valve toward
the right ventricle.

In normal persons, reclosure of the leaflets begins immediately upon reaching
their point of maximal excursion. When
tricuspid stenosis is present, the gradient
across the valve holds the leaflets in a fully
open or domed position, and the normal
initial diastolic closing movement is either
diminished or absent. As diastole progresses and the right ventricle fills, the tricuspid annulus moves superiorly and posteriorly. This annular movement draws the
leaflets in a similar direction, thereby producing movement relative to the anterior
chest wall. Independent leaflet motion,
however, does not occur until the distending pressure dissipates and the leaflets are allowed to fall backward toward a
closed position.

Figure 9–7 illustrates the systolic and
diastolic appearance of rheumatic tricuspid stenosis. During systole, the coapted
leaflets appear almost normal. Only a slight
increase in reflectivity is evident (panel
A). During diastole, however, doming of
both the anterior and posterior leaflets into
the right ventricular cavity is obvious. Because the structural deformity in this example is not prominent, the diagnosis rests
totally on the domed diastolic appearance
of the stenotic leaflets.

Direct short-axis recording of the stenotic tricuspid valve orifice has proved
more difficult than short-axis recording of
the mitral valve orifice. This difficulty occurs because of the position of the tricuspid valve orifice beneath the sternum and

its orientation relative to the anterior chest
wall. These factors combine to make positioning of the imaging plane across the
valve orifice difficult. To date, although
the tricuspid valve orifice has been recorded in a number of patients with tricuspid stenosis, there is insufficient data
to correlate the echocardiographic orifice
areas with either hemodynamic, surgical,
or pathologic measurements of tricuspid
valve area. For this reason, the accuracy
of this technique has not been confirmed.

Tricuspid Stenosis in Endomyocardial Fibrosis (Löffler's Endocarditis)

There is a group of acquired disorders—
endomyocardial fibrosis, endocardial fibroelastosis, and malignant carcinoid—
characterized by deposition of fibrinous or
fibroelastic material on the endocardial
and valvular surfaces of the right ventricular inflow tract. This deposition of fibrinous material may lead to restriction of
tricuspid leaflet motion and tricuspid stenosis. Figure 9–8 is a long-axis recording
from a young woman with Löffler's endocarditis. The tricuspid leaflets and chordae are thickened, and diastolic leaflet
doming is obvious. In addition, there is an
accumulation of echogenic material along
the anterior endocardial surface of the right
ventricle beneath the anterior tricuspid
leaflet. Although differences in the appearance of the stenotic valve in this example and of the rheumatic valve in Figure
9–7 are obvious, these lesions are uncommon, and hence, sufficient experience is
not available to permit differentiation on
an echocardiographic basis alone. The
clinical setting in which these lesions
arise, however, should suggest their cause.

LESIONS ASSOCIATED WITH TRICUSPID INCOMPETENCE

Normal closure of the tricuspid valve
depends on the integrated function of the
tricuspid leaflets, chordae tendineae, papillary muscles, and subjacent area of right

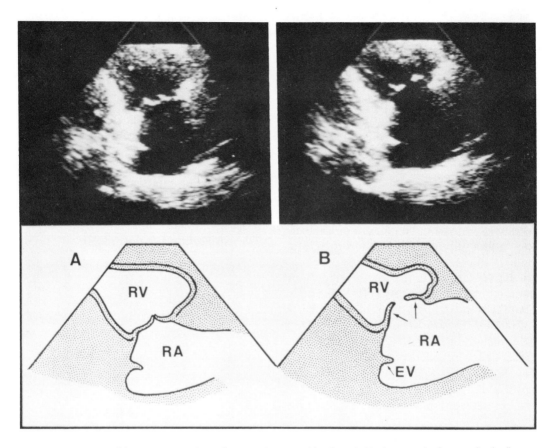

Fig. 9–7. Parasternal long-axis recording of a stenotic tricuspid valve. *A*, During ventricular systole, leaflet reflectivity is slightly increased; however, the leaflets otherwise appear normal. Right atrial dilatation is obvious. *B*, During diastole, both the anterior and posterior tricuspid leaflets arc or dome downward into the right ventricular cavity. The tricuspid orifice diameter is reduced, and reflectivity from the free edges of the stenotic leaflets is increased. The chordae extending from the ventricular surface of the posterior leaflet to the posterior papillary muscle are prominent. RV = right ventricle; RA = right atrium; EV = eustachian valve.

ventricular myocardium. Improper function of any of these components may cause the tricuspid leaflets to close improperly and may lead to valvular insufficiency. Tricuspid insufficiency is most commonly functional and occurs in the setting of right ventricular dilatation with an associated increase in tricuspid annular size, decrease in the normal systolic diminution in annular area, and inappropriate contraction of the papillary muscles.[17] Organic causes of tricuspid regurgitation include rheumatic heart disease,[14] tricuspid prolapse,[18] bacterial endocarditis,[19–21] carcinoid syndrome,[22] trauma,[17] and, more rarely, congenital disorders.[23] The congenital disorders include incomplete cusp differentiation and chordal development, which prevent normal closure[23] and Ebstein's anomaly.[24–26]

To date, echocardiography has not been proved to be a useful method for directly detecting the presence of tricuspid regurgitation. However, several indirect echocardiographic signs may be useful in inferring the presence of tricuspid valvular leakage. In addition, characteristic abnormalities of leaflet motion or configuration may be present and can aid in identifying the cause of a recognized regurgitant lesion.

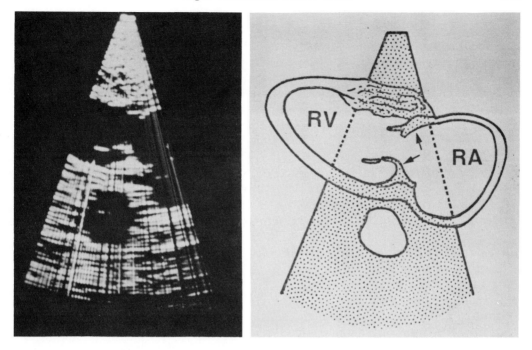

Fig. 9–8. Parasternal long-axis recording of the tricuspid valve from a patient with Löffler's endocarditis (eosinophilic endomyocardial disease) and valvular tricuspid stenosis. This frame, recorded during diastole, illustrates prominent doming of both the anterior and posterior tricuspid leaflets into the right ventricular cavity. This configuration is associated with a decrease in tricuspid orifice diameter and restriction to right ventricular inflow. A prominent accumulation of echogenic material appears along the anterior right ventricular wall just above the anterior tricuspid leaflet. The chordae tendineae from both the anterior and posterior leaflets extend toward the respective papillary muscles. The arrowheads in the accompanying diagram point to the stenotic tricuspid leaflets. The echo-free space beneath the right ventricle (RV) probably represents the descending aorta coursing behind the right heart. RA = right atrium.

Indirect Echocardiographic Methods for Detecting Tricuspid Regurgitation

The presence of tricuspid regurgitation can be indirectly inferred from (1) alterations in the right ventricular, right atrial, and inferior vena caval size, configuration, and motion pattern that result from the increased volume load on the right side of the heart and (2) characteristic changes that occur in the pattern of echocardiographic contrast flow through the right side of the heart in the presence of tricuspid insufficiency.

Tricuspid regurgitation increases the volume of blood that must be borne by all the chambers of the right side of the heart. This increased volume causes dilatation of the right ventricle, the right atrium, and the venous tributaries that drain into the right atrium. The right atrium appears to dilate early in the course of tricuspid regurgitation as does the inferior vena cava.[27] In addition to dilatation, there may be abnormal systolic expansion of the inferior vena cava due to the combined forward and regurgitant systolic flow into the vessel.

The increased volume load on the right ventricle, in addition to enlarging this chamber, also alters its shape by shifting the position of the interventricular septum toward the left ventricle.[28] This alteration causes the right ventricle to become more circular and the septum to move paradoxically during systole.

The right ventricular volume overload pattern is nonspecific (see Chap. 11), and a diagnosis of tricuspid regurgitation based on these findings must be a diagnosis of exclusion. When the cross-sectional echo-gram can exclude atrial septal defect and anomalous pulmonary venous return as diagnostic possibilities, the presence of tricuspid regurgitation may be strongly inferred. This inference is particularly relevant because pulmonary insufficiency rarely causes marked right atrial or vena caval dilatation in the absence of tricuspid regurgitation or right-heart failure. Rarer causes of right ventricular volume overload, such as ventricular septal defect with left ventricle to right atrial shunting and sinus of Valsalva aneurysmal rupture into the right side of the heart, are associated with other specific echocardiographic findings.

Tricuspid regurgitation may also alter the pattern of contrast flow through the right side of the heart producing a to-and-fro pattern of contrast movement through the tricuspid valve orifice and causing systolic regurgitation of contrast into the inferior vena cava and hepatic veins. Echocardiographic contrast injected into the upper extremity normally flows through the superior vena cava into the right atrium and then through the tricuspid orifice into the right ventricle. Slight backward or superior motion of these contrast bubbles may occur during the early part of systole because of the closing movement of the tricuspid leaflets. When tricuspid insufficiency is present, however, systolic regurgitation of the contrast medium through the incompetent valve, alternating with the normal forward contrast flow through the orifice during diastole, produces a to-and-fro pattern that is characteristic of tricuspid regurgitation.[29] Detection of this movement is based on an assessment of the overall motion of the entire contrast pool because following a single bubble back and forth through the valve orifice is almost impossible. This finding is most useful with large valvular leaks because discrimination of abnormal contrast flow patterns with lesser degrees of regurgitation may be difficult.

The second pattern of abnormal contrast flow, which is more easily detected and appears more sensitive, is the regurgitation of contrast into the inferior vena cava and hepatic veins during right ventricular systole. This phenomenon is augmented by the Valsalva maneuver and has been reported to separate patients with tricuspid regurgitation from normal persons.[29]

In patients with indwelling right ventricular catheters, detection of contrast in the right atrium following right ventricular injection is a sensitive sign of tricuspid regurgitation.

Echocardiographic Features of Specific Lesions Associated with Tricuspid Regurgitation

Tricuspid Valve Prolapse

Tricuspid valve prolapse can be defined as the anatomic displacement of one or more of the tricuspid leaflets into the right atrium during right ventricular systole. The echocardiographic diagnosis of tricuspid prolapse reflects this definition and is based on the demonstration of abnormal superior movement or arcing of one or more of the tricuspid leaflets above the plane of the tricuspid annulus at peak systolic excursion. Both tricuspid leaflet motion and the plane of the tricuspid leaflet annulus can be well defined in both the parasternal long-axis view of the right ventricular inflow tract[2] and the apical four-chamber view.[3] In the parasternal view, the anterior and posterior leaflets are visualized, whereas in the apical four-chamber view, the anterior and septal leaflets are recorded. Figure 9–9 illustrates prolapse of the tricuspid valve in the parasternal long-axis view. In this example, the anterior tricuspid leaflet arcs above the plane of the tricuspid annulus at the point of peak systolic excursion.

Isolated tricuspid prolapse occurs rarely.[30] The reported incidence of tricuspid prolapse in patients with mitral valve prolapse has varied from greater than

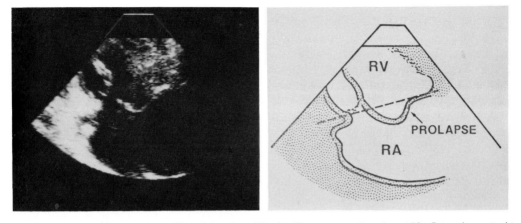

Fig. 9–9.   Parasternal long-axis recording of the tricuspid valve illustrates anterior tricuspid leaflet prolapse. In this recording, taken at the point of peak systolic superior displacement of the tricuspid valve, the anterior leaflet arcs superiorly into the right atrium (RA) beyond the plane of the tricuspid annulus. The right atrium is dilated. Clinical and hemodynamic evidence of tricuspid regurgitation was present. RV = right ventricle.

50%[31] to less than 6%.[30] Tricuspid prolapse appears to involve the septal and anterior leaflets primarily[31] and has not been noted to occur in patients with right ventricular volume overload.[30] The latter finding is in contrast to the increased incidence of mitral valve prolapse noted in the presence of right ventricular volume overload.[29,32–35] This finding is not unexpected, however, because right ventricular dilatation should increase the ventricle-valve size ratio on the right and thus retard tricuspid leaflet closure. In contrast, the altered geometry and relative decrease in size of the left ventricle should decrease this ratio on the left side, resulting in mitral valve prolapse.

Tricuspid Vegetations

Endocarditis involving the tricuspid valve is relatively infrequent and has a mean incidence of only 2% in reported series.[19] Tricuspid endocarditis is typically an acute rather than subacute process.[19] Staphylococcus aureus is the most common infecting organism.[19–21] Predisposing factors include intravenous drug abuse, alcohol abuse, virulent skin infections, and infected venous catheters.

The clinical diagnosis of tricuspid endocarditis is suggested by the triad of fever, narcotic addiction, and multiple lung lesions.[36] A pathologic murmur, which generally alerts the clinician to the possibility of endocarditis in lesions involving the left side of the heart, is frequently absent with isolated tricuspid valve involvement. In one series, the murmur was absent in 65% of patients with isolated right-sided endocarditis,[19] whereas in another series, the murmur of tricuspid insufficiency went undetected in 16 of 42 patients with proven tricuspid involvement.[21] Although significant tricuspid leaflet destruction and ruptured chordae are fairly common, the low pressure gradient between the right ventricle and right atrium may be responsible for the absence of a murmur.[20] This frequent lack of clinical signs directing attention to the tricuspid valve makes the routine echocardiographic examination of this valve imperative in instances of suspected endocarditis.

The cross-sectional echocardiographic diagnosis of tricuspid endocarditis is based on visualization of the bacterial vegetations that are characteristic of this disorder. Tricuspid vegetations generally appear as fairly large, echo-producing masses that disrupt the normally smooth, thin contour of the tricuspid leaflets.[37,38] The echoes from these vegetations have been described as thick and "shaggy" and, when leaflet destruction is present, may be associated with high frequency oscillatory motion of part of the disrupted leaflet or of the vegetations themselves.[38] Tricuspid vegetations are usually larger than corresponding left-sided lesions and tend to involve the atrial surface of the involved leaflets. In two cases, abrupt disappearance of vegetation was associated with pulmonary embolism and infarction.[37]

Figure 9–10 is an example of a large tricuspid vegetation attached to the atrial surface of the anterior tricuspid leaflet. There has been extensive destruction of the anterior leaflet and the remaining leaflet tissue has been incorporated into the mass. Consequently, visualization of discrete leaflet tissue is no longer possible. Figure 9–11 is an angiogram from the same patient and illustrates extensive contrast displacement by the large vegetative mass. Large tricuspid vegetations may be difficult to differentiate from atrial tumors. Their uniform association with the affected leaflet and their movement in unison with leaflet motion, however, aid in their identification.[37] When vegetations

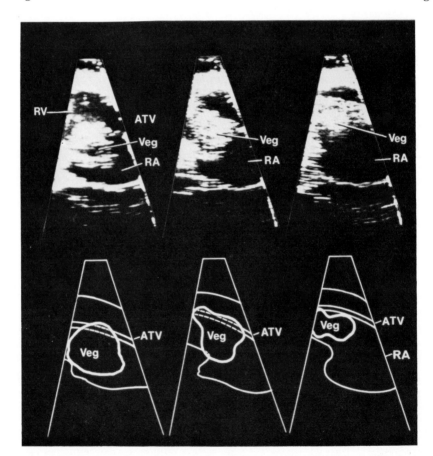

Fig. 9–10. Parasternal long-axis recording of a large tricuspid valve vegetation. The vegetation (Veg) appears as a large echo-producing mass that is attached to the atrial surface of the anterior tricuspid leaflet and moves in unison with this leaflet. In the left-hand panel, recorded during ventricular systole, the vegetative mass lies within the right atrial cavity, and the tricuspid valve is closed. In the center panel, recorded at the onset of valve opening, the vegetation shifts down into the tricuspid orifice as the leaflet opens. In the right-hand panel, recorded during mid-diastole, the vegetation is displaced into the right ventricle (RV) and almost completely fills the tricuspid valve orifice. ATV = anterior leaflet of tricuspid valve; RA = right atrium.

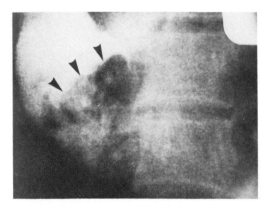

Fig. 9–11. Right atrial and ventricular angiogram from the patient discussed in Figure 9–10. The tricuspid vegetation produces a large area of contrast displacement indicated by the arrowheads in the region of the tricuspid annulus.

arise on a stalk, their motion may be more erratic. In these situations, their point of origin should aid in their recognition.

When vegetations cause extensive destruction of leaflet tissue, a portion of the leaflet may become flail and evert into the right atrium during systole.[38] Marked valvular incompetence is usually associated with a right ventricular volume overload pattern.[38]

Carcinoid Heart Disease

Malignant carcinoid tumors with hepatic metastases frequently present with a clinical syndrome characterized by episodic flushing, diarrhea, and bronchospasm.[23,29] In addition, more than half of these patients develop extensive fibrous deposits on the endocardial surfaces of the right side of the heart. These deposits interfere with normal myocardial and valvular function; as a result, heart failure is the leading cause of death. This fibrous tissue deposition appears to result from endocardial damage produced by a hormonal substance(s) secreted by the tumor. This substance(s) apparently circulates through the right side of the heart and is inactivated in the lungs because in the absence of right-to-left shunting, left-sided lesions are uncommon. Both serotonin and

kinin peptides have been implicated as the injury-inducing agent.

The reported echocardiographic features of carcinoid heart disease include: thickening and shortening of the tricuspid valve leaflets with variable degrees of diastolic leaflet immobility; failure of complete systolic leaflet coaptation; and, in one case, total freezing of leaflets in a partially open position.[40] These echocardiographic abnormalities have been noted in only five of nine cases reported to date.[40] Figure 9–12 illustrates a thickened immobile tricuspid valve in a patient with carcinoid syndrome.

Ebstein's Anomaly

Ebstein's anomaly is a congenital deformity characterized by downward displacement of all or part of a malformed tricuspid valve into the right ventricular cavity.[41,42]

The tricuspid leaflets typically attach in part to the tricuspid annulus and in part to the right ventricular endocardium either directly or by multiple thick chordae. The portion of the ventricle above the displaced tricuspid valve is thin walled and functions as a reservoir rather than contributing to the pumping ability of the right ventricle. Although an intracavitary right ventricular electrogram is recorded in this chamber, the intracavitary pressure is similar to that of the right atrium, and hence, it is referred to as "atrialized."[43–45]

The anterior tricuspid leaflet is characteristically the largest and the least affected in Ebstein's anomaly.[18,41,46,47] The septal and posterior leaflets are more deformed, and the posterior leaflet may be rudimentary or absent. The right atrium is almost always dilated, and an associated atrial septal defect is common. The degree of right ventricular dysfunction relates to (1) the degree of deformity of the tricuspid leaflets and the presence or absence of tricuspid regurgitation; (2) the size of the atrialized portion of the right ventricle that

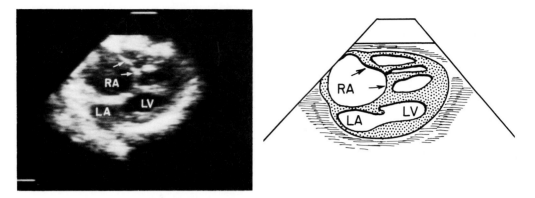

Fig. 9–12. Subcostal long-axis recording of the tricuspid valve in carcinoid syndrome. The valve leaflets (horizontal arrows) and chordae are thickened, and in this diastolic frame, there is no evidence of valve opening. In real-time, the valve appeared completely fixed and stenotic with no observable motion from diastole to systole. The right atrium is dilated.

not only fails to contribute to right ventricular contraction but may expand in an aneurysmal fashion during atrial systole, further impairing right ventricular filling; and (3) the absolute decrease in right ventricular chamber size and resulting decrease in right ventricular output.

The characteristic feature of Ebstein's anomaly (downward displacement of the malformed tricuspid valve) can be best visualized echocardiographically in the apical four-chamber view.[48] Normally, the septal leaflet of the tricuspid valve in this view inserts into the interventricular septum just below (less than 1 cm) the corresponding septal insertion of the anterior mitral leaflet. In Ebstein's anomaly, this separation increases. The ratio of the mitral valve-left ventricular apex distance to the corresponding tricuspid valve-right ventricular apex distance in normal persons and in patients with right ventricular volume overload is reported to range from 1 to 1.2 to 1 (mean 1.09 to 1) versus 1.8 to 3.2 to 1 in a group of patients with documented Ebstein's anomaly.[48]

Figures 9–13, 14, and 15 illustrate various degrees of tricuspid displacement in Ebstein's anomaly. In Figure 9–13, the septal tricuspid leaflet in a patient with hemodynamically confirmed Ebstein's anomaly and tricuspid regurgitation inserts farther below the anterior mitral leaf-

let than is normal. In Figure 9–14, the tricuspid valve is further displaced toward the apex and separates the right ventricular cavity into an atrialized chamber and a true muscular right ventricle. Figure 9–15 is a still more severe example in which the tricuspid valve is displaced well into the apical segment of the right ventricle and the atrialized portion of the ventricular chamber is much larger than the residual ventricle.

The anatomic and functional severity of Ebstein's anomaly can be assessed by determining the absolute and relative sizes of the functional right ventricle and atrialized portion of the right ventricular cavity (Fig. 9–14). The functional right ventricle extends from the right ventricular apex to the plane of the displaced tricuspid valve leaflets. The atrialized ventricle then extends from the plane of the displaced tricuspid valve to the tricuspid annulus. The tricuspid annulus is readily defined because it maintains its normal position and can be identified as a band of linear echoes that divides the right side of the heart at a level that approximates the plane of the mitral annulus and corresponds roughly to the point of mitral leaflet insertion. The right atrium then extends from the tricuspid annulus to the superior wall of the right atrial cavity. Studies comparing the length of the atrialized right ventricular

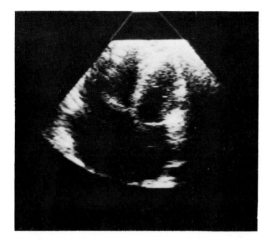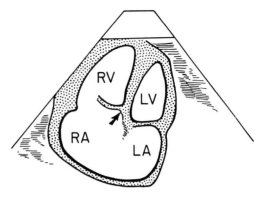

Fig. 9–13. Apical four-chamber recording illustrates minimal apical displacement of the septal tricuspid leaflet in a patient with a mild form of Ebstein's anomaly and tricuspid regurgitation. The increased separation between the anterior mitral and septal tricuspid leaflets is indicated by the arrowhead. The right atrium (RA) and right ventricle (RV) are dilated. LA = left atrium; LV = left ventricle.

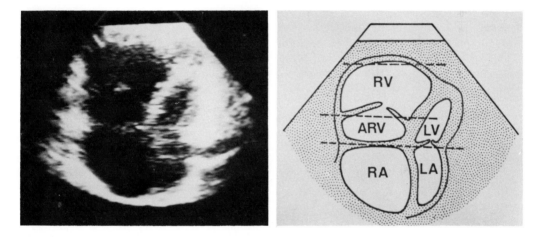

Fig. 9–14. Apical four-chamber recording illustrates a moderately severe degree of tricuspid displacement in another patient with Ebstein's anomaly. Both the displaced tricuspid leaflets and the tricuspid annulus are visible. The diagram to the right illustrates the relative sizes of the residual right ventricle (RV), extending from the right ventricular apex to the plane of insertion of the displaced tricuspid leaflets, and the atrialized right ventricle (ARV), which includes the area from the plane of insertion of the displaced tricuspid valve to the tricuspid annulus. RA = right atrium; LV = left ventricle; LA = left atrium.

chamber measured echocardiographically with that quantitated angiographically have shown a good correlation and confirm the ability of the cross-sectional echogram to define this relationship.[48]

Although the apical four-chamber view is the primary echocardiographic view for assessing Ebstein's anomaly, changes in tricuspid leaflet structure and right atrial and ventricular size can also be visualized in the parasternal long-axis and short-axis views. The long-axis view is most useful when there is associated right ventricular volume overload. In such instances, an enlarged anterior tricuspid leaflet with broad sail-like movements can be defined. Unfortunately, because the anterior leaflet is the least commonly displaced, its point of insertion into the tricuspid annulus is generally not abnormal and, hence, is non-

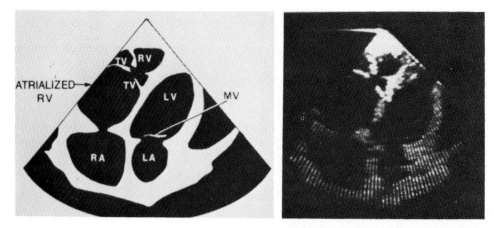

Fig. 9–15. Apical four-chamber recording illustrates an example of Ebstein's anomaly with marked apical displacement of the tricuspid valve. In this person, the atrialized portion of the right ventricle is much larger than the residual right ventricular cavity. RV = right ventricle; TV = tricuspid valve; LV = left ventricle; MV = mitral valve; RA = right atrium; LA = left atrium. (From Silverman, NH, and Schiller, NB: Apex echocardiography, a two-dimensional technique for evaluating congenital heart disease. Circulation, 57:503, 1978. Reproduced by permission of the American Heart Association.)

diagnostic. In the parasternal short-axis view, the large sail-like anterior tricuspid leaflet again predominates. When right ventricular volume overload is present, paradoxic motion of the interventricular septum may be noted.

Increased contraction of the infundibular region has also been described in milder forms. An earlier study suggested that superior, leftward displacement of the anterior mitral leaflet into the right ventricular outflow tract was a useful diagnostic sign of Ebstein's anomaly.[49] A similar pattern, however, may be seen in other forms of right ventricular volume overload associated with clockwise rotation of the base of the heart.

Cross-sectional echocardiography appears to be a far more sensitive and specific method than the M-mode echocardiogram for detecting the anatomic changes of Ebstein's anomaly. In one series, the cross-sectional echogram was diagnostic in each of 9 patients, whereas the M-mode suggested Ebstein's anomaly in only 6 of the 9 patients.[48]

THE RIGHT ATRIUM

Anatomy

The right atrium is a thin-walled (slightly thinner than the left), irregularly shaped chamber that occupies the majority of the right superior quadrant of the heart. The posterior and superior borders of the right atrium lie at the same level as, and are continuous with, those of the left atrium. The interatrial septum, which separates these two chambers, forms its left-hand margin, while inferiorly, it is bounded by the tricuspid annulus. The anterior wall, which is covered by the right atrial appendage, lies directly beneath the anterior chest wall. The free right border, which typically parallels the right side of the sternum, forms the majority of the right margin of the heart. There are four principal openings in the right atrial walls. These include (1) the orifice of the inferior vena cava, which is found along the right posterior margin of the inferior wall; (2) the insertion of the superior vena cava, which interrupts the right anterior portion of the superior wall; (3) the tricuspid orifice, which angles from anterior to posterior and superior to inferior along the inferior atrial border; and (4) the ostium of the coronary sinus, which is found posteriorly beneath the lower border of the interatrial septum and just superior to the posterior margin of the tricuspid annulus.[6,7]

Functionally, the right atrium serves as a reservoir for systemic venous blood returning to the heart during ventricular systole, as a conduit during the majority of diastolic filling, and as a contractile chamber to augment right ventricular filling just prior to tricuspid valve closure. Its volume increases throughout the systolic reservoir phase and is greatest at end-systole just prior to tricuspid valve opening.[50]

The right atrium has no natural long or short axes, and as a result, these axes, like those of the left atrium, are defined relative to the axes of surrounding structures, particularly the right ventricle. The long axis of the right atrium, therefore, is considered to lie in the same plane as that of the right ventricle and, thus, to extend from the tricuspid annulus to the superior atrial border. The short axis lies within a plane perpendicular to the long axis and runs from the interatrial septum to the free right atrial wall. Both of these axes should roughly bisect the corresponding geometric areas of the atrium.

Examining Planes and Linear Dimensions

The right atrium can be recorded in a number of the standard imaging planes or modifications thereof, including (1) the apical four-chamber view, (2) the subxiphoid long axis, (3) the parasternal long axis of the right ventricular inflow tract, and (4) a parasternal short axis at the aortic valve level, which is angled rightward to record the right atrial chamber. The primary view for recording atrial dimensions and estimating volume changes has been the apical four-chamber view (Fig. 9–16). In this image orientation, the scan plane transects the atrium from the tricuspid annulus to the superior atrial wall, with the Y axis parallel to a line running from the interatrial septum medially to the free right atrial wall laterally. Two axes or dimensions of the right atrium can be defined in the apical four-chamber view. These axes are illustrated in Figure 9–16

and include an inferior-superior dimension or long axis (D_2),* which extends from the midpoint of the tricuspid annulus to the superior border of the right atrium and should roughly bisect the geometric area of this chamber. The second dimension (D_3) is taken from the medial to lateral aspects of the atrium in a plane that is perpendicular to the long axis. Because the atrium is relatively circular in this view, this dimension should roughly bisect both the long axis and the geometric area of the atrium and represents the longest dimension that can be obtained in this plane. Other methods for obtaining the right atrial long axis have been suggested and include a maximal superior-inferior dimension[48] and a dimension from the medial insertion of the tricuspid valve drawn along the right-hand margin of the interatrial septum to the posterior atrial wall.[49] I prefer to relate these linear dimensions to the axes of the ventricle and, hence, to draw them such that they roughly bisect the atrium. This method is also consistent with the method for obtaining left atrial dimensions.

Linear dimensions used to estimate atrial size are, by convention, taken at the point of maximal atrial volume or at end-ventricular-systole. In normal persons, the superior-inferior dimension of the right atrium at end-systole has varied from 35 $\pm$ 4 mm[48] to 42 $\pm$ 1 mm.[49] The end-systolic right atrial medial to lateral dimension (short axis) appears slightly smaller, averaging 36 $\pm$ 1 mm (versus 42 $\pm$ 1 mm).[49] The normal area of the right atrium has been reported to average 13.9 $\pm$ .7 cm².[49] The change in right atrial size that occurs during systolic atrial filling is primarily due to apical displacement of the tricuspid annulus. The long axis or superior-inferior dimension, therefore, in-

*The designation of these dimensions is intended to correspond to the method used to denote the corresponding left atrial dimensions. A standardizable method for recording a right atrial anteroposterior dimension (D_1) has not yet been defined.

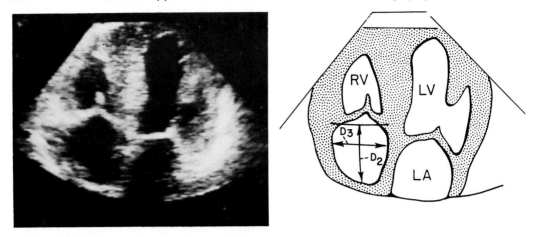

Fig. 9–16. Apical four-chamber view illustrates a method for obtaining right atrial linear dimensions. The inferior-superior dimension (D_2) is taken from the tricuspid annulus to the superior wall of the atrium. The medial-lateral dimension (D_3) is taken as the length of the line that extends from the interatrial septum to the free lateral atrial wall. This dimension roughly bisects D_2. RV = right ventricle; LV = left ventricle; LA = left atrium.

creases throughout systole, whereas the medial-lateral dimension remains fairly constant.

The right atrium has been reported to dilate in both right ventricular volume and pressure overload states.[48] This dilatation is characteristically symmetric, with an increase in both the inferior-superior and medial-lateral dimensions.[49] Figure 9–17

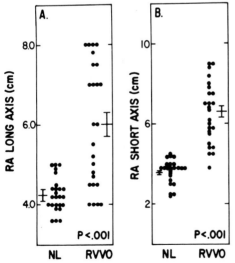

Fig. 9–17. Comparison of the means and ranges of right atrial dimensions in normal persons and patients with right ventricular volume overload. (From Bommer, W, et al.: Determination of right atrial and right ventricular size by two-dimensional echocardiography. Circulation, 60:91, 1979. Reproduced by permission of the American Heart Association.)

compares the right atrial long- and short-axis dimensions in a group of normal patients with patients with right ventricular volume overload due to both tricuspid regurgitation and atrial septal defect.

A comparable orthogonal view of the right atrium can also be recorded in the subcostal long-axis view.[4] In this orientation, the imaging plane transects the atrium from the free right atrial wall to the interatrial septum. The Y axis of the imaging plane is oriented parallel to a line running from the tricuspid annulus to the superior atrial border. The linear dimensions recorded in this plane are the same as those observed in the apical four-chamber view. In children, the right atrium may be more easily visualized in the subcostal orientation, and hence, this view offers a preferable alternative to the four-chamber view. In adults, however, the image quality is rarely as good from the subcostal transducer location, and although comparable dimensions can be obtained, the four-chamber view is clearly preferable.

The right atrium can also be recorded in a parasternal long-axis view of the right ventricular inflow tract (Fig. 9–18). In this view, the imaging plane passes obliquely through the atrium from the left anterior to the right posterior borders. Both oblique

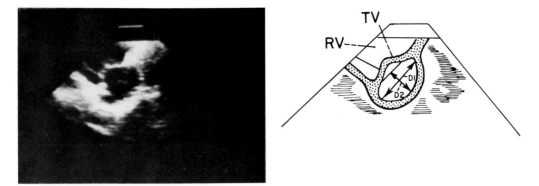

Fig. 9–18. Parasternal long-axis recording of a normal left atrium. As indicated in the accompanying diagram, both an anteroposterior dimension (D_1) and a superior-inferior dimension (D_2) can be obtained from this view. Because the plane obliquely transects the atrium, the significance of dimensions obtained in this projection remains to be established. TV = tricuspid valve; RV = right ventricle.

anteroposterior and superior-inferior dimensions of the atrium can be obtained in this projection; however, their relationship to right atrial size and their reproducibility have not been evaluated. The oblique orientation of this plane relative to the right atrium suggests that the four-chamber or subcostal views are preferable.

The parasternal short-axis view of the right atrium is even less valuable because the free right-hand border of the atrium can rarely be recorded from this transducer location. The primary role of this view is in defining the anteroposterior orientation of the interatrial septum. The aorta and anterior insertion of the interatrial septum may become displaced to the left in patients with right atrial dilatation, thereby shifting the orientation of the interatrial septum toward the left shoulder. This change in position of the aorta and interatrial septum can only be seen in the short-axis view (see Chap. 12).

The Eustachian Valve

The eustachian valve or the valve of the inferior vena cava is frequently visualized within the right atrium. This valve is formed by a fold of endocardium that arises from the lower end of the crista terminalis and stretches across the posterior margin of the inferior vena cava to become con-

tinuous with the border of the fossa ovalis.[6] The eustachian valve is most obvious in the parasternal long-axis view of the right ventricular inflow tract[51] in which it appears as a horizontal linear echo arising along the inferior border of the atrium just below the lower margin of the tricuspid annulus. The eustachian valve is evident in Figures 9–1 and 9–7. When large, the eustachian valve may show considerable (2 cm) rapid movement within the right atrial cavity[51] and has been confused on M-mode studies with right atrial catheters, vegetations, and tumors. This structure can be readily identified on cross-sectional examination, however, by its origin from the margin of the inferior vena cava and its characteristic orientation within the atrium.[51]

Right Atrial Tumors

A variety of tumors either primarily or secondarily involve the right atrium. These tumors may be intracavitary, mural, or extramural. The most common primary intracavitary tumors are the right atrial myxomas and sarcomas. Secondary extension into the right atrium may be seen with hypernephroma, sarcomas of the testes, and other less common lesions, such as the leiomyosarcoma of the inferior vena cava.

The right atrium is the site of origin of approximately 15% of cardiac myxomata. Right atrial myxomata typically arise from the right side of the interatrial septum in the region of the fossa ovalis. They may occur alone or may be associated with left atrial myxomata. Right atrial myxomata may be solitary or multiple, stationary or mobile. They may be small or may grow to almost completely fill the atrial cavity.

The echocardiographic appearance of right atrial myxomata is similar to the appearance of those arising in the left atrium. They are typically spherical or globular with well-defined borders and multiple internal reflective interfaces that give a speckled appearance to the tumor mass.[37] Right atrial myxomata are usually mobile, moving toward or into the tricuspid orifice during diastole and being thrust back into the right atrial cavity at the onset of ventricular systole. When large, they may obstruct the tricuspid orifice, thereby producing functional tricuspid stenosis. When obstructive, they interfere with the normal motion of the tricuspid leaflets because of mechanical occlusion of the tricuspid orifice and the changes they produce in the normal flow patterns through the tricuspid valve. These factors combine to hold the anterior tricuspid leaflet in a fully open position throughout diastole with a resulting loss of the normal initial diastolic closing (E–F) slope. During systole, the tumor is usually in the right atrial cavity behind and separated from the tricuspid valve. Leaflet opening, therefore, as a rule, occurs prior to movement of the tumor into the orifice. During systolic closure, leaflet movement again precedes movement of the tumor, and the leaflet appears to push the tumor out of the ventricular cavity as it closes. Systolic leaflet closure, however, ceases at the point of coaptation, whereas the momentum of the tumor typically carries it superiorly into the atrium, thereby resulting in a clear separation between the atrial surface of the tricuspid valve and the inferior tumor margin. Figures 9–19, A and B, illustrate a right atrial myxoma recorded during diastole and systole. The tumor appears as a ball-like mass of echoes lying within the right atrial cavity during systole and prolapsing downward into the tricuspid orifice during diastole.

A variety of tumors secondarily involve the right atrium by extension from the inferior vena cava. Figure 9–20 illustrates a large, echo-producing mass growing out of the inferior vena cava into the right atrium. This echogram was recorded following resection of a hypernephroma. The leading edge of the intraatrial mass was mobile and, during diastole, extended through the tricuspid orifice.

Mural right atrial tumors may arise primarily from the atrial wall or may result from secondary invasion. Figure 9–21 is an example of a metastatic tumor that has invaded the atrial and proximal ventricular walls in the region of the tricuspid annulus. In this example, the tumor is characterized by a focal increase in echo production and regional thickening of the atrial wall. Both mural and intracavitary metastatic tumors may also produce an irregular distortion in the normally smooth margins of the atrium, thereby highlighting their presence and facilitating their detection.

Venous Catheters

A variety of venous catheters can be visualized within the right ventricular inflow tract. The most common of these are transvenous pacing catheters and Swan-Ganz catheters. These catheters typically appear as elongated, thin, linear echoes that course through the inflow tract and may be detected in the right ventricle, right atrium, or right ventricular outflow tract. Their movement is comparable in timing and direction to that of the anterior tricuspid leaflet; however, it is typically damped when compared with leaflet motion. The catheter echoes may be single or associated with multiple linear reverber-

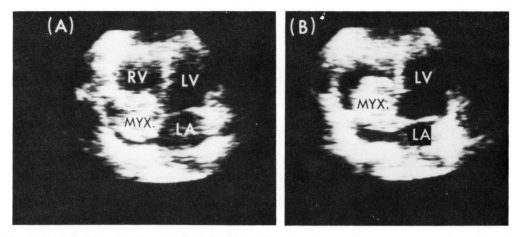

Fig. 9–19. Apical four-chamber recording of a right atrial myxoma (MYX). The tumor appears as a circular echo-producing mass with multiple internal reflections. *A,* During systole, the large echo-producing mass almost completely fills the right atrium. *B,* In diastole, the tumor prolapses through the tricuspid orifice into the right ventricle (RV). LV = left ventricle; LA = left atrium.

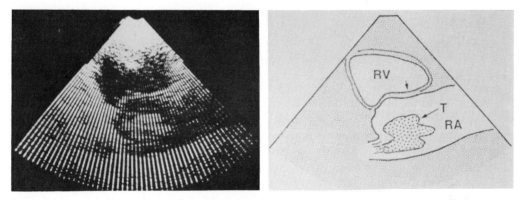

Fig. 9–20. Parasternal long-axis recording of the right ventricle (RV), right atrium (RA), and tricuspid valve illustrates a large, mobile, echo-producing mass extending into the right atrium from the inferior vena cava. The mass (T) was noted shortly after resection of a hypernephroma.

ations that can be visualized posterior to the catheter. When the catheter is visualized, the source of these reverberations is readily apparent. On occasion, reverberations from a catheter may be detected within the left side of the heart even though the right-heart catheter is not recorded. Recognition of the source of these abnormal echoes requires that the examiner be familiar with this potential artifact as well as with the clinical setting in which the study was recorded. Figure 9–22 is an example of a pacing catheter coursing through the right atrium. This catheter appears as a thin, strand-like echo arcing gradually through the posterior portion of the right atrium toward the tricuspid orifice.

Cross-sectional echocardiography may be helpful in demonstrating the position of right ventricular pacing catheters. In one study, the catheter position was demonstrated in 5 of 7 patients using a parasternal long-axis view of the right ventricle.[52] Coronary sinus catheters can also be demonstrated near the base of the atrial septum and, in the same study, were successfully identified in 3 of 5 patients.[52]

THE VENAE CAVAE

The Inferior Vena Cava

The inferior vena cava arises from the confluence of the common iliac veins an-

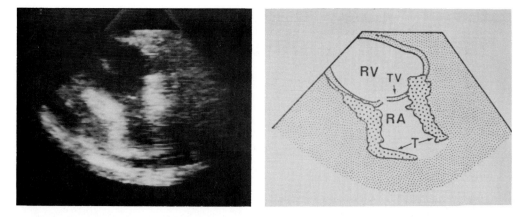

Fig. 9–21. Parasternal long-axis recording of the right ventricular inflow region from a patient with metastatic adenocarcinoma. An increase in echo density from the walls of the right atrium (RA) and tricuspid annulus is consistent with tumor infiltration (T). The area of increased echo production is indicated by the stippled area in the accompanying diagram. A pericardial effusion is also present. RV = right ventricle; TV = tricuspid valve.

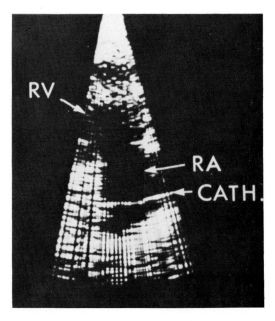

Fig. 9–22. Parasternal long-axis recording of the right atrium (RA) demonstrates a bright, thin, linear echo arising from a transvenous pacing catheter (CATH) coursing through the posterior portion of the atrial cavity. RV = right ventricle.

terior to the fifth lumbar vertebra and courses superiorly to penetrate the diaphragm and insert into the inferior border of the right atrium.[6] In the adult, this vessel extends roughly 8 inches and receives numerous tributaries, the most important of which (from an echocardiographic standpoint) are the hepatic veins. The he-patic veins insert into the anterior border of the inferior vena cava just proximal to the diaphragm.

The inferior vena cava is oriented roughly parallel to the long axis of the body. It lies to the right of the midline and is anterior to the abdominal aorta from which it must be differentiated. Echocardiographic differentiation of the inferior vena cava from the aorta is achieved by noting the absence of typical arterial pulsations, observing the insertions of the hepatic veins into its anterior border, and following its course into the right atrium.

The inferior vena cava is typically recorded in both long- and short-axis projections. Because the vessel runs parallel to the long axis of the body, these imaging-plane orientations roughly parallel the corresponding anatomic planes of the body. The inferior vena cava is recorded with the transducer placed over the anterior abdominal wall or in the subcostal region. Because only soft tissue is interposed between the vena cava and abdominal walls, this vessel is easily recorded and should be available for examination in almost every patient. Long-axis views are conventionally displayed with the superior margin of the vessel to the right of the display, whereas short-axis views are displayed as if viewed from below with the left-hand margin of the vena cava positioned to the right of the display. Figure 9–23 illustrates the long-axis appearance of the inferior vena cava in the abdominal cavity beneath the liver (A), as it courses through the diaphragm and inserts into the right atrial cavity (B), and as it relates to the other cardiac chambers (C).

In the long-axis projection, the vessel appears as a broad, linear, nonpulsatile, echo-free space with parallel margins and smooth borders. The hepatic veins join the vena cava from above, inserting at approximately a 30-degree angle. They are smaller in diameter and can be seen arising from within the hepatic parenchyma. In short axis, the inferior vena cava appears circular. The insertion points of

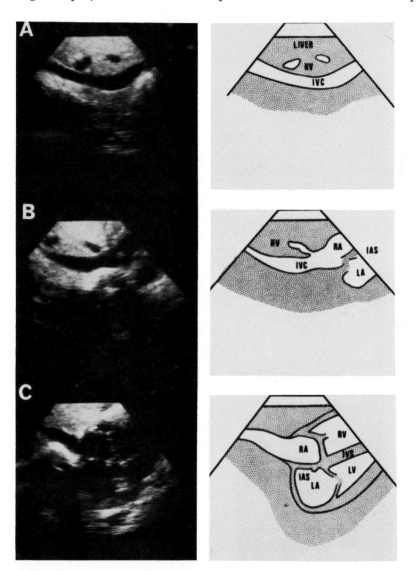

Fig. 9–23. Series of long-axis recordings of the inferior vena cava. *A,* The vessel is recorded as it courses through the abdomen beneath the liver. The two circular, echo-free areas within the hepatic parenchyma are produced by hepatic veins. *B,* Insertion of the inferior vena cava into the right atrium (RA). *C,* The relationship of the inferior vena cava to the four cardiac chambers. IVC = inferior vena cava; HV = hepatic veins; IAS = interatrial septum; IVS = interventricular septum; LA = left atrium; RV = right ventricle; LV = left ventricle.

multiple hepatic veins can frequently be recorded if the short-axis plane is positioned at the appropriate level.

Abnormalities of the vena cava that have been noted to date include (1) nonspecific dilatation of the vena cava and hepatic veins with right atrial hypertension and tricuspid valve disease, (2) inferior vena cava dilatation due to abnormal venous inflow in infants with total anomalous pulmonary venous connection to the inferior vena cava or one of its tributaries,[53] and (3) metastatic disorders extending into the right atrium via the inferior vena cava that either partially or totally occlude this vessel.

The inferior vena cava and hepatic veins frequently dilate early in the course of tricuspid valvular disorders. Inferior vena cava dilatation may also be seen with right atrial hypertension and with right ventricular failure. Figure 9–24 illustrates the long- and short-axis appearance of the inferior vena cava in a patient with cardiomyopathy and combined right and left ventricular failure. Dilatation of both the vena cava and hepatic veins is prominent, and the points of insertion of the distended hepatic veins into the vena cava are clearly evident.

Examination of the inferior vena cava may also be useful in patients with tricuspid regurgitation. This lesion produces dilatation of the inferior vena cava, and when severe, systolic expansion of the vessel may be evident. In addition, contrast injected peripherally can be observed to regurgitate into the inferior vena cava and hepatic vein during systole, thus helping to confirm this diagnosis.[29]

The Superior Vena Cava

The superior vena cava is formed by the confluence of the right and left innominate veins beneath the first intercostal space and descends vertically to join the superior border of the right atrium at the level of the third right costal cartilage.[6] The su-

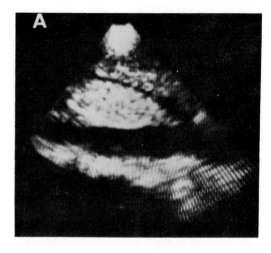

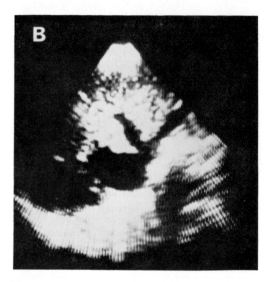

Fig. 9–24. Long- and short-axis recordings of a dilated inferior vena cava. *A*, In the long axis, the dilated vessel is recorded as it passes beneath the liver to its penetration through the diaphragm at the right-hand margin of the scan. A single hepatic vein inserts into the anterior margin of the vessel just proximal to the level of the diaphragm. *B*, In short axis, the dilated circular vessel, with two hepatic veins entering its anterior margin, can be seen.

perior vena cava can be recorded either in the parasternal long axis of the right ventricular inflow tract or in a subcostal long-axis view. Figure 9–25 illustrates the configuration of the superior vena cava in the parasternal long-axis view of the right ventricular inflow tract. In this orientation,

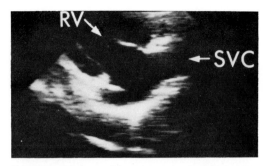

Fig. 9–25. Parasternal long-axis recording of the right ventricular inflow tract illustrates the insertion of the superior vena cava into the superior right atrial wall. SVC = superior vena cava; RV = right ventricle.

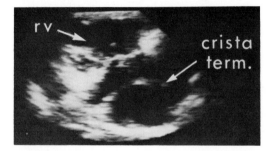

Fig. 9–26. Parasternal long-axis scan of the right ventricular inflow tract. The scan plane is angled to the right toward the lateral wall of the right atrium. In this scan position, an arcuate groove is often recorded along the lateral wall of the right atrium between the tricuspid annulus and the crista terminalis. The lateral recess of the right atrium is also evident beneath the crista terminalis. RV = right ventricle.

the vena cava courses from right to left entering the anterosuperior margin of the right atrial cavity. In the subcostal long-axis view, the superior vena cava can also be recorded entering the superior margin of the right atrium.[4] In this orientation, it lies parallel and slightly anterior to the path of the ascending aorta. The superior vena cava can also be visualized from the suprasternal notch;[2] however, the landmarks used to identify the vessel from this orientation are more difficult to define, and either the parasternal or the subcostal imaging planes appear preferable.

Few echocardiographic abnormalities of the superior vena cava have been described. This vessel dilates with the inferior vena cava in the presence of tricuspid valve disease, right atrial hypertension, or

right-heart failure. Superior vena cava dilatation has also been reported in infants with total anomalous pulmonary venous connection, which drains into the right atrium via this tributary.[53]

When there is persistence of the left superior vena cava, this anomalous vessel commonly drains into the right atrium by way of the coronary sinus. This drainage causes coronary sinus dilatation and can be detected by contrast injection into the left arm. (This anomaly is discussed further in Chapter 6.)

If the scan plane is angled farther to the right in the parasternal long-axis view, the anterior and posterior borders of the inferior and superior vena cava appear to join, forming two parallel arcuate echoes. The more anterior of these echoes is formed by the right-hand margin of the tricuspid annulus, whereas the posterior echo appears to arise from a ridge, the crista terminalis, joining the posterior borders of the two great veins (Fig. 9–26). The right atrium lies beneath the posterior margin of this ridge.

REFERENCES

1. Feigenbaum, H: Echocardiography. Philadelphia, Lea & Febiger, 1976.
2. Tajik, AJ, et al.: Two-dimensional real-time ultrasonic imaging of the heart and great vessels. Mayo Clin Proc, 53:271, 1978.
3. Silverman, NH, and Schiller, NB: Apex echocardiography. A two-dimensional technique for evaluating congenital heart disease. Circulation, 57:503, 1978.
4. Lange, LW, Sahn, DJ, Allen, HD, and Goldberg, SJ: Subxiphoid cross-sectional echocardiography in infants and children with congenital heart disease. Circulation, 59:513, 1979.
5. Gray, H: Gray's Anatomy. Edited by CM Goss. Philadelphia, Lea & Febiger, 1974, p. 589.
6. Grant, JCB, and Basmajian, JV: Grant's Method of Anatomy. Baltimore, Williams & Wilkins, 1965.
7. Hurst, JW: The Heart. New York, McGraw-Hill, 1974.
8. Friedberg, CW: Diseases of the Heart. Philadelphia, Saunders, 1966.
9. Dennis, JL, Hansen, AE, and Corpening, TN: Endocardial fibroelastosis. Pediatrics, 12:130, 1953.
10. Weyman, AE, Rankin, R, and King, HL: Loeffler's endocarditis with mitral and tricuspid stenosis. Am J Cardiol, 40:438, 1977.

11. Sapirstien, W, and Baker, CB: Isolated tricuspid stenosis. Report of a surgically treated case. N Engl J Med, 269:236, 1963.

12. Gibson, RV, and Wood, P: The diagnosis of tricuspid stenosis. Br Heart J, 17:552, 1955.

13. Hurst, JW: The Heart. New York, McGraw-Hill, 1974, p. 722.

14. Hollman, A: The anatomic appearance of tricuspid valve disease. Br Heart J, 19:211, 1957.

15. Austen, WG, DeSanctis, RW, Sanders, CA, and Scannell, JG: Surgical treatment of acquired trivalvular disease. J Thorac Cardiovasc Surg, 49:640, 1965.

16. Cooke, WT, and White, PD: Tricuspid stenosis; with particular reference to diagnosis and prognosis. Br Heart J, 3:147, 1941.

17. Friedberg, CW: Diseases of the Heart. Philadelphia, Saunders, 1966, p. 1162.

18. Osborn, JR, Jones, RC, and Jahnke, EJ: Traumatic tricuspid insufficiency: hemodynamic data and surgical treatment. Circulation, 30:217, 1964.

19. Bain, TC, Edwards, JE, Scheifley, CH, and Geraci, JE: Right-sided bacterial endocarditis and endarteritis. Am J Med, 24:98, 1958.

20. Roberts, WC, and Buchbinder, NA: Right-sided valvular infective endocarditis. Am J Med, 53:7, 1972.

21. Banks T, Fletcher, R, and Ali, N: Infective endocarditis in heroin addicts. Am J Med, 55:444, 1973.

22. Roberts, WC, and Sjoerdsma, A: The cardiac disease associated with the carcinoid syndrome. Am J Med, 36:5, 1964.

23. Reisman, M, Hipona, FA, Bloor, CM, and Talner, NS: Congenital tricuspid insufficiency: a cause of massive cardiomyopathy and heart failure in the neonate. J Pediatr, 66:869, 1965.

24. Kumar, A, Fyler, D, Miettinen, O, and Nadas, A: Ebstein's anomaly: clinical profile and natural history. Am J Cardiol, 28:84, 1971.

25. Bialostozky, D, Horwitz, S, and Espino-Vela, J: Ebstein's malformation of the tricuspid valve. A review of 65 cases. Am J Cardiol, 29:826, 1972.

26. Watson, H: Natural history of Ebstein's anomaly of tricuspid valve in childhood and adolescence. Br Heart J, 36:417, 1972.

27. Friedberg, CW: Diseases of the Heart. Philadelphia, Saunders, 1966, p. 1165.

28. Weyman, AE, Wann, LS, Feigenbaum, H, and Dillon, JC: Mechanism of abnormal septal motion in patients with right ventricular volume overload. Circulation, 54:179, 1976.

29. Lieppe, W, Behar, VS, Scallon, R, and Kisslo, JA: Detection of tricuspid regurgitation with two-dimensional echocardiography and peripheral vein injections. Circulation, 57:128, 1979.

30. DeMaria, AN, et al.: Evaluation of tricuspid valve prolapse by two-dimensional echocardiography. Am J Cardiol, 43:385, 1979.

31. Mardelli, TJ, Morganroth, J, Meixell, LL, and Vergel, J: Enhanced diagnosis of tricuspid valve prolapse by cross-sectional echocardiography. Am J Cardiol, 43:385, 1979.

32. Pocock, WA, and Barlow, JB: An association between the billowing posterior mitral leaflet syndrome and congenital heart disease particularly atrial septal defect. Am Heart J, 81:720, 1971.

33. Betriu, A, Wigle, D, Felderhof, LH, and McLoughlin, MJ: Prolapse of the posterior leaflet of the mitral valve associated with secundum atrial septal defect. Am J Cardiol, 35:363, 1975.

34. Victoria, BE, Elliot, LP, and Gessner, IH: Ostium secundum atrial septal defect associated with balloon mitral valve in children. Am J Cardiol, 33:668, 1974.

35. Leachman, RD, Corrinos, DV, and Cooley, DA: Association of ostium secundum atrial septal defects with mitral valve prolapse. Am J Cardiol, 38:167, 1976.

36. Wright, JS, and Glennie, JS: Excision of tricuspid valve with later replacement in endocarditis of drug addiction. Thorax, 33:518, 1978.

37. Come, PC, Kurland, GS, and Vine, HS: Two-dimensional echocardiography in differentiating right atrial and tricuspid valve mass lesions. Am J Cardiol, 44:1207, 1979.

38. Kisslo, J, et al.: Echocardiographic evaluation of tricuspid valve endocarditis. An M-mode and two-dimensional study. Am J Cardiol, 38:502, 1976.

39. Grahame-Smith, DG: The carcinoid syndrome. Am J Cardiol, 21:376, 1968.

40. Rakowski, H, et al.: Cardiac carcinoid: a new method of diagnosis. Circulation, (Suppl II), 57 and 58:924, 1978.

41. Edwards, JE, Carey, LS, Neufeld, HN, and Lester, RG: Congenital Heart Disease. Philadelphia, Saunders, 1965.

42. Vacca, JB, Bussmann, DW, and Mudd, JG: Ebstein's anomaly. Complete review of 108 cases. Am J Cardiol, 2:210, 1958.

43. Brown, JW, Heath, D, and Whitaker, W: Ebstein's disease. Am J Med, 20:322, 1956.

44. Ellis, K, et al.: Ebstein's anomaly of the tricuspid valve. Angiocardiographic considerations. Am J Roentgen, 92:1338, 1964.

45. Kezdi, R, and Wennemark, J: Ebstein's malformation: clinical findings and hemodynamic alterations. Am J Cardiol, 2:200, 1958.

46. Ports, TA, Silverman, NH, and Schiller, NB: Two-dimensional echocardiographic assessment of Ebstein's anomaly. Circulation, 58(2):336, 1978.

47. Sahn, DS, et al.: The comparative utilities of real-time cross-sectional echocardiographic imaging systems for the diagnosis of complex congenital heart disease. Am J Med, 62:50, 1977.

48. Kushner, FG, Lam, W, and Morganroth, J: Apex sector echocardiography in evaluation of the right atrium in patients with mitral stenosis and atrial septal defect. Am J Cardiol, 42:733, 1978.

49. Bommer, W, et al.: Determination of right atrial and right ventricular size by two-dimensional echocardiography. Circulation, 60:91, 1979.

50. Hurst, JW: The Heart. New York, McGraw-Hill, 1974, p. 94.

51. Bommer, WJ, Kwan, OL, Mason, DT, and DeMaria, AN: Identification of prominent eustachian valves by M-mode and two-dimensional echocardiography: differentiation from right atrial masses. Am J Cardiol, 45:402, 1980.

52. Reeves, WC, Nanda, NC, and Barold, SS: Echocardiographic evaluation of intracardiac pacing catheters: M-mode and two-dimensional studies. Circulation, 58:1049, 1978.

53. Bierman, FZ, and Williams, RG: Subxyphoid two-dimensional echocardiographic diagnosis of total anomalous pulmonary venous return in infants. Am J Cardiol, 43:401, 1979. (Abstract)

Chapter 10

Right Ventricular Outflow Tract

The right ventricular outflow tract extends from the crista supraventricularis to the bifurcation of the main pulmonary artery. It arises from the anterosuperior margin of the right ventricle and courses superiorly and leftward above the anterior border of the aorta. After crossing the aorta, it continues in a posterior arc along the left aortic border, bifurcating into the right and left pulmonary arteries at the level of the posterior aortic wall just above the superior margin of the left atrium. The right ventricular outflow tract has three major structural components: (1) the pulmonary valve; (2) the subvalvular conus arteriosus or infundibulum; and (3) the main pulmonary artery.

EXAMINING PLANES

The right ventricular outflow tract, like all tubular structures, is optimally recorded with the imaging plane oriented parallel to its long axis. This orientation can be achieved from either the parasternal or subcostal transducer locations.[1,2] The parasternal location appears preferable, however, because it places the area of interest in close proximity to the transducer and within the focal zone of the scan plane.

Figure 10–1 is a parasternal long-axis recording of the right ventricular outflow tract and illustrates its three major components. The subvalvular or infundibular region lies anterior to the aortic root and extends from the tricuspid annulus to the pulmonary valve. The coapted pulmonary leaflets are recorded within the outflow tract anteriorly and to the right at approximately the 1:30 o'clock position relative to the circular aorta. The pulmonary artery courses vertically along the left margin of the aorta to its point of bifurcation. The long axis of the right ventricular outflow tract is optimally recorded when the dimensions of this tubular structure are maximal throughout the region of interest. Image orientation is achieved with reference to the pulmonary valve, the proximal inflow region, and the pulmonary artery bifurcation (see Chap. 4).

A limited segment of the subvalvular portion of the right ventricular outflow tract can also be viewed in short axis from the parasternal transducer location with

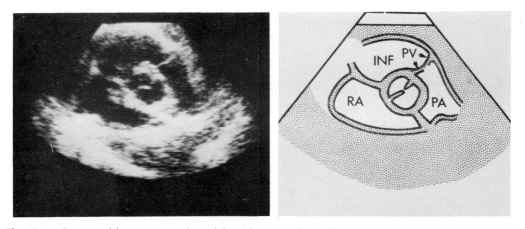

Fig. 10–1. Parasternal long-axis recording of the right ventricular outflow tract. The outflow tract extends from the crista supraventricularis, at the lefthand margin of the scan, to the bifurcation of the pulmonary artery, to the right and posteriorly. It includes the pulmonary infundibulum, the pulmonic valve, and the main pulmonary artery. INF = infundibulum; PV = pulmonary valve; PA = pulmonary artery; RA = right atrium.

the imaging plane aligned parallel to the long axis of the aorta (Fig. 10–2, A). This view, however, is difficult to standardize and has proved to be of little clinical value to date. If this plane is angled leftward, however, an orthogonal long-axis view of the pulmonary artery and valve can be obtained, and the crossing pattern of the aorta and descending pulmonary artery can be better appreciated (Fig. 10–2, B).

THE PULMONARY VALVE—NORMAL ORIENTATION AND MOTION

The pulmonary valve lies anterior, superior, and to the left of the aortic valve and, thus, is the most anteriorly positioned of the principal cardiac structures. Anatomically, the pulmonary valve has three semilunar cusps (the anterior, right, and left), which face leftward superiorly and slightly posteriorly. The pulmonary valve is best recorded from the parasternal transducer location with the imaging plane aligned parallel to the long axis of the right ventricular outflow tract and the central ray angled slightly leftward toward the left shoulder. Figure 10–3 illustrates the relationship of a 30-degree scan to the pulmonary artery and pulmonary valve. Although this type of transducer angulation

might appear unnecessary with instruments that provide larger scan areas, detection of the subtle changes noted in such disorders as pulmonary stenosis as a rule require fairly precise plane angulation and positioning of the central ray through the valve.

Figure 10–4 is a long-axis recording of a normal pulmonary valve. During diastole, the coapted pulmonary leaflets appear as a thin, linear echo lying within the pulmonary artery midway between the anterior and posterior margins of the vessel. This echo represents the line of coaptation between the anterior and one of the posterior leaflets. The cusps themselves are oriented parallel to the path of the scan plane and, thus, are rarely visualized. At the onset of systole, this single linear echo separates into two discrete linear echoes, which move rapidly away from each other toward the margins of the pulmonary artery. The echo from the posterior leaflet can usually be recorded lying parallel and in close apposition to the posterior wall of the pulmonary artery. The echo from the anterior leaflet, however, is generally lost within the dense mass of echoes originating from the anterior chest wall.[3]

A short-axis view of the pulmonary valve is far more difficult to record from the

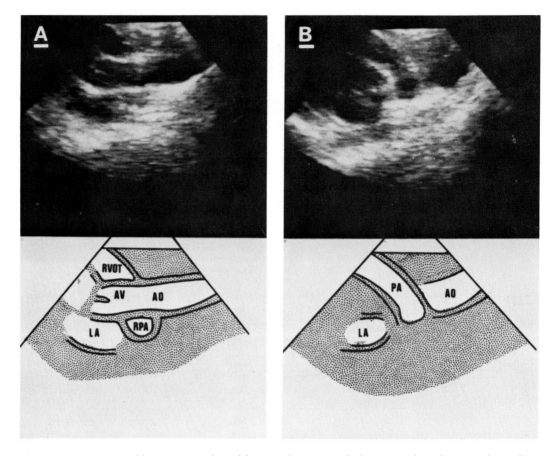

Fig. 10–2. *A,* Parasternal long-axis recording of the ascending aorta, which transects the right ventricular outflow tract (RVOT) in a plane roughly parallel to its short axis as it courses above the aortic root. The right pulmonary artery (RPA) can also be visualized beneath the aorta (AO) as it swings underneath this vessel. *B,* The plane has been angled slightly to the left to record the descending sweep of the pulmonary artery (PA). By combining these figures, the course of the pulmonary artery (across the top of the proximal aorta and down its left-hand margin to the point of bifurcation) and the return of the right pulmonary artery (beneath the aorta [AO] posteriorly at the level of the superior margin of the left atrium [LA]), can be appreciated. AV = aortic valve.

parasternal transducer location. This difficulty occurs because the pulmonary annulus in its normal orientation lies at an approximate 60-degree angle to the path of the imaging plane. Short-axis recordings of the pulmonary valve are possible in several situations, however. The most common of these occurs with large pericardial effusion and counterclockwise rotation of the base of the heart. Other conditions that shift the heart rightward can also displace the pulmonary valve beneath the parasternal window, thereby permitting short-axis recording. Figure 10–5 is a short-axis view of a normal pulmonary valve. The valve orifice in this example is oriented as if viewed from the left shoulder with the ascending aorta recorded beneath the pulmonary artery coursing to the viewer's right. Unfortunately, this type of image can be obtained so infrequently that it has more curiosity value than clinical utility.

VALVULAR PULMONARY STENOSIS

Valvular pulmonary stenosis is almost invariably congenital and is characterized by conical or dome-like fusion of the pulmonary valve cusps with a central perfo-

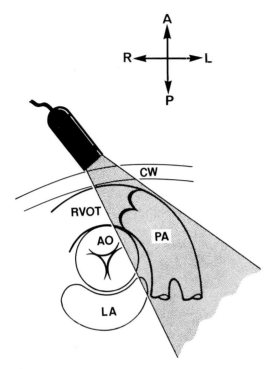

Fig. 10–3. Diagram illustrates the transducer orientation used to record the pulmonary valve. CW = chest wall; RVOT = right ventricular outflow tract; PA = pulmonary artery; AO = aorta; LA = left atrium. (From Weyman, AE, et al.: Cross-sectional echocardiographic visualization of the stenotic pulmonary valve. Circulation, 56:769, 1977. Reproduced by permission of the American Heart Association.)

ration at the apex.[4] The leaflets remain thin and pliable and can move easily toward either the right ventricle or the pulmonary artery in response to small differences in the pressures acting on their surfaces.[5] Echocardiographically, pulmonary stenosis is characterized by (1) systolic doming of the stenotic leaflets into the pulmonary artery,[3] (2) abnormal initial systolic leaflet motion,[3] and (3) opening or doming following atrial systole but before ventricular systole in more severe cases.[3,6]

Figure 10–6 illustrates the cross-sectional appearance of valvular pulmonary stenosis. During diastole, the coapted leaflets appear as a single linear echo within the pulmonary artery that is indistinguishable from that seen with a normal valve. During systole, however, the leaflets arc

into the lumen of the vessel and do not lie flat against the walls of the pulmonary artery. Consequently, a domed configuration is produced, and the pulmonary valve orifice is effectively narrowed.[3]

Figure 10–7 is a recording from a second patient with valvular pulmonary stenosis and again demonstrates the characteristic systolic doming of the pulmonary leaflets. In the majority of cases (64%), careful inspection of the valve permits doming of both the anterior and posterior leaflets to be demonstrated.[5] Only the posterior leaflet, however, must be recorded to establish the diagnosis of pulmonary stenosis. Figure 10–8 illustrates such an example. The posterior leaflet arcs into the pulmonary artery during systole and the hook-like configuration of this leaflet by itself is sufficient to establish the presence of leaflet doming and, hence, the appropriate diagnosis.

The systolic opening motion of the stenotic pulmonary valve also differs from normal. In normals, the leaflet echoes remain parallel to each other and to the walls of the pulmonary artery as they separate.[3] In patients with valvular pulmonary stenosis, the proximal portion of the leaflet echoes separates and swings through a wide arc, whereas the distal tips of the leaflets remain relatively close. This motion causes the angle between the leaflet echoes and the margins of the pulmonary artery to become increasingly obtuse, finally terminating in full leaflet doming. When viewed in real time, this abrupt tipping of the leaflet echoes as they begin to open alerts the examiner to the possible presence of pulmonary stenosis. More detailed frame-by-frame analysis is generally necessary to demonstrate the domed systolic configuration. Figure 10–9 illustrates the difference between the opening sequence of the normal and stenotic pulmonary valve.

Finally, in more severe instances, the pulmonary leaflets may shift to an open or domed position at end-diastole following

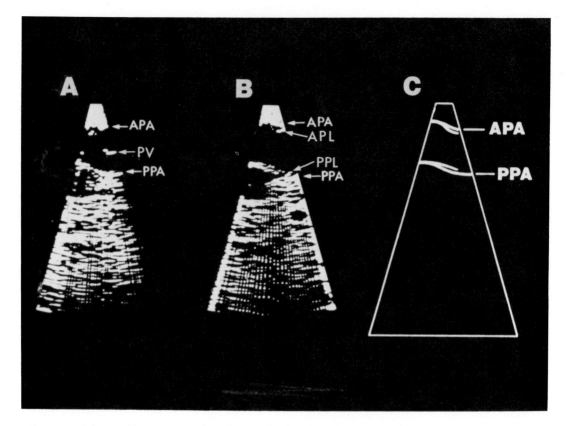

Fig. 10–4. Parasternal long-axis recording of a normal pulmonary valve. *A,* The coapted pulmonary leaflets appear as a linear echo midway between the anterior and posterior margins of the pulmonary artery. *B,* Recorded during systole, the fully open pulmonary leaflets lie parallel and close to the anterior and posterior margins of the pulmonary artery. *C,* Diagram illustrating the position of the fully open pulmonary leaflets. APA = anterior margin of the pulmonary artery; PPA = posterior pulmonary artery; PV = coapted pulmonary leaflets during diastole; APL = anterior pulmonary leaflet; PPL = posterior pulmonary leaflet. (From Weyman, AE, et al.: Cross-sectional echocardiographic visualization of the stenotic pulmonary valve. Circulation, 56:769, 1977. Reproduced by permission of the American Heart Association.)

atrial contraction but before ventricular systole (Fig. 10–10). This presystolic opening movement results from the abnormal end-diastolic pressure relationships that frequently occur in valvular pulmonary stenosis.[5,7] In this setting, the decreased compliance of the right ventricle and resulting increased force of right atrial contraction may increase peak right ventricular end-diastolic pressure to a level that exceeds simultaneous pulmonary artery pressure. This produces a positive gradient across the valve and results in presystolic valve opening or doming. This phenomenon is analogous to the enlarged A waves seen on the M-mode echocardiogram of patients with moderate or severe pulmonary stenosis.[6] The presence of this motion may be helpful in separating mild from more severe lesions.

PULMONARY VALVE ENDOCARDITIS

Infective endocarditis involving the pulmonary valve is relatively rare.[8,9] Echocardiographic visualization of pulmonary valve vegetations has been reported to date in only two cases.[10,11] Pulmonary valve vegetations have a similar appearance to vegetations involving the other cardiac valves and are described as globular or shaggy, mobile masses of echoes that ad-

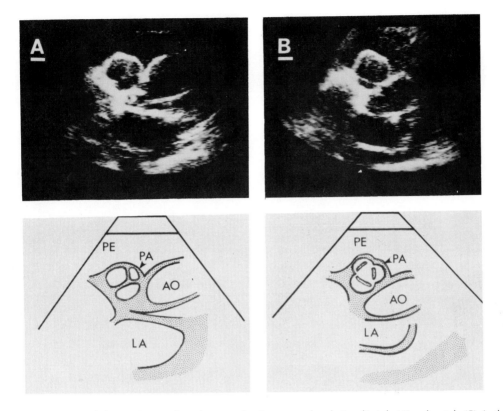

Fig. 10–5. Parasternal short-axis recording of a normal pulmonary valve during diastole (*A*) and systole (*B*). In the diastolic frame, the three commissures of the coapted semilunar pulmonary leaflets can be visualized. During systole, the leaflets separate widely, and the anterior leaflets and one posterior leaflet can be seen lying against the margins of the pulmonary arterial wall. The large echo-free area anterior to the pulmonary artery represents a large pericardial effusion. PE = pericardial effusion; PA = pulmonary artery; AO = aorta; LA = left atrium.

here to the valve leaflets. When there is disruption of the valve, the area of involvement may appear more irregular and may be associated with rapid oscillatory movement of the free edges of the damaged tissue.[10] Figure 10–11 is a parasternal long-axis recording of a pulmonary valve from one such case. In this example, a globular mass of echoes is attached to the posterior pulmonary leaflet, which was noted to move in unison with the leaflet during opening and closure.

THE SUBVALVULAR RIGHT VENTRICULAR OUTFLOW TRACT—THE CONUS ARTERIOSUS OR INFUNDIBULUM

The pulmonary infundibulum extends from the crista supraventricularis to the pulmonary valve. The crista supraventricularis is a thick, rounded, muscular ridge that lies in the angle between the body of the right ventricle and the infundibulum separating the tricuspid and pulmonary valve orifices. The infundibulum is a muscular conduit composed of two primary muscle layers. The superficial layer, which is the more complex, has a superior-inferior orientation and mechanically appears to shorten the proximal outflow tract. The deeper layer is simpler, horizontally oriented, and, on constriction, appears to narrow the outflow tract.[12]

Failure of one or more muscle groups in the infundibular region to develop results in a defect in the interventricular septum in the region separating the right and left ventricular outflow tracts, whereas hyper-

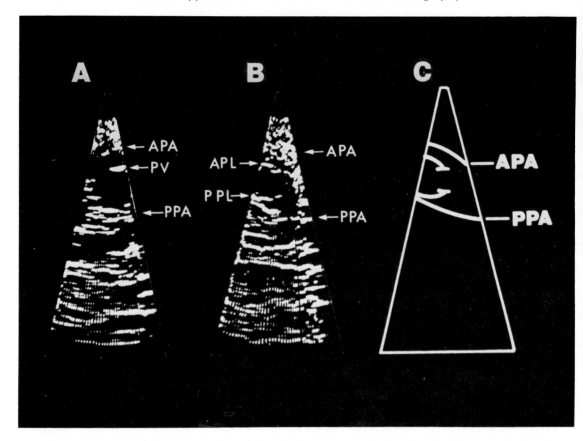

Fig. 10–6. Parasternal long-axis recording of the pulmonary artery and pulmonic valve illustrates valvular pulmonary stenosis. *A,* Recorded during diastole, the single linear echo arising from the coapted pulmonary leaflets is evident in the midportion of the artery. *B,* The domed systolic configuration of the stenotic pulmonary leaflets. *C,* A line drawing corresponding to the domed systolic appearance of the leaflets in *B.* APA = anterior margin of the pulmonary artery; PV = pulmonary valve; PPA = posterior pulmonary artery; APL = anterior pulmonary leaflet; PPL = posterior pulmonary leaflet. (From Weyman, AE, et al.: Cross-sectional echocardiographic visualization of the stenotic pulmonary valve. Circulation, 56:769, 1977. Reproduced by permission of the American Heart Association.)

trophy of these muscles may result in subvalvular obstruction.[12] This hypertrophy has been attributed either to an overgrowth of muscular tissue resulting from injury to the predifferentiated bulbar primordia or to a secondary adaptation to hemodynamic stress. The muscular hypertrophy, when present, may be confined to the area immediately beneath the valve,[13] may be located in the outflow tract farther below the valve and associated with a small subvalvular chamber,[13] or may arise in the right ventricle dividing this cavity into two chambers.[14,15] Subvalvular or infundibular pulmonary stenosis is gener-

ally associated with ventricular septal defect and is uncommon as an isolated anomaly.

INFUNDIBULAR PULMONARY STENOSIS

Infundibular pulmonary stenosis is best visualized in the parasternal long-axis view and is characterized echocardiographically by an increase in echo production from the anterior and posterior margins of the infundibulum with inward bending of the echoes from the vascular walls and narrowing of the lumen. Distal to the area of obstruction, the outflow tract

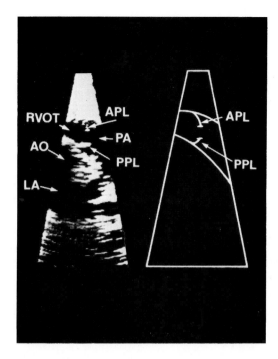

Fig. 10–7. Parasternal long-axis recording from a patient with valvular pulmonary stenosis. Again, the pulmonary leaflet echoes arc inward toward the center of the pulmonary artery, thereby producing a significant narrowing of the vascular lumen. In this example, as in Figure 10–6, both the anterior and posterior pulmonary leaflets are evident. RVOT = right ventricular outflow tract; APL = anterior pulmonary leaflet; AO = aorta; PA = pulmonary artery; PPL = posterior pulmonary leaflet; LA = left atrium. (From Weyman, AE, et al.: Cross-sectional echocardiographic visualization of the stenotic pulmonary valve. Circulation, 56:769, 1977. Reproduced by permission of the American Heart Association.)

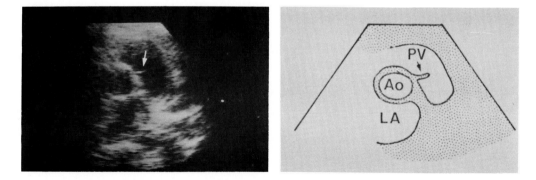

Fig. 10–8. Parasternal long-axis recording of the pulmonary artery and valve illustrates the characteristic appearance of valvular pulmonary stenosis when only one leaflet can be recorded. Although the entire valve is not visible, a diagnosis can be established based on the hook-like systolic configuration of the single leaflet. PV = pulmonary valve; AO = aorta; LA = left atrium.

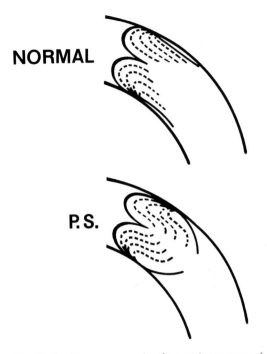

NORMAL

P.S.

Fig. 10–9. Diagram comparing the opening patterns of a normal and a stenotic pulmonary valve. In the normal valve, the leaflets move away from each other while maintaining their relative parallel orientation. In the stenotic valve, the free edges of the pulmonary leaflets angle abruptly away from each other. This motion pattern creates an increasingly more obtuse angle between the leaflet echoes as they open and highlights the presence of valvular stenosis when viewed in real time. (From Weyman, AE, et al.: Cross-sectional echocardiographic visualization of the stenotic pulmonary valve. Circulation, 56:769, 1977. Reproduced by permission of the American Heart Association.)

returns to a more normal diameter resulting in an hourglass type of deformity. Figure 10–12 is an example of isolated infundibular pulmonary stenosis and illustrates the hypertrophy of both the anterior and posterior margins of the outflow tract, which encroach upon and narrow the vascular lumen. Similar changes in outflow tract diameter have been noted in patients with tetralogy of Fallot; however, in this setting, the outflow tract deformity is frequently more extensive.

INFUNDIBULAR OBSTRUCTION IN TETRALOGY OF FALLOT

Right ventricular outflow obstruction is one of the characteristic features of tetral-

ogy of Fallot.[16] The degree of right ventricular outflow obstruction in tetralogy of Fallot is the primary determinant of right-to-left shunting and is, therefore, a major factor in determining the severity of the disorder. Right ventricular outflow obstruction in tetralogy always occurs in the infundibular area with or without coexistent valvular and/or supravalvular pulmonary stenosis.

Cross-sectional echocardiography has proved to be a useful method for recording the entire right ventricular outflow region in tetralogy of Fallot and for detecting the presence and assessing the severity of infundibular obstruction.[17] In studies performed before and after repair, an excellent correlation has been demonstrated (R = 0.93) between the cross-sectional echocardiographic and angiographic assessment of infundibular size during both diastole and systole (Fig. 10–13).In addition, the cross-sectional method proved superior to the M-mode technique in outflow tract visualization (100% versus 70%), pulmonary valve recording (90% versus 26%), and ventricular septal defect demonstration (95% versus 76%).[17] When an outflow tract diameter could be obtained by the M-mode method, this measurement correlated less well with the angiographic data (R = 0.81 versus R = 0.93) and was particularly unreliable in patients whose defects had not been repaired (R = 0.37). It has also been suggested that the noninvasive nature of the cross-sectional method might prove particularly helpful when angiographic dye appears to produce infundibular spasm and thus prevents accurate assessment of baseline outflow tract structure.[17]

THE PULMONARY ARTERY

The main pulmonary artery extends only a short distance from its origin at the pulmonary valve to its bifurcation. Throughout its course, the main pulmonary artery is oriented roughly perpendicular to the

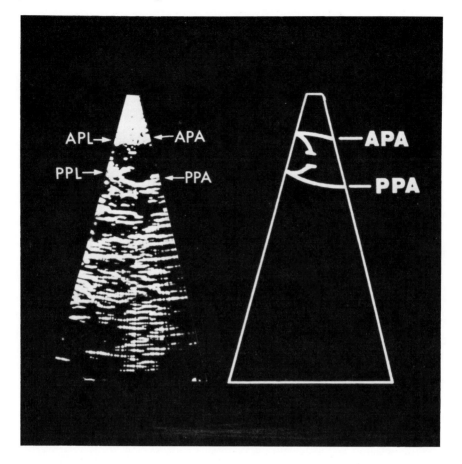

Fig. 10–10. Parasternal long-axis recording of the pulmonary artery and pulmonary valve. The recording was obtained following atrial but prior to ventricular systole. Opening or doming of the pulmonary leaflets in response to atrial contraction is evident. This presystolic opening or doming of the valve corresponds to the enlarged A waves noted in earlier M-mode studies and suggests deranged hemodynamics reflective of a more severe valvular lesion. APL = anterior pulmonary leaflet; PPL = posterior pulmonary leaflet; APA = anterior margin of the pulmonary artery; PPA = posterior pulmonary artery. (From Weyman, AE: Cross-sectional echocardiographic visualization of the stenotic pulmonary valve. Circulation, 56:769, 1977. Reproduced by permission of the American Heart Association.)

anterior chest wall, thereby making clear visualization of the arterial walls difficult. As a result, the pulmonary artery has not been extensively studied echocardiographically, and few abnormalities have been characterized. The pulmonary artery is noted to dilate in a variety of disorders, and focal constriction of the pulmonary artery is observed following surgical banding procedures. In addition, the characteristic bifurcating pattern of the pulmonary artery is particularly valuable in identifying this vessel in patients with one of the transposition complexes.

Pulmonary Artery Dilatation

Dilatation of the pulmonary artery may be observed in disorders that increase flow into the pulmonary vascular bed[18] or produce pulmonary hypertension.[19] In addition, pulmonary artery dilatation may occur as an idiopathic lesion[20–23] due to a developmental defect in pulmonary arterial elastic tissue or as a part of the complex of vascular abnormalities seen in Marfan's syndrome.[24] Post-stenotic dilatation of the pulmonary artery may also be noted in valvular pulmonary stenosis.[18]

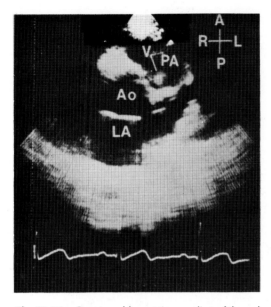

Fig. 10–11. Parasternal long-axis recording of the pulmonary valve illustrates pulmonary vegetations. The vegetations appear as globular masses of echoes attached to the anterior and posterior leaflets. These vegetations move in parallel with the leaflet motion. V = valvular vegetations; PA = pulmonary artery; AO = aorta; LA = left atrium. (From Berger, M, Delfin, LA, Jelveh, M, and Goldberg, E: Two-dimensional echocardiographic findings in right-sided infective endocarditis. Circulation, 61:855, 1980. Reproduced by permission of the American Heart Association.)

Figure 10–14 is an example of a dilated pulmonary artery. In this example, the arterial dilatation resulted from a large left-to-right shunt at the atrial level and was associated with generalized enlargement of the entire right side of the heart. The increase in size of the pulmonary artery can be appreciated by comparison to the aorta.

Pulmonary Artery Bands

Ventricular septal defects with large left-to-right shunts may lead to severe pulmonary hypertension and its associated morbidity and mortality. Experiments of nature, such as tetralogy of Fallot, have demonstrated that narrowing of the pulmonary outflow tract may control the degree of shunting through a ventricular septal defect and may exert a protective effect on the pulmonary vasculature. This prin-

ciple has been utilized surgically by placing a constricting band around the pulmonary artery in patients with large ventricular septal defects in an attempt to decrease shunting and to protect the pulmonary vascular bed.[5,26] Although the use of pulmonary artery banding has recently decreased in favor of complete repair at an early age, many of these bands are still in place and may be evident during the course of a cross-sectional study.

Echocardiographically, pulmonary artery bands appear as a focal narrowing in the proximal pulmonary artery just beyond the pulmonary valve. There may be a fairly extensive area of surrounding scar tissue, which varies the extent of the arterial narrowing produced by the band. Figure 10–15 is a recording of the right ventricular outflow tract and pulmonary artery from a child with a banded pulmonary artery. The band produces a fairly large, hourglass type of narrowing just distal to the level of the pulmonary valve. This narrowing reduces the diameter of the pulmonary artery. Distal to the band, the vessel returns to a more normal size.

GENERALIZED ABNORMALITIES OF THE RIGHT VENTRICULAR OUTFLOW TRACT

In addition to abnormalities involving specific areas of the right ventricular outflow tract, the entire outflow region may be hypoplastic or atretic in lesions, such as pulmonary atresia and pseudo truncus arteriosus (see Chap. 13), or may dilate nonspecifically because of increased flow into the pulmonary artery, such as occurs with atrial septal defect and anomalous pulmonary venous connection or with disorders that increase right ventricular volume. Figure 10–16 is an example of dilated right ventricular outflow tract from a patient with Ebstein's anomaly and right ventricular volume overload. The aortic root in this example is displaced posteriorly and appears small in comparison to the dilated right ventricular outflow tract.

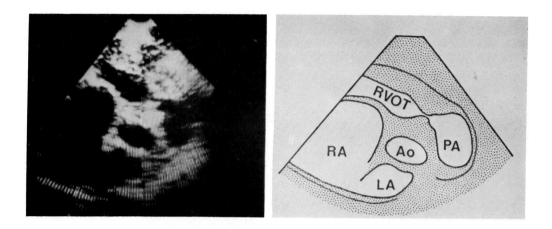

Fig. 10–12. Parasternal long-axis recording of the right ventricular outflow tract (RVOT) illustrates isolated infundibular pulmonary stenosis. Echo production from the anterior and posterior walls of the outflow tract in the infundibular region is increased, and the vascular lumen narrowed. Distal to this hourglass-shaped area of obstruction, the vessel returns to a normal diameter. Right atrial dilatation is also evident. PA = pulmonary artery; AO = aorta; RA = right atrium; LA = left atrium.

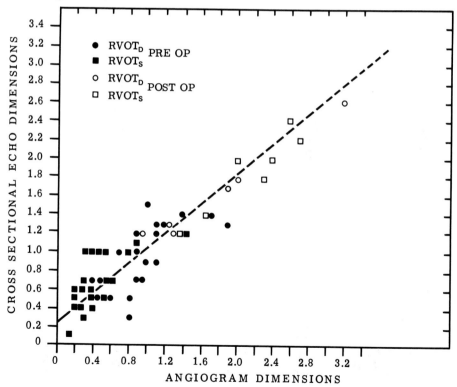

Fig. 10–13. Correlation between the cross-sectional echocardiographic and angiographic measurements of right ventricular outflow tract diameter at end-systole and end-diastole recorded prior to and following operative correction in patients with tetralogy of Fallot. (From Caldwell, RL, et al.: Right ventricular outflow tract assessment by cross-sectional echocardiography in tetralogy of Fallot. Circulation, 59:395, 1979. Reproduced by permission of the American Heart Association.)

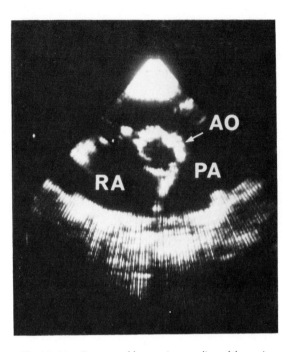

Fig. 10–14. Parasternal long-axis recording of the main pulmonary artery illustrates pulmonary artery dilatation in a patient with an atrial septal defect. PA = pulmonary artery; AO = aorta; RA = right atrium.

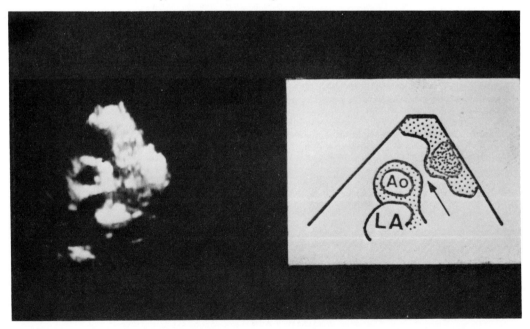

Fig. 10–15. Parasternal long-axis recording of the pulmonary artery illustrates a pulmonary artery band. The band produces an area of arterial narrowing just distal to the pulmonary valve (approximately the 2:30 position relative to the circular aorta [AO]). There is an increase in echo production from the arterial wall in the region of the band. This increase probably reflects local scarring caused by the band. Beyond the banded area, the arterial lumen returns to a more normal diameter. LA = left atrium.

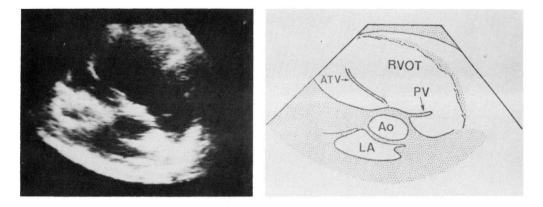

Fig. 10–16. Parasternal long-axis recording of the right ventricular outflow tract (RVOT) illustrates diffuse outflow tract dilatation. This nonspecific pattern may be seen in patients with large left-to-right shunts or with other lesions associated with the right ventricular volume overload pattern. ATV = anterior tricuspid valve leaflet; PV = pulmonary valve AO = aorta; LA = left atrium.

REFERENCES

1. Tajik, AJ, et al.: Two-dimensional real-time ultrasonic imaging of the heart and great vessels. Mayo Clin Proc, 53:271, 1978.
2. Lange, LW, Sahn, DJ, Allen, HD, and Goldberg, SJ: Subxiphoid cross-sectional echocardiography in infants and children with congenital heart disease. Circulation, 59:513, 1979.
3. Weyman, AE, et al.: Cross-sectional echocardiographic visualization of the stenotic pulmonary valve. Circulation, 56:769, 1977.
4. Friedberg, C: Diseases of the Heart. Philadelphia, Saunders, 1966.
5. Hultgren, HN, Reeve, R, Cohn, K, and McLeod, R: The ejection click of valvular pulmonic stenosis. Circulation, 40:631, 1969.
6. Weyman, AE, Dillon, JC, Feigenbaum, H, and Chang, S: Echocardiographic patterns of pulmonary valve motion in valvular pulmonary stenosis. Am J Cardiol, 34:644, 1974.
7. Reeve, R: Variations of the ejection click in valvular pulmonic stenosis. Clin Res, 14:129, 1966.
8. Roberts, WC, and Buckbinder, NA: Right-sided valvular infective endocarditis: a clinicopathologic study of twelve necropsy patients. Am J Med, 53:7, 1972.
9. Bain,RC, Edwards, JE, Scheifley, CH, and Geraci, JE: Right-sided bacterial endocarditis and endarteritis: a clinical and pathological study. Am J Med, 24:98, 1958.
10. Berger, M, Delfin, LA, Jelveh, M, and Goldberg, E: Two-dimensional echocardiographic findings in right-sided infective endocarditis. Circulation, 61:855, 1980.
11. Kramer, NE, Gill, SS, Patel, R, and Towne, WD: Pulmonary valve vegetations detected with echocardiography. Am J Cardiol, 39:1064, 1977.
12. Grant, RP, Downey, FM, and MacMahon, H: The architecture of the right ventricular outflow tract in the normal human heart and in the presence of ventricular septal defects. Circulation, 24:223, 1961.
13. Blount, SG, Vigoda, DS, and Swan, H: Isolated infundibular stenosis. Am Heart J, 57:684, 1959.
14. Lucas, RV, et al.: Anomalous muscle bundle of the right ventricle. Circulation, 25:443, 1962.
15. Gale, GE, Heimann, KW, and Barlow, JB: Double-chambered right ventricle. Br Heart J, 31:291, 1969.
16. Nadas, AS, and Fyler DC: Pediatric Cardiology. 3rd Edition. Philadelphia, Saunders, 1972.
17. Caldwell, RL, et al.: Right ventricular outflow tract assessment by cross-sectional echocardiography in tetralogy of Fallot. Circulation, 59:395, 1979.
18. Elliot, LP, and Scheibler, GL: X-ray Diagnosis of Congenital Cardiac Disease. Springfield, IL, Charles C Thomas, 1968.
19. Wood, P: The Eisenmenger syndrome or pulmonary hypertension with reversed intracardiac shunt. Br Med J, 2:701, 1958.
20. Oppenheimer, BS: Idiopathic dilatation of the pulmonary artery. Trans Assoc Am Physicians, 48:290, 1933.
21. Brenner, O: Pathology of vessels of pulmonary circulation. Arch Intern Med, 56:1189, 1935.
22. Deshmukh, M, Guvenc, S, Bentivoglio, L, and Goldberg, H: Idiopathic dilatation of the pulmonary artery. Circulation, 21:710, 1960.
23. Kaplan, BM, Schlicter, JG, Graham, G, and Miller, G: Idiopathic congenital dilatation of the pulmonary artery. J Lab Clin Med, 41:697, 1953.
24. Papaioannou, AC, Agustsson, MH, and Gasul, BM: Early manifestations of cardiovascular disorders in Marfan's syndrome. Pediatrics, 27:255, 1961.
25. Goldblatt, A, Bernhard, WF, Nadas, AS, and Gross, RE: Pulmonary artery banding—indications and results in infants and children. Circulation, 32:172, 1965.
26. Craig, TV, and Sirak, HO: Pulmonary artery banding. J Thorac Cardiovasc Surg, 45:599, 1963.

Chapter 11

Right Ventricle

The right ventricle is a structurally complex chamber that forms the majority of the anterior surface of the heart and overlies the anteromedial border of the left ventricle.[1,2] When viewed from the side, the right ventricle appears triangular, whereas in cross section, it is normally crescent shaped. Its medial wall is formed by the thick, convex, interventricular septum, whereas laterally, it is bordered by the thinner, concave, free right ventricular wall. In addition to the main right ventricular chamber, the infundibular portion of the right ventricular outflow tract is considered both structurally and functionally as a part of the right ventricle, further complicating its anatomic description.[1-4]

The inner walls of the right ventricle are irregular being lined by numerous small muscle bundles, the trabeculae carneae. In addition to forming multiple ridges along the inner surfaces of the chamber, the trabeculae occasionally cross from one wall to another. A large muscle bundle, the moderator band, is noted in approximately 60% of persons, and stretches from the lower interventricular septum to the anterior right ventricular wall, where it joins the anterior papillary muscle.[1]

Functionally, the right ventricle provides the energy to propel the systemic venous blood returning from the right atrium through the pulmonary vascular bed. Because the resistance in the pulmonary circuit is normally low, the right ventricle is not required to generate high intracavitary pressures. The shape of the right ventricle, with a large surface area relative to the intracavitary volume, is therefore ideally suited to eject large volumes of blood with minimal amounts of myocardial shortening.[4]

The right ventricle has been likened to a fireplace bellows in which the sides are large in comparison to the space between them. A slight movement of the sides toward each other causes displacement of a large volume from within.[4]

The right ventricle normally contracts by three separate mechanisms: (1) contraction of the spiral muscles, which shortens the long axis and draws the tricuspid annulus towards the apex; (2) inward movement of the right ventricular free wall, which produces the bellows effect; and (3) traction on the margins of the free right ventricular wall at their points of attachment to the left ventricle resulting from left ventricular contraction. The inward movement of the right ventricular free wall is the primary mechanism by which blood is ejected. The amplitude of this motion is not great; however, because of the shape of the right ventricle, this motion is sufficient to eject a relatively large volume.

Although the shape of the right ventricle is well suited to eject a large volume of blood with little muscular contraction, it is poorly suited to contract against high pressure. If the normal right ventricle were suddenly required to provide the intraventricular pressure developed by the left ventricle, the right ventricular myocardium would have to develop tension many times as great as that in the left ventricle.[4] As will be demonstrated later, the right ventricle frequently adapts to an acquired pressure load by altering its shape to a more efficient configuration.

The pattern of right ventricular ejection also differs from that of the left ventricle. The velocity of right ventricular ejection increases more gradually, peaks later, and decreases more slowly than that noted on the left side. Ejection also persists longer in the right ventricle. Some of this delay can be attributed to the relatively late contraction of the infundibulum, which prolongs the ejection phase of the right ventricle.

RIGHT VENTRICULAR EXAMINING PLANES AND LINEAR DIMENSIONS

The right ventricle can be recorded in (1) a parasternal long-axis view of the right ventricular inflow tract; (2) a parasternal short-axis view of the right ventricle at the tricuspid valve level; (3) the apical four-chamber view; and (4) the subcostal long-axis view of the right ventricle. In addition, portions of the right ventricle can be visualized in the subcostal long axis of the right ventricular outflow tract, and multiple short-axis cuts of the right ventricle

can be obtained from the subcostal location if necessary.

The apical four-chamber view of the right ventricle has been the most extensively studied and appears to provide the most useful information.[5] In this orientation, the imaging plane transects the right ventricle from the apex to the base, and the Y axis is oriented obliquely across the chamber from the free right ventricular wall laterally to the interventricular septum medially. This plane includes a long axis of the right ventricle from the ventricular apex to the tricuspid annulus and passes through a ventricular short axis. It also permits an area measurement, which is comparable to, but clearly not the same as, an angiographic left anterior oblique view.

It has been suggested, based on comparative measurements of right ventricular casts, that the right ventricular long axis in the four-chamber view should be drawn from the apical tip to the medial insertion of the tricuspid leaflet.[5] Figure 11–1 compares the shape of the normal right ventricle to that seen with right ventricular volume overload and marked right ventricular hypertrophy. In normal persons, the right ventricular long axis can be appropriately drawn along the right-hand margin of the interventricular septum; however, in the latter two instances, this measurement is better taken from the tip of the apex to the plane of the tricuspid annulus through the ventricular cavity. The long axis, therefore, may be best defined as the maximal distance between parallel lines passing through the tricuspid annulus and the right ventricular apex rather than drawn along the margin of the interventricular septum.

Two dimensions have also been defined that are parallel to the short-axis plane of the right ventricle.[5] These dimensions include a mid and maximal right ventricular minor dimension (short axis). The mid right ventricular dimension is measured from the right septal to the free wall endocardial intercepts of a line drawn perpendicular to and bisecting the right ven-

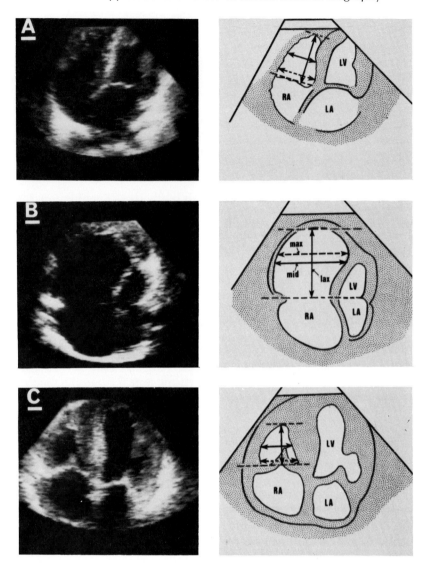

Fig. 11–1. Series of apical four-chamber recordings comparing the size and shape of the normal right ventricle (A), the volume-overloaded right ventricle (B), and the hypertrophied right ventricle (C). The variation in linear dimensions in each of these settings is indicated in the accompanying diagrams. The right ventricular long axis (lax), taken as the distance between parallel lines intersecting the right ventricular apex and tricuspid annulus, increases slightly in right ventricular volume overload (B) and may be reduced in cases of marked right ventricular hypertrophy (C). The two minor dimensions that can be obtained in this view are also indicated in the diagrams. These dimensions include a midventricular short axis (mid), which is perpendicular to and bisects the long axis (solid line), and a maximal short axis (max), which is the longest dimension that can be obtained in a plane that is perpendicular to the long axis (interrupted line). In both the normal and hypertrophied ventricle, the maximal dimension is recorded close to the tricuspid annulus. In contrast, the maximal dimension in the patient with right ventricular volume overload is positioned apical to the midventricular dimension. LV = left ventricle; RA = right atrium; LA = left atrium.

tricular long axis. The maximal dimension (short axis) is defined as the longest distance that can be measured in the four-chamber view between the septal and free wall endocardium in a plane perpendicular to the long axis. Right ventricular linear measurements can be taken at any point in the cardiac cycle. However, when a single measurement is used to express right ventricular size, it is conventionally taken at end-diastole when the ventricle is largest.[5] These dimensions are illustrated in Figure 11–1. Each of these linear dimensions and the planimetered right ventricular area have been shown to relate directly to right ventricular cast volumes. The best correlations, however, have been obtained using the maximal short-axis dimension and the planimetered area.[5]

The other standard views of the right ventricle have, to this point, proved less useful. The parasternal long axis of the right ventricular inflow tract, which is of primary value for recording the tricuspid valve, provides less information about the right ventricle. This plane transects the ventricle obliquely from its anterior to its posterolateral surfaces and, as such, is difficult to standardize. Although theoretically orthogonal to the apical four-chamber view, the apex of the ventricle is rarely recorded in this imaging plane, and hence, a ventricular area and/or reproducible dimensions are not available.

Figure 11–2 is a parasternal long axis of the right ventricle recorded at end-diastole just as the tricuspid leaflets coapt. Although the tricuspid valve is well visualized, the ventricular border is poorly recorded. The apex is not clearly visualized, and the anterior wall is interrupted by the origin of the right ventricular outflow tract. The only landmark available to standardize this view is the tricuspid valve, which is insufficient to fix the plane in space.

The parasternal short axis is likewise limited in its ability to encompass the entire ventricle (Fig. 11–3). This limitation occurs because the free wall of the right ventricle at this level lies beneath the sternum and is difficult to record consistently. When the entire ventricle is visualized, however, the parasternal short axis provides a ventricular area at the base and should permit recording of a more accurate maximal right ventricular short-axis dimension than can the apical four-cham-

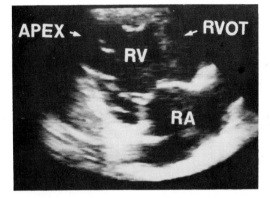

Fig. 11–2. Parasternal long-axis diastolic recording of the right ventricle (RV) and tricuspid valve. Although of primary importance in evaluating tricuspid valve motion and structure, this plane transects the right ventricular cavity obliquely; consequently, any measured right ventricular dimensions are difficult to standardize. In addition, the complete apex is rarely recorded, the anterior wall is poorly visualized, and the continuity of the anterior wall is interrupted by the origin of the right ventricular outflow tract (RVOT). This view, therefore, contains little quantitative information concerning right ventricular size or configuration. The motion of the anterior right ventricular wall and right ventricular apex, however, can be assessed, and gross changes in right ventricular contraction can be appreciated. RA = right atrium.

ber view. This occurs because of the crescent shape of the right ventricle and because the four-chamber plane may not truly pass through the maximal thickness of the crescent. The short-axis view, however, should allow this point to be defined and the measurement to be determined more appropriately. Figure 11–3 illustrates comparable parasternal short-axis recordings in a normal person and in a patient with right ventricular volume overload. In the latter example, the right ventricle is dilated and has rotated above the left ventricle such that the maximal dimension lies in a roughly anteroposterior plane. This difference in orientation can only be appreciated in the short-axis view.

The subcostal long axis of the right ventricle is often equated with, but is actually slightly oblique to the apical four-chamber view. This plane can be compared to the

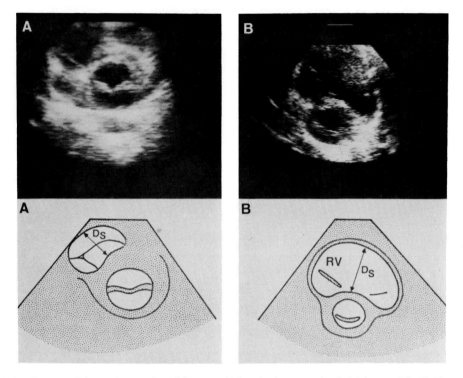

Fig. 11–3. Parasternal short-axis recording of the normal (*A*) and volume-overloaded right ventricle (*B*). The volume-overloaded ventricle (RV) is dilated and rotated clockwise relative to the normal right ventricle. The minor axis (D$_s$) shifts in the same direction, and its true position within the ventricle can be appreciated only in this short-axis view.

parasternal long axis of the left ventricle in that it passes through one of the lateral horns of the crescent rather than through its true center. This plane can be useful in defining right ventricular chamber size in infants but, to date, has played only a minor role in the examination of the adult. Measurements of the right ventricle derived from this plane vary greatly with plane elevation and are difficult to standardize, except with reference to the tricuspid valve.

Finally, the subcostal long axis of the right ventricular outflow tract should be mentioned. This plane transects the right ventricle from the free lateral wall to the pulmonary valve passing through the center of the infundibular region. This plane, therefore, should provide a long axis right ventricular dimension, which bisects the infundibulum and extends from the pulmonary valve to the free right ventricular

lateral wall. A comparable dimension taken from the RAO (right anterior oblique) right ventricular angiogram has been used in angiographic right ventricular volume calculations.[6-8] Although its value is unclear, this dimension is readily available in this view.

RIGHT VENTRICULAR VOLUME DETERMINATIONS

The right ventricle is both technically and conceptually more difficult to study in a quantitative manner than is the left ventricle. This chamber is irregular, trabeculated, and crescent shaped in cross section, thus defying description in terms of a simple geometric model. In addition, any such model would have to allow for the changes in right ventricular shape that occur with volume and pressure loads and for the contributions of the infundibular portion of the ventricle to overall chamber volume. A number of angiographic methods have been developed that, although not directly yielding right ventricular volume, show a good correlation with directly measured volumes and, when appropriately corrected, permit these volumes to be estimated. Despite the good correlations, all these methods have both theoretic and practical limitations, and as a result, there is no universally accepted method for right ventricular volume calculations.

Little information is currently available concerning the echocardiographic calculation of right ventricular volumes. Therefore, a discussion of the methods and models used to determine these volumes in other imaging formats, such as angiography, and their relationship to the available echocardiographic data would be useful because these methods and models will undoubtedly form the basis of future echocardiographic studies. The methods that have been employed to determine right ventricular volumes include (1) the Simpson's rule method; (2) the representation of the right ventricle by a simple geometric figure[7-10] or by a combination of figures;[9] and (3) the subtracting of the volume of the left ventricle and interventricular septum from the total cardiac volume to derive indirectly the right ventricular volume.[12] Because direct determination of right ventricular volume is feasible, this latter indirect method of estimation appears unnecessary[11] and is, therefore, not discussed further.

In the Simpson's rule method, the right ventricular chamber is divided into a series of slices of equal thickness. To obtain these slices, the chamber must first be imaged in two orthogonal projections, and the slices must be conventionally made perpendicular to a long axis that is common to both projections. Each slice is then assigned a geometric form, and the volume of the individual slices is calculated from the formula for the volume of that geometric figure.

Figure 11–4 illustrates how the volume of a large figure can be derived from the sum of the volumes of its components. In the original studies of the right ventricle, the slices were considered to be elliptic cylinders, and the formula for the volume of each was therefore:

$$V = \pi \left(\frac{D_1}{2}\right) \left(\frac{D_2}{2}\right) H \qquad (1)$$

The height of the elliptic cylinder, H, can be determined by dividing the measured long axis into a number of segments of even length or by arbitrarily defining the figure such that each segment has a predetermined length and the number of segments depends on the length of the long axis. D_1 and D_2 are then the distances between the contralateral borders of the image along lines drawn perpendicular to, and at specified intervals along, the long axis in each of the orthogonal imaging planes. When using the ellipsoid-cylinder formula, therefore, a total volume of the RV would equal:

$$V = \frac{\pi}{4} H \sum_{0}^{n} D_1 D_2 \qquad (2)$$

This method has consistently overestimated right ventricular volumes determined by cast studies by as much as 40%.[11] The overestimation has been related to the failure of the method to allow for the volume displaced by the trabeculae, papillary muscles, and the convex interventricular septum. The error, however, appears to be consistent, and with appropriate correlation using derived regression equations, the correlation between estimated and measured volumes has been good.

Other studies using this method have described the individual slices of the right ventricle as ellipsoids with the following formula;

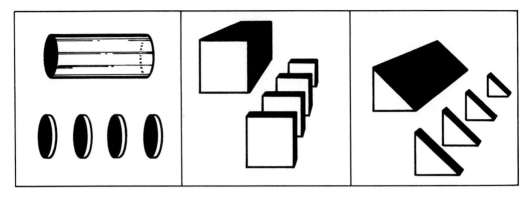

Fig. 11–4. Diagram illustrates the Simpson's rule method of volume calculation, in which the volume of a larger figure is determined from the sum of the volumes of a series of comparable smaller figures. (From Rogers, EW, Feigenbaum, H, and Weyman, AE: Echocardiography for quantitation of cardiac chambers. *In* Progress in Cardiology. Edited by PN Yu, and JF Goodwin. Philadelphia, Lea & Febiger, 1979.)

$$V = \frac{\pi}{3} H \sum_{o}^{n} D_1 D_2 \qquad (3)$$

or as rectangles, where

$$V = H \sum_{o}^{n} L\, W \qquad (4)$$

As might be expected, each of these methods overestimates actual volume but, again, shows excellent correlation coefficients.

From an echocardiographic standpoint, the right ventricular long axis can readily be defined from the apical four-chamber view. In addition, one area is available in this view. A second orthogonal plane with a common long axis, however, is difficult to record. The parasternal long axis would be a potential orthogonal imaging plane; however, visualization of the apex is rarely possible in this view, and the area recorded is difficult to standardize. The subcostal long axis is not orthogonal, but is rather almost parallel. The parasternal short-axis view is orthogonal, but the common axis with the apical four-chamber view is a short axis. These theoretic problems might be overcome by taking multiple short axes at sequential levels of the right ventricle, as is done with the left ventricle; however, the appropriate internal

references are lacking in the right-sided chamber.

The complexity of the Simpson's rule method has led to the evaluation of a series of simpler geometric figures as possible models from which right ventricular volumes might be calculated. These figures include the prolate ellipse,[9,10] the parallelepiped,[10] the prism,[7] and the pyramid with a triangular base.[8] The ellipse has been examined as a basis for right ventricular volume calculations in several angiographic studies.[9,10] Volumes are calculated using the formula:

$$V = \frac{4}{3}\pi \left(\frac{D_1}{2}\right) \times \left(\frac{D_2}{2}\right) \times \left(\frac{L}{2}\right) \qquad (5)$$

where

$$D \text{ is } \frac{4A}{\pi\, L\, \max}$$

and L max equals the longer of the two major axes. The areas in these examples were derived from the frontal and lateral radiographic projections of right ventricular casts. This method again overestimated measured right ventricular volume; however, in each instance, an excellent correlation with measured volumes was obtained, and reasonably accurate estimates of calculated volume were possible after appropriate correction.

In an attempt to allow for the two-chamber configuration of the right ventricle, a modification of this method has also been examined in which the right ventricular inflow chamber is expressed as an ellipse and the outflow chamber is considered separately as a cylinder.[9] The total right ventricular volume then is the sum of the volume of the outflow chamber (V_O) and the inflow chamber (V_I), where

$$V_o = (\pi r^2_o L) \qquad (6)$$

and

$$V_I = \frac{4}{3} \pi r^2 \frac{LL}{2} \qquad (7)$$

This method uses only the lateral angiogram and divides the right ventricle at the level of the superior aspect of the tricuspid valve into inflow and outflow segments. This approach again yielded a good correlation with measured volumes; however, it was associated with a greater percent error than was the simple area-length method.[9] The additional calculations, therefore, did not appear warranted.

Because the right ventricle is obviously not a true ellipse, three other figures have been examined as possible geometric models because they appear to correspond more closely to the actual right ventricular shape. These figures are illustrated in Figure 11–5. The first is the parallelepiped or three-dimensional parallelogram. The volume of this figure is simply expressed by:

$$V = \text{length} \times \text{width} \times \text{height} \qquad (8)$$

When derived from angiographic images, imaginary rectangles are constructed with surface areas identical to those of the ventricular images recorded in the frontal and lateral planes and with lengths equal to a superior-inferior dimension in the lateral plane. The area of the right ventricle can then be equated with length times width in the frontal plane, whereas the height

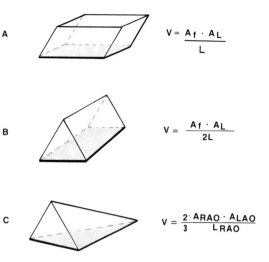

Fig. 11–5. Diagram illustrates the simple geometric figures that have been used to represent the right ventricle and the formulas for their volumes. *A*, The three-dimensional parallelogram or the parallelepiped. *B*, The prism. *C*, The pyramid with a triangular base. V = volume; A_f = angiographic area in the frontal projection; A_L = angiographic area in the lateral projection; L = length; A_{RAO} = angiographic area in the right anterior oblique projection; A_{LAO} = angiographic area in the left anterior oblique projection. (From Rogers, EW, Feigenbaum, H, and Weyman, AE: Echocardiography for quantitation of cardiac chambers. *In* Progress in Cardiology. Edited by PN Yu, and JF Goodwin. Philadelphia, Lea & Febiger, 1979.)

can be determined by dividing the area in the lateral projection by the maximal length. The angiographic volume, therefore, is expressed by:

$$V = \frac{(\text{Area}_{\text{Frontal}}) \times (\text{Area}_{\text{Lateral}})}{LL} \qquad (9)$$

This method has been used in both in vitro comparisons to right ventricular casts[10] and in pediatric studies with good correlations consistently observed.[13]

The next figure whose shape has been compared with that of the right ventricle is the prism with a triangular base. The volume of such a prism is expressed as:

$$V = \text{Area}_{\text{Triangle}} \times \text{Height}$$

$$\text{or} \quad \frac{L\ (\text{Base}) \times W\ (\text{Base})}{2} \times H \qquad (10)$$

By assuming that the frontal and lateral angiographic projections form the sides of the triangular prism, the volume can then be calculated from:

$$V = \frac{Area_{Frontal} \times Area_{Lateral}}{2L} \qquad (11)$$

This method, as with the previous figures, correlates well with cast-determined volumes, but in this instance, the model slightly underestimated the actual measured volume.[7]

The final figure is the pyramid with the triangular base. In this model, the triangular base is assumed to be formed by the base of the right ventricle (including the right ventricular outflow tract), whereas the long axis or height of the pyramid is the long axis of the right ventricle from the base to the apex. The volume of such a figure is expressed by:

$$V = Area_{Base} \times \frac{H}{3} \qquad (12)$$

The base of the pyramid cannot be directly visualized angiographically; however, this value can be calculated from the RAO and LAO projections of the right ventricle using the formula:

$$V = \frac{2}{3} \text{ area RAO} \times \text{area LAO}$$

$$\div \text{ length (RAO)} \qquad (13)$$

The validity of this method has also been confirmed in vitro and applied to patients with coronary artery disease. This method has also been adapted to single-plane ventriculograms and, therefore, represents the first method for right ventricular volume calculations that does not require biplane images.[14] By assuming that the area of the LAO projection approximates two thirds of the area in the RAO projection, the formula can be simplified to:

$$V = 0.4 \frac{(\text{area RAO}^2)}{L \text{ RAO}} + 3.9 \qquad (14)$$

These single-plane volumes have been shown to correlate well with biplane volumes.

This lengthy discussion of right ventricular volume calculations using shadowing methods may appear inappropriate in an echocardiographic text. The evolution of left ventricular echocardiographic volume data, however, has extensively used angiographic models and concepts. Consequently, the echocardiographic methods for determining right ventricular volumes will probably follow this same path. This discussion, therefore, should outline the options available.

The only cross-sectional echocardiographic study reported to date has used angiographic models and concepts.[15] In this report, right ventricular stroke volume was calculated from systolic and diastolic right ventricular volumes using the formula for a pyramid with a triangular base:

$$V = \text{area} \times \frac{H}{3}$$

Echocardiographically, the area of the base can be directly measured in cross section, whereas the length is available in the apical four-chamber view. The right ventricular stroke volume in this study unfortunately did not correlate well with the left ventricular stroke volume, which, in the absence of intracardiac shunts, can be assumed to approximate the right ventricular measurement. The reader can assume, however, that this or other models will eventually yield reliable volume data that can be used to serially assess the performance of the right ventricle.

None of these methods allows for the change in right ventricular shape that occurs during volume loading. The Simpson's rule method should be more appropriate in the dilated ventricle, where the individual slices more truly approximate

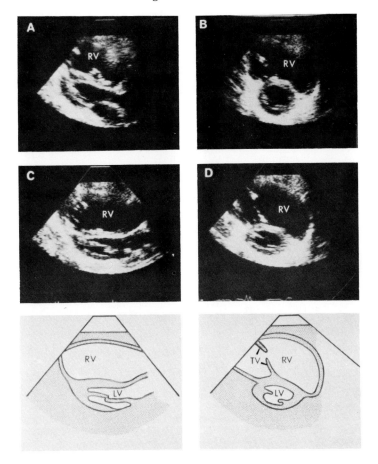

Fig. 11–6. Parasternal long- and short-axis recordings of the right ventricle (RV) illustrate right ventricular volume overload. In the long-axis projection, the ventricle is expanded in both the anteroposterior and the apex-to-base dimensions. The right ventricle occupies the cardiac apex, and the left ventricle (LV) and the interventricular septum are displaced posteriorly. In the short-axis view, the right ventricle is enlarged and rotated in a clockwise direction above the left ventricle. During diastole (C and D), the interventricular septum is displaced posteriorly, and the left ventricle is flattened in its short-axis configuration. During systole (A and B), the septum shifts anteriorly or paradoxically, and the ventricle becomes more circular. The diagrams at the bottom of the figure correspond to the diastolic frames, C and D.

an elliptic cylinder or an ellipse. In the normal right ventricle, however, this method fails to account for the invagination of the septum, which cannot be appreciated by using the shadow techniques. The other figures do not allow for changes in ventricular shape, and their correlation with right ventricular volume, therefore, would be expected to change depending on the size of the ventricle.

RIGHT VENTRICULAR VOLUME OVERLOAD

Volume overload of the right ventricle may be seen with a variety of conditions, including atrial septal defect,[7,9] partial or total anomalous pulmonary venous connection, tricuspid regurgitation, and pulmonary insufficiency. Less common causes include ventricular septal defect with left ventricle to right atrial shunting and sinus of Valsalva aneurysm rupture into the right atrium. Note that ventricular septal defect without a ventriculoatrial communication is not typically a cause of right ventricular volume overload.[7]

Right ventricular volume overload can alter both the size and the shape of the right ventricle. Figure 11–6 is an example

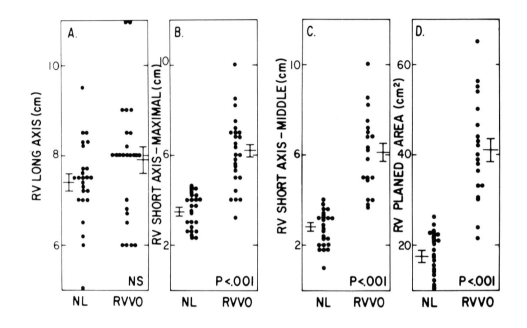

Fig. 11–7. Comparison of the means and averages for right ventricular long axis, maximal short axis, midventricular minor dimension, and planimetered right ventricular area in normals (NL) with patients with right ventricular volume overload (RVVO). (From Bommer, W, et al.: Determination of right atrial and ventricular size by two-dimensional echocardiography. Circulation, 60:91, 1979. Reproduced by permission of the American Heart Association.)

of a massively dilated right ventricle recorded in both parasternal long- and short-axis projections during diastole and systole. In the long axis, the dilated ventricle expands in both an anteroposterior and superior-inferior direction. The right ventricular apex is distal to the left ventricular apex, and the right ventricular cavity is much larger than the left. In short axis, the right ventricle is no longer crescent shaped but appears more oval. During diastole, the interventricular septum is displaced toward the left ventricular cavity, further smoothing the posterior surface of the ventricle. With systolic contraction, however, the increase in left ventricular systolic pressure pushes the septum in toward the

right ventricle and makes the left ventricle more circular.[16] It has been demonstrated in the apical four-chamber view, that the right ventricular mid and maximal short-axis dimensions and the planed right ventricular area are greater in patients with right ventricular volume overload than in normal patients (Fig. 11–7).[5] It has been further suggested that the right ventricular long axis does not increase significantly in right ventricular volume overload.[5] However, as illustrated in Figures 11–6 and 11–1,B, some increase in the long axis does occur in more severe cases. However, the percent increase in the right ventricular long axis does not approach the percent increase in the short-axis dimensions.

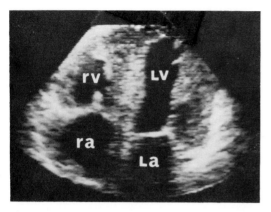

Fig. 11–8. Apical four-chamber recording illustrates diffuse cardiac infiltration and right ventricular hypertrophy in a patient with hereditary amyloidosis. RV = right ventricle; RA = right atrium; LV = left ventricle; LA = left atrium.

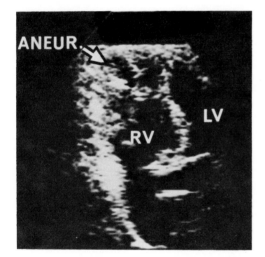

Fig. 11–9. Apical four-chamber recording illustrates aneurysmal dilatation of the right ventricular apex in a patient with a large anteroapical left ventricular myocardial infarct and clinical evidence of associated right ventricular infarction. During the real-time study, the right ventricular apex and anterior wall were dyskinetic. ANEUR. = aneurysm; RV = right ventricle; LV = left ventricle.

RIGHT VENTRICULAR HYPERTROPHY

The right ventricle may hypertrophy in a variety of conditions that increase the resistance against which the ventricle must pump. Such conditions include valvular pulmonary stenosis, infundibular pulmonary stenosis, tetralogy of Fallot, and long-standing pulmonary hypertension. Right ventricular hypertrophy is generally assessed by determining the thickness of the right ventricular free wall. Although the interventricular septum may also hypertrophy with right ventricular pressure overloads, the septum is primarily a functional component of the left ventricle, and septal hypertrophy is therefore more commonly associated with disorders of the left ventricle. In addition, the septum may hypertrophy independently in such conditions as IHSS, thereby making its value minimal as a predictor of right ventricular wall thickness.

Although the right ventricular free wall may be viewed in many projections, it probably is best recorded from the parasternal transducer location with the beam directed toward the left ventricle. This orientation places the endocardial and epicardial interfaces perpendicular to the beam axis and in the near field of the transducer and should provide the best resolution. Because the right ventricle lies immediately beneath the anterior chest wall, precise near-gain adjustment is necessary to separate this structure from the highly reflective chest wall. An alternative view is the subcostal long axis, in which a wide extent of the posterior right ventricular free wall is available for examination. This view may be particularly useful in infants and children with congenital heart disease because this region of the heart is more accessible. The normal right ventricular wall thickness is 5 mm. Wall thickness greater than 5 mm is indicative of right ventricular hypertrophy. In addition to right ventricular pressure loads, an increase in right ventricular wall thickness may also be noted in cardiac amyloidosis.[17] In a series of 6 patients with clinically significant infiltrative amyloid, the mean right ventricular wall thickness was 7.5 mm with a range of 5 to 10 mm.[17] Fig-

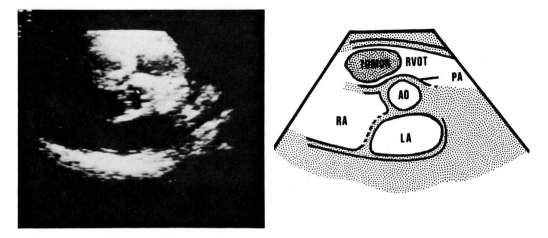

Fig. 11–10. Parasternal short-axis recording of the right ventricle illustrates a large tumor mass above the anterior tricuspid leaflet and extending into the right ventricular outflow tract (RVOT). PA = pulmonary artery; AO = aorta; LA = left atrium; RA = right atrium.

ure 11–8 is a recording from a patient with hereditary amyloidosis and diffuse infiltration of the myocardium and the cardiac valvular tissue. There is an increase in both right and left ventricular wall thickness as well as thickening of the atrial walls and interatrial septum.

RIGHT VENTRICULAR INVOLVEMENT IN ISCHEMIC HEART DISEASE

Right Ventricular Infarcts

Isolated right ventricular infarction is rare; however, ischemic dysfunction of a part of the right ventricular free wall in association with left ventricular infarction is not uncommon.[18–20] Right ventricular infarction is suggested clinically by hypotension and neck vein distention with little or no pulmonary congestion in patients with inferior-posterior infarcts.

Echocardiographically, right ventricular infarction is characterized by enlargement of the right ventricle and by an increase in the right ventricle/left ventricle end-diastolic dimension ratio (greater than .05).[21,22] In one study, segmental wall motion abnormalities were noted in five patients with right ventricular infarction. These abnormalities included hypokine-

sis of the right ventricular free wall,[3] akinesis of the free wall with paradoxic apical motion,[1] and anterolateral aneurysm.[1] Figure 11–9 is an apical four-chamber recording that illustrates aneurysmal dilatation of both the right and left ventricular apices in a patient with a large anterior wall infarction.

Right Ventricular Tumors

Right ventricular tumors are uncommon, and the echocardiographic experience with these lesions is therefore limited. The most commonly observed right ventricular tumor appears to be the myxoma.[23–25] Right ventricular involvement with rhabdomyoma of the interventricular septum[26] and malignant melanoma[23] also have been reported. Right ventricular tumors appear to originate primarily from the interventricular septum[23,24] and may expand to involve the tricuspid valve, restricting its motion;[23] prolapse into the right ventricular outflow tract, causing outflow obstruction;[24] or produce mechanical right ventricular failure as a result of cavity obliteration.[23] The wide spectrum of clinical presentations of these tumors and their relative rarity make their clinical detection difficult. Echocardiographic evaluation of the right side of the heart in patients with suspected right ventricular tumors is therefore particularly important.

When a right ventricular tumor is present, the ventricle is characteristically enlarged,[23,24] and paradoxic septal motion may be recorded.[23] The tumor itself appears as a large cluster or mass of echoes within the ventricular cavity and/or in the outflow tract above the anterior tricuspid leaflet. The tricuspid orifice is typically uninvolved unless the tumor extends through the tricuspid valve from below.

These tumors are frequently mobile and move toward or into the outflow tract during systole. Figure 11–10 is an example of a large intracavitary right ventricular tumor positioned in the outflow tract above the anterior tricuspid leaflet. The borders of the tumor are well demarcated, and little movement of the mass was noted.

REFERENCES

1. Grant, JCB, and Basmajian, JV: Grant's Method of Anatomy. Baltimore, Williams & Wilkins, 1968.
2. Gray, H: Gray's Anatomy. 29th Ed. Edited by CM Goss. Philadelphia, Lea & Febiger, 1973.
3. Hurst, JW: The Heart. New York, McGraw-Hill, 1974.
4. Rushmer, RF: Cardiovascular Dynamics. Philadelphia, Saunders, 1970.
5. Bommer, W, et al.: Determination of right atrial and ventricular size by two-dimensional echocardiography. Circulation, 60:91, 1979.
6. Gentzler, RD, Briselli, MF, and Gault, JH: Angiographic estimation of right ventricular volume in man. Circulation, 50:324, 1974.
7. Fisher, EQ, DuBrow, IW, and Hastreiter, AR: Right ventricular volume in congenital heart disease. Am J Cardiol, 36:67, 1975.
8. Ferlinz, J, Gorlin, R, Cohn, PF, and Herman, MV: Right ventricular performance in patients with coronary artery disease. Circulation, 52:608, 1975.
9. Graham, TP, Jarmakami, JW, Atwood, GF, and Canent, RV: Right ventricular volume determinations in children. Circulation, 47:144, 1973.
10. Arcilla, RA, Tsai, P, Thilenius, OG, and Ranniger, K: Angiographic method for volume estimation of right and left ventricles. Chest, 60:446, 1971.
11. Goerke, RJ, and Carlsson, E: Calculation of right and left ventricular volumes. Invest Radiol, 2:360, 1967.
12. Reedy, T, and Chapman, CB: Measurement of right ventricular volume by cineangiofluorography. Am Heart J, 69:221, 1963.
13. Thilenius, OG, and Arcilla, RA: Angiographic right and left ventricular volume determination in normal infants and children. Pediatr Res, 8:67, 1974.
14. Ferlinz, J: Measurement of right ventricular volumes in man from single plane cineangiograms. Am Heart J, 94:87, 1977.
15. Chaudry, KR, et al.: Biplane measurements of left and right ventricular volumes using wide-angle cross-sectional echocardiography. Am J Cardiol, 41:391, 1978.
16. Weyman, AE, Wann, LS, Feigenbaum, H, and Dillon, JC: Mechanism of abnormal septal motion in patients with right ventricular volume overload. Circulation, 54:179, 1976.
17. Child, JS, Krivokapich, J, and Abbasi, AS: Increased right ventricular wall thickness on echocardiography in amyloid infiltrative cardiomyopathy. Am J Cardiol, 44:1391, 1979.
18. Workma, WB, and Hellerstein, HK: The incidence of heart disease in 2000 autopsies. Ann Int Med, 28:51, 1948.
19. Wade, WP: The pathogenesis of infarction of the right ventricle. Br Heart J, 21:545, 1959.
20. Laurie, W, and Woods, JD: Infarction in the right ventricle of the heart. Acta Cardiol, 18:399, 1963.
21. Sharpe, DN, et al.: The non-invasive diagnosis of right ventricular infarction. Circulation, 57:483, 1978.
22. D'Arcy, BJ, et al.: Real-time two-dimensional echocardiography in right ventricular infarction. Am J Cardiol, 45:436, 1980.
23. Ports, TA, Schiller, NB, and Strunk, BL: Echocardiography of right ventricular tumors. Circulation, 56:439, 1977.
24. Roelandt, J, et al.: Ultrasonic demonstration of right ventricular myxoma. J Clin Ultrasound, 5:191, 1977.
25. DeMaria, AN, et al.: Unusual echographic manifestations of right and left heart myxomas. Am J Med, 59:713, 1975.
26. Farooki, ZQ, Henry, JG, Arciniegas, E, and Green, E: Ultrasonic pattern of ventricular rhabdomyoma in two infants. Am J Cardiol, 34:842, 1974.

Chapter 12

Interatrial and Interventricular Septa

The interatrial and ventricular septa partition the fetal atrioventricular canal and thereby provide the framework for the separation of the pulmonary and systemic circulations in the fully developed heart.[1,2] In addition, these membranes form a significant portion of the muscular walls of the atria and ventricles and contribute to their contractile function. Normally, the septa appear to favor, both geometrically and functionally, the left-sided cardiac chambers, which bear the major work load of the heart. A variety of disorders, however, alter the configuration, motion, and structural integrity of the septa. These abnormalities form the basis of this chapter.

Before discussing the septa individually, it is important to note that each of these membranes is situated between dynamic chambers in which intracavitary pressures and volumes are continuously changing.[3] The observed shape and movement of the respective septa, therefore, are dependent on the relative magnitude and timing of events acting on their opposite surfaces.[4,5] In addition, loss of structural integrity of a part of one septum may affect the shape and movement of the other,[6]

whereas more complex lesions may involve both.[7] For these reasons, although the shape, motion, and integrity of both the interatrial and interventricular septa are considered separately, all of these factors are of necessity interrelated.

THE INTERATRIAL SEPTUM

Anatomy

Anatomically, the interatrial septum is a thin, muscular membrane that separates the right and left atrial chambers.[1,2] It stretches from the posteromedial margin of the aortic root posteriorly and slightly rightward to the common posterior atrial wall and from the midportion of the superior atrial border to its junction with the upper margin of the interventricular septum. An oval depression in the midportion of the septum, the fossa ovalis, corresponds to the position of the foramen ovale in the fetal heart.[1,2]

Development

Embryologically, the interatrial septum develops in several stages (Fig. 12–1). Ini-

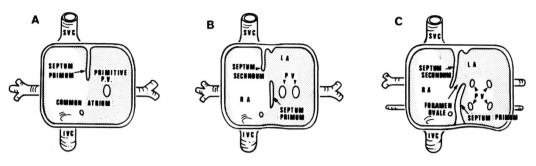

Fig. 12–1.   Diagram illustrates the development of the interatrial septum. *A,* The primitive septum primum initially grows downward from the superior border of the common atrium. *B,* Prior to reaching the floor of the atrium, the septum primum separates from its original point of attachment to the atrial roof. A second membrane, the septum secundum, then grows downward from the superior border of the atrium to the right of the septum primum. *C,* In the fetal heart, the free edge of the septum secundum overlaps the superior border of the septum primum, thereby forming a flap valve, the foramen ovale, which permits blood flow from the right to the left atrium.

tially, an anteroposterior partition, the septum primum, grows downward from the superior border of the primitive common atrial chamber and divides the chamber into right and left halves (Fig. 12–1, A).[1] Before its lower end reaches the anterior and posterior endocardial cushions, which have already fused and divide the common primitive atrioventricular canal into the mitral and tricuspid orifices, its connection with the superior margin of the atrium is severed (Fig. 12–1, B). Consequently, the superior border of the septum primum is free. A second partition, the septum secundum, then grows downward from the atrial roof to the right of the septum primum until their edges overlap.[1,2] These overlapping membranes form a flap valve between the two atria (Fig. 12–1, C). Prior to birth, right atrial pressure exceeds left atrial pressure, thereby holding this valve open and permitting blood flow from right to left. After birth, with the establishment of the normal pulmonary circulation, the pressure gradient between the right and left atria is reversed, closing the flap valve. When closed, the free edge of the septum secundum becomes the crescentic upper margin of the foramen ovale. In about 75% of individuals, the opposed surfaces of the two septa fuse.[1] In the remaining 25%, the opposed surfaces fail to fuse; as a result, the foramen is patent anatomically but closed physiologically. In these situations, should right atrial hypertension develop, the flap valve will reopen and physiologic right-to-left shunting will occur.

Examining Planes

The interatrial septum can be visualized using four principal echocardiographic views. These views include (1) a parasternal short axis at the aortic level (Fig. 12–2, A);[8,9] (2) the apical four-chamber view (Fig. 12–2, B);[10,11] (3) a subcostal long axis optimized to the interatrial septum (Fig. 12–2, C);[12,13] and (4) a right parasternal long-axis of the interatrial septum (Fig. 12–2, D).[4,5]

In the parasternal short-axis view, the imaging plane transects the interatrial septum from its anterior insertion into the aortic root to its posterior junction with the common atrial wall. The Y axis of the imaging plane is perpendicular to the superior-inferior or long axis of the septum.

Figure 12–2, A, illustrates the appearance of the interatrial septum in this orientation. The septum normally arises from the posterior aortic wall at approximately the 7 o'clock position. It then courses vertically (posteriorly) and slightly rightward through a gradual arc curving away from the left atrium. It usually joins the posterior atrial wall at a point almost directly beneath the medial margin of the aorta.

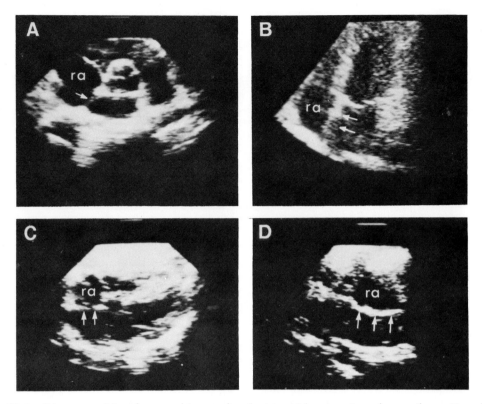

Fig. 12–2. Primary examining planes used in recording the interatrial septum. In each case, the position of the interatrial septum is indicated by the arrows. *A,* The parasternal short-axis view at the aortic valve level. *B,* The apical four-chamber view. *C,* The subcostal long-axis view optimized to the interatrial septum. *D,* The right parasternal long axis of the interatrial septum. ra = right atrium.

Success in recording the atrial septum in this plane has varied from 83[8] to 90%.[9] Because the path of the ultrasonic beam is normally parallel to the plane of the septum, echo "dropout" in the midportion of the septum occurs frequently, and was noted in 50% of normal patients in one study.[9]

This problem can be partially alleviated by shifting the transducer leftward on the chest and angling the imaging plane back toward the septum. This change in transducer position frequently shifts the orientation of the scan plane sufficiently to permit complete septal recording. This view is primarily important for recording the relative anteroposterior and medial-lateral orientation of the septum and for defining the changes in septal orientation that occur in the presence of right and left

atrial volume overloads. Septal defects can also be recorded; however, the high incidence of false-positives makes other views preferable for that purpose.

The apical four-chamber view is probably the most useful plane for imaging the interatrial septum in the adult. In this orientation, the imaging plane transects the septum from its inferior junction with the interventricular septum to its superior border. Figure 12–2, *B,* illustrates the configuration of the septum in this view. Normally, the atrial septum is not a straight line extension of the interventricular septum, but is displaced slightly toward the left atrium.[11] This view is ideal for determining the relative sizes of the atria and also for permitting visualization of septal defects.[10,11,14] Unfortunately, the path of the imaging plane in the four-chamber view is also parallel to the interatrial septum and makes complete recording difficult.[11,12] In addition, when this plane is angled posteriorly, echo dropout is commonly noted in the region of the fossa ovalis.[11] Anterior plane angulation more frequently results in complete septal visualization without thinning or dropout; however, this plane orientation bypasses the location of the typical ostium secundum defect. Thus, both false-positive and false-negative atrial septal defects can be produced using this view, and septal echo dropout as an isolated finding must be interpreted with caution.

The subcostal long axis is theoretically the ideal view for recording the interatrial septum.[12,13] In this orientation, the septum is perpendicular to the path of the scan plane and can be visualized throughout its superior-inferior extent (see Fig. 12–2, C). With this view, the interatrial septum was adequately displayed in one study in 87 of 88 infants with a variety of congenital disorders,[13] whereas in a second study, satisfactory imaging was obtained in each of 118 consecutive infants and children.[12] In adults, this plane is more difficult to utilize because of the distance of the interatrial septum from the transducer face. When the septum can be recorded from this transducer location, it should be considered the optimal plane for evaluating its structural integrity.

An additional plane has recently been described and has proved useful for evaluating interatrial septal motion.[4,5] This plane, which is termed here the *right* parasternal long axis of the interatrial septum (see Fig. 12–2, D), is recorded with the transducer located to the right of the sternum in the third, fourth, or fifth intercostal spaces. The Y axis of the imaging plane then appears to be aligned parallel to the superior-inferior axis of the interatrial septum, and the plane is then angled sharply to the left until it passes through the septum from right to left atria. This orientation should result in the imaging plane transecting the anterior third of the septum along a line running from the interventricular septum to the superior atrial border.

Spatial Orientation of the Interatrial Septum

The normal spatial orientation and shape of the interatrial septum can be altered by changes in the relative volumes and pressures within the right and left atria. Changes in both septal orientation and shape can be appreciated and have been described in each of the standard septal imaging planes.[4,5,8,13] Figure 12–3, A through D, compares the normal short-axis configuration of the interatrial septum with that seen in left and right atrial volume overloads and right atrial hypertension. Normally, the septum bows slightly toward the right atrium (Fig. 12–3, A). As the left atrial volume increases, the anteroposterior length of the septum also increases, and it bows more prominently toward the right atrium (Fig. 12–3, B).

As a rule, when the left atrial dilatation is chronic (i.e., in mitral stenosis), the percent change in atrial volume from diastole to systole is small, and there is prominent septal bowing toward the right atrium during both diastole and systole. When the left atrial volume overload is acute (i.e., with chordal rupture), the cyclic change in left atrial volume may be great with the septum bowing toward the right atrium at end-systole but returning to a more normal, flat or even slightly convex orientation relative to the left atrium at end-diastole.[5]

When there is a right atrial volume overload, the structures at the base of the heart rotate in a clockwise direction and the interatrial septum becomes more horizontally positioned and tends to bow inward toward the left atrium (Fig. 12–3, C). This convexity is present at end-diastole and increases during systolic right atrial filling, thereby resulting in paradoxic mo-

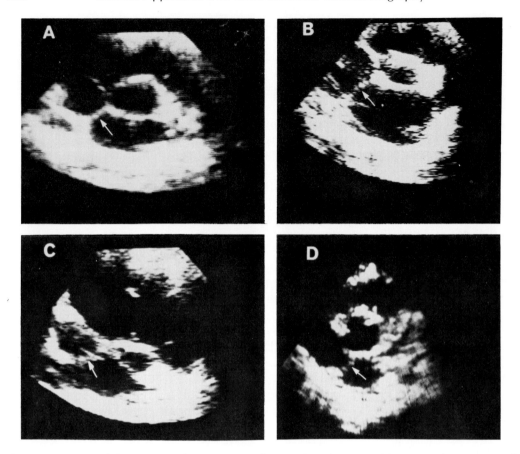

Fig. 12–3. Parasternal short-axis recordings comparing the normal configuration of the interatrial septum (*A*) with that in left atrial volume overload states (*B*), right ventricular volume overload (*C*), and right atrial hypertension (*D*). The interatrial septum in each instance is indicated by the oblique arrow.

tion of the interatrial septum. Right atrial hypertension reverses the normal curvature of the septum, displacing it toward the left atrium without significantly increasing its length (Fig. 12–3, *D*).

Interatrial Septal Motion

The interatrial septum is a relatively thin membrane that separates two dynamic chambers. Motion of the septum, therefore, would be expected to reflect the relative pressures to which it is exposed during various phases of the cardiac cycle.[3,5] When viewed in short axis, the normal curvature of the septum causes the structure to appear confluent with the other borders of the left atrium and, hence, to

form a part of this chamber. This septal orientation may reflect the fact that left atrial pressure normally exceeds that in the right atrium and, therefore, represents the major influence on septal configuration.[3] Detailed studies of atrial septal movement, however, suggest a more complex relationship. These studies have been conducted primarily from the *right parasternal transducer* location. As a result, the imaging plane transects the septum at approximately the 10:30 o'clock position relative to the short axis of the left atrium.[4,5] The motion recorded in this view, therefore, is comparable to that along a vector oriented roughly midway between the anteroposterior (D_1) and medial-lateral (D_3) axes of the left atrium. Because the largest component of motion in this plane normally is due to the anteroposterior expansion of the atrium, this component should predominate.

Figure 12–4 illustrates the imaging plane orientation used to record septal motion in the right parasternal view as well as the normal septal motion pattern. These M-mode recordings are taken from the midpoint of the septum, where maximal movement has been observed. Septal events are identified at eight points la-

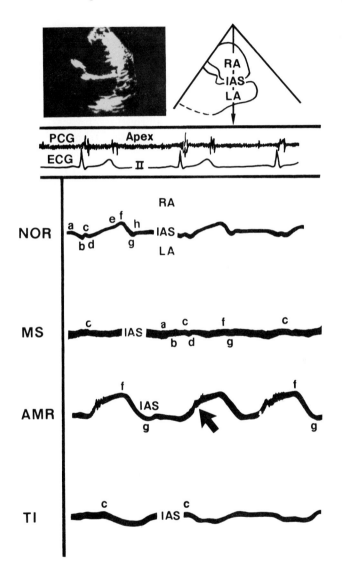

Fig. 12–4. (Upper panel) Cross-sectional scan of the interatrial septum (IAS) recorded from the right parasternal transducer location. As indicated in the accompanying diagram, the imaging plane transects the septum from right atrium (RA) to left (LA). The Y axis is aligned parallel to the long axis of the septum. (Lower panels) Serial redrawn M-mode recordings depict the "M-mode" pattern of the septal motion sampled from the midseptum (area indicated by the vertical arrow in the upper right-hand diagram). NOR = normal; MS = mitral stenosis; AMR = acute mitral regurgitation; TI = tricuspid insufficiency. The arrowhead in the example of acute mitral regurgitation points to an area of early, systolic, high-frequency, septal fluttering produced by the turbulent jet of blood (from the regurgitant lesion) that strikes the septum. (Redrawn from Tei, C: Echocardiographic analysis of interatrial septal motion. Am J Cardiol, 44:472, 1979.)

beled a through h. These points can be related to specific points in the cardiac cycle. The initial downward movement toward the left atrium (a) has been attributed to right atrial contraction, which normally precedes left atrial contraction and thus may reverse or decrease the left-to-right pressure gradient.[5] This downward movement is followed by a series of small movements (b,c,d) that have been related to the pressure fluctuations that result from the dissociation between left and right atrial and ventricular contraction and ejection.[5] The septum then moves anteriorly toward the right atrium as the left atrium fills (d,e). At the end of atrial filling, rightward movement increases slightly (e,f). The increase has been explained by the fact that the tricuspid valve opens before the mitral valve, thus increasing the left-to-right gradient and shifting the septum further toward the right atrium.[5] During rapid left ventricular filling, the septum moves inward toward the left atrium (f,g), and little movement occurs during mid-diastole. These characteristic movements are diminished with chronic left atrial volume overload (MS); exaggerated with acute left atrial volume overload (AMR); and may show a reversal in direction with right atrial volume overload (TI). These patterns are summarized in Figure 12–4. Although there appears to be a great deal of information in the analysis of septal motion, the role of this type of measurement in the clinical setting remains to be defined.

Atrial Septal Defects

Uncomplicated atrial septal defect is one of the more common forms of congenital heart disease, representing from 7 to 15% of all cases in children. It is the most common congenital lesion (excluding the bicuspid aortic valve) encountered after the age of 20.[15]

Atrial septal defects are classified on the basis of their position in the septum and their embryologic origin.[15–17] The most common is the ostium secundum type, which represents roughly 70% of all defects in the atrial septum.[16] Ostium secundum defects are located in the region of the fossa ovalis and result from incomplete development of the septum secundum.

Ostium primum defects are less common (approximately 20%) and are positioned in the lower portion of the septum in continuity with the atrioventricular valves. Ostium primum defects result from incomplete fusion of the septum primum with the endocardial cushions and are considered a partial form of the common atrioventricular canal.

Defects positioned high in the interatrial septum in close proximity to the entrance of the superior vena cava are termed sinus venosus defects. These defects constitute 6 to 8% of all defects in the atrial septum and are frequently associated with anomalous drainage of the pulmonary veins.[16]

Two other less common types of atrial septal defects have been described anatomically but have not been reported echocardiographically. These include defects positioned posteriorly in close proximity to the entrance of the inferior vena cava and, even more rare, defects at the site of origin of the coronary sinus, which are usually associated with a persistent left superior vena cava that connects to the left atrium.[17]

Echocardiographically, atrial septal defects are usually suspected on the basis of the nonspecific changes they produce in right ventricular and right atrial size and in interventricular septal motion (the right ventricular volume overload pattern).[18–21] Their presence can then be confirmed either by direct echocardiographic visualization of the defect[7–9,12,13,22,23] or by abnormalities in the pattern of echocardiographic contrast flow through the atria that result from the defect.[24–26]

The right ventricular volume overload pattern occurs in atrial septal defect because of the characteristic tendency for shunt flow to occur from left to right.[27–31] Left-to-right shunting predominates because the major determinants of the degree and direction of shunting are (1) the size of the defect and (2) the relative compliances of the ventricles. Because the thin-walled right ventricle is normally more compliant than the thicker left ventricle, predominant shunting is toward the right and imposes an increased volume load on the right atrium and ventricle. Increased right ventricular diastolic volume also displaces the interventricular septum posteriorly toward the left ventricle. During systole, the increased left ventricular pressure shifts the interventricular septum anteriorly or paradoxically as a result of the reestablishment of a more normal ventricular shape[6] and/or the anterior displacement of the centroid of the left ventricle.[32]

Right ventricular dilatation is almost invariably noted in patients with an uncomplicated atrial septal defect.[18–21] Likewise, paradoxic ventricular septal motion has been reported in M-mode studies in the majority of patients with atrial septal defect.[18–21] It also has been noted to develop experimentally with shunts measuring as small as 500 ml and to resolve following cessation of the abnormal flow pattern.[33] In cross-sectional studies, the reported incidence of abnormal septal motion, however, has varied from 38[34] to 100%.[6,35] The relatively low incidence reported in the former study may be due to the fact that septal movement was examined at the papillary muscle level (where this abnormality is less evident). The right ventricular volume overload pattern is illustrated in Chapter 11, Figure 11–6; paradoxic interventricular septal motion is illustrated and discussed later in this chapter.

Direct visualization of atrial septal defects can be achieved in each standard view of the interatrial septum. Defects appear as discontinuities or areas of focal dropout in the normal linear band of echoes arising from the interatrial septum.[8–13] In ostium secundum defects, this area of dropout is located in the midportion of the septum (Fig. 12–5), whereas with ostium primum defects, the dropout is located in the lower atrial septum just superior to the crest of the interventricular septum and insertions of the atrioventricular valves (Fig. 12–6). Studies to date suggest that areas of focal echo dropout can be observed almost uniformly in patients with atrial septal defect, providing that the septum itself is recorded.[8,9,11–13] Although false-negatives can theoretically occur when the cross-sectional plane transects the interatrial septum at a level above or below the defect, they have not presented a problem provided that the full extent of the septum is examined. False-positives, however, are a major problem and are particularly common in the short-axis and apical views in which the scan plane is oriented parallel to the path of the septum. Although the reported incidence of false-positives has ranged from 27% for the apical view to 50% for the short-axis view,[9] an apparent false-positive can be produced in almost every patient at some time during the study.

One sign that helps to differentiate true defects from false-positives is the characteristic echo broadening that is frequently noted at the margins of a true defect. Echo broadening is caused by the more highly reflective blood-tissue interface at the defect margin and is illustrated in Figure 12–7. Because of the high incidence of false-positive defects noted in the apical and short-axis views, the subcostal imaging plane, which places the interatrial septum perpendicular to the path of the scan plane, has been stressed as the view of choice for recording the interatrial septum. Using this transducer location, the sensitivity and specificity of the technique have improved markedly,[12,13] and in infants, differentiation of patent foramen ovale from true ostium secundum atrial septal defect has also been possible in the majority of cases.[13]

When direct anatomic visualization of a

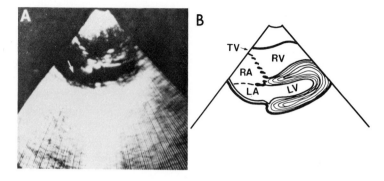

Fig. 12–5. Subcostal long-axis recording of an ostium secundum atrial septal defect. *A,* The position of the defect is indicated by the vertical arrow. *B,* The expected position of the septum is indicated by the interrupted horizontal line. A small segment of septum primum extending superiorly from the atrioventricular ring to the margin of the defect is apparent. TV = tricuspid valve; RV = right ventricle; RA = right atrium; LA = left atrium; LV = left ventricle.

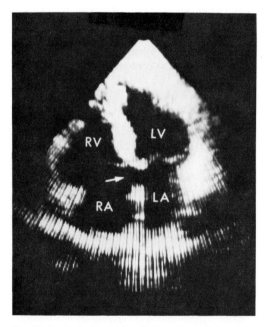

Fig. 12–6. Apical four-chamber recording illustrates an ostium primum atrial septal defect. The defect extends from the plane of the atrioventricular ring superiorly to the lower border of the septum secundum and is indicated by the horizontal arrow. RV = right ventricle; LV = left ventricle; RA = right atrium; LA = left atrium.

defect cannot be achieved or when the question of a false-positive remains, echocardiographic contrast can be utilized to confirm the diagnosis.[24–26] The contrast technique involves the injection of such substances as saline or indocyanine green (Cardio-Green) dye, which contain mul-

tiple microbubbles, into a peripheral arm vein and following the path of contrast flow through the right side of the heart. Normally, contrast passes through the right atrium into the right ventricle and then out into the pulmonary arterial system. The microbubbles are totally filtered out at the pulmonary capillary level, and no contrast should flow into the left side of the heart. In normal persons, the contrast completely fills the right atrium and outlines the borders of the interatrial septum. This sharply defined contrast margin can be used to confirm the presence of the dividing membrane and to rule out a false-positive defect even when the interatrial septum itself is not visualized (Fig. 12–8). When an atrial septal defect is present with right-to-left shunting, contrast can be seen immediately flowing into the left atrium, thereby confirming the presence and location of the defect and the direction of the shunt.[24,26] Even in patients with predominant left-to-right shunts, mixing at the atrial level frequently results in the recording of microbubbles in the left atrium, thus providing defect confirmation. When right-to-left shunting is not present, however, observation of the displacement of the contrast-containing blood from the right atrial side of the septal defect by non-contrast-containing blood flowing through the defect from left to right (the negative

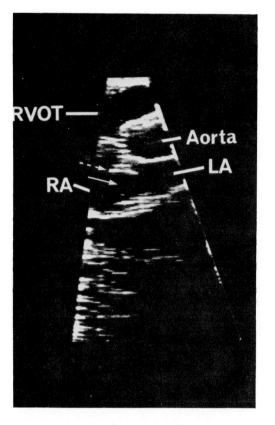

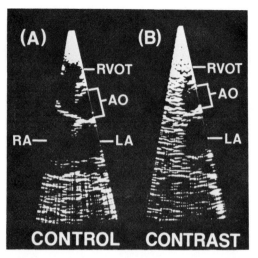

Fig. 12–8. Parasternal short-axis recordings of the interatrial septum prior to (A) and following (B) peripheral contrast injection. A, The septum is incompletely recorded, suggesting an atrial septal defect. B, Following contrast injection, the right atrium is completely opacified, and its medial boundary is clearly demarcated. This pattern confirms the integrity of the interatrial septum, although this membrane itself is never recorded. RVOT = right ventricular outflow tract; AO = aorta; LA = left atrium; RA = right atrium.

Fig. 12–7. Parasternal short-axis recording illustrates an ostium secundum atrial septal defect (horizontal arrow). The anterior margin of the defect is artifactually broadened, thereby giving the appearance of an inverted "T." The broadened defect margin is indicated by the interrupted arrow. RVOT = right ventricular outflow tract; LA = left atrium; RA = right atrium.

contrast effect) can be utilized to confirm the presence of the defect.[25] The use of echocardiographic contrast is discussed in more detail in Chapter 13.

Patent Foramen Ovale

The foramen ovale is an opening in the midportion of the fetal atrial septum at the junction of the septum primum and septum secundum. This foramen is normally covered by a thin flap of septum primum. Prior to birth, it is kept open by flow from the right to left atrium. After birth, the establishment of the normal pulmonary circulation increases the left atrial pressure and presses the flap of septum primum against the foramen ovale closing the opening. This flap may then fuse with the septum secundum to close the orifice permanently or may remain separate such that the orifice can reopen if the left-to-right pressure gradient should reverse.

Several studies in infants have demonstrated that the foramen ovale and covering flap of septum primum can be visualized from a subcostal transducer location.[12,13] Movement of this flap has also been observed in response to cyclic cardiac and respiratory motion.[12,13] In the majority of infants with right-sided volume overload, the septal flap has been observed to bulge into the left atrium while the remainder of the atrial septum remains flat.[13] This configuration is usually associated with a right-to-left shunt. A small associated defect may be seen at the superior aspect of the formen ovale and has been attributed to separation of the superior rim of the septum primum from the septum secundum.[13]

In infants with left ventricular volume and pressure overloads, the entire atrial septum and the thinner, septum primum-covered foramen ovale bow into the right atrium.[13] Frequently, a small area of echo dropout is noted at the superior margin of the foramen ovale and has been associated with incompetence of the flap.

Effects of Balloon Atrial Septostomy and Surgical Septectomy on the Interatrial Septum

Enlargement of the foramen ovale is frequently necessary in infants with transposition of the great vessels to permit increased mixing of blood at the atrial level. This enlargement is usually achieved by balloon atrial septostomy (tearing a larger hole in the septum by pulling an inflated balloon through the foramen ovale) or, when this is unsuccessful, by surgical septectomy. The septostomy defect is located in the midportion of the septum, and the rhythmic movement of blood through the defect can be observed to impart corresponding motion to the torn margins of the septum primum.[13] Successful septostomies have been reported to produce defects that occupy more than 30% of the total septal length, whereas smaller defects (less than 30%) are frequently associated with persistent desaturation and require early surgical intervention.[36] The surgical septectomy defect is larger and includes both the original defect and the surgically created defect in the posterior septum. Figure 12–9 summarizes the principal atrial septal defect locations and associated patterns of septum primum movement relative to the foramen ovale in each of these disorders.

Atrial Septal Aneurysms

Infants with either right ventricular inflow or outflow obstruction often require

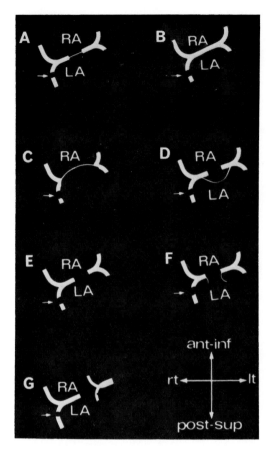

Fig. 12–9. Diagram summarizes the position and appearance of the atrial septum, recorded from the subcostal transducer location, in a variety of common disorders. RA = right atrium; LA = left atrium. A, Normal, undeviated interatrial septum shows thinning in the region of the foramen ovale. The horizontal arrow indicates the position of insertion of the right pulmonary vein. B, Normal septal position with septal thickening in the region of the septum primum. C, Deviation of the interatrial septum toward the right atrium with left atrial volume overload. This configuration is analogous to the short-axis recording illustrated in Figure 12–3, B. D, Right ventricular volume overload with opening of the flap valve of septum primum covering the foramen ovale. E, Ostium secundum atrial septal defect illustrates the absence of septal echoes in the region of the foramen ovale. F, Flail remnants of septum primum at the margins of an atrial septal defect created by balloon atrial septostomy. G, Ostium primum atrial septal defect located in the inferior portion of the septum and bounded inferiorly by the atrioventricular valves. (From Bierman, FZ, and Williams, RG: Subxiphoid two-dimensional imaging of the interatrial septum in infants and neonates with congenital heart disease. Circulation, 60:80, 1979. Reproduced by permission of the American Heart Association.)

patency of the interatrial septum, either in the form of an atrial septal defect or a patent foramen ovale, to survive. When there is restricted right-to-left shunting, aneurysmal dilatation of the interatrial septum may develop, and the thinned septum may bulge prominently into the left atrium.[37,38] These septal aneurysms may grow to a point where they partially obstruct the mitral orifice. Figure 12–10 is an example of such an aneurysm in a patient with tricuspid atresia.

With left atrial hypertension, similar aneurysmal dilatation of the septum may occur with bulging into the right atrium. Figure 12–11 is an example of a larger atrial septal aneurysm that partially fills the right atrium. In this example, contrast has been injected into the opposite atrial chamber to highlight the presence of the lesion.

Atrial Septal Thickness

An abnormal increase in the thickness of the interatrial septum has been noted in three settings. In adults, an abnormally thick septum may be seen in amyloidosis in association with increased thickening of the other walls of the heart and cardiac valves. Figure 12–12 is a subcostal long-axis view of the interatrial septum from a patient with hereditary amyloidosis and demonstrates this generalized increase in cardiac and interatrial septal thickness.

In infants, apparent thickening of the interatrial septum due to loss of the normal central thinning characteristic of the foramen ovale has been reported in two cases and, in both, was associated with torrential pulmonary blood flow and left ventricular volume overload.[13]

The most common cause of an apparently thickened atrial septum, however, is a surgical patch covering a repaired atrial septal defect. These patches appear thicker and more highly reflective than the normal septum and do not show the same elastic motion that is characteristic of the normal septum. Figure 12–13 illustrates the increase in reflectivity and width of a surgical patch covering a defect in the atrial septum.

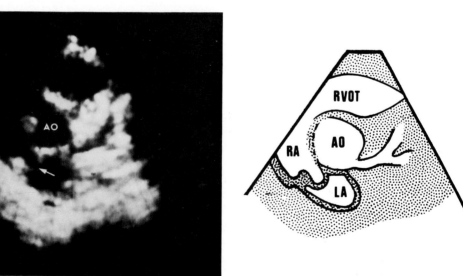

Fig. 12–10. Parasternal short-axis recording of the interatrial septum demonstrates a septal aneurysm in a patient with tricuspid atresia. The aneurysm (arrow) is produced by the chronically elevated right atrial pressure, which distends the interatrial septum and causes it to bulge into the left atrium (LA). RVOT = right ventricular outflow tract; RA = right atrium; AO = aorta.

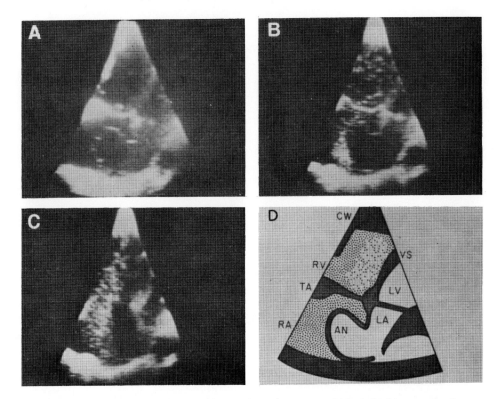

Fig. 12–11. Apical four-chamber recording of an atrial septal aneurysm (AN). *A,* In this example, the aneurysm bulges into the right atrium (RA). *B* and *C,* Contrast has been injected peripherally and fills the right atrium, outlining the aneurysm. *D,* Diagram illustrates the relationship of the aneurysm to surrounding structures. CW = chest wall; VS = ventricular septum; RV = right ventricle; LV = left ventricle; TA = tricuspid annulus; LA = left atrium. (From Nanda, NC: Contrast echocardiography. *In* Progress in Cardiology. Edited by PN Yu, and JF Goodwin. Philadelphia, Lea & Febiger, 1979.)

THE INTERVENTRICULAR SEPTUM

Anatomy

The interventricular septum is a thick, triangular, muscular wall that separates the left and right ventricles.[1] Normally, this septum is both an anatomic and a functional component of the left ventricle and comprises roughly one third of the muscle mass of that chamber.[1] Its radius of curvature is similar to that of the free wall of the left ventricle; consequently, it is concave toward the left ventricle and convex toward the right. The majority of the septum is muscular with the exception of a small membranous segment located at its superior border just beneath the right and noncoronary cusps of the aortic valve.

Development

Embryologically, the interventricular septum develops from three different sources.[39] The major component, the muscular septum, originates as a median partition along the floor of the common ventricle. This partition grows superiorly as the ventricles enlarge. It has the form of a crescentic plate with two horns that join the respective dorsal and ventral endocardial cushions. For a short time, the primitive interventricular septum is an incomplete partition that only partially divides the common ventricle. The remaining communication between the ventricles, situated above the superior margin of the muscular septum, is called the interventricular foramen. This foramen is bounded

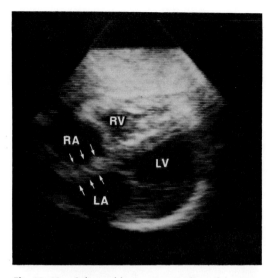

Fig. 12–12. Subcostal long-axis recording of the inter-atrial septum in hereditary amyloidosis. An increase in atrial septal thickness is associated with generalized hypertrophy of the cardiac valves and the ventricular myocardium. The thickened interatrial septum is indicated by the arrowheads. RA = right atrium; RV = right ventricle; LV = left ventricle.

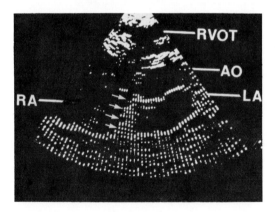

Fig. 12–13. Parasternal short-axis recording of the interatrial septum illustrates a septal patch. The patch (arrowheads) is thicker and more highly reflective than the normal septum. The movement of the patch is restricted, and the normal diastolic decrease in anteroposterior septal length is diminished. RVOT = right ventricular outflow tract; AO = aorta; LA = left atrium; RA = right atrium.

(1) inferiorly by the interventricular septum; (2) anterosuperiorly by the proximal bulbar septum, which continues downward from the longitudinally dividing bulbus; and (3) posterosuperiorly by the fused middle portion of the endocardial cush-

ions. Final closure of the interventricular foramen is the result of tissue proliferation from each of these sources, but especially from the endocardial cushions. The resulting thin membrane that completes this partition is the membranous septum.[39]

Examining Planes

The interventricular septum is primarily recorded in (1) the parasternal long-axis view of the left ventricle; (2) a parasternal short axis, which can be swept from the cardiac apex to the basal insertion of the septum into the atrioventricular groove; (3) the apical four-chamber view; and (4) the subcostal long-axis views (Fig. 12–14, A through D). Portions of the septum can also be recorded in the apical long-axis view, and serial short-axis scans can be obtained from the subcostal transducer location. The long and short axes of both interventricular and interatrial septa are defined relative to those of the surrounding chambers.

The parasternal long-axis view transects the interventricular septum between the 11 and 12 o'clock positions (relative to the left ventricular short axis) along a line from its junction with the anterior aortic root to a point just proximal to its apical termination. This plane is ideally suited for (1) evaluating septal motion in an anteroposterior direction; (2) relating septal motion to aortic root motion, which is normally in the opposite direction; and (3) defining the hinge point at which these oppositely directed movements intersect.[40] This plane also permits the junction of the interventricular septum and anterior aortic root to be recorded and larger defects in the membranous or bulbar septum to be visualized (particularly those associated with aortic over-riding). Finally, this view is useful for defining diffuse and/or focal abnormalities of interventricular septal thickness.

The parasternal short-axis view displays the anteroposterior arc of the septum and,

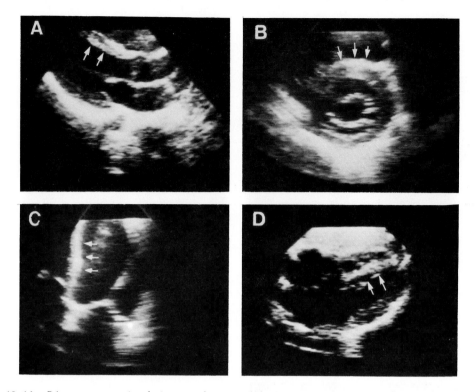

Fig. 12–14. Primary cross-sectional views used to record the interventricular septum. *A,* Parasternal long-axis view. *B,* Parasternal short-axis view. *C,* Apical four-chamber view. *D,* Subcostal long-axis view. The position of the interventricular septum in each frame is indicated by the arrowheads.

as such, is the primary plane for recording changes in septal position and configuration as well as for detecting relative changes in left and right ventricular shape. Parasternal short-axis recordings can be taken at any level from the base of the left ventricle to the apical extreme of the septum; however, changes in ventricular shape are most obvious at the base. This view is useful for visualizing the apically positioned interventricular septal aneurysms and septal defects associated with acute myocardial infarction and for recording the membranous aneurysms associated with congenital defect closure. The circumferential extent of septal involvement in ischemic heart disease is also best defined using this plane.

In the four-chamber view, the interventricular septum is visualized from the cardiac apex to its insertion into the interatrial septum at the base of the right and left ventricles. This plane is ideal for recording septal defects in the region of the atrioventricular canal as well as for recording the larger defects in the muscular septum. Muscular defects that are located toward the apex of the ventricle and associated with acute myocardial infarction can, on occasion, also be recorded in this plane. The four-chamber view is also useful for defining the superior-inferior extent of dyssynergy in the midseptal plane.

The subcostal long-axis view of the interventricular septum is ideal for visualizing defects in the muscular portion of this membrane. In this view, the imaging plane is perpendicular to the path of the interventricular septum, and hence, defects should be clearly visualized. Because of the difficulty in locating small defects in the muscular septum, rotating the plane 90 degrees and sweeping the interventricular septum from apex to base may be necessary. This combination of subcostal planes should provide the most detailed evaluation of the interventricular septum and should offer the greatest sensitivity for detection of muscular defects.

Interventricular Septal Thickness, Thickening, and Scar

The normal thickness of the interventricular septum (mean, 9 mm; range, 7 to 12 mm) is approximately the same as that of the left ventricular free wall[41] (mean, 10 mm; range, 7 to 12 mm) and roughly 3 times that of the right ventricle.[1] The thickness of the septum is conventionally measured during mid-diastole between the rapid phase of diastolic relaxation and atrial contraction.[41] During systolic contraction, septal thickness normally increases. The peak systolic thickness of the septum can be compared to the diastolic measurement, and a percent thickening or thinning can be determined. The thickening characteristics of the septum can then be related to local myocardial performance.[41–43]

The diastolic thickness of the septum may increase with the rest of the left ventricle in response to chronic pressure loads, such as systolic hypertension or left ventricular outflow obstruction. Septal thickness may also increase in some of the infiltrative myopathies, including amyloidosis and hemochromatosis.

An increase in septal thickness disproportionate to that of the remainder of the left ventricle may also be noted. This increase is most frequently described in patients with idiopathic hypertrophic subaortic stenosis and has been considered the anatomic basis for that disorder.[44–46] The septum may also hypertrophy disproportionately to the left ventricular free wall in association with right ventricular hypertrophy[46] and a number of other nonspecific disorders. As a result, its diagnostic value as an isolated finding is limited.[46] Most of the specific causes of septal

hypertrophy are discussed in detail elsewhere (see Chap. 7) and, therefore, are only mentioned in this section.

An abnormally thin septum is less common and, when noted, suggests septal scar formation following myocardial infarction.[47] The criteria for septal scar include (1) a mid-diastolic septal thickness of less than 7 mm; (2) an increase in echo production from the thinned septal area in comparison either to surrounding, more normal areas of septum or to the opposite ventricular wall; and (3) myocardium in the scarred area that is 30% thinner than adjacent areas. Using these criteria, scar was detected echocardiographically in 52 of 182 patients with coronary artery disease and was confirmed either pathologically or surgically in 95% of patients.[47]

Surprisingly, in the absence of frank scar formation, the diastolic thickness of the septum remains within the normal range in most patients with both acute and chronic coronary artery disease and in congestive cardiomyopathy.[41,47]

In addition to baseline measurements of septal thickness, the thickening characteristics of the septum may provide useful information concerning regional left ventricular function. Left ventricular thickening may be determined at specific points along the ventricular wall or along serial radii drawn around the ventricular circumference.[48] Thickening measurements are particularly useful because they are generally independent of motion and are less critically dependent on the centroid placement in radial systems.

M-mode studies have shown that normal septal thickening averages 36% (range 14 to 57%). Septal thickening has been reported to increase slightly in some patients with atrial septal defect[41] and was likewise noted to increase in 20% of patients with inferior wall infarcts.[41]

Septal thinning apparently occurs only with acute ischemia and has been reported in 30% of patients with acute infarcts.[41] Experimentally, systolic thinning is noted more frequently. In one study, systolic thinning was observed in 30 of 37 animals following acute coronary occlusion; reduced thickening was present in the remaining 7 animals.[42] This difference in clinical and experimental data probably represents the more precise sampling from the center of the ischemic region that can be achieved in the experimental setting. Figure 12–15 compares the normal pattern of septal motion and thickening to the decreased thickness and thickening seen in acute ischemic disease.

Decreased systolic thickening without actual thinning is frequently noted in patients with coronary artery disease and a history of prior myocardial infarction. It is also seen in patients with congestive cardiomyopathy. Abnormal thickening, however, is less common in patients *without* prior infarct histories despite the angiographic presence of coronary artery disease.[41]

A decrease in percent septal thickening has also been reported in idiopathic hypertrophic subaortic stenosis.[49,50] In view of the marked increase in baseline septal thickness, however, these abnormal changes may be less reflective of septal function.

Interventricular Septal Motion

The unique position of the interventricular septum between the right and left ventricles causes both septal orientation and movement to be dependent on the relative forces acting on its opposite surfaces. Normally, the interventricular septum is oriented and contracts such that it forms an integral part of the left ventricle, and its function in this context is discussed in Chapter 8. On occasion, however, the relative dynamics of the right and left ventricles may alter the movement and/or configuration of the septum such that it

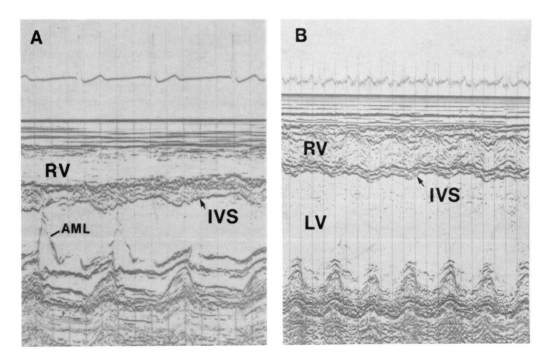

Fig. 12–15. M-mode recordings compare the normal pattern of interventricular septal motion, thickness, and thickening (A) to the decreased thickness, thickening, and excursion noted in a patient with acute anterior wall infarction (B). IVS = interventricular septum; RV = right ventricle; LV = left ventricle.

functions either in part or totally independent of the left ventricle or, at the extreme, as part of the right ventricle. Any analysis of septal movement may be further complicated by the fact that the septum may be primarily influenced by one chamber or set of forces during one portion of the cardiac cycle and by a completely different dynamic milieu at another. It is not surprising, therefore, that a number of different patterns of abnormal septal motion have been observed and that a number of clinical settings have been noted in which abnormal motion can occur.[51]

To recognize and understand the factors that underlie the various abnormal patterns of septal motion, one must first become familiar with the general mechanisms by which septal movement occurs. The septum can move (1) in response to the contraction and relaxation of the septal musculature; (2) as a result of motion of the left ventricle in space; and (3) in response to factors that change the position of the septum relative to the two ventricles and, therefore, change the shape of the ventricles themselves.

Before considering septal motion further, two additional points must be noted. First, this motion is considered relative to a fixed external reference (i.e., the anterior chest wall or transducer face). As discussed in Chapter 8, analysis of endocardial motion relative to the centroid of the left ventricle would be preferable; however, this type of motion analysis is not currently practical in most laboratories, and the principles discussed in this section should apply irrespective of the reference used.

Secondly, motion does not always imply function. Thus, infarcted or scarred muscle may be pulled in a normal direction by surrounding normally contracting areas,[47] whereas normally contracting muscle may appear to move abnormally through one of the mechanisms discussed later.[6,52] As described in the preceding section, however, normal muscle thickens when it contracts, and its function can be inferred from its thickening characteristics. Once its functional status is determined, the reasons for a particular pattern of movement can then usually be elucidated.

Normal Septal Motion

Normal motion of the interventricular septum can best be appreciated in the short-axis view of the left ventricle at the mitral valve level. In this view, the left ventricle appears circular, and the septum forms an arc representing approximately two fifths of its circumference. Normal systolic contraction of the septal musculature displaces this arc inward toward its center of curvature, thereby contributing to the overall decrease in left ventricular circumference and cavity area. This direction of contraction is mandated by the concave orientation of the septum relative to the ventricular cavity because, if any muscle or series of muscles is fixed at both ends and positioned in an arc, muscular contraction must, by geometric necessity, displace the arc toward its center of curvature.

Figure 12–16, B, illustrates diagrammatically the normal short-axis contraction sequence of the left ventricular endocardium from end-diastole to end-systole. Figure 12–16, A, is a comparable M-mode recording from contralateral points on the septum and posterior wall. In each of these figures it is evident that the systolic excursion of the septum and that of the posterior wall are not equal. The difference in excursion is attributable to the second factor determining net septal motion (i.e., the spatial displacement of the left ventricle). Figure 12–17, A, illustrates the relative effects of myocardial contraction and the spatial motion of the heart on the recorded excursion of individual points on the anterior (septal) and posterior endocardial surfaces of the left ventricle. Because both of these compo-

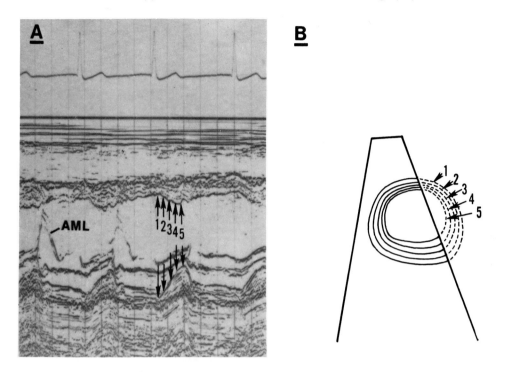

Fig. 12–16. *A,* M-mode recording of a normal left ventricle illustrates the patterns and the relative amplitudes of motion of the septum and posterior wall during normal ventricular contraction and relaxation. The vertical arrows indicate five selected points during the contraction sequence from end-diastole (1) to end-systole (5). *B,* A corresponding diagram illustrates the position of the left ventricular endocardium, viewed in short axis, at corresponding points in the contraction sequence. AML = anterior mitral leaflet.

nents of motion have amplitude and direction, they can be represented as vectors. Thus, in this figure, a contraction vector (C) represents the amplitude and direction of endocardial motion resulting from active muscular contraction. Because both the anterior and posterior walls move inward toward the center of curvature of the ventricle, the contraction vectors of each wall are equal in amplitude but opposite in direction.

Also, a spatial vector (S) represents the overall motion of the left ventricle in space and has the same amplitude and direction relative to both the anterior and posterior walls. The net vector (N) represents the sum of the spatial and contraction vectors and, thus, the actual motion perceived from the anterior chest wall.

Normally both the anterior and posterior walls contract equally (Fig. 12–17, A); however, because the ventricle as a whole

moves anteriorly in space, the spatial vector is added to the posterior wall contraction vector and is subtracted from the septal contraction vector. The net septal motion, therefore, is less than the corresponding posterior wall motion.

During diastole, this sequence is reversed, the septum moves anteriorly or away from the center of the left ventricle, and its radius of curvature increases. Spatial movement of the left ventricle is posterior and, therefore, is again subtracted from the absolute septal displacement, thereby decreasing apparent or recorded septal motion.

Throughout the normal contraction and relaxation sequences, the ventricle retains its circular configuration, and the radius of curvature of the septum corresponds to that of the free wall. Changes of ventricular shape or septal position, therefore, do not affect normal contraction.

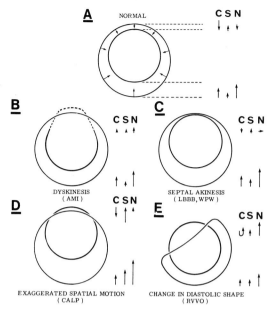

Fig. 12–17. Series of diagrams depicts the factors (expressed as vectors) that determine recorded interventricular septal motion. C = the contraction vector; S = spatial vector, which corresponds to the overall spatial movement of the heart; N = the net vector or sum of the spatial and contraction vectors. *A*, Normal contraction. *B*, Septal dyskinesis, as in anterior wall myocardial infarction (AMI). *C*, Septal akinesis, as in a left bundle branch block or Wolff-Parkinson-White syndrome. *D*, Abnormal septal motion due to exaggerated anterior displacement of the left ventricle in space, as in congenital absence of the left pericardium (CALP) or large pericardial effusion. *E*, Abnormal septal motion due to a change in ventricular shape and septal position, as occurs in right ventricular volume overload (RVVO).

Abnormal Septal Motion

Abnormal septal motion may fall into one of three categories: (1) exaggerated or abnormally increased septal motion (septal hyperkinesis); (2) diminished or absent septal motion (hypokinesis or akinesis); or (3) paradoxic septal motion. Paradoxic septal motion is defined as motion that is opposite to the normally expected direction of septal movement. Thus paradoxic systolic motion is anterior rather than posterior, whereas paradoxic diastolic motion is posterior rather than anterior. Dyskinetic motion may be classified as paradoxic, but the converse is not always true because dyskinesis implies an abnormal-

ity of muscular function that is not inherent in the concept of paradoxic motion.

Exaggerated Septal Motion

Exaggerated septal motion occurs in two primary settings: (1) left ventricular volume overload and (2) compensatory hypercontraction in response to reduced function elsewhere in the ventricle. In left ventricular volume overload states, the primary increase in septal motion is due to an increase in muscular contraction. Note, however, that the amplitude of septal excursion frequently exceeds the corresponding motion of the posterior wall. This is the reverse of the normal relationship and suggests that the spatial vector has shifted and that systolic motion of the centroid of the left ventricle is now posterior. Consequently, the spatial vector is added to the septal contraction vector.

Exaggerated septal motion occurring as a compensation for reduced motion elsewhere is most frequently seen in ischemic heart disease and has been noted in as many as 65% of patients with acute inferior wall infarction.[41] Exaggerated septal motion also commonly occurs in children with anomalous origin of the left coronary artery and produces a characteristic left ventricular contraction pattern. This pattern includes hyperkinesis of the basal septum in association with extensive anterolateral hypokinesis. This prominent dissociation in regional motion draws attention to the underlying abnormality and is the primary echocardiographic sign suggestive of anomalous coronary artery (see Chap. 14). Likewise, in adult patients with diffuse ischemic disease and severe left ventricular dysfunction, a small area of the basal septum is frequently hyperdynamic. This small area of preserved function permits the segmental or ischemic cause of the dysfunction to be defined and a generalized cardiomyopathy to be excluded.

Diminished Septal Motion

Decreased septal excursion can be observed in a variety of disorders, including ischemic heart disease, various forms of cardiomyopathy, and infiltrative disease of the septum, and as a result of delayed or asynchronous septal contraction caused by abnormal electrical activation. In each of these disorders, the decrease in septal movement represents a decrease in the contraction vector (Fig. 12–17, C). The spatial motion of the ventricle is rarely abnormal, and the position or shape of the interventricular septum is not markedly distorted. In the majority of these cases, there is corresponding hypofunction of other areas of the ventricle. (These specific disorders are discussed more extensively in the general discussion of the left ventricle in Chapter 8.) In some patients, however, diminished septal motion may represent one end of a spectrum in which severe expression is characterized by paradoxic septal motion. The operative factors in this situation are discussed in the next section.

Paradoxic Septal Motion

If contraction of the normal concave interventricular septum must be inward toward the diastolic center of septal curvature (or posteriorly relative to the anterior chest wall), paradoxic motion must be passive and can theoretically occur in only one of three ways: (1) as a result of septal dyskinesis; (2) as a result of exaggerated motion of the entire left ventricle in space; or (3) as a result of a change in septal shape or configuration from diastole to systole.

Both mechanisms (1) and (3) may be associated with a change in ventricular shape. However, in the former, the affected muscle does not function normally, whereas in the latter, a normally functioning septum is compelled to move in an abnormal direction by a shift in its spatial configuration.

Paradoxic movement of the septum is generally viewed as a systolic phenomenon because systole is the portion of the cardiac cycle during which the functional activity of the septum occurs. There is generally also a diastolic component which, in the instances of dyskinesis and exaggerated motion of the ventricle in space, merely reflects return of the septum to the normal basal position. When septal and ventricular shape change, however, the diastolic abnormality may be predominant, and the paradoxic systolic movement is merely a secondary response. *As a general rule, any movement of the septum that is more rapid than the peak velocity of normal systolic muscular contraction is passive and is associated with some change in septal position and, hence, ventricular shape.*

In several situations, paradoxic septal motion may be confined to a specific portion of the cardiac cycle (usully diastole) and may not be associated with any alteration in systolic motion or function.

Septal dyskinesis (systole). Septal dyskinesis resulting from myocardial ischemia is the simplest situation and is illustrated in Figure 12–17, B. In this setting, the septum fails to contract actively and is pushed outward by the developing left ventricular intracavitary pressure. The "contraction vector," therefore, is anterior or paradoxic. The ischemic muscle is stretched, and the wall either fails to thicken normally or thins slightly, indicating that the muscle is functioning abnormally. The left ventricle moves anteriorly in space, and the spatial vector is anteriorly directed and normal in amplitude. The spatial vector, therefore, is added to the anterior or paradoxic movement of the ischemic region and to the normal anteriorly directed contraction vector of the posterior wall, thereby increasing the apparent movement of both regions.

A similar, though less dramatic example, occurs with septal akinesis or hypokinesis (Fig. 12–17, C). In this setting, septal contraction is diminished or absent, and the contraction vector is also absent or decreased. The anterior motion of the left ventricle in space, however, persists. When the anterior spatial motion equals the diminished septal contraction, no motion is perceived relative to the anterior chest wall. When the contraction vector exceeds the spatial vector, slight or hypokinetic movement may be noted, whereas spatial motion in excess of septal contraction results in paradoxic septal motion relative to the external reference point.

Paradoxic septal motion as a result of exaggerated motion of the left ventricle in space. Exaggerated motion of the left ventricle in space is apparent in such conditions as moderate or large pericardial effusion and congenital absence of the left pericardium in which the normal pericardial restraint on the heart is lost. In these disorders, although contraction of both the anterior and posterior walls is normal, the increase in spatial cardiac movement is so marked that the spatial vector greatly exceeds contraction, and net septal motion is, therefore, anterior or paradoxic (Fig. 12–17, D). The fact that the septal musculature is contracting normally despite its abnormal movement in space can be determined by the normal pattern of systolic muscular thickening.

This mechanism has also been postulated to at least partially underlie the paradoxic septal motion noted following open-heart surgery.[53] Studies of the overall excursion of the posterior wall epicardium suggest exaggerated anterior motion of the entire heart in space with resulting paradoxic septal motion. This has been related to sternal adhesions, which fix the anterior right ventricular wall and cause the heart to assume a "tear drop" shape during diastole and an exaggerated anterior motion during systole as it returns to a more normal configuration. Postoperative septal motion is obviously a complex situation, and other mechanisms, such as septal ischemia, may be contributory in individual situations. However, this observation does partially clarify one aspect of this multifactorial problem.

Paradoxic septal motion due to changes in left ventricular shape. Paradoxic motion of the interventricular septum resulting from a change in left ventricular shape may affect both the systolic and diastolic phases of the cardiac cycle or be confined to diastole alone. Functionally, isolated paradoxic diastolic septal motion (and by inference and abnormal shape change) should affect only ventricular compliance, whereas paradoxic systolic and diastolic motion may affect both compliance and systolic function.

Paradoxic systolic and diastolic motion. The final method by which the interventricular septum can move paradoxically during systole is through the rearrangement of a shape abnormality that originated during the diastolic filling phase.[6] This phenomenon occurs most frequently in right ventricular volume overload and is diagrammed in Figure 12–17, E, and illustrated in Figure 12–18. In this example, there is marked right ventricular volume overload due to pulmonary insufficiency. During diastole, the increased right ventricular volume displaces the interventricular septum away from the right ventricle and causes it to bow inward toward the left ventricle (Fig. 12–18, A and B). At the onset of systole, the left ventricular intracavitary pressure rises rapidly and exceeds simultaneous right ventricular intracavitary pressure. This positive left-to-right pressure gradient shifts the septum toward a more normal orientation, which is concave toward the left ventricle, and causes the left ventricle to return to a more circular configuration (Fig. 12–18, C). This rearrangement of ventricular shape has the effect of thrusting the septum into the right ventricular cavity (paradoxically) and might theoretically contribute to right ventricular ejection.

Figure 12–19, A, is an M-mode recording that demonstrates this type of paradoxic septal motion. Figure 12–19, B, il-

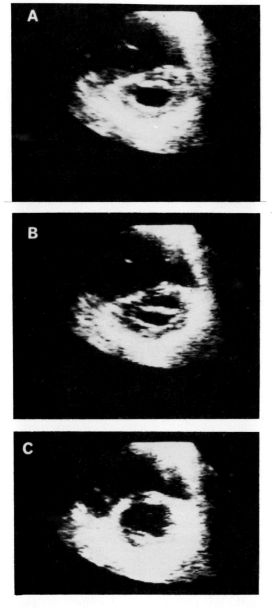

Fig. 12–18. Short-axis, cross-sectional recording of the left ventricle at the mitral valve level illustrates the variation in ventricular shape and septal position from diastole to systole. Such variation is characteristic of a right ventricular volume overload. *A*, Recorded during initial diastole. The right ventricle is dilated, and the septum is displaced to the left and flattened. The mitral valve is fully open. *B*, Recorded later in diastole. The left ventricular cavity area is slightly larger. The mitral valve is in a resting position, and the septum remains flattened and displaced to the left. *C*, Recorded during ventricular systole. The left ventricle is more circular, the mitral valve is closed, and the septum has shifted to the right (paradoxically) and is now more convex toward the right ventricle.

lustrates the left ventricular endocardial contraction sequence underlying this motion. These companion figures suggest that the primary rearrangement in shape occurs early in systole during isovolumic contraction and is associated with an abrupt upward movement of the interventricular septum. During the later phases of systole, anterior movement of the ventricle continues as a result of an exaggeration of the spatial vector. The fact that the septal myocardium functions normally can again be ascertained by observing the preserved pattern of septal thickening.

Several points should be emphasized about this type of systolic change in ventricular shape. First, as previously mentioned, the primary abnormality is diastolic not systolic. The apparent abnormal systolic motion merely represents a rearrangement or normalization of left ventricular shape that corrects a distortion that occurred during diastole because of the unequal filling of the two ventricles. Second, the degree of distortion appears to have some relationship to both the degree and the type of right ventricular volume overload. In patients with isolated right ventricular volume overloads, such as tricuspid insufficiency and pulmonary insufficiency, the septum appears to be more markedly displaced, and the left ventricle appears more distorted. The septal distortion may not be as great in the right ventricular volume overload associated with atrial septal defect. It has been suggested that the atrial septal defect itself may play a protective role because as the right ventricle becomes deformed, right ventricular compliance decreases. As a result, more blood is preferentially shunted into the left ventricle and further septal deformity is retarded. Third, although the relative effects of pressure and volume on the abnormal septal configuration remain to be defined, the diastolic deformity is apparently related to differences in right and left ventricular volumes. In systole, however, the degree to which the septum returns to

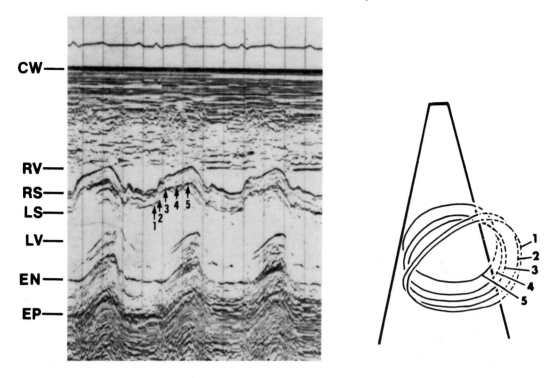

Fig. 12–19. M-mode recording illustrates paradoxic septal motion in a patient with right ventricular volume overload. An abrupt, initial, anterior (paradoxic) motion of the septum corresponds to the change in ventricular shape that occurs in early systole. This initial rapid movement is followed by a more gradual continued anterior or paradoxic septal motion. The septal muscle thickens normally, indicating preservation of myocardial function. Diagram illustrates the corresponding short-axis motion from end-diastole (1) to end-systole (5). CW = chest wall; RV = right ventricle; RS = right septal interface; LS = left septal interface; LV = left ventricle; EN = endocardium; EP = epicardium. (From Weyman, AE, et al.: Mechanism of abnormal septal motion in patients with right ventricular volume overload. Circulation, 54:179, 1976. Reproduced by permission of the American Heart Association.)

normal appears to relate roughly to the relative pressures in the two ventricles. Thus, with right-sided systolic hypertension, the septum appears to retain much of its abnormal diastolic configuration and to remain flattened during systole.[54] When right-sided systolic pressures are lower, greater normalization is evident, and the left ventricle becomes more circular during systolic contraction.

A shift in septal position has also been noted during Müller's maneuver (forced inspiration against a closed airway).[55] This maneuver causes a transient increase in right ventricular loading and is associated with a leftward shift in interventricular septal position. In this setting, the septum also transiently fails to return to a normal systolic configuration, thereby implying

an altered systolic relationship between the two chambers.[55] Finally, the degree of deformity is greatest at the base of the heart and decreases toward the apex. This predominant basal deformity is illustrated in Figure 12–20 and can be explained by the simple relationship: force = pressure × area. Because the area at the base is greatest, it has the greatest force acting upon it and should, therefore, show the greatest degree of deformity.

Paradoxic diastolic septal motion. Isolated paradoxic diastolic septal motion is seen in several conditions, the most common of which are mitral stenosis and aortic insufficiency.

MITRAL STENOSIS. Isolated paradoxic diastolic septal motion occurs most prominently in patients with mitral stenosis.[56]

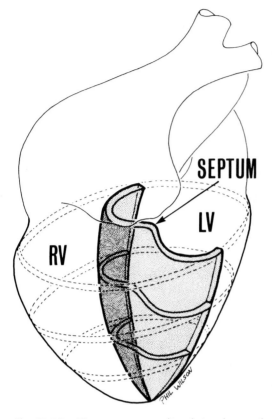

Fig. 12–20. Diagram compares the relative degree of septal displacement at the base and apex of the heart in right ventricular volume overload states. As illustrated, the degree of septal displacement and corresponding change in left ventricular shape is relatively greater at the base and gradually decreases toward the apex. RV = right ventricle; LV = left ventricle. (From Weyman, AE, et al.: Mechanism of abnormal septal motion in patients with right ventricular volume overload. Circulation, 54:179, 1976. Reproduced by permission of the American Heart Association.)

Figure 12–21 is an M-mode recording from a patient with mitral stenosis. In this example, the septum moves abruptly, paradoxically or posteriorly, at the onset of diastole. This motion is more rapid than the peak rate of normal septal contraction and, thus, according to the concepts discussed previously, should be passive. Such movement also results in a decrease in the transverse diameter of the left ventricle when the ventricle should be actively filling. This disparity suggests that the geometric shape of the ventricle must be changing in order for one of the minor ven-

tricular axes to decrease while ventricular volume is increasing.

Figure 12–22 contains a series of short-axis cross-sectional scans of the left ventricle from initial diastole to end-diastole from a patient with mitral stenosis. This figure illustrates this predicted change in shape. At end-systole, the ventricle is circular. At the onset of diastole, however, the septum abruptly shifts inward toward the center of the left ventricular cavity. The orientation of the septum and the shape of the left ventricle consequently change. As diastolic filling progresses, the septum gradually shifts away from the center of the left ventricular cavity and returns toward a more normal position. By end-systole, the ventricular shape is circular, and systolic contraction proceeds in a normal sequence and direction.

The initial diastolic shift in the position of the septum in mitral stenosis has been demonstrated to result from an inequality in filling of the two ventricles during early diastole.[56] This inequality occurs because the stenotic mitral valve delays left ventricular filling, whereas the right ventricle fills at a normal rate. This produces a relative right ventricular volume overload and shifts the septum to the left. Because the volume that can be accepted by one ventricle at any given filling pressure has been shown to be related directly to the degree of filling of the other, the initial diastolic compliance of the right ventricle may increase because of the partially empty left ventricle.[57] This may create not only a relative but also an absolute right ventricular volume overload. As the left ventricle slowly fills, the cavity expands, and the septum returns toward a more normal position. Left ventricular filling, however, occurs when the right ventricle is already fully distended. Left ventricular compliance, therefore, may be relatively decreased, and a greater filling pressure may be required to introduce a normal diastolic volume.

The degree of initial diastolic septal dis-

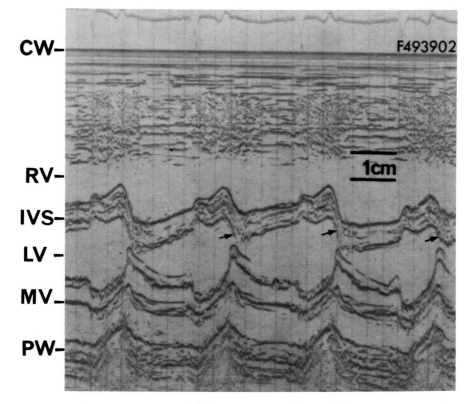

CW–

F493902

1cm

RV–

IVS–

LV –

MV–

PW–

Fig. 12–21. M-mode recording of the left ventricle (LV) and the interventricular septum (IVS) from a patient with mitral stenosis illustrates prominent initial paradoxic diastolic septal motion (arrows). This motion corresponds to mitral valve (MV) opening and exceeds the peak posterior excursion of the septum during systolic contraction. CW = chest wall; RV = right ventricle; PW = posterior wall.

placement in mitral stenosis has been shown to relate to the severity of the stenotic lesion and to be absent with tricuspid stenosis.[56] Figure 12–23 shows the relationship between varying rates of the left ventricular filling and the severity of this paradoxic septal movement. Figure 12–24 compares the right and left ventricular angiographic filling rates for each quarter of diastole (normalized to 100%) to septal motion in a patient with both mitral stenosis and a right ventricular volume overload. In each example the interdependence of septal motion on right and left ventricular filling patterns is evident.

AORTIC INSUFFICIENCY. Another disorder associated with a unique pattern of paradoxic diastolic septal motion is aortic insufficiency. In aortic insufficiency there is frequently an abrupt anterior movement of the septum at end-systole followed by a second downward or paradoxic displacement at the onset of ventricular diastole (Fig. 12–25). Both of these movements are more rapid than can be accounted for by active contraction and, therefore, should be passive. It has been suggested that the initial upward movement is due to the regurgitant flow through the aortic valve, which begins immediately following aortic valve closure. This flow causes the left ventricular cavity to expand during left-sided isovolumic relaxation prior to tricuspid valve opening. Once the tricuspid valve opens and right ventricular filling begins, the septum is then displaced toward the left ventricle. This paradoxic septal displacement may appear unusual in the setting of a left ventricular volume overload; however, one must remember

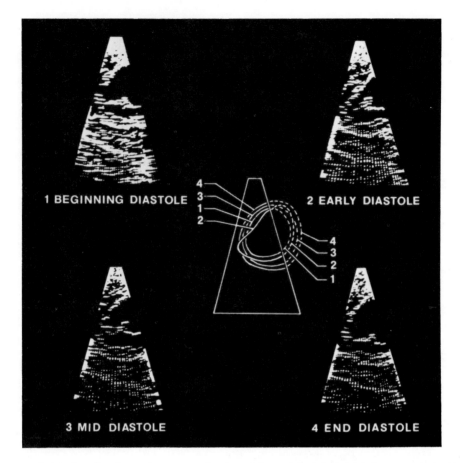

Fig. 12–22. Serial, diastolic, short-axis, cross-sectional recordings of the left ventricle from a patient with mitral stenosis and prominent septal motion abnormality. At end-systole or beginning-diastole (frame 1), the left ventricle has a relatively circular configuration. In the initial portion of diastole, immediately after opening of the mitral valve (frame 2), the position of the interventricular septum shifts away from the right ventricle and toward the left ventricle. This movement alters the shape of the left ventricle during initial diastole. Throughout the remainder of diastole (frames 3 and 4), the left ventricle gradually fills, and septal position shifts back toward the right ventricle and away from the left ventricle. At end-diastole, the ventricle has returned to its normal circular configuration. Systolic contraction then proceeds in a normal fashion. In the center panel, the relative positions of the endocardial surface of the left ventricle are outlined from end-systole to end-diastole. Between positions 1 and 2, left ventricular diastolic shape changes abruptly. In positions 3 and 4, the ventricle gradually returns toward its normal circular configuration. (From Weyman, AE, et al.: Mechanism of paradoxical early diastolic septal motion in patients with mitral stenosis: a cross-sectional endocardiographic study. Am J Cardiol, 40:691, 1977.)

that the total left ventricular volume in aortic insufficiency accumulates throughout diastole. Initial diastolic inflow, therefore, may represent a relatively smaller than normal percentage of end-diastolic ventricular volume. Thus, there may be a comparative right ventricular volume overload in initial diastole because the initial right ventricular inflow represents a greater percentage of end-diastolic right ventricular volume than does the comparable initial left ventricular inflow.

Left Bundle Branch Block

These principles can be used to approach other abnormalities of septal motion. In left bundle branch block, for example, a characteristic feature is an abrupt downward or posterior movement of the interventricular septum almost coincident with the onset of the QRS complex (the so-called septal beak).[58,59] This movement is usually small and occurs at a rate be-

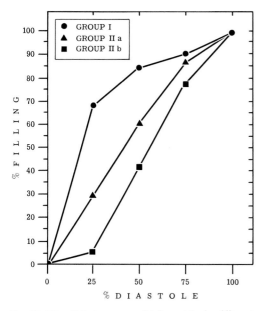

Fig. 12–23. Relative rates of left ventricular filling in normal patients (group I), patients with mitral stenosis with minimal septal motion abnormality (group IIa), and patients with mitral stenosis with more severe septal motion abnormality (group IIb). The rate of diastolic filling of the left ventricle is significantly different between group I and groups IIa and IIb at each of the first three quarters of diastole. In addition, the difference between group IIa and IIb is significant in the first quarter of diastole. (From Weyman, AE, et al.: Mechanism of paradoxical early diastolic septal motion in patients with mitral stenosis: a cross-sectional echocardiographic study. Am J Cardiol, 40:691, 1977.)

analyzing the various components of abnormal septal motion when it is encountered. Although most of these phenomena have been described and are best depicted using the M-mode format, they can be seen interrupting the normally symmetric contraction and relaxation sequence of the left ventricle during cross-sectional studies. An understanding of the mechanisms underlying these abnormal movements therefore appears warranted.

Ventricular Septal Defects

Ventricular septal defect is the most common congenital malformation of the heart occurring in between 1.3 and 2.4% of live births.[60] These defects may occur as isolated lesions, may form an integral part of a more complex anomaly, such as tetralogy of Fallot or truncus arteriosus, or may be associated with, but not anatomically related to, other cardiac anomalies.[61] Isolated ventricular septal defects represent approximately 23% of all instances of congenital heart disease, but ventricular septal defects are present in approximately 50% of all congenital anomalies of the heart.[60]

Isolated Ventricular Septal Defect

Anatomically, ventricular septal defects are conventionally divided at the level of the crista supraventricularis into supracristal and infracristal defects. The supracristal defects lie immediately below the pulmonary valve, and the valve typically forms the superior margin of the defect. They appear in an area of the interventricular septum that is normally closed by downward growth of the bulbar septum and represent incomplete development of this membrane. Viewed from the left side of the heart, they are positioned immediately inferior to the commissure between the left and right aortic cusps.[60] Infracristal defects, as a group, are found inferior and posterior to the crista and can be subdivided into those that encompass or are contiguous with the membranous septum

yond that which is associated with active contraction. If one assumes that, because of the conduction delay, isovolumic contraction in the right ventricle precedes isovolumic contraction in the left ventricle, this motion may represent passive movement of the septum in response to the unopposed initial increase in right ventricular pressure. Once the left ventricle contracts, this minimal derangement of shape is rapidly corrected, and septal motion then depends on the relative magnitudes of the contraction and spatial vectors.

Discussion of all the possible ways in which the septum can move paradoxically or abnormally is clearly beyond the scope of this text. Hopefully, however, these simple principles will aid the reader in

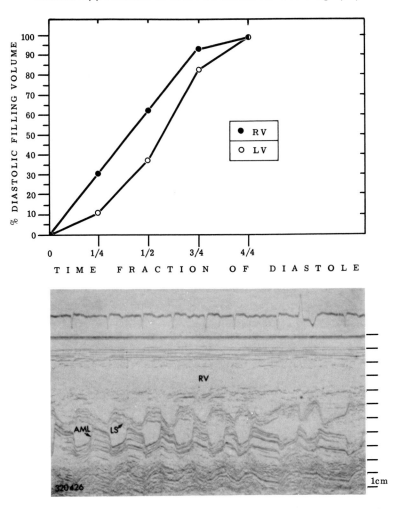

Fig. 12–24. Top, Comparative right and left ventricular filling rates (at each quarter of diastole) normalized to 100% filling in a patient with combined mitral stenosis and right ventricular overload. Bottom, An M-mode echocardiographic recording from the same patient illustrates the abnormal septal motion that occurs as a result of this discrepancy in relative ventricular filling.

(the membranous septal defects), those within the muscular septum that are completely surrounded by muscular tissue (muscular septal defects), and those that arise in the site that the defect would occupy if it were part of an endocardial cushion malformation.

The most common of these defects is the membranous defect. Although referred to as membranous because of their anatomic association with the membranous septum, these defects generally include a portion of the muscular septum. This loss of muscular tissue may constitute the major por-

tion of the lesion.[61] When viewed from the left side of the heart, membranous defects lie beneath the commissure between the right and noncoronary aortic cusps. Muscular defects may arise anywhere in the muscular septum. They may be small or large, single or multiple. On occasion, the septum may be thin and may contain multiple sieve-like fenestrations. In other instances, small sinusoidal passages may be threaded among the septal trabeculae. From a functional standpoint, multiple small defects appear to have the same significance as do single large defects.[62,63]

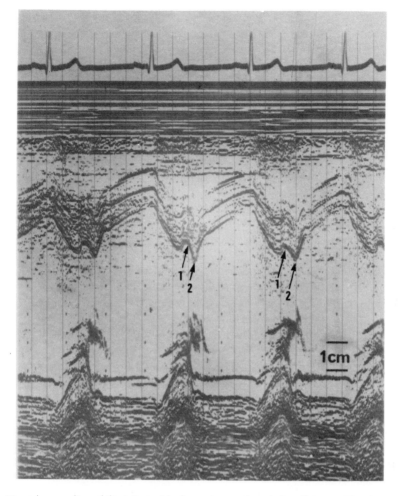

Fig. 12–25. M-mode recording of the interventricular septum and aortic insufficiency. The characteristic pattern in these cases is an abrupt anterior motion of the septum at end-ventricular systole (arrow 1) followed by a rapid downward or paradoxic motion of the septum at the onset of ventricular diastole (vertical arrow 2).

Most ventricular septal defects are clinically apparent, and the echocardiographic examination, therefore, is directed toward defining their location, size, and association with other lesions. Nonspecific assessment of the presence of the defect based on the sequelae of the left-to-right shunt (the left ventricular volume overload pattern), therefore, is of secondary diagnostic importance. In contrast, the atrial septal defect is itself clinically silent, and its presence must be initially inferred from the effects of the lesion on the right ventricle and atrium (the right ventricular volume overload pattern).[6,18–20]

Once recorded, however, the echocardiographic appearances of defects in both the atrial and ventricular septa are similar and are characterized by a focal discontinuity or area of "dropout" in the normally continuous linear band of echoes arising from the intact septum.

Echocardiographic ventricular septal defect recording can be achieved in a variety of imaging planes; however, the parasternal long-axis, the apical four-chamber, and the subcostal long-axis views are the most commonly used for this purpose. Supracristal defects are probably best visualized in a parasternal short-axis view because of their atypical leftward position.

Success rates for visualization of isolated ventricular septal defects have ranged from 74[64] to 88%[65] in prospective studies and from 88[66] to 100%[67] in patients with known ventricular septal defect. False-negatives have been noted primarily in patients with small defects[64-66] and/or as a result of failure to visualize a second lesion in a patient with multiple defects. Failure to record at least one large ventricular septal defect, however, has been reported.[64] The smallest defect that has been visualized to date measured 2 mm.[67]

The relative value of individual views in recording defects has varied in reported series. In one study, for example, 91% of recorded defects were visualized in the parasternal long-axis view,[66] whereas in another, only 46% were apparent in this view.[67] Similarly, from the subcostal location, reported success rates have varied from 42[67] to 88%.[65] This wide variability undoubtedly reflects the large anatomic variation in defect size and location. However, in general, the subcostal views are more successful in infants and children, whereas the parasternal and apical views are more useful in adults with complicated lesions.

False-positives have also been noted in as many as 12% of normal persons.[64,67] False-positives are encountered more frequently in the apical four-chamber view; 70% of false-positives occur in this one plane.[67] The highest specificity has been noted in the subcostal view (92% in one series and 100% in another). Importantly, when the long-axis, apical four-chamber, and subcostal views were all recorded, no false-positives were imaged consistently in all views.[67]

The apparent size of the defect may also vary in different views. This variance has been attributed to the asymmetric anatomic shape of many defects and to the resulting variations in the defect diameter presented to a particular imaging plane.

Defect size also decreases from diastole to systole. A mean decrease of almost 50% has been reported.[67] In individual patients, a decrease in defect size of as much as 90% has been noted.[67]

Because of the wide variability in patient size, the absolute dimensions of a ventricular septal defect have little meaning. Therefore, defect size is customarily normalized by relating it to the aortic root diameter (VSD/AO).[61,68] Using this ratio, a weak but consistent relationship between echocardiographic defect size and shunt flow, QP/QS, has been observed.[67]

Figure 12–26 is an example of a large ventricular septal defect recorded in the parasternal long-axis view. In this figure, a prominent area of discontinuity between the superior border of the interventricular septum and the anterior aortic root is evident. Figure 12–27 is a second recording of a ventricular septal defect visualized in the apical four-chamber view. This defect is positioned again at the superior margin of the muscular septum and separates the septum from its normal point of junction with the interatrial septum.

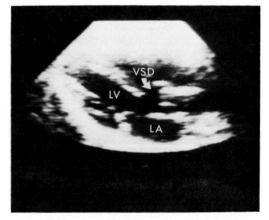

Fig. 12–26. Parasternal long-axis recording of the left ventricle (LV) illustrates a large ventricular septal defect (VSD). The defect extends from the superior border of the muscular septum to the anterior margin of the aortic root and includes a portion of the muscular septum. LA = left atrium.

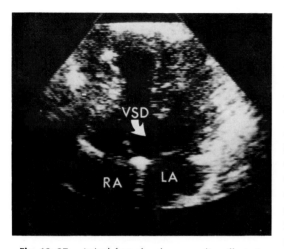

Fig. 12–27. Apical four-chamber recording illustrates a large ventricular septal defect (VSD) extending from the superior border of the muscular septum to the plane of insertion of the atrioventricular valves. RA = right atrium; LA = left atrium.

Ventricular Septal Defects Forming an Integral Part of More Complex Congenital Anomalies

Ventricular septal defects may form an integral part of a variety of complex congenital anomalies of the heart, including tetralogy of Fallot, truncus arteriosus, double outlet right ventricle, D- and L-transposition, and endocardial cushion defects.[60,61] These defects can be generally subdivided into those that are associated with aortic overriding or malposition and those that arise in the region of the closing endocardial cushions. The latter defects are considered in the section on endocardial cushion malformations and, therefore, are not discussed further here.

Defects associated with aortic overriding occur in either the bulbar or the membranous septa. When the lesion involves primarily the bulbar septum, as in truncus arteriosus, it is typically high, anterior, and limited by the semilunar valves of the truncus superiorly and the crest of the ventricular septum posteriorly. When it involves the membranous septum, as in tetralogy of Fallot, the bulbar septum extending below the semilunar valve is present and limits the defect superiorly. These defects are usually large, easily recognized, and are best recorded in the parasternal long-axis view of the left ventricle.

Figure 12–28 is an example of a large ventricular septal defect associated with truncus arteriosus. In this example, the large separation between the superior margin of the interventricular septum and the anteriorly positioned anterior border of the aortic root is clearly evident. The presence of these defects is highlighted by the associated aortic overriding. Success rates for defect recording are better for this group (93 to 95%)[67,69] than those reported for isolated defects.

Ventricular Septal Aneurysms

Two primary types of aneurysms involve the ventricular septum: the discrete membranous ventricular septal aneurysms, which develop as part of the natural process of closure of congenital ventricular septal defects, and the large septal aneurysms, which complicate acute myocardial infarction and underlie ventricular septal perforation. This section deals with the small, congenital, ventricular septal aneurysm. The infarct-associated aneurysms are discussed under complications of acute myocardial infarction in Chapter 8.

Studies of the natural history of ventricular septal defects suggest a continuing rate of spontaneous closure throughout childhood.[70–72] Aneurysm formation has been well documented as one mechanism by which this defect closure occurs.[73–75] The initial formation of a ventricular septal aneurysm is frequently associated with partial defect closure and decrease in the size of the left-to-right shunt. After complete closure, the aneurysms may remain as the only evidence of a prior defect. In addition to suggesting the presence of an earlier defect, the aneurysm may also offer a possible nidus for infection in bacterial endocarditis. Membranous ventricular aneurysms are generally visualized in the

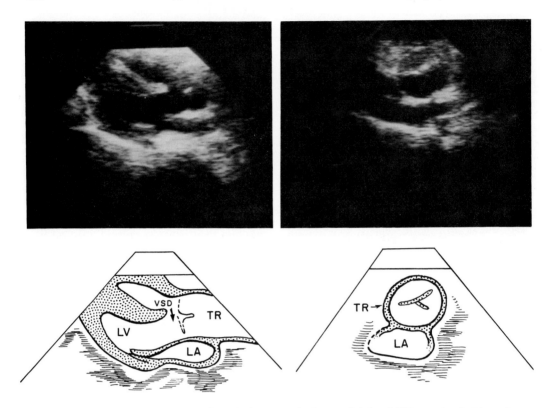

Fig. 12–28. Parasternal long-axis recording of a large ventricular septal defect (VSD) associated with aortic overriding in a patient with truncus arteriosus. The defect is indicated by the vertical arrow. RA = right atrium; LA = left atrium.

right ventricular outflow tract, anterior to the junction of the anterior aortic root and muscular septum. They are typically small, thin walled, and show little mobility. They can usually be recorded in either a parasternal long-axis view of the left side of the heart or a short-axis view of the left ventricular outflow tract recorded below the level of the aortic valve. Figure 12–29 illustrates a membranous ventricular septal aneurysm recorded in both long and short axes. In each recording, the thin-walled aneurysm is seen protruding from the anterior margin of the septum into the right ventricular outflow tract.

Endocardial Cushion Defects

Endocardial cushion defects are complex developmental abnormalities that characteristically involve both the inter-atrial and interventricular septa. Embryologically, the endocardial cushions arise early in the development of the fetal heart as local thickenings in the dorsal and ventral surfaces of the common atrioventricular canal. They grow rapidly, projecting deeply into the canal, and soon fuse to form a septum (the septum intermedium) that divides the canal into the mitral and tricuspid orifices. The fused endocardial cushions, in addition to dividing the atrioventricular canal, also provide a framework to which the advancing atrial septum primum and upwardly developing interventricular septum can attach. They further contribute to the final closure of the interventricular foramen and the septum primum and to the development of the anterior mitral and septal tricuspid leaflets.[76,77]

The endocardial cushions, therefore, are

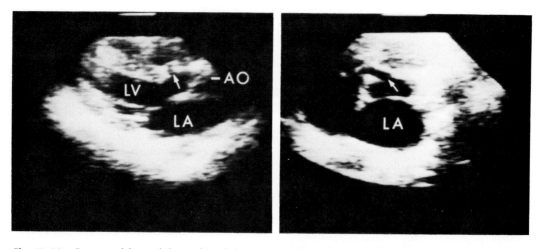

Fig. 12–29. Parasternal long- (left panel) and short-axis (right panel) recordings illustrate a small membranous ventricular septal aneurysm. The aneurysm is situated anterior to the interventricular septum, is thin walled, and protrudes into the right ventricular outflow tract just proximal to the junction of the membranous septum and anterior aortic root (the arrow points to the aneurysm). LV = left ventricle; LA = left atrium; AO = aorta.

situated at a critical location within the fetal heart, and developmental faults in these cushions may cause abnormalities in the interatrial septum, the interventricular septum, and the atrioventricular valves either individually or in various combinations. These developmental abnormalities have been described in many ways; however, in this section, they will be discussed in a format that parallels the echocardiographic features by which they can be separated. These types of defects therefore include (1) the complete form of the endocardial cushion defect, (2) the partial endocardial cushion defect, and (3) the ventricular septal defect of the endocardial cushion type. A cleft in the anterior mitral leaflet is considered an integral part of the endocardial cushion deformity and, hence, may be seen in each of these conditions.

In the complete form of endocardial cushion defect, the dorsal and ventral cushions fail to develop completely, and the converging crescentic borders of the atrial septum primum and interventricular septum have nothing with which to fuse. This lack of fusion results in a defect in the atrial septum just above the normal position of the atrioventricular valves and in a corresponding defect in the superior margin of the interventricular septum. The cushions also fail to close the mitral and tricuspid orifices and to make their appropriate contributions to the anterior mitral and septal tricuspid leaflets. These atrioventricular valves, therefore, are continuous at the midline and form a common AV valve, which extends through the large atrioventricular defect normally closed by the developing cushions.

The complete form of endocardial cushion defect has been further subdivided pathologically into three types based on the division and pattern of attachment of the anterior mitral leaflet.[78] In type A, the anterior leaflet is divided at its midportion and attaches by thin, long chordae just to the right of the crest of the interventricular septum. In type B, the anterior leaflet is again divided; however, in this type, both medial segments are attached to a single papillary muscle situated high in the right ventricular cavity adjacent to the interventricular septum. The final type, C, is characterized by an undivided, unattached, anterior leaflet that is usually associated with a membranous ventricular septal defect.

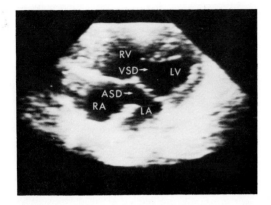

Fig. 12–30. Subcostal long-axis recording illustrates an atrioventricular canal defect. In this example, a moderately large ventricular septal defect (VSD) appears at the base of the septum, separating the superior septal margin from the plane of insertion of the atrioventricular valves. There is also a large ostium primum atrial septal defect (ASD). The atrioventricular valve extends through this extensive area of incomplete atrial and ventricular partitioning. RV = right ventricle; LV = left ventricle; RA = right atrium; LA = left atrium.

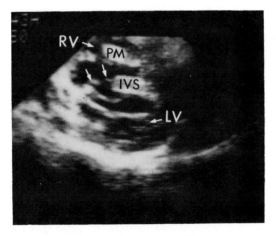

Fig. 12–31. Parasternal short-axis recording of the right (RV) and left (LV) ventricles in a patient with an atrioventricular canal defect. The insertion of the atrioventricular valve into the margin of the interventricular septum (IVS) is illustrated (arrowheads). In addition, there is a hypertrophied right ventricular papillary muscle (PM), a clearly defined ventricular septal defect, and a cleft in the anterior mitral leaflet. In this example, only the medial portion of the left anterior leaflet is recorded.

The various components of the endocardial cushion defects are complex and frequently lie at unusual orientations relative to each other. As a result, multiple echocardiographic views are typically

required to characterize the disorder completely.[79]

The apical four-chamber view is probably the best view for visualizing the defects in the atrial and ventricular septa. Figure 12–30 is an example of a patient with an endocardial defect and illustrates both the atrial and ventricular septal defects and their relationship to the atrioventricular valves. In this example, the ventricular septal defect can be observed at the superior margin of the interventricular septum just beneath the common AV valve. The companion defect in the septum primum is also evident distal to this valve. It has been reported that this view permits differentiation of the type of AV valve structure and points of anterior leaflet attachment and, thus, subclassification of the defects.[79] Figure 12–31 is an example of a type A defect in which the common anterior leaflet appears to divide and to attach directly to the crest of the interventricular septum.

The long-axis view is useful for defining the anterior relationship of the common AV valve within the left ventricular outflow tract and the anteriorly directed orientation of the mitral orifice.[79]

The short-axis view of the mitral valve permits visualization of the characteristic cleft as well as definition of the relative sizes of the right and left ventricles and the characteristic pattern of interventricular septal motion.

Partial Endocardial Cushion Defect

The partial endocardial cushion defect (ostium primum atrial septal defect with cleft mitral valve) is likewise best demonstrated in the apical four-chamber view. In this view, the defect can be seen directly above the attachments of the mitral and tricuspid leaflets into the crest of the interventricular septum (see Fig. 12–26). The superior border of the defect frequently appears to be widened by the increased reflectivity at the blood-tissue interface (the so-called "t" sign).

In long axis, the right ventricle is characteristically dilated because of the left-to-right shunting through the defect. The anterior mitral leaflet is frequently displaced anteriorly into the outflow tract, and the mitral orifice is directed more anteriorly toward the interventricular septum. In short axis, the cleft in the anterior mitral leaflet, which is characteristic of AV canals, is again noted. The cleft mitral valve is illustrated in Chapter 5 and is characterized by loss of the normal fish-mouthed configuration of the two mitral leaflets with conversion to a triangular pattern caused by the division of the anterior leaflet. The cleft has been noted to be typically eccentric and located toward the anteromedial portion of the anterior leaflet.[79]

Isolated Ventricular Septal Defect of the Endocardial Cushion Type

The final variation of the endocardial cushion malformation is the ventricular septal defect that is located in the region normally formed by the developing cushions and associated with a cleft mitral valve.[80] This defect appears similar to that noted in the complete canal and extends from the superior margin of the interventricular septum to the line of junction of the atrioventricular valves. In contrast to the complete defect, however, the interatrial septum distal to the junction of the AV valves is intact.

The cross-sectional method appears to be a highly reliable means of detecting endocardial cushion defects and of defining their type and associated AV valve structure. Accurate demonstration of specific features of these complex lesions has been achieved in as many as 96% of surgically confirmed cases.[79]

REFERENCES

1. Grant, JCB, and Basmajian, JV: Grant's Method of Anatomy. Baltimore, Williams & Wilkins, 1965.
2. Bloor, CM: Cardiac Pathology. Philadelphia, Lippincott, 1978.
3. Braunwald, TE, Fishman, AP, and Cournand, A: Time relationship of dynamic events in the cardiac chambers, pulmonary artery and aorta in man. Circ Res, 4:100, 1956.
4. Tei, C, et al.: Real-time cross-sectional echocardiographic evaluation of the interatrial septum by right atrium-interatrial septum-left atrium direction of ultrasonic beam. Circulation, 60:539, 1979.
5. Tei, C, et al.: Echocardiographic analysis of interatrial septal motion. Am J Cardiol, 44:472, 1979.
6. Weyman, AE, Wann, LS, Feigenbaum, H, and Dillon, JC: Mechanism of abnormal septal motion in patients with right ventricular volume overload. Circulation, 54:179, 1976.
7. Hagler, DJ, et al.: Real-time wide angle sector echocardiography: atrioventricular canal defects. Circulation, 59:140, 1979.
8. Dillon, JC, et al.: Cross-sectional echocardiographic examination of the interatrial septum. Circulation, 55:1, 1977.
9. Schapira, JN, Martin, RP, Fowles, RE, and Popp, RL: Single and two-dimensional echocardiographic features of the interatrial septum in normal subjects and patients with an atrial septal defect. Am J Cardiol, 43:816, 1979.
10. Silverman, NH, and Schiller, NB: Apex echocardiography. A two-dimensional technique for evaluating congenital heart disease. Circulation, 57:503, 1978.
11. Tajik, AJ, et al.: Two-dimensional real-time ultrasonic imaging of the heart and great vessels. Mayo Clin Proc, 53:271, 1980.
12. Lange, LW, Sahn, DJ, Allen, HD, and Goldberg, SJ: Subxiphoid cross-sectional echocardiography in infants and children with congenital heart disease. Circulation, 59:513, 1979.
13. Bierman, FZ, and Williams, RG: Subxiphoid two-dimensional imaging of the interatrial septum in infants and neonates with congenital heart disease. Circulation, 60:80, 1979.
14. Kushner, FG, Lam, W, and Morganroth, J: Apex sector echocardiography in evaluation of the right atrium in patients with mitral stenosis and atrial septal defect. Am J Cardiol, 42:733, 1978.
15. Friedberg, CK: Diseases of the Heart. Philadelphia, Saunders, 1966.
16. Hurst, JW: The Heart. New York, McGraw-Hill, 1978.
17. Perloff, JK: The Clinical Recognition of Congenital Heart Disease. Philadelphia, Saunders, 1978.
18. Diamond, MA, et al.: Echocardiographic features of atrial septal defect. Circulation, 43:129, 1971.
19. McCann, WD, Harbold, NB, and Giuliani, BR: The echocardiogram in right ventricular overload. JAMA, 221:1243, 1972.
20. Tajik, AJ, Gau, GT, Ritter, D, and Schattenberg, TT: Echocardiographic pattern of right ventricular diastolic volume overload in children. Circulation, 46:36, 1972.
21. Pernod, J, Terdjman, M, Kermarec, J, and Haguenauer, G: Myocardial contraction. Study by ultrasonic echography (results in 200 normal patients). Nouv Presse Med, 2:2393, 1973.
22. Matsumoto, M: Ultrasonic features of interatrial

septum: its motion analysis and detection of its defect. Jpn Circ J, 37:1383, 1973.

23. Nimura, Y, et al.: Interatrial septum in ultrasonocardiotomogram and ultrasoundcardiogram. Med Ultrasonics, 9:58, 1971.

24. Seward, JB, Tajik, AJ, Spangler, JG, and Ritter, DG: Echocardiographic contrast studies: initial experience. Mayo Clin Proc, 50:163, 1975.

25. Weyman, AE, et al.: Negative contrast echocardiography: a new method for detecting left-to-right shunts. Circulation, 59:498, 1979.

26. Valdes-Cruz, LM, Pieroni, DR, Roland, JM, and Varghese, PJ: Echocardiographic detection of right-to-left shunts following peripheral vein injections. Circulation, 54:558, 1976.

27. Dow, JW, and Dexter, L: Circulatory dynamics in atrial septal defect. J Clin Invest, 29:809, 1950.

28. Dexter, L: Atrial septal defect. Br Heart J, 18:209, 1956.

29. Hull, E: Cause and effects of flow through defects of atrial septum. Am Heart J, 38:350, 1949.

30. Mathew, R, Thilenius, OG, and Arcilla, RA: Comparative responses of right and left ventricles to volume overload. Am J Cardiol, 38:209, 1974.

31. Rowe, GG, et al.: Atrial septal defect and the mechanism of shunt. Am Heart J, 61:369, 1961.

32. Pearlman, AJ, et al.: Determinants of ventricular septal motion. Circulation, 54:84, 1976.

33. Kerber, RE, Dippel, WF, and Abbound, FM: Abnormal motion of the interventricular septum in right ventricular volume overload. Experimental and clinical echocardiographic studies. Circulation, 48:86, 1973.

34. Lieppe, W, Scallion, R, Behar, VS, and Kisslo, JA: Two-dimensional echocardiographic findings in atrial septal defect. Circulation, 56:447, 1977.

35. Schreiber, TL, Weyman, AE, Feigenbaum, H, and Stewart, J: Effects of atrial septal defect repair on left ventricular geometry and degree of mitral valve prolapse. Circulation, 61:888, 1980.

36. Williams, RG, and Bierman, FZ: Evaluation of balloon atrial septostomy by subxiphoid two-dimensional echocardiography. Am J Cardiol, 43:401, 1979.

37. Freedom, R, and Rowe, R: Aneurysm of the atrial septum in tricuspid atresia: diagnosis during life. Am J Cardiol, 38:265, 1976.

38. Sahn, DJ, Allen, HD, Anderson, R, and Goldberg, SJ: Echocardiographic diagnosis of atrial septal aneurysm in an infant with hypoplastic right heart syndrome. Chest, 73:227, 1978.

39. Goor, OA, Edwards, JE, and Lillehei, CW: The development of the interventricular septum of the human heart: correlative morphogenetic study. Chest, 58:453, 1970.

40. Hagan, AD, et al.: Ultrasound evaluation of systolic anterior septal motion in patients with and without right ventricular volume overload. Circulation, 50:248, 1974.

41. Corya, BC, et al.: Systolic thickening and thinning of the septum and posterior wall in patients with coronary artery disease, congestive car-

diomyopathy, and atrial septal defect. Circulation, 55:109, 1977.

42. Kerber, RE, Marcus, ML, Ehrhardt, J, and Abbound, FM: Effect of increases in afterload on the systolic thickening of acutely ischemic myocardium: an experimental echocardiographic study. Acta Med Scand, 205(627):142, 1978.

43. Kerber, RE, Martins, JB, and Marcus, ML: Effect of acute ischemia, nitroglycerin and nitroprusside on regional myocardial thickening, stress and perfusion. Circulation, 60:121, 1979.

44. Henry, WL, Clark, CE, and Epstein, SE: Asymmetric septal hypertrophy: the unifying link in the IHSS disease spectrum: observations regarding its pathogenesis, pathophysiology and course. Circulation, 47:827, 1973.

45. Henry, WL, Clark, CE, and Epstein, SE: Asymmetric septal hypertrophy: echocardiographic identification of the pathognomonic anatomic abnormality of IHSS. Circulation, 47:225, 1973.

46. Maron, BJ, and Epstein, SE: Hypertrophic cardiomyopathy: recent observations regarding the specificity of three hallmarks of the disease: asymmetric septal hypertrophy, septal disorganization and systolic anterior motion of the anterior mitral leaflet. Am J Cardiol, 45:141, 1980.

47. Rasmussen, S, Corya, BC, Feigenbaum, H, and Knoebel, SB: Detection of myocardial scar tissue by M-mode echocardiography. Circulation, 57:230, 1978.

48. Garrison, JB, et al.: Quantifying regional wall motion and thickening in two-dimensional echocardiography with a computer. Aided contouring system. In Proceedings of Computers in Cardiology. Edited by H Ostrow and K Ripley. Long Beach, CA, IEEE, 1977.

49. Rossen, RM, Goodman, DJ, Ingham, RE, and Popp, RL: Ventricular septal thickening and excursion in idiopathic hypertrophic subaortic stenosis. Circulation, 50:29, 1974.

50. Smith, ER, and Flemington, CS: Systolic muscle thickening and excursion in patients with asymmetric septal hypertrophy. Circulation, 52:141, 1975.

51. Feigenbaum, H: Echocardiography. Philadelphia, Lea & Febiger, 1976.

52. Kerber, RE, et al.: Correlation between echocardiographically demonstrated segmental dyskinesis and regional myocardial perfusion. Circulation, 52:1097, 1975.

53. Kerber, RE, and Duty, D: Abnormalities of interventricular septal motion following cardiac surgery. Cross-sectional echocardiographic studies. Am J Cardiol, 41:372, 1978.

54. Lieppe, W, Scallion, R, Behar, VS, and Kisslo, JA: Two-dimensional echocardiographic findings in atrial septal defect. Circulation, 56:447, 1977.

55. Brinker, JA, et al.: Leftward septal displacement during right ventricular loading in man. Circulation, 61:626, 1980.

56. Weyman, AE, et al.: Mechanism of paradoxical early diastolic septal motion in patients with mitral stenosis: a cross-sectional echocardiographic study. Am J Cardiol, 40:691, 1977.

57. Taylor, RR, Covell, JW, Sonnenblick, EH, Ross, J: Dependence of ventricular distensibility on filling of the opposite ventricle. Am J Physiol, 213:711, 1967.

58. McDonald, IG: Echocardiographic demonstration of abnormal motion of the interventricular septum in left bundle branch block. Circulation, 48:272, 1973.

59. Dillon, JC, Chang, S, and Feigenbaum, H: Echocardiographic manifestations of left bundle branch block. Circulation, 49:876, 1974.

60. Keith, JD, Rowe, RD, and Vlad, P: Heart Disease in Infancy and Childhood. New York, Macmillan, 1978.

61. Beca, LM, et al.: Anatomic and pathologic studies in ventricular septal defect. Circulation, 14:349, 1956.

62. Saab, NG, Burchell, HB, DuShane, JW, and Titus, JL: Muscular ventricular septal defects. Am J Cardiol, 18:713, 1966.

63. Perloff, JH: The clinical recognition of congenital heart disease. Philadelphia, Saunders, 1970.

64. Cheatham, JP, Latson, LA, and Gutgesell, HP: Ventricular septal defect in infancy: detection by two-dimensional echocardiography. Circulation, 60(II):112, 1979.

65. Bierman, FZ, and Williams, RG: Prospective diagnosis of ventricular septal defects in infants by subxyphoid two-dimensional echocardiography. Circulation, 60(II):112, 1979.

66. Seward, JB, Tajik, AJ, Hagler, DJ, and Mair, DD: Visualization of isolated ventricular septal defect by wide-angle two-dimensional sector echocardiography. Circulation, 58(II):202, 1978.

67. Canale, JM, et al.: Factors affecting real-time cross-sectional echocardiographic imaging of perimembranous ventricular septal defects. Circulation, 63:689, 1981.

68. Selzer, A: Defect of the ventricular septum: summary of twelve cases and review of the literature. Arch Intern Med, 84:798, 1949.

69. Caldwell, RL, et al.: Right ventricular outflow tract assessment by cross-sectional echocardiography in tetralogy of Fallot. Circulation, 59:395, 1979.

70. Freedom, RM, et al.: The natural history of the so-called aneurysm of the membranous ventricular septum in childhood. Circulation, 49:375, 1974.

71. Hoffman, JIE, and Rudolph, AM: The natural history of ventricular septal defects in infancy. Am J Cardiol, 16:634, 1965.

72. Bloomfield, K: The natural history of ventricular septal defects in patients surviving infancy. Circulation, 29:914, 1964.

73. Lambert, ME, et al.: Natural history of ventricular septal defects associated with ventricular septal aneurysms. Am Heart J, 88:566, 1974.

74. Varghese, PJ, and Rowe, RD: Spontaneous closure of ventricular septal defects by aneurysmal formation of the membranous septum. J Pediatr, 75:700, 1969.

75. Miora, KP, et al.: Aneurysm of the membranous ventricular septum: a mechanism for spontaneous closure of ventricular septal defect. N Engl J Med, 283:58, 1970.

76. Van Mierop, LHS, Alley, RD, Kausel, HW, and Stanahan, A: The anatomy and embryology of endocardial cushion defects. J Thorac Cardiovasc Surg, 53:71, 1962.

77. Campbell, M, and Missen, GAK: Endocardial cushion defects. Common atrioventricular canal and ostium primum. Br Heart J, 19:403, 1957.

78. Rastelli, G, Kirklin, JW, and Titus, JL: Anatomic observations on complete form of persistent common atrioventricular canal with special reference to atrioventricular valves. Mayo Clin Proc, 41:296, 1966.

79. Hagler, DJ, et al.: Real-time wide-angle sector echocardiography: atrioventricular canal defects. Circulation, 59:140, 1978.

80. Newfeld, HN, et al.: Isolated ventricular septal defect of the persistent common atrioventricular canal type. Circulation, 23:685, 1961.

Chapter 13

Complex Congenital Heart Disease—
A Diagnostic Approach

The evaluation of the patient with complex congenital heart disease is one of the most challenging and rewarding areas in cross-sectional echocardiography. The echocardiographer's approach to these patients should be like the clinician's approach to the physical examination in that the echocardiographic examination must be conducted in an organized and orderly fashion. The precise sequence in which the examination is conducted is not as important as are the presence of order and the compilation of sufficient data to answer all of the relevant diagnostic questions. Without such an organized approach, even the most experienced observer frequently becomes fascinated by one or two striking abnormalities and fails to record all the information necessary to describe completely the anatomic and functional characteristics of a particular lesion.

This chapter describes an approach we have found helpful in examining these patients. With this method, the examination is conducted to answer a series of questions. These questions are directed toward determining (1) ventricular number, size, orientation, and identity; (2) great vessel orientation and identity; (3) the pattern by which the great vessels are connected to the ventricular chambers; (4) the presence and direction of intracardiac shunts; and (5) the presence, location, and severity of outflow obstruction.

The information necessary to answer these questions is contained in views that are comparable to the standard imaging planes. In the patient with complex congenital heart disease, however, the primary cardiac structures used to align these planes may be far removed from their normal position or relationships, and the appearance and identity of structures within these views may be greatly dissimilar to those that are normally encountered. Therefore, here more than in any other circumstance, these planes must be aligned relative to specific intracardiac structures rather than to groups of structures or external references.

The relative importance of individual examining planes is also significantly different from their importance in the routine examination and differs still further depending on whether an adult or child is studied. In the routine examination, for example, the majority of information is obtained from the parasternal long-axis view. In the patient with complex congenital heart disease, in contrast, the parasternal short-axis, apical four-chamber, and subcostal views provide more information. In the adult, the parasternal short-axis and apical four-chamber views, which define the orientation of the interventricular septum, AV valve structure, and great vessel orientation, are of primary importance, whereas in the child, almost the entire examination can usually be recorded from the subcostal transducer location. Despite these generalities, standard views, as a rule, are less meaningful when examining the malformed, malpositioned heart, and for this reason, the examination is directed toward answering specific questions rather than toward obtaining a series of routine views.

VENTRICULAR NUMBER, SIZE, ORIENTATION, AND IDENTITY

Is there an interventricular septum?

The first goal in examining the patient with complex congenital heart disease is to determine whether there is one ventricular chamber or two separate ventricular chambers. This is determined by the presence or absence of an interventricular septum. The normal interventricular septum is best visualized in the parasternal short-axis, apical four-chamber, and subcostal long- and short-axis views (see Chap. 12). The same views are used in the patient with complex congenital disease to confirm or exclude the presence of a septum.

Figure 13–1 compares the appearance and orientation of the interventricular septum in the normal biventricular heart to the single large chamber and the complete

absence of septum, which characterize the single ventricle. In both the apical four-chamber and subcostal long-axis views, the interatrial septum helps to define the expected point of insertion and orientation of the interventricular septum and further highlights the absence of this structure. On occasion, as illustrated in Figure 13–1, *F*, single or multiple large papillary muscles may give the appearance of a rudimentary septum, particularly in the subcostal long-axis view. These papillary muscles can be distinguished from a rudimentary septum in short axis by the demonstration of ventricular cavity surrounding the papillary muscle head. It might also be expected that chordal origin could be used to differentiate a papillary muscle from septum. However, this differential point may be misleading because, in certain disorders, such as the atrioventricular canal, chordae may arise directly from the interventricular septum.

In some patients, a rudimentary muscular shelf can be observed extending outward from the ventricular wall in a position that, if further extended, would roughly bisect the large ventricular chamber. Figure 13–2 illustrates the short-axis appearance of such a muscular shelf. These rudimentary septa are important anatomically because they differentiate the biventricular heart with a large ventricular septal defect from a single ventricle. From a functional standpoint, however, these rudimentary septa appear to have little significance.[1]

Finally, when confronted with a single ventricle, one must determine whether an outflow chamber is present.[1,2] These outflow chambers represent the infundibular portion of the right ventricle and, when the great vessels are transposed, are always found at the base of the anteriorly positioned aorta. In the uncommon situation in which the great vessels are normally oriented, the outflow chamber will be associated with the anterior pulmonary artery.[1] Figure 13–3 illustrates the appear-

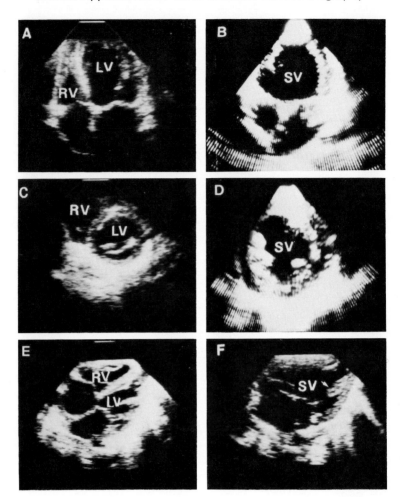

Fig. 13–1. Series of recordings compares the appearance and orientation of the interventricular septum of the normal biventricular heart with the single, large chamber and complete absence of the septum, which characterize the single ventricle (SV). *A,* Apical four-chamber recording illustrates the division of the normal heart into two separate ventricles by the interventricular septum. *B,* Apical four-chamber view of a single ventricle. There is no septum and only one large chamber. *C,* Normal appearance of the two ventricles and interventricular septum in the parasternal short-axis view. *D,* Large, circular, single ventricle in short-axis view. *E,* Subcostal long-axis (four-chamber) views of a normal heart. *F,* Subcostal long-axis recording of a single ventricle in which a large papillary muscle arises from the posterolateral ventricular wall (oblique arrow). LV = left ventricle; RV = right ventricle.

ance of an outflow chamber at the base of the anteriorly positioned aorta in a patient with a single ventricle and transposition of the great vessels.

What is the relative size of the two ventricles, and are they both morphologically intact?

Once the presence of two ventricular chambers has been established, the next step is to determine their relative size and structural integrity. Normally, the two ventricles are approximately equal in size. Marked disproportion in ventricular size may occur because the larger ventricle is subject to an abnormal volume load, because flow into the smaller ventricle is obstructed, or because the smaller ventricle is hypoplastic. Figure 13–4 compares the appearance of the left and right ventricles of three infants younger than 2 months in age. Panel *A* is recorded from a normal infant and illustrates the appropriate size

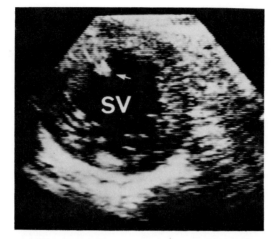

Fig. 13–2. Parasternal short-axis view records a single large ventricular chamber (SV) with a rudimentary interventricular septum arising from the ventricular wall at roughly the 11:00 position (horizontal arrow).

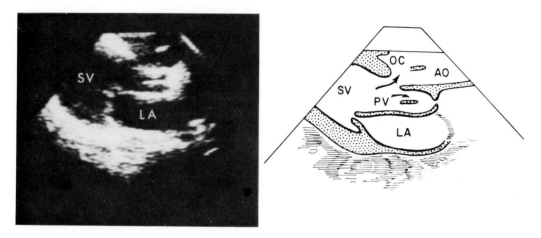

Fig. 13–3. Parasternal long-axis recording from a patient with a single ventricle and D-transposition of the great vessels illustrates the appearance of a subaortic outflow chamber. The longer curved arrow illustrates the path of blood flow from the single ventricle (SV) into the anteriorly positioned aorta (AO). The apparent abrupt termination of the posteriorly positioned pulmonary artery is due to a pulmonary artery band positioned just above the pulmonary valve (PV). OC = outflow chamber; LA = left atrium.

and configuration of the left and right ventricles. In panel B, the left ventricle is much smaller than the right, and the interventricular septum is displaced posteriorly. The aortic root is also considerably smaller than normal. In this example, the decrease in left ventricular size was the result of reduced left ventricular inflow because of a supravalvular membrane or cor triatriatum. Panel C is a recording from a patient with a hypoplastic left ventricle with as-sociated mitral and aortic hypoplasia. The size of the left ventricle in panels B and C is below the lower limit of normal for a patient of such age, and because the obstructing membrane in the patient with cor triatriatum cannot be appreciated in this view, it was initially questioned whether this might not also be an example of a hypoplastic left heart. A truly hypoplastic left ventricle, however, can usually be differentiated from a ventricle that is abnor-

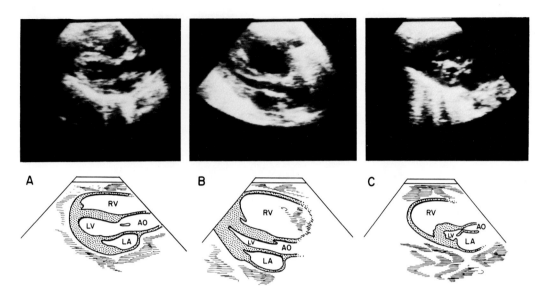

Fig. 13–4. Parasternal long-axis recordings of the left (LV) and right (RV) ventricles from (A) a normal infant, (B) an infant with a marked reduction in left ventricular size due to right ventricular volume overload and obstructed left ventricular inflow, and (C) an infant with a hypoplastic left ventricle. AO = aorta; LA = left atrium.

mally small because of reduced inflow or compression by a dilated right ventricle by examining atrioventricular valve structure. In the hypoplastic ventricle, the associated atrioventricular valve is characteristically smaller, structurally deformed, and moves poorly, if at all. In the morphologically normal ventricle, the atrioventricular valve is normally formed and typically moves freely despite the reduced ventricular size and/or limited inflow from the left atrium. Figure 13–5 is a comparable example of the hypoplastic right ventricle and fixed immobile tricuspid valve of tricuspid atresia. In this example, the interatrial septum is absent, and hence, there is a common atrium.

How are the ventricles positioned in the chest?

The position of the ventricles within the thorax and their relationship to one another may vary widely in patients with complex congenital heart disease. The spatial relationship of the ventricles is best defined in the parasternal short-axis view. This view permits both the relationship of the ventricles to one another and, by noting the position of the transducer and path of the scan plane during the recording, their position within the chest to be defined.

Which is the morphologic right and which is the morphologic left ventricle?

In many instances in which the ventricles are malpositioned or ventricular inversion is suspected, one must determine which is the morphologic right ventricle and which is the morphologic left ventricle. Normally, the ventricles are differentiated by their position, their shape, and the thickness of their muscular walls. In complex congenital heart disease, however, all these features may be misleading. In Figure 13–6, A, for example, there is a large, circular, anterior ventricle and a smaller, flat, posterior ventricle. The walls of both ventricles are thick, and the septum, in real time, appeared to contract with the anterior ventricle. The identity of these ventricles can be established by determining which ventricle contains the mitral valve and which contains the tricuspid valve because the mitral valve is always associated with the anatomic left ventricle

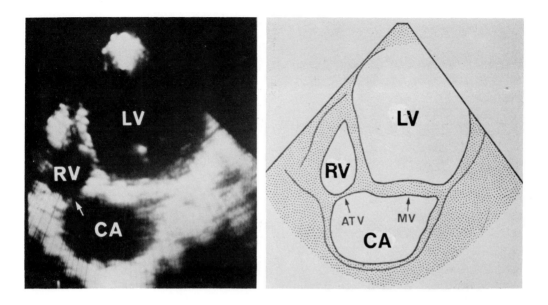

Fig. 13–5. Apical four-chamber view illustrates tricuspid atresia. The left ventricle (LV) is dilated, and the right ventricle (RV) is small. During diastole, tricuspid valve movement was not apparent, whereas the mitral valve orifice (MV) was large. Interatrial septum was not present. ATV = atretic tricuspid valve, CA = common atrium. The vertical white arrow points to the tricuspid valve.

and the tricuspid valve with the anatomic right ventricle.

Four features distinguish the tricuspid valve and anatomic right ventricle from the mitral valve and associated left ventricle. The simplest method for distinguishing the mitral valve from the tricuspid valve is to determine the number of leaflets the valve contains. (The tricuspid valve normally has three leaflets, whereas the normal mitral valve has only two.)[3,4] Figure 13–6, B, illustrates this leaflet structure. The atrioventricular valve associated with the anterior ventricle, in this example, has three distinct leaflets and, therefore, must be an anatomic tricuspid valve. The posterior valve is not as well visualized but, by exclusion, can be assumed to be the mitral valve. By this simple method, the anterior ventricle can be determined with surety to be the anatomic right ventricle, whereas the posterior ventricle then becomes the anatomic left ventricle. Thus, if either the mitral or tricus-

pid valves can be visualized and if the number of leaflets in that valve can be determined, the identity of the second atrioventricular valve and associated ventricle can be inferred. Confusion occasionally arises when there is a cleft mitral valve; however, in these instances, there are still only two commissures and the systolic configuration is that of an anatomic mitral valve.

Figure 13–7 is a second example in which the two atrioventricular valves are side by side and no interventricular septum is recorded. In this example, the left-sided atrioventricular valve has three clearly defined commissures and, therefore, is the anatomic tricuspid valve, whereas the right-sided valve has only two commissures and, therefore, is the mitral valve. (In this example, right and left are used to refer to the patient's rather than the viewer's right and left). By identifying atrioventricular valve structure, the ventricles in this example can be determined to be inverted.

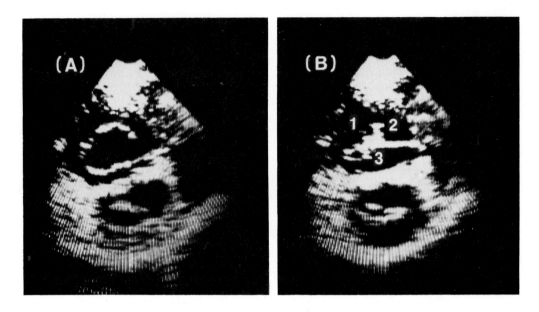

Fig. 13–6. Parasternal short-axis scans of a biventricular heart. *A,* A large circular anterior ventricle and a smaller, flattened posterior ventricle. The walls of both ventricles are thick, and in this diastolic frame, both atrioventricular valves are open. *B,* During systole, the trileaflet tricuspid valve can be observed within the anterior ventricle (1,2,3). It can thereby be confirmed that the anterior ventricle is the morphologic right ventricle, and the posterior ventricle must be the anatomic left ventricle.

The second method for identifying the atrioventricular valves is through their relative level of insertion into the interventricular septum. The septal leaflet of the tricuspid valve normally inserts slightly inferior (apical) (5 to 10 mm) to the insertion of the anterior mitral leaflet.[5] This occurs because the mitral atrioventricular groove is normally slightly superior to the tricuspid groove. The anterior leaflet of the mitral valve, therefore, inserts into the left atrioventricular sulcus near the superior end of the membranous septum, whereas the septal leaflet of the tricuspid valve inserts near the midportion of the membranous septum.[5]

Figure 13–8 illustrates the relative points of septal insertion of the mitral and tricuspid valves in the normal patient (A) and in a patient with ventricular inversion (B). The relative position of leaflet insertion is frequently easier to define than the number of valve leaflets and is not affected by a cleft mitral valve.[6] When the tricuspid valve inserts more than 10 mm inferior to the mitral valve, Ebstein's anomaly should be considered.

The third feature that differentiates the morphologic right and left ventricles is the number and orientation of the papillary muscles associated with each chamber. The anatomic left ventricle usually has two papillary muscles of relatively equal size that arise from the medial and lateral walls of the ventricle at the junction of the apical and middle thirds of the chamber. These muscles lie parallel with, and slightly below, the line of mitral leaflet coaptation. The right ventricle, in contrast, normally contains three papillary muscles that vary in size and site of origin. Figure 13–9 compares the two-papillary-muscle configuration of the anatomic left ventricle to the three papillary muscles that typify the anatomic right ventricle.

The final feature that distinguishes the

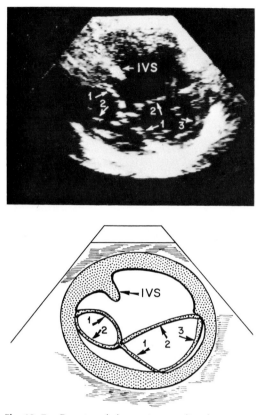

Fig. 13–7. Parasternal short-axis recording from a patient with a large ventricular septal defect and ventricular inversion. The left-sided AV valve in this example (the valve to the viewer's right) has three distinct leaflets and commissures, indicating that this valve is a tricuspid valve. The right ventricle, therefore, is to the patient's left. The right-sided atrioventricular valve (the valve to the viewer's left) is a two-leaflet or mitral valve, and the chamber to the patient's right (the viewer's left) is the anatomic left ventricle. IVS = interventricular septum.

anatomic right ventricle is the large muscular moderator band.[6] The moderator band is found only in the right ventricle where it stretches from the lower interventricular septum to the anterior right ventricular wall at which point it joins the base of the anterior papillary muscle. The moderator band, within an inverted right ventricle, can be appreciated in Figure 13–8, *B*.

GREAT VESSEL ORIENTATION AND IDENTITY

Are the great vessels normally related or transposed?

The second step in evaluating a patient

with complex congenital heart disease is to determine the orientation and identity of the great vessels. Customarily, great vessel orientation is defined first because, if the vessels are normally oriented, their identity can be presumed. Normally oriented vessels cross obliquely as they exit from the right and left ventricles. The right ventricular outflow tract lies anterior to the aorta and intersects it at approximately a 45-degree angle. After crossing the aorta, it then curves posteriorly as the main pulmonary artery and continues posteriorly and superiorly to its point of bifurcation into the right and left pulmonary arteries. These normal relationships are best illustrated in the subcostal long-axis view of the right ventricular outflow tract (Fig. 13–10). Because the great vessels normally cross at their origin, an imaging plane aligned parallel to the short axis of one great vessel is, of necessity, oblique to the short axis or more closely parallel to the long axis of the other crossing vessel.[7] The vessel that the imaging plane transects parallel to its short axis appears circular by definition, whereas the vessel that is transected obliquely appears as an elongated oval or has a more "sausage-like" shape.[7] Similarly, if the plane is oriented parallel to the long axis of one vessel, it must be oblique to the short axis of the other. Thus, as illustrated in Figure 13–10, a plane passing through the long axis of the right ventricular outflow tract and pulmonary artery is slightly oblique to the short axis of the aorta when these vessels cross normally.

When the great vessels are transposed, they maintain a parallel orientation as they leave the heart. When vessels are parallel, any plane that is oriented such that it passes through the short axis of one vessel must, of necessity, be parallel to the short axis of the second.[5] Both the aorta and pulmonary artery therefore appear circular in short axis when the vessels exit the heart in a parallel fashion.[7–10] Figure 13–11, *A* through *C*, illustrates this double-circle

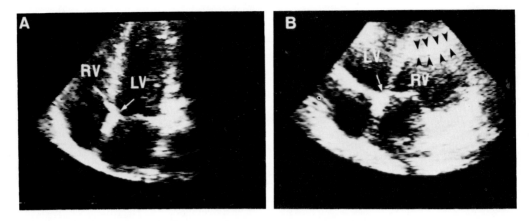

Fig. 13–8. Apical four-chamber views illustrate normal ventricular orientation (*A*) and ventricular inversion (*B*). Differentiation of the right (RV) and left ventricles (LV) can be achieved by determining the identity of the tricuspid and mitral valves. The septal leaflet of the tricuspid valve has an apical or inferior point of insertion into the ventricular septum, relative to the insertion point of the mitral valve. The superior insertion point of the mitral valve is indicated by the oblique arrow in panel *A*. When the ventricles are inverted (*B*), the mitral valve and anatomic left ventricle reverse their position, and the right-sided AV valve then has a relatively superior point of insertion into the interventricular septum (oblique arrow, *B*).

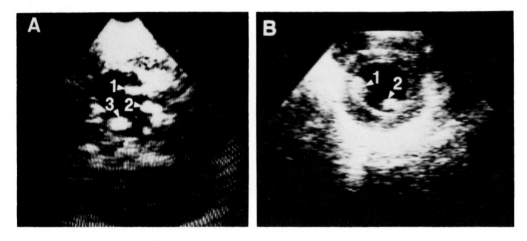

Fig. 13–9. Short-axis scans illustrate the characteristic three-papillary-muscle configuration of the right ventricle (*A*) and the two papillary muscles, which typify the left ventricle (*B*).

appearance of the transposed vessels in patients with D-transposition (*A*), L-transposition (*B*), and double-outlet right ventricle (*C*). Although the double-circle configuration can be uniformly demonstrated in patients with transposition of the great vessels, a similar configuration can, on occasion, be produced in patients with normally crossing great vessels. Figure 13–12 illustrates two examples in which normally crossing great vessels are recorded such that they both appear circular. Panel

A is a recording from a patient with primary pulmonary hypertension in whom the pulmonary artery is dilated and is significantly larger than the aorta. When the imaging plane was aligned parallel to the short axis of the pulmonary artery, a configuration looking much like D-transposition of the great vessels was produced. Figure 13–12, *B*, is a second example in which the short-axis great vessel appearance looks similar to that of L-transposition. In this example, the origin of the great

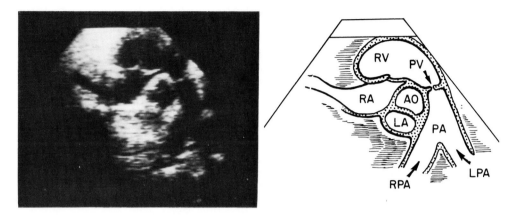

Fig. 13–10. Subcostal long-axis recording of the right ventricular outflow tract illustrates the normal crossing pattern of the great vessels. The pulmonary artery (PA), viewed in the long axis, crosses the aorta (AO) and then sweeps posteriorly to its bifurcation into the left (LPA) and right pulmonary arteries (RPA). Because the vessels cross at their origin, the same plane transects the aorta oblique to its short axis, and this vessel appears roughly circular. RV = right ventricle; PV = pulmonary valve; RA = right atrium; LA = left atrium.

vessels was also normal, and the vessel that is anterior and to the left is the pulmonary artery. When the examination is easily performed and the pulmonary artery and aorta are readily identified, these patterns cause little confusion. In limited examinations, however, they may lead to incorrect diagnoses. In such situations, the observation that the anterior vessel is the pulmonary artery makes the presence of one of the transposition complexes unlikely.

The final great vessel pattern is produced by the truncus arteriosus. When a truncus is present, orientation of the short-axis imaging plane through the base of the ventricle results in the display of a single, large, circular vessel. Figure 13–13 illustrates the appearance of the truncus arteriosus in both the long-axis and parasternal short-axis views.

Figure 13–14 summarizes the different short-axis configurations of the great vessels. In the left-hand panel, the normally crossing vessels are oriented such that when the imaging plane is aligned parallel to the short axis of the aorta, it must be oblique to the short axis of the pulmonary artery or must more closely approximate its long axis. The aorta, therefore, appears circular, whereas the pulmonary artery

looks like an oval or curved cylinder crossing anteriorly above the aorta. The center panel depicts the configuration observed when the great vessels exit the heart in a parallel or transposed orientation. Here, the imaging plane is parallel to the short axis of both the aorta and the pulmonary artery, and thus, they both appear circular. Finally, the right-hand panel illustrates the single large circular vessel characteristic of the truncus arteriosus.[7]

In the less common situation in which the examining plane can be passed directly through the long axes of both great vessels, their parallel orientation can be directly defined. Figure 13–15 illustrates this parallel orientation in both the parasternal long-axis (A) and subcostal long-axis (B) views. In A, there is a large anterior aorta and a slightly smaller posterior pulmonary artery. The aorta originates from the anterior ventricular chamber and the pulmonary artery from the posterior chamber. The larger aorta courses more superiorly into the neck and, by varying the imaging plane, can be observed to give rise to the neck vessels. The smaller posterior vessel appears to terminate more quickly and, by following its branching pattern in short axis, could be identified as the pulmonary artery. Panel B is an example of a

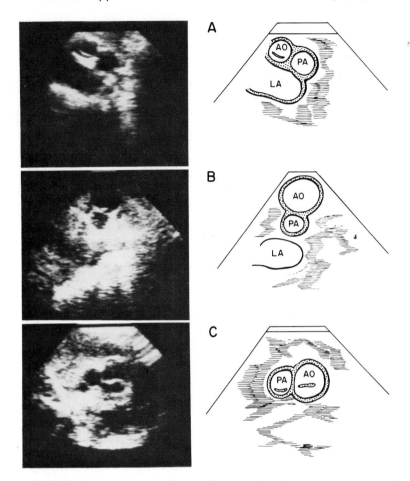

Fig. 13–11. Parasternal short-axis recordings illustrate the typical double-circle appearance of the great vessels when they leave the heart parallel to one another. *A,* A recording from a patient with a D-transposition of the great vessels in which the anterior aorta is positioned to the patient's right. *B,* An example of an L-transposition in which the anterior aorta is to the patient's left. *C,* An example of a double-outlet right ventricle in which the two great vessels lie side by side. AO = aorta; PA = pulmonary artery; LA = left atrium.

double-outlet right ventricle with an L-loop in which both great vessels exit from the left-sided ventricle, which is the anatomic right ventricle. Here, again, the parallel orientation of the great vessels (with the two semilunar valves positioned at an identical level) confirms that the great vessels are transposed.

If there are two great vessels, which is the aorta and which is the pulmonary artery?

Once the relationship of the great vessels has been defined, the examiner must then determine which is the aorta and which is the pulmonary artery. When the great vessels cross at their origin, the anterior vessel is always the pulmonary artery and the posterior vessel is always the aorta. When the great vessels are transposed and one vessel is anterior to the other, the anterior vessel is almost invariably the aorta, and the posterior vessel, the pulmonary artery. When the great vessels lie beside one another, as illustrated in Figure 13–16, *A,* identification of the aorta and pulmonary artery may be more difficult. When there is a question, the great vessels can be identified by following their course superiorly and observing their branching patterns and distribu-

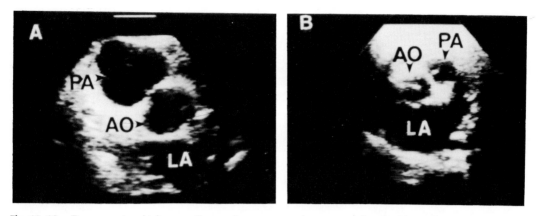

Fig. 13–12. Two cases in which normally crossing great vessels present with a double-circle configuration that might be confused for transposition. *A,* The anterior vessel is positioned to the patient's right and simulates D-transposition. *B,* The anterior vessel is to the left, simulating an L-transposition. In each case, however, the anterior vessel is the pulmonary artery (PA), which makes the diagnosis of transposition highly unlikely. AO = aorta; LA = left atrium.

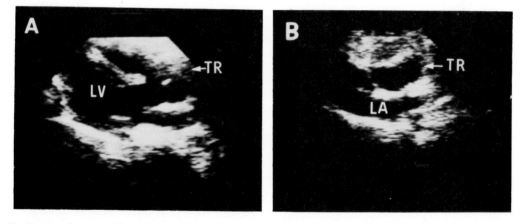

Fig. 13–13. Parasternal long- (*A*) and short-axis (*B*) views of a patient with truncus arteriosus (TR). In the parasternal long-axis view (*A*), a single, large vessel overrides a large ventricular septal defect. In short axis (*B*), the vessel appears as a single large circle without evidence of either a second parallel vessel or an anterior crossing vessel. LA = left atrium.

tion.[11] The vessel that courses posteriorly into the thorax and bifurcates is always the pulmonary artery, whereas the vessel that courses into the neck and gives off multiple branches to the upper extremities is always the aorta.[11]

Figure 13–16, *B* and *C,* illustrates the characteristic features of the aorta and pulmonary artery in the parasternal long-axis view. In *B,* the larger of the two transposed vessels can be observed to curve anteriorly and to continue toward the neck. If the scan is continued superiorly, branches to the upper extremities can be identified. The anterior path and superior extension of this vessel suggest that it is the aorta. In addition, the left pulmonary artery can be visualized just superior to the left atrium, crossing beneath the larger aorta. In *C,* the scan plane has been aligned parallel to the long axis of the smaller vessel. At its origin, there is stenosis of the semilunar valve and an additional area of supravalvular narrowing. Distal to the area of stenosis, the vessel dilates transiently and then appears to end abruptly. This ap-

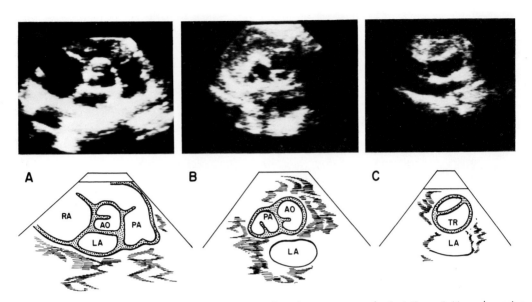

Fig. 13–14. Parasternal short-axis recordings summarize the primary great vessel orientations. *A*, Normal crossing pattern. The aorta (AO) appears as a single circle, and the cylindric pulmonary artery (PA) courses above and to the right of the aortic root. *B*, Transposed great vessels in which both the aorta (AO) and the pulmonary artery (PA) are transected parallel to their short axes and, therefore, appear circular. *C*, The single large circle that characterizes the truncus arteriosus (TR). LA = left atrium; RA = right atrium.

parent point of vessel termination actually represents the bifurcation of a pulmonary artery and illustrates a second general rule: when the scan plane is aligned such that it follows the long axis of transposed great vessels superiorly, the vessel that appears to end first is the pulmonary artery.

The course and branching pattern of the great vessels can frequently be better visualized from the subcostal transducer location than from the anterior chest wall. Figure 13–17 contrasts the appearance of a normal aortic arch arising from the left-sided ventricle (*A*) with that of a left-sided or transposed pulmonary artery in a patient with D-transposition of the great vessels (*B*). The normal aorta courses leftward in a gradual arc after leaving the left-sided ventricle and gives off several small branches to the upper extremities. The pulmonary artery (*B*), in contrast, follows a straighter path and bifurcates after several centimeters into two large vessels of approximately equal size.

VENTRICULAR-GREAT VESSEL RELATIONSHIPS

How are the great vessels and ventricles connected?

The third step in approaching the patient with complex congenital heart disease is to define the interrelationship of the ventricles and the great vessels. The relationship of the great vessels to the ventricular chambers is defined relative to the plane of the interventricular septum. There are two general methods for determining the relationship of the great vessels to the septal plane: the short-axis approach, in which the short-axis orientation of the septum and great vessels relative to the transducer are compared,[12] and the long-axis method, in which the scan plane is simultaneously directed through the long axes of both great vessels and the septum. In the short-axis approach, the short-axis plane of the interventricular septum is first defined. Without changing the orientation of the scan plane, the transducer is then angled superiorly to determine the spatial

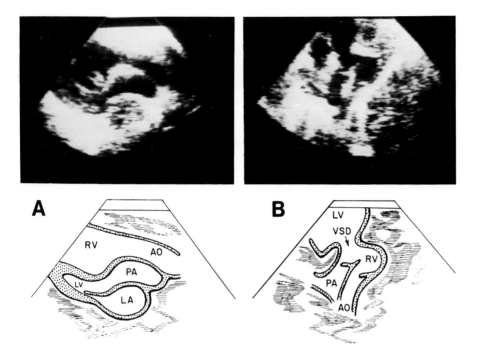

Fig. 13–15. Parasternal and subcostal long-axis views of parallel transposed great vessels recorded with the scan plane simultaneously directed through the long axis of both vessels. *A*, D-transposition with an anterior aorta (AO) and posterior parallel pulmonary artery (PA). *B*, Double-outlet right ventricle (RV) and ventricular inversion again illustrate the parallel orientation of the two great vessels as they exit from the left-sided cardiac chamber. LV = left ventricle; LA = left atrium; VSD = ventricular septal defect.

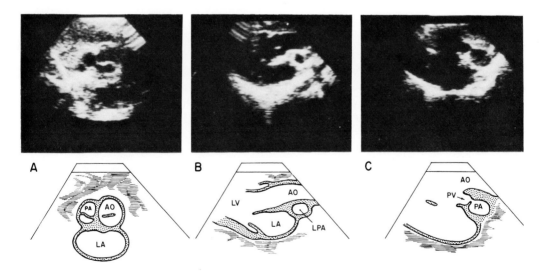

Fig. 13–16. *A*, Short-axis recording of transposed, side-by-side vessels. *B*, Long-axis recording demonstrates that the larger vessel courses anteriorly and superiorly toward the neck and therefore is the aorta (AO). This conclusion can further be confirmed by the presence of the left pulmonary artery (LPA) sweeping beneath this anterior vessel. *C*, Long-axis scan of the smaller vessel which angles posteriorly and bifurcates, thereby indicating that it is the pulmonary artery (PA). Systolic doming of the pulmonary valve (PV) and associated supravalvular narrowing are apparent. LV = left ventricle; LA = left atrium.

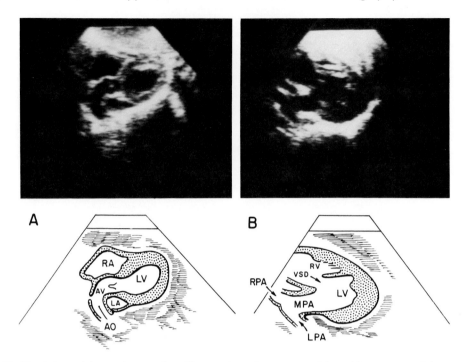

Fig. 13–17. Subcostal long-axis recordings illustrate how the course and branching patterns of the aorta and pulmonary artery can be used to identify these vessels. *A,* The aorta (AO) arises normally from the left ventricle (LV) and then sweeps to the left, giving off smaller branches to the neck. *B,* Unlike the aorta, a transposed pulmonary artery courses directly superiorly and bifurcates into two branches of equal size. RPA = right pulmonary artery; LPA = left pulmonary artery; AV = aortic valve; LA = left atrium; RA = right atrium; MPA = main pulmonary artery; VSD = ventricular septal defect; RV = right ventricle.

orientation of the great vessels. The relationship of the great vessels to the septal plane can then be determined by marking the plane of the septum on the video screen,[12] superimposing photographic outlines of the septum and great vessels or simply scanning rapidly back and forth from one area to the other to visually establish their relative positions.

Figure 13–18 compares the most common septal-great vessel relationships. Diagram *A* depicts the normal pattern in which the great vessels cross at their origin, and the plane of the septum approximates the superior border of the aorta. The aorta, in this example, is positioned below the septal plane and the pulmonary artery above the plane of the septum. In *B* (tetralogy of Fallot), the great vessels cross normally at their origin, and the pulmonary artery is above the aorta. Because of aortic overriding, the septal plane lies well below the anterior margin of the aorta. In *C,* the double-outlet right ventricle, the great vessels are transposed; consequently, both appear circular in short axis and both originate from the right ventricle, anterior and to the right of the plane of the interventricular septum. In a double-outlet left ventricle, both great vessels would arise from the left ventricle or beneath the plane of the interventricular septum. The final example *(D)* illustrates the relationship of the great arteries to the septum in D-transposition. Here, again, the great vessels appear circular in short axis because they are transposed. The aorta in D-transposition is anterior to the plane of the interventricular septum and the pulmonary artery is posterior to the septal plane.

In the long-axis method, the scan plane is oriented such that it passes through the long axis of the great vessels and interventricular septum simultaneously and,

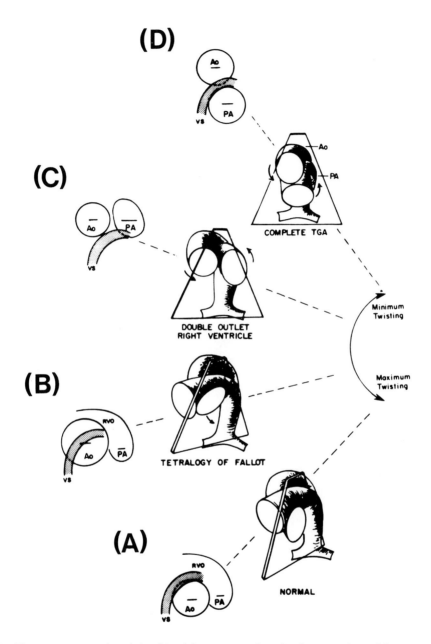

Fig. 13–18. Diagrams compare the relationship of the great vessels to the short-axis plane of the interventricular septum in the more common complex congenital anomalies. *A,* The normal pattern. The great vessels cross at their origin, and the septal plane is at roughly the same level as the anterior margin of the aorta. *B,* In tetralogy of Fallot, aortic overriding occurs, and the anterior margin of the aortic root is displaced above the plane of the septum. *C,* The double-outlet right ventricle in which the aorta and pulmonary artery are parallel and arise above the septal plane. *D,* In D-transposition of the great vessels, both vessels appear circular because they leave the heart parallel to one another. The septal plane is below the anterior aorta and above the posterior pulmonary artery. (From Henry, WL, et al.: Cross-sectional echocardiography in the diagnosis of congenital heart disease. Circulation, 56:267, 1977. Reproduced by permission of the American Heart Association.)

thereby, permits direct visualization of their relationship. Figure 13–19 illustrates three examples, recorded in the subcostal long-axis view, in which the relationship of the great vessels to the interventricular septum can be directly appreciated. In A, a single, large vessel straddles the plane of the septum at its origin and curves superiorly and leftward into the neck, thereby indicating that this vessel is the aorta. No pulmonary artery is evident. This example, which illustrates aortic overriding, was obtained from a patient with pulmonary atresia. In B, both great vessels are parallel as they leave the ventricles and, therefore, are transposed. The left-sided great vessel, which bifurcates in this example, is the pulmonary artery and arises totally to the left of the interventricular septum. The right-sided aorta, in contrast, originates from the right-sided ventricle. The septum is intact, and because the aorta is to the patient's right and the vessels are transposed, this pattern must represent D-transposition. In the final example (C), both great vessels again are parallel or transposed and both arise from the left-sided ventricular chamber. A defect in the interventricular septum is present, but both vessels are clearly positioned to the left of the septal plane. In this example, the ventricles are also inverted and, therefore, represent an example of a double-outlet right ventricle with an L-loop. Simultaneous visualization of the great vessels and septum obviously is the preferable method for determining the pattern in which they are connected. Unfortunately, the vessels are not always aligned such that these long-axis relationships can be recorded, and as a result, the short-axis method remains the primary basis for determining these patterns.

PRESENCE AND LOCATION OF INTRACARDIAC SHUNTS

Are there any intracardiac shunts present, and what is the direction of shunt flow?

The fourth step in the evaluation of the

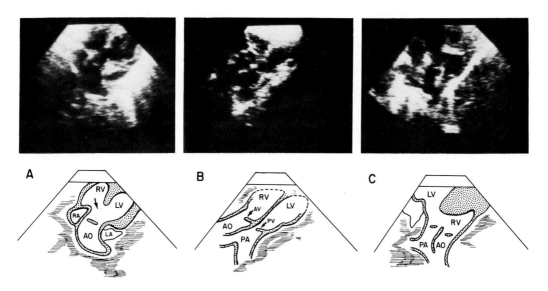

Fig. 13–19. Illustrative examples in which the relationship of the great vessels to the interventricular septum can be directly visualized in long axis. A, A recording from a patient with pulmonary atresia where the large aorta (AO) overrides the plane of the interventricular septum. B, An example of D-transposition in which the great vessels are parallel as they leave the right (RV) and left (LV) ventricles and originate from opposite sides of the interventricular septum. C, A recording from a patient with double-outlet right ventricle and ventricular inversion where both great vessels arise from the left-sided chamber or from the left of the septal plane. RA = right atrium; LA = left atrium; AV = aortic valve; PV = pulmonary valve.

patient with complex congenital heart disease is to determine whether there are any intracardiac shunts and, if present, to determine their location and the direction of shunt flow. Intracardiac shunts occur when there is a defect in one of the walls of the heart or great vessels that separate the left and right sides of the circulation or there is an arteriovenous communication that bypasses the pulmonary or myocardial capillary beds. The most common and best-studied intracardiac shunts are those associated with defects in the atrial or ventricular septa. The direct visualization of defects in the interventricular and interatrial septa is discussed in detail in Chapter 12. The demonstration of such an apparent defect depends on an absence of echoes arising from a particular portion of the heart, and as a result, false-positives are frequent. Furthermore, when a defect is recorded, it is usually not possible to determine the direction of shunt flow from the image alone. This section, therefore, is concerned with the documentation of the presence and direction of abnormal blood flow through these apparent defects.

The presence and direction of abnormal blood flow through a defect in the interatrial or interventricular septum can usually be demonstrated by the use of echocardiographic contrast. The echocardiographic contrast effect is the result of multiple intense reflections arising from microbubbles that develop during the injection of a variety of media into the vascular stream. The gaseous material within these microbubbles is a strong, omnidirectional, ultrasonic reflector, and the reflections arising from these microbubbles can be used to follow their path and, by inference, to follow the path of the blood with which the bubbles mix as it passes through the heart.[13–16] A variety of substances have been used to produce this contrast effect, including saline, indocyanine green (Cardio-Green) dye, rapidly reinjected blood, and, more recently, polysaccharide-encapsulated microballoons

or microbubbles. These contrast-producing agents can be injected into a peripheral vein or directly into the heart via a catheter. When injected peripherally, the microbubbles normally follow the path of blood flow into the right atrium and then continue through the tricuspid valve into the right ventricle and then into the pulmonary artery.

Figure 13–20 is a short-axis scan at the aortic root level that illustrates the normal pattern of contrast flow through the right side of the heart. Panel A is recorded prior to peripheral vein contrast injection and illustrates the normal, relatively echo-free appearance of the blood pool within each of the cardiac chambers. Following the injection of indocyanine green (Cardio-Green) dye (B), multiple bright echoes fill the right atrium and right ventricular outflow tract. These echoes are recorded as the contrast medium flows through the right side of the heart and disappear after the microbubbles are completely cleared from the right side of the circulation. The aorta and left atrium, in this example, are echo free because the microbubbles producing the contrast effect are too large to pass through the pulmonary capillary bed and, consequently, are trapped at this level.

The pattern of contrast flow in patients with intracardiac shunts varies depending on the location and the direction of the shunt. When there is a right-to-left shunt at either the atrial or ventricular level, a portion of the peripherally injected contrast travels with the shunted blood and appears on the left side of the heart in the chamber into which the shunt empties.[15–17] When the right-to-left shunt is at the atrial level, contrast is initially visualized in the left atrium and then flows through the mitral valve into the left ventricle. When the right-to-left shunt is at the ventricular level, contrast initially appears in the left ventricle, and no contrast is evident in either the left atrium or mitral valve orifice.

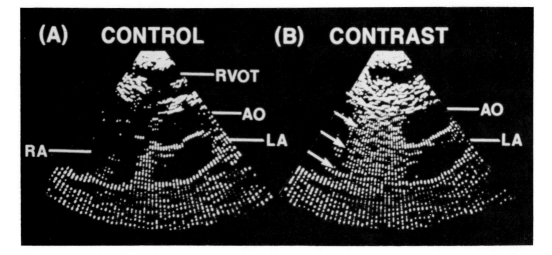

Fig. 13–20. Parasternal short-axis recordings of the left (LA) and right atria (RA) prior to (A) and following peripheral contrast injection (B). The contrast (horizontal arrows in B) creates a dense cloud of echoes, which completely opacifies the right atrium and right ventricular outflow tract (RVOT) as they pass through the right heart. The aorta (AO) and left atrium remain echo-free because the microbubbles are filtered out in the pulmonary capillary bed and do not cross to the left side of the heart. (From Weyman, AE, et al.: Negative contrast echocardiography: a new method for detecting left to right shunts. Circulation, 59:498, 1979. Reproduced by permission of the American Heart Association.)

Figure 13–21 illustrates the patterns of contrast flow through a defect in the interatrial septum. Panel A illustrates the preinjection appearance of the right and left atria and the atrial septal defect (vertical arrow). In panel B, recorded immediately following contrast injection, there is opacification of both the right and left atria due to contrast flow through the defect. In this example, contrast was injected into the left atrium, and flow was from left to right. A similar pattern would have been observed if a right-to-left shunt had been present and contrast had been injected into the right side of the circulation. Detection of contrast on the left side of the heart following right-sided injection is highly specific for a right-to-left shunt, and when this pattern of contrast flow is evident, no further study is necessary to confirm the presence of the shunt.[16–20]

Detecting a predominant left-to-right shunt using the echocardiographic contrast method may prove more difficult. Left-to-right shunts may be detected in two ways. In patients with a predominant left-to-right shunt in whom there is a small right-to-left component, some passage of contrast across the plane of the atrial or ventricular septum may be observed during the period of right-to-left shunting.[19,20] Alternatively, when no right-to-left shunting is apparent, a left-to-right shunt can still be inferred from the area of "negative contrast," which occurs when noncontrast-containing blood passing from left to right through the septal defect displaces the contrast-containing blood from the right side of the lesion.[20,21]

Figure 13–21, C, is an example of this negative contrast phenomenon. This recording was obtained following peripheral injection of contrast material and demonstrates a large accumulation of contrast within the right ventricular cavity. There is no contrast, however, within the right atrium to the right of the atrial septal defect. This occurs because the contrast-containing blood entering the atrium from the superior vena cava is displaced above and below the level of the atrial septal defect. The atrium to the immediate right side of the defect, therefore, appears free of contrast because flow into this area is pre-

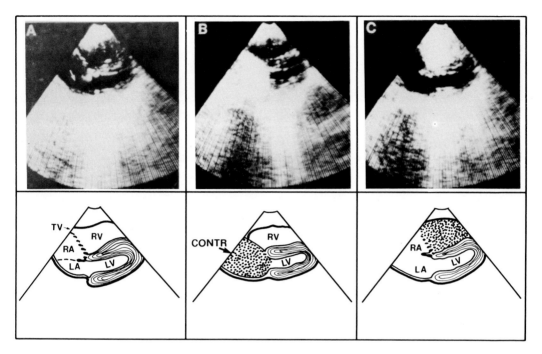

Fig. 13–21. Subcostal long-axis recordings illustrate the patterns of contrast flow through the left and right atria in a patient with an atrial septal defect and predominant left-to-right shunting. *A,* The defect is indicated by the vertical arrow. *B,* Contrast has been injected into the left atrium and flows from left to right through the defect, indicating the presence of a left-to-right shunt. Contrast flow in the opposite direction is observed when contrast is injected into the right atrium and the patient has a right-to-left shunt. *C,* Contrast has been injected peripherally, and a cloud of bubbles can be seen in the right ventricle but not in the right atrium. The contrast is displaced from the right atrial side of the interventricular septum by noncontrast-containing blood that flows from left to right through the defect, thereby producing an area of "negative contrast." TV = tricuspid valve; RV = right ventricle; RA = right atrium; LA = left atrium; LV = left ventricle. (From Weyman, AE, et al.: Negative contrast echocardiography: a new method for detecting left to right shunts. Circulation, 59:498, 1979. Reproduced by permission of the American Heart Association.)

dominantly composed of noncontrast-containing blood entering the right atrium through the atrial septal defect.

When a catheter is already present in the peripheral venous system or within the heart, use of contrast is further facilitated. On occasion, a catheter is placed in such a fortuitous manner that a shunt can be directly detected. Figure 13–22, *A,* is a recording from a young infant with an atrial septal defect in whom there is left-to-right shunting at the atrial level. In this example, an umbilical vein catheter has inadvertently been passed through the right atrium and the atrial septal defect and lies along the superior border of the left atrium. In *B,* recorded while the catheter was being flushed, a stream of bubbles flows from the

tip of the catheter through the atrial septal defect into the right atrium. This pattern of contrast flow confirms the presence of the atrial septal defect and indicates that predominant shunting is from left to right. Combining both direct visualization of defects in the interatrial and interventricular septum with an assessment of the pattern, location, and direction of shunt flow as evidenced by the pattern of contrast flow through and around these lesions should represent an accurate and minimally invasive method for determining the direction and location of intracardiac shunting in patients with complex congenital disease.

Contrast can also be used more simply to confirm or to exclude a defect in pa-

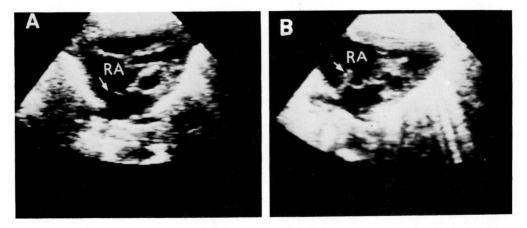

Fig. 13–22. Subcostal long-axis recording obtained from a patient with a hypoplastic left ventricle and an atrial septal defect (vertical arrow.) *A,* An umbilical vein catheter has been passed through the defect and lies along the superior wall of the left atrium. *B,* As the catheter is flushed, a stream of bubbles flows from the tip of the catheter back through the defect from the left atrium to the right (RA). This pattern of contrast flow serves to confirm the presence of the defect and indicates that the direction of the shunt is from left to right.

tients with echo "dropout" in the inter-atrial or interventricular septum. Figure 13–23, *A,* illustrates an example in which echoes could not be recorded from a portion of the interatrial septum, thereby simulating an atrial septal defect. Following peripheral contrast injection (*B*), the right atrium is completely opacified, and the separation between right and left atria is clearly demonstrated. The separation of the contrast within the right atrium from the echo-free blood pool of the left atrium serves to confirm the integrity of the septum even though the membrane itself cannot be visualized.

LOCATION AND PRESENCE OF OUTFLOW OBSTRUCTION

The final step in evaluation of the patient with complex congenital heart disease is to determine the presence and location of left or right ventricular outflow obstruction. The general appearance of individual obstructive lesions in patients with complex congenital disease is similar to that observed in patients with isolated lesions. In patients with complex disease, however, the degree of outflow tract deformity tends to be more marked, and ob-

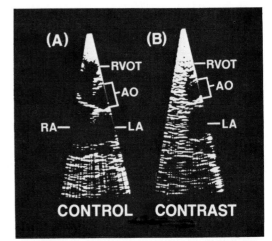

Fig. 13–23. Parasternal short-axis recordings of the right (RA) and left atria (LA) obtained prior to and following peripheral contrast injection. *A,* Recorded prior to contrast injection, an apparent defect in the interatrial septum is noted. *B,* Following contrast injection, the atrium is homogenously opacified, and the contrast pool outlines the position of the interatrial septum even though the septum itself cannot be visualized. No contrast flows from right to left, and displacement of contrast from the right side of the apparent defect does not occur. Contrast, therefore, can be used to confirm the integrity of the septum, even when the membrane itself cannot be visualized. (From Weyman, AE, et al.: Negative contrast echocardiography: a new method for detecting left to right shunts. Circulation, 59:498, 1979. Reproduced by permission of the American Heart Association.)

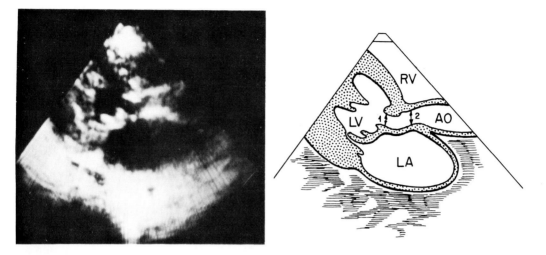

Fig. 13–24. Parasternal long-axis recording of the left ventricular outflow tract illustrates subvalvular aortic stenosis and aortic root hypoplasia. The two areas of maximal narrowing are indicated by the vertical arrows in the accompanying diagram. RV = right ventricle; LV = left ventricle; AO = aorta; LA = left atrium.

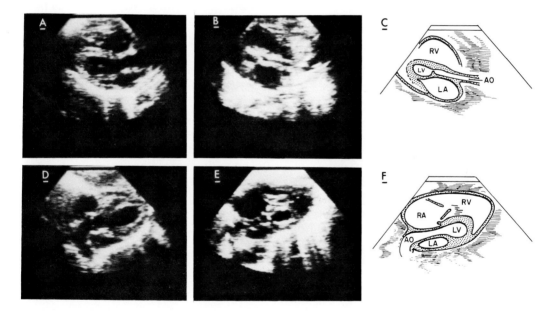

Fig. 13–25. Series of illustrations compares the normal configuration of the aortic root in the parasternal long-axis (A) and subcostal long-axis (D) views with that of a hypoplastic aorta (B & E). These recordings were obtained from children of comparable size. The accompanying diagrams (C & F) correspond to the parasternal long-axis (B) and the subcostal long-axis (E) recordings of the hypoplastic vessel. RV = right ventricle; LV = left ventricle; LA = left atrium; AO = aorta; RA = right atrium.

struction at multiple levels is common. Further, when the vessels are transposed or malpositioned, the location of the obstructing lesions may be far removed from that which might be expected if the great vessels were normally oriented. Figure 13–24, for example, illustrates a complex type of left ventricular outflow obstruction in which there is an elongated area of subvalvular narrowing consistent with a subvalvular tunnel and an extensive area of aortic annular hypoplasia. Distal to this

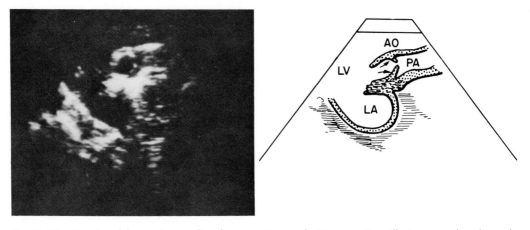

Fig. 13–26. Parasternal long-axis recording from a patient with D-transposition illustrates combined annular, valvular, and supravalvular narrowing of the posterior pulmonary artery (PA). The pulmonary valve is domed and obviously stenotic. The overall size of the vessels is reduced, and there is further narrowing at the annulus and in the supravalvular area. AO = aorta; LV = left ventricle; LA = left atrium.

prolonged area of obstruction, the aorta begins to dilate to a more normal diameter. There is also marked left ventricular hypertrophy, and the left atrium is dilated. Figure 13–25 is another example of severe left ventricular outflow obstruction in a patient with a normally oriented great vessel and aortic hypoplasia. Figure 13–25, A and B, compares the normal parasternal long-axis appearance of the left ventricular outflow tract to the severely deformed hypoplastic outflow tract. In the hypoplastic aorta, diffuse outflow tract narrowing begins in the subvalvular region and continues superiorly into the aortic arch. The aortic valve is deformed, and valvular motion is restricted. Panels D and E compare the appearance of this hypoplastic aortic arch to the normal aortic arch in the subcostal long-axis view. Again, obstruction involving the entire sweep of the vessel can be appreciated. When the great vessels are transposed, similar patterns of outflow obstruction can be appreciated. Figure 13–26, for example, illustrates a small pulmonary artery with narrowing at the annulus, doming of the pulmonary valve indicating stenosis at the valvular level, and a decrease in vascular size distal to the area of valvular stenosis in a patient with D-transposition of the great vessels.

The individual components of these complicated outflow lesions are not greatly dissimilar to those that characterize isolated obstruction at each level; however, their appearance in groups or in series is more characteristic of the complicated malformation.

If a patient with complex congenital disease is approached in this fashion, the examiner should be able to piece together all the components of the lesion. Once the various elements of a particular disorder are recorded, it is a relatively simple matter to determine the pathologic entity with which one is dealing.

REFERENCES

1. Perloff, JK: The Clinical Recognition of Congenital Heart Disease. Philadelphia, Saunders, 1980.
2. Seward, JB, Tajik, AJ, Hagler, DJ, and Mair, DD: Cross-sectional echocardiography in common ventricle utilizing 80° phased array sector scanning. Circulation, 55–56:III–41, 1977.
3. Sahn, DJ, et al.: The comparative utilities of real-time cross-sectional echocardiographic imaging systems for the diagnosis of complex congenital heart disease. Am J Med, 63:50, 1977.
4. Henry, WL, et al.: Evaluation of A-V valve morphology in congenital heart disease by real-time cross-sectional echocardiography. Circulation, 52:120, 1975.
5. Tajik, AJ, et al.: Two-dimensional real-time ultrasonic imaging of the heart and great vessels: technique, image orientation, structure identi-

fication and validation. Mayo Clin Proc, 53:271, 1978.

6. Hagler, DJ, et al.: Wide angle two-dimensional echocardiographic criteria for ventricular morphology. Am J Cardiol, 45:466, 1980. (Abstract)

7. Henry, WL, et al.: Differential diagnosis of anomalies of the great arteries with real-time two-dimensional echocardiography. Circulation, 51:283, 1975.

8. King, DL, Steeg, CN, and Ellis, K: Demonstration of transposition of the great arteries by cardiac ultrasonography. Radiology,107:181, 1973.

9. Sahn, DJ, Terry, R, O'Rourke, R, and Friedman, WF: Multiple crystal cross-sectional echocardiography in the diagnosis of cyanotic congenital heart disease. Circulation, 50:230, 1974.

10. Foale, RA, Stefanine, L, Richards, AF, and Somerville, J: Two-dimensional echocardiographic features of corrected transposition. Am J Cardiol, 45:466, 1980.

11. Bierman, FZ, and Williams, RG: Prospective diagnosis of D-transposition of the great arteries in neonates by subxyphoid, two-dimensional echocardiography. Circulation, 60:1496, 1979.

12. Henry, WL, Maron, BJ, and Griffith, JM: Cross-sectional echocardiography in the diagnosis of congenital heart disease: identification of the relations of the ventricles and great arteries. Circulation, 56:267, 1977.

13. Gramiak, R, Shah, DM, and Kramer, DH: Ultra-sound cardiography: contrast studies in anatomy and function. Radiology, 92:939, 1969.

14. Feigenbaum, H, et al.: Identification of ultrasound echoes from the left ventricle using intracardiac injections of indocyanine green. Circulation, 41:615, 1970.

15. Seward, JB, Tajik, AJ, Spangler, JG, and Ritter, PG: Echocardiographic contrast studies: initial experience. Mayo Clin Proc, 50:163, 1975.

16. Seward, JB, Tajik, AJ, Hagler, DJ, and Ritter, DG: Peripheral venous contrast echocardiography. Am J Cardiol, 39:202, 1977.

17. Valdes-Cruz, LM, Pieroni, DR, Roland, JMA, and Varghese, DJ: Echocardiographic detection of intracardiac right-to-left shunts following peripheral vein injection. Circulation, 54:558, 1976.

18. Serrnys, PW, VanDenBrand, M, Hugenholtz, PG, and Roelandt, J: Intracardiac right-to-left shunts demonstrated by two-dimensional echocardiography after peripheral vein injection. Br Heart J, 42:429, 1979.

19. Fraker, TD, Harris, PJ, Behar, VS, and Kisslo, JA: Detection and exclusion of interatrial shunts by two-dimensional echocardiography and peripheral venous injection. Circulation, 59:379, 1979.

20. Gilbert, BW, Drobac, M, and Rakowski, H: Contrast two-dimensional echocardiography in inter-atrial shunts. Am J Cardiol, 45:402, 1980. (Abstract)

21. Weyman, AE, et al.: Negative contrast echocardiography: a new method for detecting left-to-right shunts. Circulation, 59:498, 1979.

Chapter 14

Coronary Arteries

Cross-sectional echocardiographic visualization of the left main coronary artery was first described in 1976.[1] The same report also noted that areas of left main coronary narrowing and aneurysmal dilatation similar to those seen at angiography could be recorded in selected patients. Subsequently, a number of studies have confirmed the ability of the cross-sectional technique to visualize both the proximal left[2–10] and right[7,8,11] coronary arteries, have defined in more detail the normal and pathologic echocardiographic anatomy of these vessels,[2] and have evaluated the role of this technique in directly visualizing areas of proximal coronary stenosis.[2–6,10]

The potential significance of noninvasive visualization of even the most proximal portion of the coronary arteries is enormous. Coronary artery disease represents the most important threat to the adult cardiac population today. Although the atherosclerotic process may strike any portion of the coronary tree, it most commonly affects the proximal segments of these vessels.[12] In addition, lesions affecting the proximal coronaries generally are associated with the greatest pathologic im-

port and are the most amenable to surgical correction. Even if direct visualization of stenotic lesions does not prove consistently possible, the ability to exclude the presence of obstructing lesions of only the left main coronary artery would be of great clinical value. Therefore, although this area of study is embryonic, it is discussed in some detail in the hopes of indicating its potential and emphasizing the current problems and limitations.

CORONARY ANATOMY

Anatomically, the left and right coronary arteries arise from their corresponding sinus of Valsalva just superior to the insertions of the aortic leaflets. Figure 14–1 diagrammatically illustrates the relationship of these arteries to the aortic root and surrounding structures. This diagram corresponds to an imaging plane passing through the aortic root roughly parallel to its short axis just above the aortic annulus. In this projection, the left coronary artery originates from the posterolateral wall of the aorta near the base of the left coronary cusp of the aortic valve.

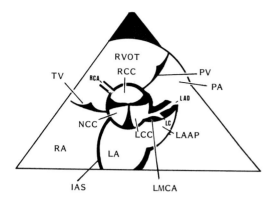

Fig. 14–1. Diagram of a short-axis view of the aortic root illustrates the relative positions of origin of the left and right coronary arteries. The left main coronary artery (LMCA) arises from the aortic root at approximately the 4 o'clock position and courses laterally and slightly anteriorly. After traveling approximately 1 cm, it bifurcates into a left anterior descending (LAD) and a left circumflex (LC) branch. The right coronary artery (RCA) arises from approximately the 10 o'clock position and courses to the right and anteriorly. The three aortic cusps, the right coronary (RCC), the left coronary (LCC), and the non-coronary (NCC), insert slightly inferior to the origins of the coronary arteries; however, they are included for orientation. Likewise, the pulmonary valve (PV) is directly superior to the origin of the coronaries and is included to indicate its relative position. RA = right atrium; LA = left atrium; LAAP = left atrial appendage; IAS = interatrial septum; RVOT = right ventricular outflow tract; PA = pulmonary artery; TV = tricuspid valve.

The left main segment of the left coronary artery is a relatively short vessel that extends leftward from the ostium approximately 1 cm before dividing. Angiographically, the left main segment has been reported to range from 4 to 15 mm (mean of 10.5 mm),[13] whereas pathologically, left main coronary length has varied from 0 to 40 mm (mean of 9.5 mm).[14,15] Significantly, from the standpoint of echocardiographic visualization, the left main coronary extends less than 2 cm in more than 95% of patients. The diameter of the left main segment ranges from 5 to 10 mm.[15] In the majority of patients (66%), the left main coronary bifurcates into a left anterior descending branch, which courses leftward and anteriorly, and a left circumflex branch, which runs posteriorly following the path of the mitral annulus (see Fig. 14–1). Frequently (31%), however, a third

vessel, the intermediate or diagonal branch, also arises at this dividing point, whereas on occasion (2.4%), a fourth branch is present.[16]

The left main coronary artery normally lies in a relatively fixed anatomic position in relationship to the left ventricle and great vessels. It is bordered anteriorly by the right ventricular outflow tract as it crosses the root of the aorta, superiorly by the descending portion of the pulmonary artery (the pulmonic valve lies superior and to the left of the left main coronary artery), inferiorly by the superior margin of the left ventricle, and posteriorly by a portion of the left atrium. The left main coronary immediately abuts the posterior wall of the pulmonary artery, and hence, anomalous insertion of this vessel into the pulmonary artery involves a shift in its ostial position of only a few millimeters.

The right coronary artery originates from the anteromedial border of the aortic root at a level parallel with or slightly superior to the origin of the left coronary artery (see Fig. 14–1). It initially courses slightly anteriorly and rightward along the superior margin of the right ventricular outflow tract and then almost directly rightward parallel to the anterior chest wall until it disappears into the atrioventricular groove beneath the right atrial appendage. No anatomic landmarks in the right coronary system compare to the bifurcation of the left main coronary artery. It is more difficult, therefore, to define the precise position of abnormalities in the right coronary system except with reference to the ostium. Likewise, fewer external anatomic references are available to help to locate the origin of the right coronary artery or to determine its path. The right ventricular outflow tract defines its inferior boundary; however, no structures either anterior or superior to the vessel are useful in further defining its position in space.

EXAMINING PLANES

Two echocardiographic examining planes have been utilized to record the coronary arteries: (1) a parasternal long axis of the left and right coronary arteries (this plane is comparable to a parasternal short axis of the aortic valve but is rotated to be specifically aligned parallel to the long axis of the vessels to be examined) and (2) an apical long axis of the left main coronary artery.

To record the left main coronary artery from the parasternal transducer location, the imaging plane is initially aligned parallel to the short axis of the aorta at the aortic valve level. The artery is then located by angling the imaging plane in a superior-inferior arc to define the superior margin of the left ventricle and the descending portion of the pulmonary artery. These reference points represent the upper and lower limits of the area in which the left main coronary artery should lie.[1] During the course of the sweep, a relatively dense mass of echoes originating along the left, inferior border of the aorta and extending leftward beneath the right ventricular outflow tract can be visualized. This mass of echoes corresponds to the dense echoes normally seen behind the pulmonary artery during routine examination of the pulmonary artery and valve and has been termed the atriopulmonic sulcus.[17] The left main coronary artery lies within this mass of echoes. After locating the area in which the left main coronary lies, the examiner rotates the transducer clockwise approximately 30 degrees in an attempt to align it parallel to the long axis of the left main coronary segment. The probe is then swept back and forth within the previously described boundaries. The aorta is maintained in the left-hand margin of the scan until the coronary ostium or left main coronary itself is located. Fine changes in the rotation of the transducer are required to align the scan plane parallel to the long axis of this vessel. Although this process is difficult to describe, the area of the left main coronary artery is relatively easy to locate, and with expe-

rience, the entire process can be accomplished in minutes.

The right coronary artery is recorded from the parasternal location using the same basic imaging plane as is used to record the left coronary artery. Location of the right coronary artery is more difficult, however, because of the lack of well-defined anatomic landmarks bracketing the vessel.

The right coronary artery lies slightly superior to the plane of the left main coronary and requires superior angulation of the imaging plane. The right coronary is generally located by angling the imaging plane in a superior-inferior arc from the aortic valve upward to the superior portion of the right coronary sinus of Valsalva while focusing on the right superior margin of the aortic root until an interruption in the aortic wall at the base of the right coronary cusp is visualized. This interruption usually appears between the 10 and 11 o'clock positions relative to the short axis of the aorta. Fine positioning of the plane parallel to the long axis of the right coronary can then be achieved by alternately rotating the plane in a clockwise-counterclockwise pattern until the parallel linear echoes from the right coronary are optimally recorded.

The short-axis examining plane appears optimal for recording both the left and right coronary arteries because it places these vessels perpendicular to the path of the scan plane and, likewise, positions them in the near field of the transducer.

The left coronary artery also can be recorded from the cardiac apex.[3,4] When recording the vessel from the cardiac apex, the transducer is located over the apical impulse, and the central ray of the beam is angled superiorly and anteriorly to record the aortic root. The plane is initially aligned in a two-chamber view of the heart and is then rotated clockwise until the coronary ostium and left main coronary are visualized. This imaging plane views the left coronary in an orthogonal orientation to the short-axis scan and, hence, may permit better detection of lesions that are poorly visualized from the anterior chest wall. This imaging plane has the theoretic disadvantages of placing the structures to be examined in the far field of the scan plane where the lateral resolution is poorer and the penetration of the sound beam is diminished. In addition, the anatomic landmarks that are utilized from the apex are less well defined than those that are available from the left sternal border. Recording of the right coronary artery from the apex has not been described.

NORMAL ECHOCARDIOGRAPHIC ANATOMY

Figures 14–2 and 14–3 illustrate the normal echocardiographic appearance of the left and right coronary arteries. The left coronary ostium normally appears as a funnel-shaped structure that originates from the posterolateral wall of the aorta between the 4 and 5 o'clock positions.[1] The vessel then continues laterally as two parallel linear echoes separated by a distance of several millimeters. After coursing laterally beneath the posterior wall of

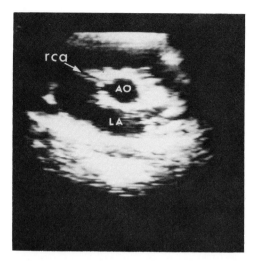

Fig. 14–3. Cross-sectional echogram of the proximal right coronary artery. This scan plane is aligned roughly parallel to a short axis of the aorta. It is then repositioned to record the long axis of the right coronary artery arising from the aorta at approximately the 10 o'clock position and coursing anteriorly and to the right. The vessel appears as two parallel linear echoes with an echo-free space interposed. rca = right coronary artery; AO = aorta; LA = left atrium.

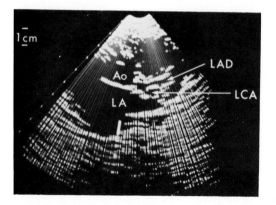

Fig. 14–2. Long-axis cross-sectional echogram of the proximal left coronary artery system. The left main coronary artery can be seen originating from a posterolateral wall of the aorta at approximately the 4 o'clock position. It then courses laterally roughly 1 cm and bifurcates into left anterior descending and left circumflex branches. AO = aorta; LA = left atrium; LAD = left anterior descending coronary artery; LCA = left circumflex coronary artery.

the pulmonary artery for approximately 1 cm, the parallel linear echoes arising from the left main coronary segment bifurcate into two pairs of parallel echoes, one of which continues laterally and anteriorly while the other courses more posteriorly (Fig. 14–2). In vitro studies have confirmed that the anteriorly coursing pair of linear echoes originates from the left anterior descending branch of the left coronary artery, whereas the posterior pair arises from the left circumflex branch.[2]

Throughout the cardiac cycle, there is both anteroposterior and superior-inferior motion of the aortic root. Because the left main coronary segment is attached to the aorta, it follows this motion. At end-diastole, the aorta is in its most posterior position. At this point, the left main coronary artery generally follows a lateral and slightly anterior course after leaving the aorta. During systole, the aorta moves anteriorly and reaches its most anterior position at approximately end-systole. From this aortic position, the left main coronary segment generally pursues an almost directly lateral course. The superior-inferior motion of the vessel follows the motion of the base of the heart. During systolic contraction, the base of the heart moves inferiorly, while during diastole, it moves superiorly. The left coronary artery, therefore, is in its most anterior and inferior position at end-systole and at its most posterior and superior position at end-diastole.

The normal appearance of the proximal right coronary artery is illustrated in Figure 14–3. The ostium of the proximal right coronary lies at approximately the 10 o'clock position. The right coronary ostium, in general, is less well defined and not as funnel shaped as that of the left coronary. The right coronary artery appears again as two parallel linear echoes that leave the aortic root and course almost directly rightward with a slight degree of anterior angulation. The spatial motion of the right coronary artery follows that of the aortic root and is similar in timing and direction to that of the left coronary artery.

The fact that these parallel linear echoes represent the coronary vessels has been confirmed in several ways. The first method was by direct injection of contrast into the vessels during cardiac catheterization.[1] Figure 14–4 is an example of such a study. In the left-hand panel (A), the left main coronary artery is visualized prior to contrast injection. In B, indocyanine green (Cardio-Green) dye is injected directly into the left main coronary and opacifies the area between the two parallel linear echoes, thereby confirming their identity as a coronary vessel. In addition, the coronaries have been visualized during extensive studies of excised hearts, and their ostia have been recorded during serial catheter insertions and multiple contrast injections.[2] Finally, experiments of nature, such as coronary aneurysms, have been detected within the coronary arteries, and their presence has been used to confirm

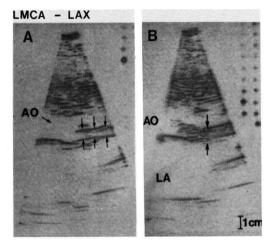

Fig. 14–4. *A,* A cross-sectional recording of a normal left main coronary artery (LMCA). The artery, which appears as two parallel linear echoes (indicated at the tips of the vertical arrows), arises from the inferolateral border of the aorta (AO) and extends slightly anteriorly and to the left. The relatively echo-free space between these linear echoes represents the lumen of the vessel. *B,* Recording from the same patient during injection of indocyanine green dye (Cardio-Green) directly into the left main coronary artery. The dye produces a cloud of echoes that completely fills the space between the original parallel linear echoes confirming that this is the arterial lumen. The near-field echoes seen in this and subsequent recordings are frequently recorded over the pulmonary artery, and their precise origin is unclear. AO = aorta; LA = left atrium; LAX = long axis. (From Weyman, AE, et al.: Noninvasive visualization of the left main coronary artery by cross-sectional echocardiography. Circulation, 54:169, 1976. Reproduced by permission of the American Heart Association.)

that the structures from which they originate are the coronary vessels.[1,7,8]

The reported frequency with which various segments of the coronary arteries have been visualized echocardiographically is summarized in Table 14–1. The ostium of the left coronary has been recorded in between 90 and 99% of adult patients with coronary artery disease[5,10] and in nearly all pediatric patients.[9] The left main coronary segment has been slightly more difficult to visualize, and success rates have varied from 58 to 99% of adult patients (mean 78%).[10,11] The bifurcation has been detected in 62% of normal patients and in 57% of patients with coronary obstruction.[4] More recently, detection of the bi-

TABLE 14–1
REPORTED SUCCESS RATES IN IMAGING VARIOUS SEGMENTS OF THE CORONARY SYSTEM

		LCA				PRCA
	N	Ostium	LMCA	Bifurcation/LAD	Circ.	PRCA
Ogawa[3]	35	—	27 (77%)	—	12 (34%)	—
* Chen[4]	32	—	—	17 (53%)	—	—
Rogers[5]	100	90 (90%)	—	—	—	—
Friedman[6]	53	—	42 (79%)	—	—	—
*Yoshikawa[7]	37	37 (100%)	29 (78%)	—	—	17 (46%)
Aronow[10]	93	—	54 (58%)	—	—	—
Rink[11]	72	71 (99%)	71 (99%)	—	—	—
Total	422	198 (95%)	223 (77%)	17 (53%)	12 (34%)	17 (46%)

N = number of patients examined
LCA = left coronary arterial system
LMCA = left main coronary artery
LAD = left anterior descending coronary artery
PRCA = proximal right coronary artery
Circ. = circumflex coronary artery
* = success rates not specifically stated, percentages derived from data presented.

furcation has improved to 75% in prospectively examined patients.[18] The circumflex branch is the most difficult of the vessels on the left side to record being noted in only 34% of cases in one study.[3] The right coronary artery is uniformly more difficult to visualize than is the left. The success rate for right coronary recording was reported in only one study and, in that instance, was 46%.[7]

In more general terms, the coronary arteries are relatively small structures arising from the larger aorta. In patients in whom the aorta and aortic root can clearly be recorded, the coronary arteries can as a rule also be detected. Conversely, when the aorta and aortic root cannot be well defined, it is usually not possible to record the coronaries. As a result, the coronaries are relatively easier to evaluate in normal persons and pediatric patients (in whom the echocardiographic examination is simpler) than in patients with coronary artery disease in whom the study in general is more difficult.

A number of other technical considerations must be kept in mind when attempting to record the left main coronary artery or other segments of the coronary tree. First, several structures in the area of the left coronary artery produce horizontal linear echoes. To be sure one is visualizing the left coronary, one must record its origin from the aorta and the continuity between the lumens of the two vessels. Second, because the artery does not remain in the field of vision throughout the cardiac cycle but rather moves in and out of the plane of the cross-sectional scan, analysis of a number of still frames may be required to locate the few frames that clearly depict the left main coronary structures. Thus, high-quality still frames are an obvious requirement. Finally, the left main coronary artery, although relatively short, may curve such that it cannot be recorded in its entirety in one examining plane. Slight changes in transducer angulation, therefore, may be required to record the coronary ostium, the body of the left main coronary, and the bifurcation. Thus, individual areas of the vessel may need to be evaluated separately.

CORONARY ARTERY STENOSIS

Atherosclerosis is by far the most common cause of coronary artery stenosis. Atherosclerotic coronary lesions are characterized by a focal accumulation of lipids, fibrous tissue, and, frequently, calcium deposits, which both deform the arterial wall and narrow the vascular lumen.[19]

Two characteristic echocardiographic abnormalities have been noted in patients with atherosclerotic coronary artery disease that correspond to the pathologic nature of the process. These abnormalities are (1) a focal decrease in echocardiographic lumen size and (2) an increase in the local reflectivity of the vascular walls. The luminal narrowing is typified by an increase in the echoes from either the anterior or the posterior margins of the vessel with loss of their normal parallel orientation and either a decrease or total disruption of the continuous echo-free space characteristic of the vascular lumen. Figure 14–5 is an echocardiogram from a patient with a left main coronary lesion and illustrates this type of abnormality. Figure 14–6 is the corresponding angiogram demonstrating the relationship in both configuration and location to the angiographic obstruction.

The abnormal increase in echo intensity occurs at specific points along the vessel that are presumed to represent areas of increased reflectivity due to the abnormal histologic composition of the atherosclerotic lesions. This increased reflectance may occur with or without associated vascular narrowing.

The true sensitivity and specificity of these criteria for detecting coronary lesions are difficult to assess. Although a number of studies have addressed these questions, each has utilized different types

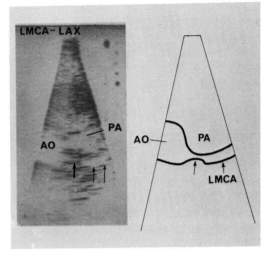

Fig. 14–5. Cross-sectional echogram from a patient with obstruction of the proximal left main coronary artery (LMCA). A fairly extensive area of luminal narrowing begins just distal to the coronary ostium and produces almost complete obliteration of the arterial lumen (large vertical arrow). A relatively normal arterial lumen is recorded distal to the area of obstruction (small, vertical arrows). PA = pulmonary artery; AO = aorta; LAX = long axis. (From Weyman, AE, et al.: Noninvasive visualization of the left main coronary artery by cross-sectional echocardiography. Circulation, 54:169, 1976. Reproduced by permission of the American Heart Association.)

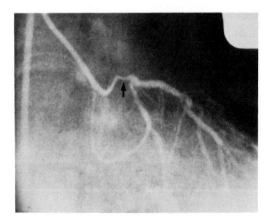

Fig. 14–6. Coronary cineangiogram corresponding to the cross-sectional study illustrated in Figure 14–5. Narrowing of the left main coronary segment is significant, extending from the catheter tip to directly proximal to the bifurcation of the left main coronary artery. (From Weyman, AE, et al.: Noninvasive visualization of the left main coronary artery by cross-sectional echocardiography. Circulation, 54:169, 1976. Reproduced by permission of the American Heart Association.)

of instrumentation, examining techniques, criteria for diagnosing coronary lesions, and/or methods of image processing. Despite these limitations, there is enough consistency in the results to suggest some general patterns. Thus, lesions in the left main coronary are the easiest to record and have been the most extensively studied.

Table 14–2 summarizes the available data on visualization of left main coronary artery lesions using the criteria of luminal narrowing and increased regional reflectivity. Because these numbers are derived from a small group of preliminary reports, they serve only to indicate general trends and cannot in themselves be considered significant.[1,3,4,6,10,11] They do suggest, however, that left main coronary lesions can be detected in the majority of patients. False-negatives have been reported in only one study,[6] whereas false-positives occur

TABLE 14–2
COMPARISON OF ECHOCARDIOGRAPHIC AND ANGIOGRAPHIC DETECTION OF LEFT MAIN CORONARY STENOSIS USING STANDARD ECHOCARDIOGRAPHIC SIGNAL PROCESSING

		STANDARD ECHO		
LMCA		+	−	
ANGIO	+	33	8	41
	−	18	154	172
		51	162	

Sens. $\dfrac{33}{41} = 80\%$

Spec. $\dfrac{154}{172} = 89\%$

Pred. V. $\dfrac{33}{51} = 64\%$

with fairly high frequency. The highest sensitivity appears to be achieved by using *both criteria together.* When luminal narrowing was used alone in one study, only four of eight left main coronary lesions were detected, whereas when the combination of luminal narrowing and increased echo intensity was used, all eight lesions were visualized.[4] Using echo intensity alone results in false-positives because increased reflectivity appears to occur in many patients with coronary artery disease but without stenotic lesions of the left main coronary segment.[11]

Other areas of the proximal coronaries are more difficult to record and have been less extensively studied. In one report, however, the left anterior descending branch of the left coronary artery was visualized in 27 of 35 patients. In 20 normal patients, there was no interruption of the vascular lumen, whereas in 7 patients with echocardiographic luminal interruptions, 5 patients had proximal left anterior descending (LAD) disease and 2 had insignificant LAD lesions in corresponding areas.[3]

To determine with confidence that an area of luminal narrowing represents a stenotic lesion, one must visualize the lumen of the vessel both proximal and distal to the narrowed area. If the lumen is not visible distal to the area of apparent stenosis, the vessel may merely have curved out of the scan plane so that the plane crosses the vascular wall and, thus, the lumen is no longer recorded. When lesions occur near the bifurcation, viewing the distal vessel may be more difficult, and a higher incidence of false-positives must be accepted.[18]

In addition, no intracardiac structure is ever completely echo free. Fine transient echoes are frequently seen in the left ventricle, left atrium, and aorta. Transient echoes that appear to fill the arterial lumen may also be seen in the proximal coronaries. Intra-arterial echoes must be fixed in position, consistent from cycle to cycle, and of greater intensity than surrounding structures to be considered indicative of a lesion.

The detection of changes in luminal diameter and the variation in intensity of the echoes from the arterial wall obviously require clear visualization of the vessels. Direct visualization of the coronary arteries is difficult for several reasons:

1. The coronary vessels are near the limits of resolution of currently available cross-sectional echocardiographic equipment when they are of normal size. When the lumen becomes further narrowed by atherosclerotic changes, a clear definition of the change in caliber may be difficult to appreciate.

2. There are variations in normal coronary anatomy that are well recognized and may simulate obstructive lesions.

3. The vessels move throughout the cardiac and respiratory cycles and, hence, only pass through the plane of the ultrasonic beam transiently, thereby making their identification and visualization even more difficult.

RECENT TECHNICAL IMPROVEMENTS THAT FACILITATE CORONARY VISUALIZATION

Several recent technical advances have helped to overcome some of the problems related to vascular movement and have partially obviated the need for direct visualization of changes in luminal size.

Difficulties in vascular imaging due to movement of the vessel in and out of the plane of the cross-sectional scan can be at least partially overcome by the use of the strobe mode available in some commercial instruments.[11] This mode of operation permits the examiner to select frames from any desired point in the cardiac cycle. Once the portion of the cardiac cycle at which the vessel is best visualized has been determined, the strobe mode can be activated and only those frames that are likely to contain useful data are recorded. In this

fashion, sequential frames from a number of cardiac cycles that should lie in a plane of optimal visualization are available for analysis, thus shortening the examining time and increasing the efficiency of data analysis.

The second development that has aided coronary evaluation is the use of variable function amplification systems to highlight the abnormally high intensity echoes returning from areas of atherosclerosis.[5,6] The method of operation of one of these amplification circuits is illustrated in Figure 14–7. In this format, the low-intensity echoes that enter the system (*A*) are subject to logarithmic amplification, which increases their intensity to a detectable level and compresses them into a uniform field of gray. The midrange echoes (*B*) are linearly amplified and displayed over three

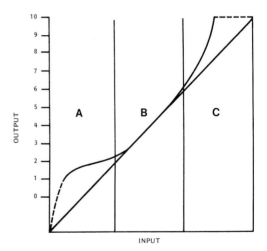

Fig. 14–7. Diagram illustrates the type of variable signal processing used to highlight the increased reflectivity from presumed atherosclerotic lesions in the coronary system. *A*, Logarithmic compression amplifies the low range signals so that they are included in the lowest shades of gray on the digital output scale. *B*, The midrange signals are displayed in a linear fashion, whereas in *C*, exponential processing of the high-intensity signals causes subsequent display over the final four to five shades of gray in the digital output. This processing enhances the more highly reflective signals and presents them in sharper contrast to the lower intensity of background echoes. (From Rogers, EW, et al.: Possible detection of atherosclerotic coronary calcification by 2-D echocardiography. Circulation, 62:1046, 1980. Reproduced by permission of the American Heart Association.)

shades of gray as indicated on the output scale. The high-intensity echoes can be variably amplified in a series of selectable formats from log to exponential. In C, an exponential amplification format is indicated. Exponential amplification increases the amplitude of the higher-intensity echoes and displays them over the final four shades of gray. This amplification format accentuates the higher-intensity reflected signals and presents them in sharp contrast to the more uniform, logarithmically compressed, lower-amplitude reflections. Figure 14–8 compares a bistable image of a normal left main coronary to a processed image from the same patient.

In preliminary clinical studies employing this type of signal processing, areas of increased reflectivity or high-intensity echoes were frequently noted in the region of the proximal left coronary artery in patients with atherosclerotic coronary artery disease. The high-intensity echoes were, therefore, felt to indicate the corresponding presence of an atherosclerotic lesion. Figure 14–9 compares the processed image from a patient with normal coronaries with a corresponding image from a patient with atherosclerotic disease, which demonstrates high-intensity echoes in the region of the proximal left coronary system.

Two prospective studies have subsequently examined the relationship of these high-intensity echoes to atherosclerotic disease.[5,6] Table 14–3 summarizes the results of these studies in detecting atherosclerotic lesions in the left main coronary artery. They suggest that high-intensity echoes are highly sensitive indicators of

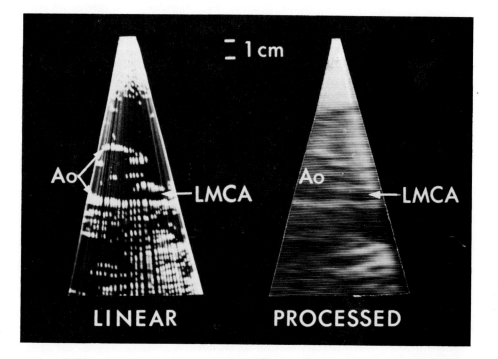

Fig. 14–8. (Left) An unprocessed (or linear) scan of the long axis of the left main coronary artery (LMCA) in a normal patient. The margins of the aortic root (Ao) are indicated, and leaflets can be seen within the aorta. (Right) A digitally processed scan from the same patient. In this panel, the background echoes have been amplified and form a fairly homogeneous field of gray. The specular echoes from the margins of the aorta and coronary artery are still visible; however, they stand out in less contrast when compared to the linear image. (From Rogers, EW, et al.: Possible detection of atherosclerotic coronary calcification by 2-D echocardiography. Circulation, 62:1046, 1980. Reproduced by permission of the American Heart Association.)

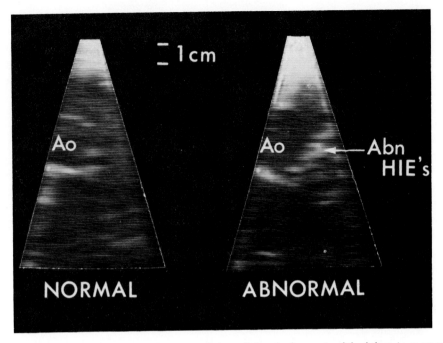

Fig. 14–9. Processed scans from two patients recorded parallel to the long axis of the left main coronary artery. In the normal patient, the region of the left main coronary is relatively echo free. In the right-hand panel, recorded from a patient with atherosclerotic disease of the proximal left coronary system, abnormal high-intensity echoes (Abn HIE) are noted in the region of the left coronary artery. AO = aorta. (From Rogers, EW, et al.: Possible detection of atherosclerotic coronary calcification by 2-D echocardiography. Circulation, 62:1046, 1980. Reproduced by permission of the American Heart Association.)

left main coronary lesions. (High-intensity echoes were recorded in each of 27 patients with left main coronary artery lesions.) This increased sensitivity when compared to standard image processing, however, results in a loss in specificity. False-positives may be due to the presence of atherosclerotic lesions elsewhere in the proximal left coronary system or to lesions that do not produce stenosis and, therefore, cannot be detected angiographically. They may likewise indicate other abnormalities that increase local reflectivity, such as valvular or annular calcification or increased epicardial fat overlying the left coronary artery.[2] Despite this lack of specificity, the absence of false-negatives raises hope that the addition of this type of signal processing may aid in making the cross-sectional method a useful screening procedure for the exclusion of underlying diseases of the proximal coronary system.

This type of imaging has the major additional advantage that it requires only that the coronary ostium be identified to roughly orient the imaging plane within this region. The vessel itself need not be clearly visualized nor must changes in the vascular lumen be detected.

The use of high-intensity echoes to detect coronary lesions in areas of the proximal left coronary system other than the left main segment has likewise shown great promise. Thus, of 53 patients with significant stenotic lesions in the left coronary system, 50 demonstrated high-intensity echoes (94%) in the region of the proximal left coronary artery. In contrast, of 37 patients without angiographic lesions in this area, only 13 demonstrated high-intensity echoes.[5]

It has been suggested that these high-intensity echoes might be related to the presence of calcification in the athero-

TABLE 14–3

COMPARISON OF ECHOCARDIOGRAPHIC AND ANGIOGRAPHIC DETECTION OF LEFT MAIN CORONARY LESIONS USING VARIABLE FUNCTION SIGNAL PROCESSING

	ANTILOG ECHO		
LMCA	+	−	
ANGIO +	27	0	27
−	54	63	117
	81	63	

Sens. $\dfrac{27}{27}$ = 100%

Spec. $\dfrac{63}{117}$ = 54%

Pred. V. $\dfrac{27}{81}$ = 33%

sclerotic lesions. Although high-intensity echoes are almost invariably noted in patients with fluoroscopically calcified coronary arteries, many patients with high-intensity echoes and angiographic stenosis do not appear to have calcified coronaries. In the group of 53 patients with stenotic lesions of the proximal left coronary system, only 30 had fluoroscopic evidence of coronary calcification, whereas 50 had high-intensity echoes. Thus, high-intensity echoes appear to be far more sensitive as detectors of coronary artery disease than are coronary calcifications. When fluoroscopic calcification and high-intensity echoes were observed together (N = 28), significant coronary stenoses were invariably present.[5]

The effects of calcific valvular heart disease and valve prostheses on the genesis of high-intensity echoes have been less well studied. In a group of eight patients with calcific valvular disease (seven aortic and one mitral), high-intensity echoes were noted in six. Three of these patients had angiographic coronary artery stenoses, whereas three were nomal. In the two other patients in whom high-intensity echoes were not recorded, angiographic studies were normal. In an additional patient with an aortic prosthesis, high-intensity echoes were not noted in the coronary region.[5] Figure 14–10 illustrates the presence of high-intensity echoes in both the aortic valve and proximal coronary regions from a patient with combined valvular and coronary disease.

CORONARY ARTERY ANEURYSMS

Aneurysms of the coronary arteries may be single, multiple, fusiform, or saccular.[20] They involve predominantly the left coronary artery. Generally, coronary aneurysms are asymptomatic and, thus, are unsuspected unless complicated by thrombosis, rupture, or embolism from the aneurysm itself.[21] The majority of coronary artery aneurysms are associated with atherosclerotic disease; however, they may also occur in patients with polyarteritis, syphilis, infection, rheumatic disease, or following trauma. Recent reports suggest a high incidence of coronary aneurysms in children with the mucocutaneous lymph node syndrome.[7,8,22–24]

Cross-sectional echocardiographic recording of aneurysms located within the proximal coronary systems has been demonstrated.[1,7,8] These aneurysms appear echocardiographically either as an abrupt focal separation in the echoes from the anterior and posterior walls of the coronary artery or as a diffuse increase in the diameter of the vessel, producing a large echo-free space between the arterial margins. Figure 14–11 illustrates the angiographic appearance of a single saccular aneurysm recorded in a patient with atherosclerotic coronary artery disease. The aneurysm lies at the distal portion of the

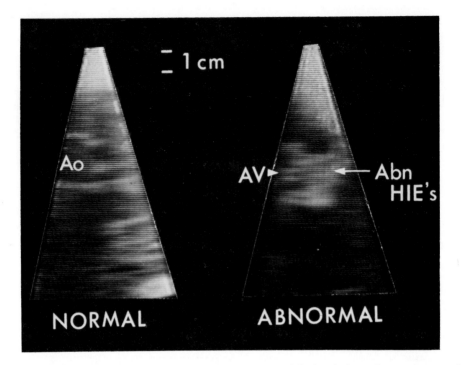

Fig. 14–10.   Processed scans from a normal patient and a patient with both valvular and coronary artery disease. In the normal example, as in the previous studies, the specular echoes from the margins of the aorta (Ao) and left main coronary can be vaguely recognized against the relatively homogeneous background. On the right, however, abnormal high-intensity echoes (Abn HIE) are seen both from the aortic valve (AV) region and from the area of the left coronary artery in the patient with combined aortic stenosis and proximal coronary artery disease. (From Rogers, EW, et al.: Possible detection of atherosclerotic coronary calcification by 2-D echocardiography. Circulation, 62:1046, 1980. Reproduced by permission of the American Heart Association.)

left main coronary artery and involves the origins of the left anterior descending and left circumflex branches. Figure 14–12 is a cross-sectional recording of the same patient and illustrates the large, well-circumscribed, echo-free space characteristic of the saccular arterial aneurysm. In addition, the left main coronary segment, with its origin from the aortic root and entrance into the proximal margin of the aneurysm, can be appreciated. Figure 14–13 demonstrates multiple aneurysms involving the proximal portions of both the right and left coronary arteries in a patient with the mucocutaneous lymph node syndrome.[7] In this example, there are extensive areas of luminal dilatation just distal to the ostia of both coronary vessels. The communication of both vessels with the aneurysm and the aortic root is detectable.

Although a number of aneurysms in the proximal coronary arteries have been recorded, there have been no reports describing aneurysms beyond the first 4 to 5 cm of the coronary tree. Likewise, the sensitivity of the cross-sectional technique in recording coronary aneurysms has not been evaluated. The smallest reported aneurysm that has been recorded, however, has been in the 4- to 5-mm range.[8]

ANOMALOUS ORIGIN FROM THE PULMONARY ARTERY

The left, right, or both coronary arteries may originate anomalously from the pulmonary trunk.[21] The pulmonary trunk, as indicated in Figure 14–1, lies immediately adjacent to the proximal segments of both the left and right coronary systems so that

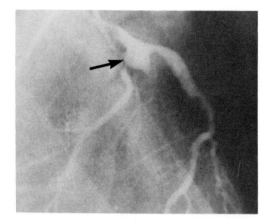

Fig. 14–11. Coronary cineangiogram demonstrates a large aneurysm involving the distal portion of the left main coronary segment (horizontal arrow). Both the anterior descending and the circumflex coronary arteries arise from the aneurysm. (From Weyman, EW, et al.: Noninvasive visualization of the left main coronary artery by cross-sectional echocardiography. Circulation, 54:169, 1976. Reproduced by permission of the American Heart Association.)

anomalous insertion of either vessel involves displacement of the coronary ostia by only a few millimeters. When both coronary arteries arise from the pulmonary trunk, survival beyond the neonatal period is generally not possible because normal pulmonary artery pressure is inadequate to perfuse the left ventricular myocardium. Abnormally arising right coronary arteries, in contrast, are generally asymptomatic and are frequently undetected. Anomalous origin of the left coronary artery, therefore, is the condition most frequently encountered by the echocardiographer. When the left coronary artery arises from the pulmonary trunk, the pressure in the left coronary system is much lower than that in the right, which maintains its normal continuity with the aorta and, hence, is perfused at systemic pressures. This pressure gradient between the pulmonary and systemic circulations typically leads to a reversal of flow in the left coronary system, producing, in effect, an arteriovenous fistula. Once retrograde flow is established in the left coronary artery, intracoronary anastomoses develop

that effectively bypass the capillary bed, resulting in myocardial ischemia in the area of ventricle supplied by the anomalously inserted artery.

The manifest disorder in anomalous left coronary artery, therefore, is left ventricular failure secondary to extensive myocardial ischemia. As a result, children with anomalous left coronary artery are generally referred to the echocardiographic laboratory in the hopes of defining a cause for their left ventricular dysfunction. The differential diagnosis in these instances rests between a congestive cardiomyopathy, myocarditis, or an anomalous coronary artery. Suspicion is directed toward an anomalous coronary artery when an ischemic pattern of left ventricular contraction is observed. This ischemic pattern is usually characterized by an extensive area of anterolateral hypokinesis or akinesis, myocardial thinning, and decreased systolic muscular thickening. The area of hypofunction is made more obvious by a characteristic area of compensatory hyperfunction generally observed at the base of the septum in a region supplied by the normal coronary artery.

Children with a congestive cardiomyopathy, in contrast, show dilatation of the left ventricle with diffuse hypokinesis. Myocarditis may produce either diffuse or focal left ventricular dysfunction. When a selected area of the left ventricle is involved, however, it is rarely isolated to the anterolateral wall and is rarely associated with hyperfunction of the remainder of the ventricle. Figure 14–14 diagrammatically contrasts the patterns of short-axis ventricular contraction seen in the normal infant with those observed with cardiomyopathy and anomalous left main coronary artery.

The observation of a pattern consistent with left ventricular ischemia in an infant or small child, therefore, should alert the examiner to the possibility of the presence of an anomalously arising coronary artery. This diagnosis may be confirmed by di-

LMCA – LAX

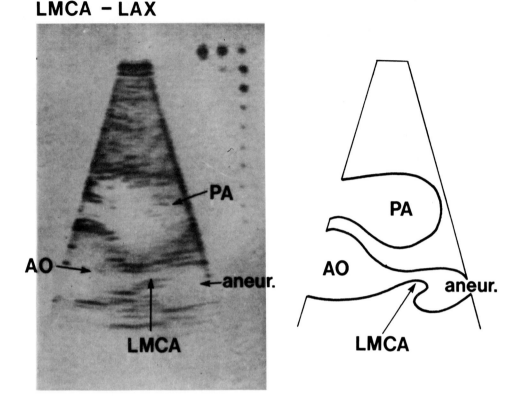

Fig. 14–12. Cross-sectional echocardiogram corresponds to the cineangiogram illustrated in Figure 14–11. The left main coronary artery (LMCA) appears to arise from the inferolateral margin of the aorta (AO) and to extend laterally to communicate with a large, circular, echo-free space representing the aneurysm. PA = pulmonary artery. (From Weyman, AE, et al.: Noninvasive visualization of the left main coronary artery by cross-sectional echocardiography. Circulation, 54:2, 169, 1976. Reproduced by permission of the American Heart Association.)

rectly examining the coronary arteries. Anomalous origin of a coronary vessel is characterized by (1) failure to demonstrate a connection between the abnormally arising vessel and the aortic lumen and, of equal importance, (2) dilatation of the opposite normally inserting vessel. In some situations, the insertion of the anomalous coronary into the pulmonary trunk may be seen; however, this feature of the disorder is more difficult to demonstrate and is not required to confirm the diagnosis.

Figure 14–15 is a cross-sectional echogram from a patient with an anomalous left coronary artery. The prominent feature of this example is the dilated right coronary artery. The left coronary artery is not visualized, which is unusual for a child of this age. Figure 14–16 is a second example from another patient with an anomalous left coronary artery. Here, again, the right coronary artery is dilated. In panel B, fragments of the left coronary artery can be seen, but it is never continuous with the aortic lumen. Figure 14–17 demonstrates serial cross-sectional recordings of the area of expected origin of the left coronary artery in a third patient with an anomalously arising vessel. In panel B, there is apparent connection of the left coronary artery with the aortic lumen. This apparent connection, however, is evident in only this one frame and is not evident in either the preceding (A) or subsequent (C,D) frames. It appears that for a vessel to be considered to arise normally from the aorta it must be

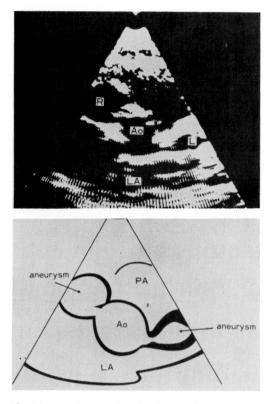

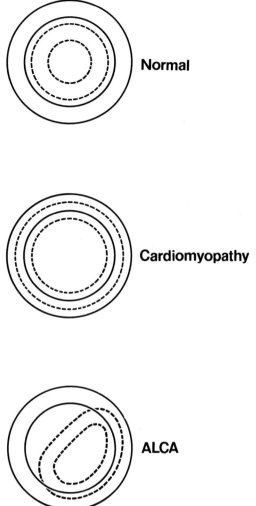

Fig. 14–13. Cross-sectional echogram from a patient with the mucocutaneous lymph node syndrome demonstrates large aneurysms of both the left main (L) and the proximal right (R) coronary arteries. The origins of both the left main and the proximal right coronary arteries, as well as their communications with the aneurysms, are evident. AO = aorta; LA = left atrium; PA = pulmonary artery. (From Yoshikawa, J, et al.: Cross-sectional echocardiographic diagnosis of coronary artery aneurysms in patients with the mucocutaneous lymph node syndrome. Circulation, 59:133, 1979. Reproduced by permission of the American Heart Association.)

demonstrated to be continuous with the aortic lumen on multiple consecutive frames.[9] Figure 14–18, A through D, is a series of cross-sectional scans from a patient with anomalous origin of the right coronary artery that was recorded while sweeping the transducer from the superior margin of the right coronary sinus to the aortic annulus. In these sequential frames, the right coronary artery initially appears along the right anterior margin of the aorta, coursing leftward and posteriorly toward the aorta (A). It then curves anteriorly around the anterior margin of the aortic

Fig. 14–14. Diagram compares the contractile patterns of the left ventricle in normal infants with those seen in infants with congestive cardiomyopathy and anomalous left coronary artery (ALCA). The outer solid rings indicate the position of the endocardium and epicardium at end-diastole, whereas the inner interrupted circles indicate the corresponding endocardial and epicardial positions at end-systole. Normally, the ventricle contracts symmetrically with both the endocardial and the epicardial interfaces moving toward the centroid of the ventricle. Epicardial motion in this normal example is exaggerated for effect. In children with cardiomyopathy, symmetric decrease in contractile motion of the entire ventricle occurs, whereas in patients with anomalous left coronary artery, hypokinesis or akinesis of the anterolateral wall of the ventricle with compensatory hyperfunction of the septal area at the base of the left ventricle is apparent. This pattern in an infant or young child is highly suggestive of anomalous coronary artery and should direct the examiner to study the coronary ostia.

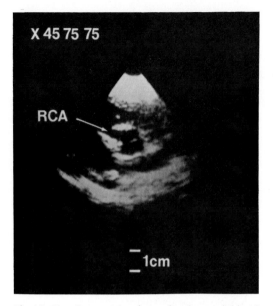

Fig. 14–15. Cross-sectional recording from a child with anomalous left coronary artery. There is marked dilatation of the right coronary artery (RCA), which must now bear the entire circulation to the heart. The left coronary artery, which is not visualized in this recording, was not evident on multiple sweeps through the aortic root level. (Illustration courtesy of Dr. RL Caldwell.)

root, where its lumen appears to be continuous with that of the pulmonary artery (B). It continues above the aorta in C and D; however, the normal connection of the right coronary artery with the aorta is never visualized.

Finally, Figures 14–19, A and B, are pre- and postoperative recordings from another child with anomalous left coronary artery. In the preoperative study, the left coronary artery can be visualized arising from the inferior border of the pulmonary artery. In the postoperative study, the reinserted left coronary artery is continuous with the aorta but arises at a level anterior to its normal position.

To date, we have been able to demonstrate the absence of a normal coronary insertion into the aorta in each of five patients with anomalous left coronary arteries and in one patient with an anomalous right coronary artery.[9] The primary echocardiographic feature of anomalous coronary insertion, however, is still left ven-

tricular dysfunction. Although direct visualization of the coronary arteries is useful in determining the cause of the ischemic left ventricular pattern, the diagnosis of an anomalous coronary artery cannot be supported in the absence of abnormal left ventricular motion.

Dilatation of the opposite coronary artery appears to be a consistent feature in anomalous coronary insertion, and disproportionate dilatation of one coronary artery suggests either a coronary AV fistula, aneurysmal involvement of the dilated vessel, or anomalous insertion of the contralateral vessel.

ANOMALOUS ORIGINS FROM THE AORTA

Anomalous sites of origin of either the right or the left coronary artery from the aorta are reported in roughly 0.5% of patients undergoing coronary cineangiography. Anomalous origin of the left circumflex coronary artery from the right sinus of Valsalva or the right coronary artery is noted most commonly, followed by anomalous origin of both the left circumflex and left anterior descending coronary arteries from one of these sites. Anomalous origin of the right coronary artery occurs less frequently.[25] Aberrantly arising left coronary arteries can be further subdivided into those in which the abnormal vessel passes (1) above both the aorta and right ventricular outflow tract, (2) beneath the aorta, or (3) between the two great vessels. When the anomalous arterial connection passes above or below the great vessels, longevity appears normal, and the anomalous vessel is usually detected as an incidental finding. When an anomalous arterial branch connecting the left circumflex and left anterior descending systems with the aorta courses between the infundibulum and the anterior aortic wall, a significant incidence of sudden death has been reported.[25] Sudden death occurs most commonly in young males and makes the

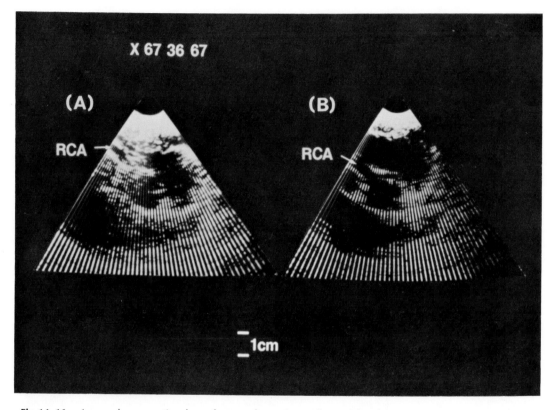

Fig. 14–16. A second cross-sectional scan from another patient with anomalous left coronary artery. In this example, the markedly dilated right coronary artery (RCA) is again visible in the upper left-hand margin of both scans. In *B*, fragments of left coronary artery can be seen, but the artery is never observed to be in continuity with the aortic lumen. (Illustration courtesy of Dr. RL Caldwell.)

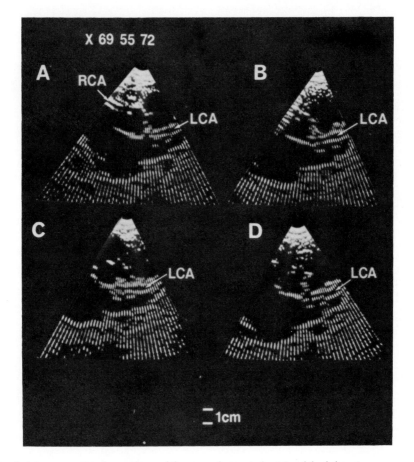

Fig. 14–17. Serial cross-sectional recordings of the area of expected origin of the left main coronary artery (LCA) in a third patient with an anomalously arising left coronary. This figure clearly illustrates the close proximity of the left main coronary system to the pulmonary artery. *A,* No continuity between the left coronary artery and aorta is evident. *B,* The left coronary artery appears to connect directly to the aortic root. *C & D,* This continuity is no longer apparent. It has been stated that a vessel can be considered to arise normally from the aorta only when it is demonstrated to be continuous with the aortic lumen on three consecutive frames. The difficulties inherent in this type of assessment, however, should be obvious, making the need for abnormal left ventricular function and a dilated right coronary artery (RCA) even more valuable as integral components of this total disease complex.

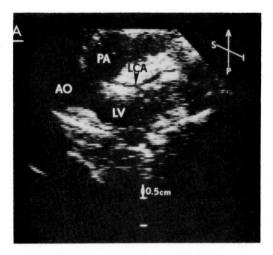

Fig. 14–18. Serial cross-sectional scans from the superior margin of the right coronary sinus of Valsalva to the aortic annulus in a patient with an anomalously arising right coronary artery (rca). *A,* The right coronary can be visualized in the upper left-hand margin of the scan (horizontal arrow) coursing to the left and posteriorly. *B,* The right coronary bends slightly to the left, whereas in *C,* it crosses the top of the aortic root. *D,* The right coronary continues over the top of the aortic root. In both *C* and *D,* the right coronary appears to be continuous with the lumen of the pulmonary artery. At no point is it observed to connect with the aortic root. LCA = left coronary artery. (Illustration courtesy of Dr. RL Caldwell.)

detection of this pattern particularly important.

Figure 14–20 is an example of such an anomalous coronary artery. In this figure, the left coronary system arises from the right coronary artery just distal to the coronary ostium. The anomalous left coronary artery then courses rightward and slightly posteriorly between the infundibulum and aorta. After passing beyond the lateral margin of the aorta, it bifurcates into the left anterior descending and left circumflex branches. This study was performed retrospectively following coronary cineangiography, but demonstrates the potential of the echocardiographic method for visualizing this type of lesion.

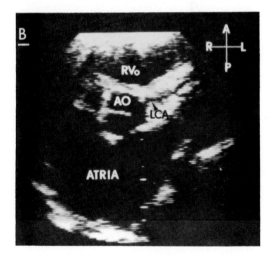

Fig. 14–19. Pre- and postoperative recordings of an anomalous left coronary artery (LCA). *A,* The anomalous vessel before the operation originates from the inferior border of the pulmonary artery (PA). *B,* After the surgical procedure, the anomalous left coronary artery has been reinserted into the aortic root. However, the point of origin is abnormally high, and the vessel courses to the left at an angle more anterior than usual. AO = aorta; LV = left ventricle; RVO = right ventricular outflow tract. (From Fisher, EA, et al.: Two-dimensional echocardiographic visualization of the left coronary artery in anomalous origin of the left coronary artery from the pulmonary artery. Pre and postoperative studies. Circulation, 63:698, 1981. Reproduced by permission of the American Heart Association.)

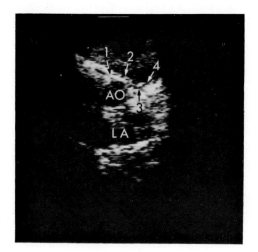
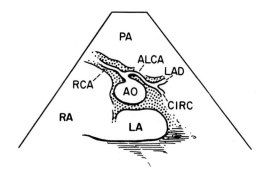

Fig. 14–20. Parasternal recording with the scan plane aligned oblique to the short axis of the aorta and left atrium illustrates an anomalous left coronary artery (ALCA) arising from the right coronary artery (RCA). Arrow #1 points to the origin of the anomalous left coronary artery from the proximal right coronary. The left coronary then courses between the aorta and right ventricular infundibulum (arrow #2). After crossing beneath the pulmonary artery, it then bifurcates (arrow #3) into the left anterior descending (#4) and circumflex branches.

REFERENCES

1. Weyman, AE, et al.: Noninvasive visualization of the left main coronary artery by cross-sectional echocardiography. Circulation, 54:169, 1976.
2. Rogers, EW, et al.: Evaluation of coronary artery anatomy in vitro by cross-sectional echocardiography. (Abstract). Am J Cardiol, 43:386, 1979.
3. Ogawa, S, et al.: A new approach to noninvasive left coronary artery visualization using phased array cross-sectional echocardiography. Circulation, 58:II-188, 1978.
4. Chen, CC, et al.: Differential density and luminal irregularities as criteria to detect disease in the left main coronary artery by apex phased array cross-sectional echocardiography. (Abstract). Am J Cardiol, 43:386, 1979.
5. Rogers, EW, et al.: Possible detection of coronary atherosclerosis by cross-sectional echocardiography. Circulation, 58:II-56, 1978.
6. Friedman, MJ, et al.: High frequency, high resolution cross-sectional (2D) echo for evaluation of left main coronary artery disease (LMCAD): is resolution alone enough? (Abstract). Circulation, 60:II–596, 1979.
7. Yoshikawa, J, et al.: Cross-sectional echocardiographic diagnosis of coronary artery aneurysms in patients with the mucocutaneous lymph node syndrome. Circulation, 59:133, 1979.
8. Hiraishi, S, Yashiro, K, and Kusano, S: Noninvasive visualization of coronary arterial aneurysm in infants and young children with mucocutaneous lymph node syndrome with two-dimensional echocardiography. Am J Cardiol, 43:1225, 1979.
9. Caldwell, RL, et al.: Cross-sectional echocardiographic differentiation of anomalous left coronary artery from primary myocardiopathy. (Abstract). Circulation, 58:II-202, 1978.
10. Aronow, WS, Chandraratna, PAN, Murdock, K, and Milholland, H: Left main coronary artery patency assessed by cross-sectional echocardiography and coronary arteriography. (Abstract). Circulation, 60:II-145, 1979.
11. Rink, LD, et al.: Improved echocardiographic technique for examining the left main coronary artery. (Abstract). Am J Cardiol, 45:435, 1980.
12. Yoshikawa, J, et al.: Ultrasonic features of anomalous origin of the left coronary artery from the pulmonary artery. Jpn Heart J, 19:46, 1978.
13. Penther, PH, et al.: The length of the left main coronary artery, pathologic features. Am Heart J, 94:705, 1977.
14. Fox, C, Davies, MJ, and Webb-Peploe, MM: Length of left main coronary artery. Br Heart J, 35:795, 1973.
15. James, TM: Anatomy of the Coronary Arteries. Hagerstown, MD, Harper & Row, 1961.
16. Baraldi, G, and Scamaggoni, G: Coronary Circulation in the Normal and the Pathologic Heart. Washington, DC, U.S. Government Printing Office, 1967.
17. Gramiak, R, Nanda, NC, and Shah, PM: Echocardiographic detection of pulmonary valve. Radiology, 102:153, 1972.
18. Rink, LD, et al.: Echocardiographic Detection of Left Main Coronary Artery Obstruction. Circulation, 65:719–724, 1982.
19. Roberts, W: Coronary heart disease. A review of abnormalities observed in the coronary arteries. Cardiovasc Med, 2:29, 1977.

20. Hurst, JW: The Heart. 3rd Edition. New York, McGraw-Hill, 1974.

21. Perloff, JK: The Clinical Recognition of Congenital Heart Disease. Philadelphia, Saunders, 1970.

22. Fujiwara, H, and Hamashima, Y: Pathology of the heart in Kawasaki disease. Pediatrics, 61:100, 1978.

23. Asai, T, Kuguti, H, Watanabe, T, and Kusakawa, S: Cardiac lesions in Kawasaki's disease—indications for coronary angiography. Jpn J Pediatr, 29:1086, 1976.

24. Haba, S, et al.: The relationships of coronary artery aneurysm to clinical symptoms and therapy in patients with mucocutaneous lymph node syndrome. Report presented to Japanese Pediatric Society, Tokyo, 1978.

25. Liberthson, RR, et al.: Aberrant coronary artery origin from the aorta: diagnosis and clinical significance. Circulation, 50:774, 1974.

Chapter 15

Pericardial Diseases

The pericardium is a thick, fibrous membrane that covers the external surface of the heart and separates it from other intrathoracic structures.[1,2] A pair of serous membranes, the visceral and parietal pericardia, are interposed between this outer fibrous covering and the external border of the heart. The parietal pericardium lines the outer fibrous capsule, whereas the inner, visceral pericardium or epicardium directly overlies the external surface of the heart. Between the two serous membranes is the pericardial cavity. This cavity is normally a potential space and contains only enough fluid to allow the serous membranes to slide smoothly over one another and, thus, to permit free motion of the heart within the pericardial sac.[1,2]

The pericardial space is limited superiorly by sleeve-like attachments of the pericardium to the great arteries just distal to their origins. Posteriorly, the pericardial space is also fixed at the insertions of the pulmonary veins and venae cavae. This posterior series of venous attachments forms a U-shaped arc that is concave inferiorly and creates a blind cul-de-sac behind the left atrium (the oblique pericar-

dial sinus). Between the superior margin of this venous arc and the arterial attachments is a pericardium-lined passage, the transverse sinus (Fig. 15–1). In a variety of disease states, fluid may exude into the pericardium, thereby enlarging the pericardial cavity. The pericardial cavity can expand medially, laterally, and apically; however, it is restrained posteriorly at the

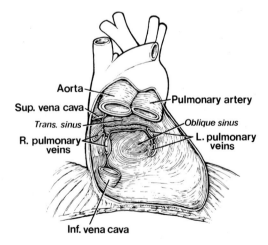

Fig. 15–1. Diagram illustrates the arterial and venous pericardial attachments. (Adapted from Goss, CM (Ed.): Gray's Anatomy of the Human Body. 29th Ed. Philadelphia, Lea & Febiger, 1973.)

480

atrial level by the venous pericardial attachments and superiorly by the arterial attachments limiting fluid accumulation in these areas.

CROSS-SECTIONAL EVALUATION OF THE PERICARDIUM

Because the pericardium covers the entire external surface of the heart, portions of these membranes are recorded in all the standard cross-sectional cardiac imaging planes. Similarly, a thorough evaluation of the pericardium involves a detailed study that uses multiple views from different vantage points. Fortunately, most disorders of the pericardium are associated with pericardial effusion or involve the pericardium diffusely. Increased pericardial fluid tends to collect initially behind the posterior wall of the left ventricle just distal to the atrioventricular groove. In this location, the fluid is easily recorded in the parasternal long-axis view of the left ventricle. This view is, therefore, the primary imaging plane used to evaluate the pericardium. Generalized pericardial thickening or fibrosis can also typically be appreciated in the long-axis view and even such characteristically focal disorders as neoplastic invasion of the pericardium appear to have a predilection for this region. As a result, when the pericardium appears normal in the parasternal long-axis and routine short-axis views of the left ventricle, a high index of suspicion is necessary to pursue the examination of the pericardium further.[3]

When fluid is present behind the left ventricle or when a localized disorder is suspected, a more extensive examination is necessary to determine the location and extent of these abnormalities.[4] This examination includes the following:

1. The parasternal long-axis view.

2. Serial short-axis scans from the base of the heart to the apex. These scans permit the medial and lateral aspects of the left ventricle to be examined and the extent of fluid accumulation in these areas to be defined.

3. An apical study in the four-chamber orientation and, from this transducer position, a sweep of the scan plane downward toward the patient's left hip until the apical portion of the pericardial space is imaged. This sequence allows the magnitude of apical fluid accumulation to be determined and any intrapericardial abnormality in the apical region to be recorded.

4. With the transducer at the apex and the Y axis of the imaging plane in an anteroposterior orientation, angulation of the scan plane medially to visualize the posteromedial and anteromedial pericardial recesses and laterally to visualize the posterolateral and anterolateral recesses of the pericardial space.

5. Placement of the transducer in the subcostal position to evaluate the pericardium surrounding the right ventricular free wall.[4]

This detailed examining sequence is both difficult to describe and to perform; however, it may be necessary to record localized intrapericardial fibrous bands, thrombi, focal tumor implants, or areas of loculated effusion.[4] As discussed in the section on congenital heart disease, when the examination is complex, it must be performed in a routine standardized fashion so that atypically positioned or unusual abnormalities are not overlooked.

THE NORMAL PERICARDIUM

The normal epicardium and pericardium are in almost direct contact with only a thin fluid layer separating their opposing surfaces. Echocardiographically, these contiguous layers appear as a single, highly reflective, linear band of echoes that completely surrounds the external surface of the heart. This single echo layer is generally referred to as the epicardium although it originates from the combined epicardial and pericardial interfaces.[5] Figure

15–2, A, is a long-axis recording of a normal left ventricle illustrating the bright, single, linear epicardial echo covering the external surface of the posterior ventricular wall. The epicardial echo also extends over the external surface of the left atrium; however, the atrial walls are usually so thin that appreciation of this layer as separate is difficult.

The reflections from the epicardial interface are normally so dominant that they can be separated from other less intense

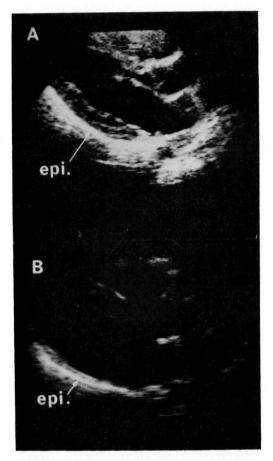

Fig. 15–2. *A,* Long-axis recording of a normal left ventricle illustrates the single dominant linear epicardial echo, which normally covers the external surface of the posterior left ventricular wall (epi = epicardium). *B,* A similar long-axis recording from the same patient with marked damping of the output signal. In this example, the surrounding, less intense echoes are markedly reduced, and the stronger pericardial-epicardial interface stands out in greater contrast.

echoes in the same area by either decreasing the strength of the transmitted pulse (damping) or decreasing the receiver gain.[5] Each of these maneuvers serves to decrease the amplitude of the surrounding less intense endocardial and myocardial echoes while still permitting visualization of the stronger epicardial-pericardial reflection. Figure 15–2, B, is a second long-axis recording with an input signal that is more heavily damped. In this figure, the epicardial echo is still well visualized, but now stands out in even greater contrast to the surrounding less visible echoes.

PERICARDIAL EFFUSION

The amount of fluid in the pericardial cavity may increase in a variety of disorders, including pericardial inflammation, neoplastic invasion of the pericardium, hypothyroidism, mediastinal irradiation, and trauma.[6] In addition, disorders that increase cardiac work without directly involving the pericardium may also increase pericardial fluid.[5]

Pericardial effusion is detected on the cross-sectional echogram by (1) separation of the visceral and parietal pericardial surfaces (epicardium and pericardium) with an "echo-free" space interposed between these two reflective interfaces; (2) decrease in the motion of the parietal pericardium; and (3) swinging of the entire heart within the pericardial sac when the effusion is large.

Separation of the epicardium and pericardium occurs because the increase in pericardial fluid enlarges the pericardial space, thereby changing it from a potential space to a fluid-filled cavity. The single linear echo from the normally contiguous pericardial membranes consequently divides into two discrete linear echoes. Each echo arises from one of the now separate borders of the fluid-filled pericardial space. The degree of separation of these echoes, as expected, is related to the amount of fluid accumulated. The fluid itself is relatively echo free and appears as a clear space between the epicardial and pericardial echoes.[3–5]

The location and distribution of fluid varies with the size of the effusion. Figure 15–3, A through C, are long-axis recordings from three patients with different sizes of effusions. With small effusions (less than 100 ml),[3,5,7] the fluid tends to be localized behind the posterior left ventricular wall just distal to the atrioventricular ring. As a rule, no fluid is detectable anteriorly, laterally, or apically. On occasion, an anterior, echo-free space is noted in patients with a small posterior effusion; however, this echo-free space is not typically caused by pericardial fluid and is not continuous with the pericardial space. Its exact cause is unclear; however, epicardial fat or accumulated connective tissue have been suggested.[3]

At normal gain settings, small effusions may be obscured by the multiple, low-intensity reflections frequently recorded from the region posterior to the left ventricle or by echoes arising from the pericardial fluid itself. Decreasing the receiver gain or damping the output signal usually reduces these extraneous echoes to a point where the stronger epicardial and pericar-

dial reflections become clearly visible. Figure 15–3, A, is a recording from a patient with a small pericardial effusion illustrating the typical echo-free space behind the left ventricular posterior wall.

With moderate effusions (100 to 500 ml), more fluid accumulates posteriorly; however, in these instances, fluid is also found laterally, apically, and anteriorly and, thus, is more evenly distributed around the heart.[3] Figure 15–3, B, is a recording from a patient with a moderate pericardial effusion. In this example, the damping has been increased to highlight the pericardial and epicardial echoes. A more extensive clear space is noted behind the left ventricle with greater apical extension. This fluid is limited superiorly by the venous pericardial attachments behind the left atrium and, hence, does not spread in a superior direction. Figures 15–4, A and B, are short-axis and subcostal long-axis recordings from a second patient with a moderately large effusion and illustrate the pattern of fluid spread medially and rightward around the free wall of the right ventricle.

With large effusions (greater than 500 ml), fluid continues to accumulate posteriorly (Fig. 15–3, C); however, in these in-

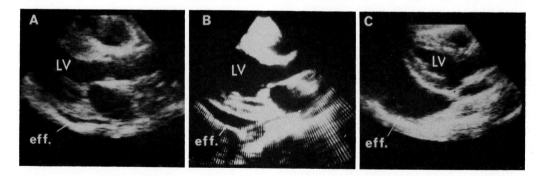

Fig. 15–3. Long-axis, cross-sectional recordings from three patients with pericardial effusions of varying size and distribution. *A,* A small pericardial effusion, which is characterized by a discrete echo-free space behind the posterior wall of the left ventricle separating the epicardium and pericardium. This echo-free space is narrow and extends only from the atrioventricular ring to the midposterior ventricular wall. *B,* A larger pericardial effusion in which the characteristic echo-free space between the posterior left ventricular wall and pericardial interface is larger, and the fluid extends farther toward the cardiac apex. *C,* A large pericardial effusion with an extensive accumulation of fluid posteriorly and apically. The fluid is limited at the atrioventricular ring and fails to extend behind the left atrium because of the venous attachments of the pericardium in this region. Eff = pericardial effusion; LV = left ventricle.

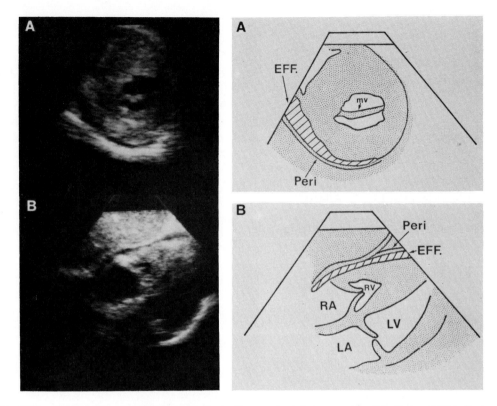

Fig. 15–4. *A,* Short-axis recording from a patient with a moderately large pericardial effusion (EFF) indicates the posterior and rightward extension of the fluid. *B,* Subcostal recording from the same patient illustrates the pattern of fluid spread medially and to the right around the free wall of the right ventricle (RV). LA = left atrium; LV = left ventricle; MV = mitral valve; Peri = pericardium; RA = right atrium.

stances, there is relatively greater expansion of the pericardial space laterally, apically, and anteriorly.[3] Figures 15–5, *A* and *B,* are long- and short-axis recordings from a patient with a large effusion and illustrate the typical anterior, lateral, and apical accumulations of this excess fluid.

When the pericardium and epicardium are in their normal, closely apposed position, they characteristically move in unison following the movement of the external surface of the heart. During systole, this motion is inward (toward the center of the heart), whereas during diastole, motion is outward (away from the center of the heart). As fluid increases in the pericardial space and the membranes separate, the motion of the pericardial layer gradually decreases as an increasingly greater area of contact with the epicardium is lost.

The epicardium, in contrast, which remains attached to the external surface of the heart, continues to move in unison with the cardiac border. This dissociation between the movements of the pericardium and epicardium helps to draw attention to the presence of pericardial effusion.[5]

In patients with large fluid accumulations, the entire heart may swing dramatically within the pericardial space. This movement occurs in both an anteroposterior and a medial-lateral direction and may include an exaggerated twisting of the heart around its long axis.[8] These abnormal swings may be confined to a single cardiac cycle or may spread over two or more cycles. This swinging motion has been related to the electrocardiographic phenomenon of electrical alternans, and a

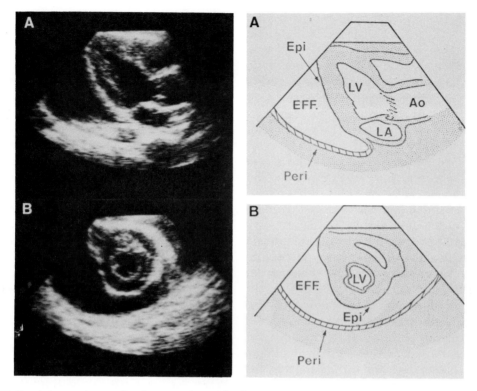

Fig. 15–5. *A,* Long-axis recording from a patient with a large pericardial effusion (EFF) illustrates the apical and posterior fluid spread. *B,* Short-axis recording from the same patient illustrates the extensive anterior medial and lateral fluid accumulation. Epi = epicardium; Peri = pericardium; LV = left ventricle; AO = aorta; LA = left atrium.

clear association can be demonstrated between the position of the heart within the pericardial sac at the onset of electrical systole and the amplitude of the externally recorded QRS deflection.[9–11]

An additional unusual motion pattern noted by ourselves and others[3] in patients with large effusions is a striking undulant motion of the anterior right ventricular wall in the region of the right ventricular outflow tract. This motion, on occasion, may be so pronounced that the right ventricular anterior wall may actually invaginate into the outflow tract during diastole. The significance of this phenomenon and its relationship to hemodynamic events, however, remain unclear to date.

EFFECTS OF POSITIONAL CHANGE ON PERICARDIAL FLUID DISTRIBUTION

The effects of positional change on the distribution of fluid in the pericardial space have also been examined.[3] It has been noted that with moderate and large effusions there is a redistribution of fluid toward the cardiac apex after 2 minutes in the sitting position.[3] This redistribution does not occur in patients with small effusions, and absence of this characteristic fluid shift has been observed in patients with compartmentalization of the pericardium by fibrous bands and with loculated pericardial effusions.[4] Demonstration of an apical shift in pericardial fluid, therefore, may be useful prior to pericardiocentesis to exclude entrapment or loculation of fluid.

INTRAPERICARDIAL FIBROUS BANDS

Intrapericardial adhesions or fibrous bands have been reported in a small group of patients with moderate or large effusions.[4] These bands have been observed most commonly in patients with chronic or recurrent effusion associated with malignancy and irradiation and with chronic renal failure. They have also been noted, however, with acute infectious pericarditis and following trauma.[4] The characteristics of these bands are illustrated in Figure 15–6. They typically appear as a series of dense, linear, strand-like echoes that frequently seem to connect the parietal and visceral pericardial surfaces and to divide the pericardial space into a series of compartments. These bands frequently have segments that do not stretch completely across the pericardial space and demonstrate an undulant motion synchronous with the movement of the heart.

When these bands are present, fluid shifts in response to changes in position are typically absent. This may imply that these bands are associated with loculation of the pericardial fluid or alternatively that they simply retard fluid movement by preventing further local separation of the pericardial membranes without causing actual loculation.

Echo-producing fibrinous bands similar to those described in the pericardium may also be seen with chronic extrapericardial fluid collection. Figure 15–7 is a recording from a patient with a large extrapericardial inflammatory pulmonary cyst located immediately adjacent to the left pericardial border. This cyst contained several filamentous bands that projected into the cavity of the cyst and demonstrated an undulating motion that was apparently in response to the motion of the heart (Fig. 15–8).

LOCULATED PERICARDIAL EFFUSION

The intrapericardial bands described in the preceding section appear to arise within fluid spaces that are evenly or symmetrically distributed around the heart. When the pericardial fluid is localized to

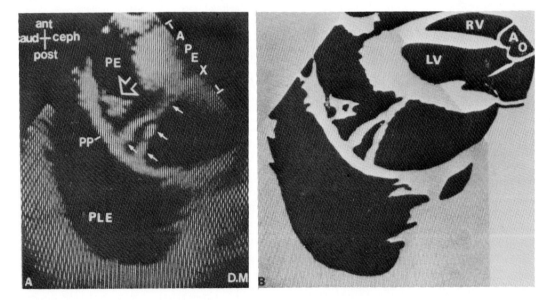

Fig. 15–6. Long-axis cross-sectional scan taken in the region of the cardiac apex illustrates both pericardial and pleural effusion. A series of intrapericardial fibrinous bands (horizontal arrows) extends from the visceral pericardium to the parietal pericardium. B, Diagram relating the position of the fibrinous bands to the left ventricular long axis. PE = pericardial effusion; PLE = pleural effusion; PP = parietal pericardium; LV = left ventricle; RV = right ventricle; AO = aorta. (From Martin, RR, Bowden, R, Filly, K, and Popp, RL: Intrapericardial abnormalities in patients with pericardial effusion; findings by two-dimensional echocardiography. Circulation, 61:568, 1980. Reproduced by permission of the American Heart Association.)

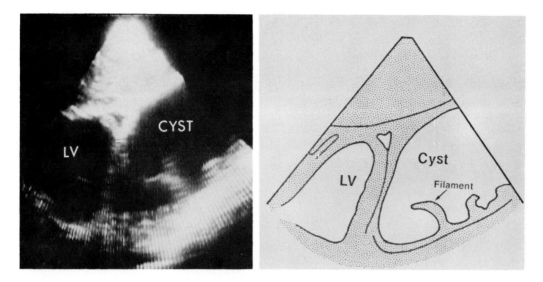

Fig. 15–7. Apical recording from a patient with a large extrapericardial inflammatory cyst. A small portion of the left ventricular apex (LV) is evident in the left portion of the figure. The large, fluid-filled cyst with mobile fibrous filaments is recorded to the right of the scan.

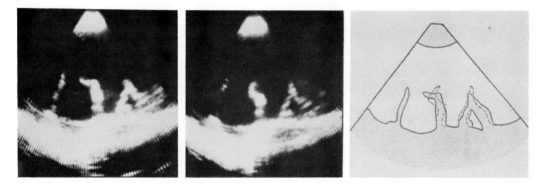

Fig. 15–8. Direct recording of the inflammatory cyst shows the mobility of these filaments. The diagram to the right indicates the position and undulant motion of the filaments during different points in the cardiac cycle.

a specific area of the heart, it may be more difficult to detect. Nevertheless, several cases have been reported in which an isolated anterior effusion, as well as a posterolateral effusion, was visualized and its distribution clearly defined.[12]

PERICARDIAL THICKENING AND ADHESIONS

Chronic pericardial inflammation and effusion may evolve to pericardial fibrosis and chronic thickening with adhesion between the visceral and parietal pericardial layers.[13] Echocardiographically, pericardial fibrosis is characterized by (1) separation between the pericardial and epicardial layers, which is fairly constant around the entire external surface of the heart; (2) an increase in echo production from the fibrous tissue between these two membranes; and most importantly, (3) parallel motion of the visceral and parietal layers, which implies that they are adherent.[5]

Figure 15–9 is an example of a patient with a thickened, adherent pericardium. Panel *A* is a short-axis recording that demonstrates the fairly even separation be-

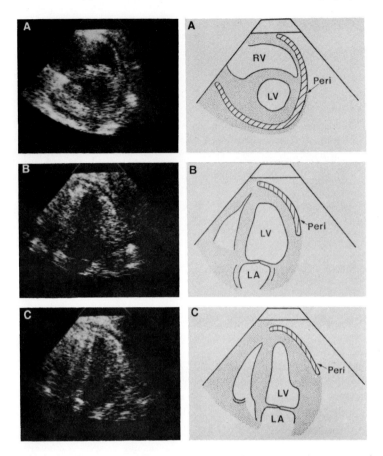

Fig. 15–9. *A,* Short-axis recording from a patient with a thickened adherent pericardium (Peri). Relatively symmetric separation of the visceral and parietal pericardia is apparent around the entire external margin of the left (LV) and right ventricles (RV). *B & C,* Diastolic and systolic frames illustrate the lack of systolic separation between the parietal and visceral pericardia, suggesting that these layers are adherent. LA = left atrium.

tween the pericardial and epicardial layers around the anterior, lateral, and posterior extremes of the cardiac border. Panels *B* and *C* are diastolic and systolic frames recorded in the apical four-chamber view. These images demonstrate failure of the separation between the membranes to increase during systole, thus suggesting that they are adherent.

PERICARDIAL CALCIFICATION

Pericardial calcification may develop as a further degenerative change complicating chronic pericardial inflammation.[13] Pericardial calcification is nonspecific and may be observed in patients with bacterial,

tuberculous, or traumatic pericarditis and, on occasion, may occur without demonstrable cause.[13] The calcium may form discontinuous plates or may completely surround the heart. It tends to involve both the parietal and visceral layers of the pericardium and is generally associated with pericardial adhesions and partial or complete obliteration of the pericardial space. Pericardial calcification appears echocardiographically as an increase in the reflectivity of the pericardial membranes. This increase in reflectivity may be focal or generalized and is not typically associated with free fluid in the pericardium.

Figure 15–10 is a recording from a patient with extensive pericardial calcifica-

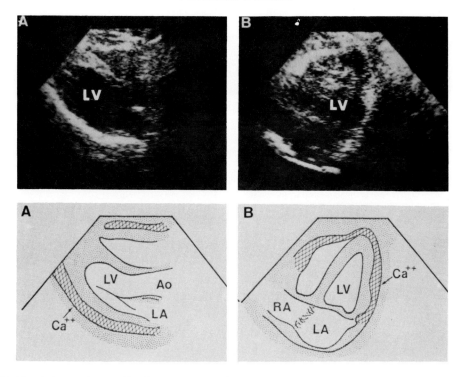

Fig. 15–10. *A,* Long-axis recording from a patient with a densely calcified pericardium (Ca^{++}). *B,* Four-chamber view of the same heart. In this example, a marked increase in reflectivity from the calcified pericardium is apparent in both projections. LV = left ventricle; LA = left atrium; AO = aorta; RA = right atrium.

tion. In this example, there is an increase in the intensity and width of the pericardial echo in all the standard views. Unfortunately, this increase in reflectivity cannot be differentiated from dense fibrosis, and when this differentiation is considered essential, a roentgenographic examination is probably preferable. When calcium is noted on a roentgenogram of the chest, however, the axial resolution of the echogram may aid in defining its location.

NEOPLASTIC INVOLVEMENT OF THE PERICARDIUM

The pericardium is a frequent site of tumor spread in a variety of neoplastic disorders. Pericardial infiltration is most commonly seen with carcinoma of the lung and breast; however, it may also occur with malignant melanoma, lymphoma, and leukemia.[13] With the exception of renal fail-ure, by far the most common cause of an unsuspected moderate or large pericardial effusion is malignancy. In many instances, this association remains only statistical until the primary tumor site is defined, pericardial fluid is directly analyzed, or the pericardium itself is biopsied. In other instances, however, tumor implants can be directly visualized on the parietal or visceral pericardial surfaces. When present, the area of neoplastic infiltration is typically more highly reflective than are surrounding regions and disrupts the normal smooth borders of the pericardium.

Figure 15–11, *A,* is a recording from a patient with a metastatic adenocarcinoma with extensive tumor invasion of the epicardium. Panel *A* is a long-axis recording that demonstrates tumor within the pericardial space beneath the posterior wall of the left ventricle just distal to the atrioventricular ring. In addition to the encroachment on the pericardial space, tu-

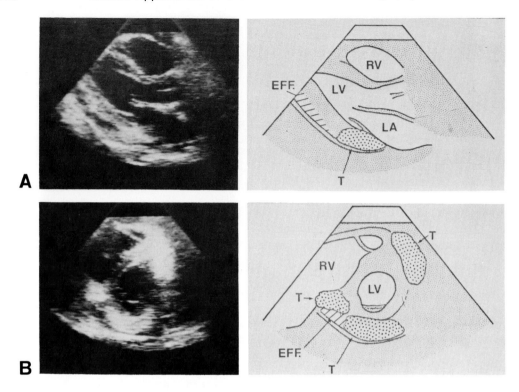

Fig. 15–11. *A*, Long-axis recording from a patient with metastatic adenocarcinoma with extensive tumor invasion (T) of the myocardium and pericardium. In this view, tumor invasion is evident at the base of the posterior wall in the region of the atrioventricular ring with extension into the pericardial space. The stipple in the accompanying diagram indicates the area of tumor involvement. *B*, Short-axis recording from the same patient illustrates extensive areas of tumor involvement (T) of the anterolateral left ventricle (LV) in the region of the anterior interventricular groove of the posterior ventricular wall and of the posterior interventricular groove in the region of the posterior right ventricular (RV) free wall. These areas of tumor involvement are indicated by the stippled areas in the diagram to the right. Accompanying pericardial effusion is evident in both *A* and *B*. LA = left atrium; Eff = effusion.

mor can also be appreciated invading the left ventricular myocardium. Figure 15–11, *B*, is a short-axis recording that illustrates the multiple bright echoes produced by these malignant implants anterolaterally in the region of the anterior interventricular groove, posteriorly beneath the cavity of the left ventricle, and medially beneath the tricuspid ring. In each of these views, the tumor is easily visualized because of the associated presence of pericardial effusion. In the areas where the tumor directly invades the left ventricular wall, the normal linear epicardial echoes are no longer evident and are replaced by the less well-defined masses of tumor echoes.

CARDIAC TAMPONADE

Cardiac tamponade, by definition, is an impairment of the diastolic filling of the heart caused by an abnormal rise in intrapericardial pressure. This rise in the pericardial pressure may occur as a result of the rapid accumulation of a small amount of intrapericardial fluid, such as occurs in the catheterization laboratories following laceration of the heart, or may develop more slowly with gradual accumulation of large amounts of fluid, as in chronic uremic pericarditis. The inability of the heart to fill normally produces a compensatory rise in venous filling pressure and a fall in systemic arterial pressure. There is also an increase in the normal inspiratory fall in arterial pressure (the so-called paradoxic pulse).[13] The cross-sectional echocardiographic correlates of these hemodynamic abnormalities have not been studied in detail. In general, however, a diagnosis of tamponade is difficult to support without echocardiographic demonstration of effusion, and in our experience, if patients with acute cardiac perforation are excluded, tamponade rarely occurs in patients without moderate or large effusion.[14] Although no specific cross-sectional features indicate the presence of tamponade, short-axis studies of the left and right ventricles have shown a generalized decrease in right ventricular chamber size,[15] an inspiratory increase in right ventricular cross-sectional area, and a corresponding inspiratory decrease in left ventricular area associated with a leftward shift in the position of the interventricular septum.[3] These observations are consistent with the dimensional changes noted on M-mode studies and may underlie the inspiratory drop in left ventricular stroke volume and systemic arterial pressure.[16,17]

RELATIONSHIP OF PERICARDIAL EFFUSION TO PERICARDITIS

Many patients with chest pain or other features of pericarditis are referred for echocardiographic study in hope of demonstrating pericardial effusion or thickening. The association between effusion and pericarditis, however, is imprecise. In a large, uremic population, 27% of patients without clinical evidence of pericarditis were nonetheless found to have a pericardial effusion echocardiographically.[14] More importantly, 33% of patients with clinical evidence of pericarditis and a pericardial friction rub on auscultation did not have a demonstrable pericardial effusion.[14] The size of the effusion, however, did appear to have some prognostic significance because surgical intervention was necessary only in patients with moderate or large effusions.[14]

RELATIONSHIP OF CROSS-SECTIONAL AND M-MODE ECHOCARDIOGRAPHY IN THE DETECTION OF PERICARDIAL EFFUSION

The relative abilities of the cross-sectional and M-mode techniques to detect pericardial effusion have not been examined in detail. In studies reported to date, both of these methods have been uniformly successful in recording effusions in a small group of patients.[3] In our experience, however, the M-mode method may be slightly more sensitive in detecting small effusions. Although, theoretically, the axial resolution of both the M-mode and cross-sectional formats should be comparable, the degradation in axial discrimination, which results when the cross-sectional images are transformed to the video format, may occasionally make small effusions difficult to appreciate. From the standpoint of eliminating false-positives, however, the cross-sectional method appears to be clearly preferable. Many of the sources of false-positive pericardial effusion noted on M-mode recordings, such as mitral annular calcification,[18–20] dissection of a large dilated left atrium behind the posterior wall of the left ventricle,[21] and differentiation from pleural effusion,[22] have presented little difficulty in cross-sectional studies.[3,12] Once these structural abnormalities can be viewed in a spatially oriented format, these potential sources of false-positive effusions can be fairly easily identified and eliminated. In addition, true appreciation of the distribution of pericardial effusion, the presence of intrapericardial masses, and areas of loculation can be achieved only in the cross-sectional format and serve to support the primary role of this type of display.

REFERENCES

1. Gray, H: Anatomy of the Human Body. 29th Edition. Edited by CM Goss. Philadelphia, Lea & Febiger, 1973.
2. Gardner, E, Gray, DJ, and O'Rahilly, R: Anatomy.

A regional study of human structure. 4th Edition. Philadelphia, Saunders, 1975.

3. Martin, RP, Rakowski, H, French, JW, and Popp, RL: Localization of pericardial effusion with wide-angle phased array echocardiography. Am J Cardiol, 42:904 1978.

4. Martin, RP, Bowden, R, Filly, K, and Popp, RL: Intrapericardial abnormalities in patients with pericardial effusion. Findings by two-dimensional echocardiography. Circulation, 61:568, 1980.

5. Feigenbaum, N: Echocardiography. 2nd Edition. Philadelphia, Lea & Febiger, 1976.

6. Hurst, JW: The Heart. 3rd Edition. New York, McGraw-Hill, 1974.

7. Horowitz, MS, et al.: Sensitivity and specificity of echocardiographic diagnosis of pericardial effusion. Circulation, 50:239, 1974.

8. Matsuo, H, et al.: Rotational excursion of the heart in massive pericardial effusion studied by phased-array echocardiography. Br Heart J, 41:513, 1979.

9. Feigenbaum, H, Zaky, A, and Grabhorn, L: Cardiac motion in patients with pericardial effusion: a study using ultrasound cardiography. Circulation, 34:611, 1966.

10. Gabor, GE, Winsberg, F, and Bloom, HS: Electrical and mechanical alternation in pericardial effusion. Chest, 59:341, 1971.

11. Yuste, P, Torres-Carballada, MA, and Miguel Alonso, JL: Mechanism of electric alternance in pericardial effusion. Study with ultrasonics. Arch Inst Cardiol Mex, 45:197, 1975.

12. Friedman, MJ, Sahn, DJ, and Haber, K: Two-dimensional echocardiography and B-mode ultra-sonography for the diagnosis of loculated pericardial effusion. Circulation, 60:1644, 1979.

13. Friedberg, CK: Diseases of the Heart. Philadelphia, Saunders, 1966.

14. Luft, FC, Gilman, JK, and Weyman, AE: Pericarditis in the patient with uremia: clinical and echocardiographic evaluation. Nephron, 25:160, 1980.

15. Schiller, NB, and Botvinick, EN: Right ventricular compression as a sign of cardiac tamponade. Circulation, 56:774, 1977.

16. D'Cruz, IA, Cohen, HC, Prabhu, R, and Glick, G: Diagnosis of cardiac tamponade by echocardiography. Change in mitral valve motion and ventricular dimensions with special reference to paradoxical pulse. Circulation, 52:460, 1975.

17. Settle, HP, et al.: Echocardiographic study of cardiac tamponade. Circulation, 56:951, 1977.

18. Hirschfeld, DS, and Emilson, BB: Echocardiogram in calcified mitral annulus. Am J Cardiol, 36:354, 1975.

19. Gabor, GE, Mohr, BD, Goel, PD, and Cohen, G: Echocardiographic and clinical spectrum of mitral annular calcification. Am J Cardiol, 38:836, 1976.

20. D'Cruz, IA, et al.: Clinical manifestations of mitral annulus calcification with emphasis on its echocardiographic features. Am Heart J, 94:367, 1977.

21. Ratshin, RA, Smith, MK, and Hood, WP: Possible false-positive diagnosis of pericardial effusion by echocardiography in presence of large left atrium. Chest, 65:112, 1974.

22. Goldberg, BB, Ostrum, BJ, and Isard, JJ: Ultrasonic determination of pericardial effusion. JAMA, 202:103, 1967.

Appendix A

A Modified Segmental System for Describing Left Ventricular Function

A segmental system for describing regional left ventricular function was presented in Chapter 8. It was noted, however, that this particular system was not optimal for three reasons: the segments were too large to appropriately depict the variety of regional wall motion abnormalities encountered clinically; the large segments tended to displace certain lesions from their actual anatomic locations; and the segment boundaries lacked readily identifiable markers, making individual segments difficult to define during the examination or when studies were being reviewed in real time. This format was presented because there was no general agreement on a better system and because it formed the basis for much of the data in the literature.

Recently, we have devised a format that has proven flexible enough to readily describe the variety of functional abnormalities encountered in the ischemic population. This format also contains a sufficient number of anatomic references to permit identification of individual segments in real time.

In this format, as in the earlier method, the left ventricle is divided along its long axis into three regions of roughly equal length, using the papillary muscles as a landmark (Fig. A–1). These regions are the basal region, which includes that portion

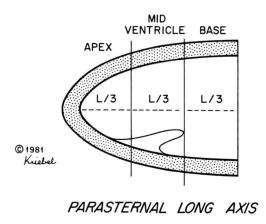

Fig. A–1. Diagram illustrating the division of the left ventricular long axis into three segments of roughly equal length, using the tips and bases of the left ventricular papillary muscles as a fixed anatomic reference.

493

of the ventricular wall lying between the tips of the papillary muscles and the plane of the mitral annulus; the mid-ventricular region, which extends from the tips of the papillary muscles to the most apical portion of the papillary muscle base; and the apical region, which is the portion of the ventricle from the tip of the cardiac apex to the most caudal or apical portion of the base of the papillary muscles. The anterior margins of these regions can be defined more precisely as the septal intercepts of lines drawn perpendicular to the ventricular long axis and intersecting the tips and bases of the papillary muscles. Since this system is intended to divide the ventricle into three parts of roughly equal length, an acceptable alternative in those views in which the papillary muscles are not visualized, but the entire long axis of the ventricle is recorded (Fig. A–2), is to simply divide the ventricular long axis into three parts of equal length.

To identify specific segments around the ventricular circumference at each of these levels, the ventricle is then subdivided using short-axis planes through the mid-

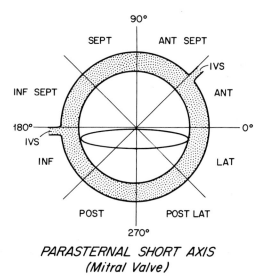

PARASTERNAL SHORT AXIS
(Mitral Valve)

Fig. A–3. Diagram illustrating the division of the left ventricular short axis into eight segments at the mitral valve level. The 0° reference in this system is taken as a line that is drawn through the center of the left ventricle parallel to the medial and lateral commissures of the mitral valve.

portion of each long-axis region. The short-axis planes used to define these segments are the parasternal or subcostal long-axis views at the mitral valve level, the papillary muscles, and the cardiac apex (Figs. A–3, A–4, A–5). Eight segments are identified in the short-axis view at the mitral valve level, eight at the papillary muscle level, and four at the cardiac apex for a total of 20 segments. The ventricular segments within each region are determined using a radial-coordinate system in which each radius has at least one fixed anatomic point of reference. The point of origin of this system (0° reference) is taken as the free wall intercept of a line drawn parallel to the two mitral commissures and/or the tips of the two papillary muscles, and passing through the center of the ventricular cavity (Figs. A–3, A–4).

When extended to the left, this line also intersects the ventricular wall near the posterior junction of the right ventricular free wall with the interventricular septum. It is important to note that this 0° reference is aligned only with reference to the left

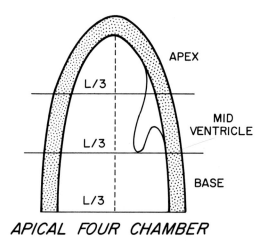

APICAL FOUR CHAMBER

Fig. A–2. Diagrammatic representation of the left ventricle in the apical four-chamber view. Since the format described in Figure A–1 divides the ventricle into three regions of roughly equal length, a simple alternative in those views in which the papillary muscles are not visualized would be to divide the ventricular long axis into thirds.

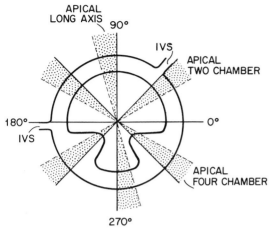

PARASTERNAL SHORT AXIS
(Papillary Muscle)

Fig. A–4. Diagram illustrating the division of the left ventricle at the papillary muscle level into eight segments along with the orientation in which the three primary apical views transect these segments.

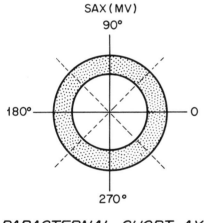

PARASTERNAL SHORT AXIS
(Apex)

Fig. A–5. Diagram illustrating the division of the left ventricular apex into quadrants.

ventricle and is depicted as horizontal (Figs. A–3, A–4, A–5) only for illustrative simplicity. Within the chest of the supine patient, this reference line would be rotated approximately 30° counterclockwise from the horizontal. The orthogonal dimension in this system (90 to 270°) passes through the center of the left ventricular

cavity and is perpendicular to the plane of the mitral commissures. At the papillary muscle level, it passes between the medial and lateral papillary muscles.

Each of these quadrants is then subdivided into octants as illustrated in Figures A–3 and A–4. At the mitral valve level, the 45° radius should intersect the junction of the interventricular septum and the anterior wall anteriorly, and the 135° radius should separate the inferior third of the interventricular septum from the anterior two thirds. At the papillary muscle level, the 235° radius should pass through the center of the medial papillary muscle, while the 315° radius should pass through the center of the lateral papillary muscle.

In this system, the interventricular septum is divided into three segments at the base and the mid-ventricular level. These segments are termed the anterior septum, the mid-septum, and the inferior septum.

The free wall of the left ventricle is divided into five segments at the mitral valve and papillary muscle level (Figs. A–3, A–4). These five segments are the *inferior segment*, which extends from the posterior junction of the interventricular septum with the left ventricular free wall to the middle of the medial papillary muscle (180 to 225°); the *infero-posterior segment*, which extends from the middle of the medial papillary muscle (225° radius) to a point bisecting the two papillary muscles (270° radius); the *postero-lateral segment*, which extends from a point bisecting the two papillary muscles to the middle of the lateral papillary muscle (315° radius); the *lateral segment*, which extends from the middle of the lateral papillary muscle (315°) to the 0° reference; and the *anterior segment*, which extends from the 0° reference to the anterior insertion of the interventricular septum into the left ventricular free wall (45°). One can distinguish segments at the base of the ventricle from those at the mid-ventricular level by using the prefix basal (i.e., the basal anterior segments).

At the ventricular apex, the ventricle is divided into quadrants. The anterior quadrant extends from the 0 to 90° radii; the septal quadrant, from 90 to 180°; the inferior quadrant from 180 to 270°; and the lateral quadrant from 270 to 0°. Segments at the apical level can be distinguished by using the prefix apical.

This system has a number of advantages over the one described in Chapter 8. It divides the ventricle into a sufficient number of segments so that functional abnormalities, while not falling clearly within any one segment, can be conveniently described by combinations of two or more segments. The reference lines used to divide the individual segments have at least one, if not two, anatomic references that can be identified at the point at which they transect the ventricular wall, making it unnecessary to actually construct the coordinate system in order to visually define the margins of the segment. The system can be conveniently applied to computer segmental algorithms that tend to naturally divide the ventricle by binary expansion. This format also permits utilization of most of the data currently available in the literature.

When segmental wall motion abnormalities are identified, they can be displayed on a target diagram, such as that illustrated in Figure A–6. In this display, the inner ring of the target depicts the cardiac apex, the middle ring depicts the mid-ventricle, and the outer ring illustrates the ventricular base. The ventricle is, therefore, displayed as if viewed from the top of the apex looking toward the base. The

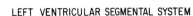

LEFT VENTRICULAR SEGMENTAL SYSTEM

Fig. A–6. Target diagram illustrating the position of the individual segments around the ventricle. The inner concentric ring in this figure depicts the cardiac apex, the middle ring corresponds to the mid-ventricle, and the outer ring corresponds to the ventricular base. The ventricle, therefore, is displayed as if viewed from the tip of the apex looking toward the base. The bars at the 1:30 and 9:00 positions indicate the insertions of the right ventricular free wall into the interventricular septum (exact nomenclature of segments is not established).

bars at the 1:30 and 9:00 positions indicate the anterior and posterior insertions of the right ventricular free wall into the interventricular septum. The nomenclature used to describe these segments is arbitrary. In this system, the term "base" is used to indicate that the individual segment occurs at the base of the ventricle, while the term "apex" is used to indicate an apical segment. Absence of a prefix or suffix indicates that the segment is in the middle of the ventricle.

Appendix B

Normal Cross-Sectional Echocardiographic Measurements in Adults

Despite the large volume of cross-sectional echocardiographic data published in recent years, few normal cross-sectional echocardiographic values are available in the literature. Undoubtedly, development of these values has been delayed by the lack of accepted standards for making these measurements, the large number of potential measurements available, which makes the selection of particular structures or areas for measurement difficult, and the acceptability of normal M-mode values for most of the major dimensions required in routine study analysis. Despite these difficulties, it is obvious that normal cross-sectional values in both the adult and child must be developed and made generally available.

In the following pages, we provide a series of normal cross-sectional values for most of the cardiac structures recorded in the primary echocardiographic views. These values were obtained from an adult patient group that ranged in age from 15 to 62 years, in weight from 118 to 190 pounds, and in body-surface area from 1.55 to 2.10 cm². In several cases, the same structure is measured in several views. When this occurs, the preferable view is indicated and the alternative measurements are included in order to provide some baseline values in those patients in whom the primary view is unobtainable. In addition, since there are no accepted standards for the point at which measurements should be taken, in many cases, we have provided several alternatives (for example, the left atrial antero-posterior dimension at the aortic valve level, which is comparable to the M-mode point of measurement and the largest dimension in the antero-posterior plane). All linear dimensions and area measurements are made using the inner-edge method, which is consistent with that discussed throughout the text. All these measurements were made in the Cardiac Ultrasound Laboratory at the Massachusetts General Hospital and in some cases, may differ slightly from values given in the text, which were taken from the literature. These data were obtained largely through the efforts of Dr. Marco Triulzi.

NORMAL CROSS-SECTIONAL VALUES*

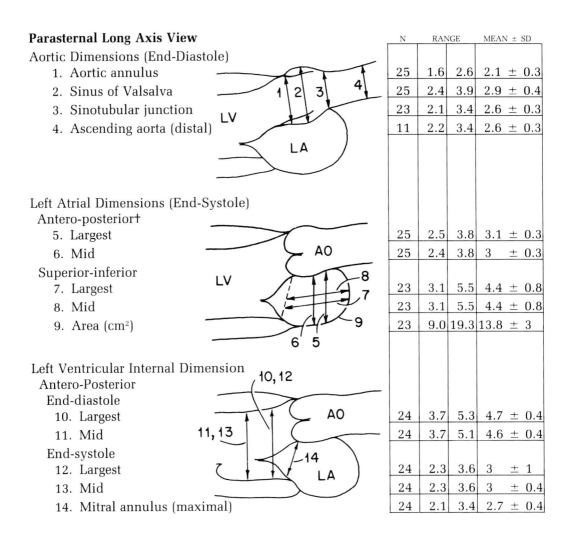

Parasternal Long Axis View	N	RANGE		MEAN ± SD
Aortic Dimensions (End-Diastole)				
1. Aortic annulus	25	1.6	2.6	2.1 ± 0.3
2. Sinus of Valsalva	25	2.4	3.9	2.9 ± 0.4
3. Sinotubular junction	23	2.1	3.4	2.6 ± 0.3
4. Ascending aorta (distal)	11	2.2	3.4	2.6 ± 0.3
Left Atrial Dimensions (End-Systole)				
Antero-posterior†				
5. Largest	25	2.5	3.8	3.1 ± 0.3
6. Mid	25	2.4	3.8	3 ± 0.3
Superior-inferior				
7. Largest	23	3.1	5.5	4.4 ± 0.8
8. Mid	23	3.1	5.5	4.4 ± 0.8
9. Area (cm²)	23	9.0	19.3	13.8 ± 3
Left Ventricular Internal Dimension				
Antero-Posterior				
End-diastole				
10. Largest	24	3.7	5.3	4.7 ± 0.4
11. Mid	24	3.7	5.1	4.6 ± 0.4
End-systole				
12. Largest	24	2.3	3.6	3 ± 1
13. Mid	24	2.3	3.6	3 ± 0.4
14. Mitral annulus (maximal)	24	2.1	3.4	2.7 ± 0.4

*All linear dimensions are in cm, and areas are in cm².
†Indicates the preferable view for obtaining a particular measurement.

Parasternal Short Axis View at the Level of the Great Vessels

	N	RANGE		MEAN ± SD	

Left Atrial Dimensions (End-Systole)
Antero-Posterior

	N	RANGE		MEAN ± SD
15. Mid	23	2.3	3.7	3 ± 0.5

Medial-lateral†

16. Largest	25	3.1	5.3	4.1 ± 0.7
17. Mid	25	3.0	5.3	4.1 ± 0.7
18. Area (cm²)	25	7.2	13	10.8 ± 2.5

Pulmonary Artery Dimensions (End-Diastole)†

19. RV outflow tract	23	1.9	2.2	2.7 ± 0.4
20. Valvular	21	1.1	2.2	1.8 ± 0.2
21. Supravalvular	20	1.5	2.5	1.9 ± 0.3
22. Right PA	17	0.8	1.6	1.3 ± 0.3
23. Left PA	9	1	1.4	1.2 ± 0.8

†Indicates the preferable view for obtaining a particular measurement.

Parasternal Short Axis Views at the Ventricular Level

Right Ventricle at the Level of Tricuspid Valve
Septal free wall (largest dimension)

Left Ventricle
Area (cm²)

Papillary Muscles
Area (cm²)

Interpapillary Muscle Measurements
Tip

Base

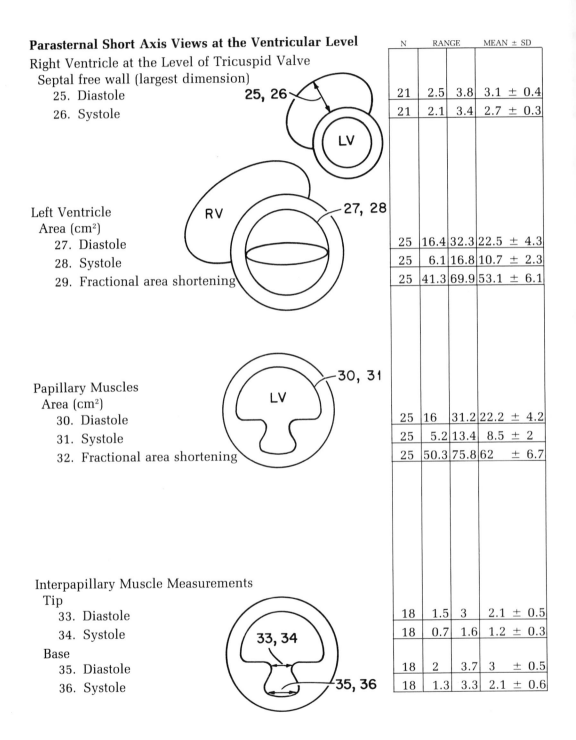

	N	RANGE		MEAN ± SD
25. Diastole	21	2.5	3.8	3.1 ± 0.4
26. Systole	21	2.1	3.4	2.7 ± 0.3
27. Diastole	25	16.4	32.3	22.5 ± 4.3
28. Systole	25	6.1	16.8	10.7 ± 2.3
29. Fractional area shortening	25	41.3	69.9	53.1 ± 6.1
30. Diastole	25	16	31.2	22.2 ± 4.2
31. Systole	25	5.2	13.4	8.5 ± 2
32. Fractional area shortening	25	50.3	75.8	62 ± 6.7
33. Diastole	18	1.5	3	2.1 ± 0.5
34. Systole	18	0.7	1.6	1.2 ± 0.3
35. Diastole	18	2	3.7	3 ± 0.5
36. Systole	18	1.3	3.3	2.1 ± 0.6

Apical Four-Chamber View

Left Atrial Dimensions (End-Systole)
  Superior-inferior dimension†
    37. Largest
    38. Mid
  Medial-lateral
    39. Largest
    40. Mid
    41. Area (cm²)
    42. Mitral valve annulus

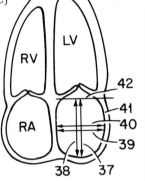

N	RANGE		MEAN ± SD
25	3.3	5.2	4.3 ± 0.6
25	3.1	5.1	4.2 ± 0.6
25	2.9	4.4	3.6 ± 0.4
25	2.5	4.4	3.5 ± 0.5
25	10.2	17.8	14.7 ± 2.2
25	1.9	3.1	2.4 ± 0.3

Right Atrial Dimension (End-Systole)
  Superior-inferior dimension
    43. Largest
    44. Mid
  Medial-lateral
    45. Largest
    46. Mid
    47. Area (cm²)
    48. Tricuspid annulus

N	RANGE		MEAN ± SD
24	3.4	4.9	4.2 ± 0.4
24	3.4	4.9	4.1 ± 0.4
24	3.1	4.5	3.7 ± 0.4
24	2.9	4.5	3.7 ± 0.4
24	11.3	16.7	14 ± 1.5
21	1.7	2.8	2.2 ± 0.3

†Indicates the preferable view for obtaining a particular measurement.

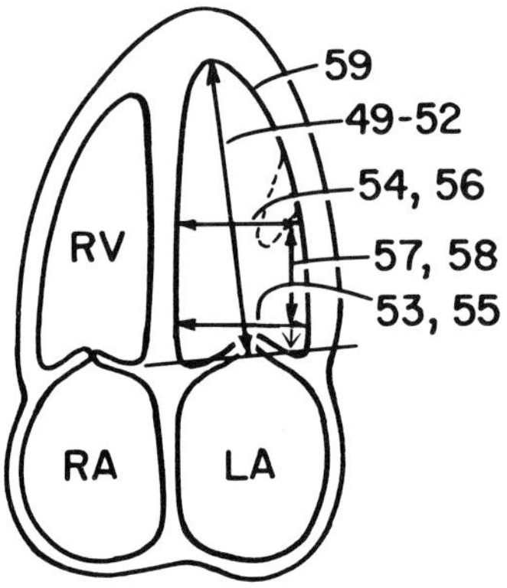

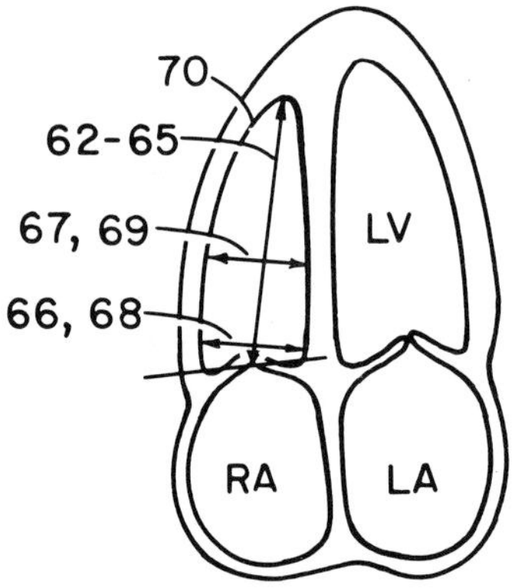

	N	RANGE		MEAN ± SD

Left Ventricular Dimensions
 Length
  Diastole

	N	RANGE		MEAN ± SD
49. Largest	25	7	8.4	7.5 ± 1
50. Mid	25	7	8.4	7.6 ± 0.4

  Systole

51. Largest	25	4.6	6.4	5.6 ± 0.5
52. Mid	25	4.6	6.4	5.6 ± 0.5

 Medial-lateral
  Diastole

53. Largest	25	3.7	5.4	4.6 ± 0.4
54. Mid	25	3.3	5.2	4.3 ± 0.6

  Systole

55. Largest	25	2.8	4.3	3.5 ± 0.4
56. Mid	25	2.4	4.2	3.1 ± 0.4

Papillary Muscle—MV

57. Diastole	9	2.2	3.6	3 ± 0.4
58. Systole	9	1.6	2.6	2.2 ± 0.3

Left Ventricular Area (cm^2)

59. Diastole	25	21.2	40.2	31.2 ± 5.3
60. Systole	25	8	21.1	14.2 ± 3.3
61. Fractional area contraction	25	40.1	67.9	54.4 ± 7.6

Right Ventricular Dimensions
 Length
  Diastole

62. Largest	23	5.8	7.8	6.7 ± 0.6
63. Mid	23	5	7.8	6.6 ± 0.6

  Systole

64. Largest	23	4.3	5.9	5 ± 0.5
65. Mid	23	4.3	5.9	5 ± 0.5

 Medial-lateral
  Diastole

66. Largest	23	3.3	4.3	3.6 ± 0.4
67. Mid	23	2.5	4.2	3.3 ± 0.5

  Systole

68. Largest	23	2.2	3.6	2.9 ± 0.4
69. Mid	23	2	3.2	2.6 ± 0.3

 Area (cm^2)

70. Systole	21	12	22.7	18.6 ± 3.3
71. Diastole	21	5.4	14.6	9.9 ± 2
72. Fractional area contraction	21	30	59.5	46.1 ± 8.5

Apical Two-Chamber View

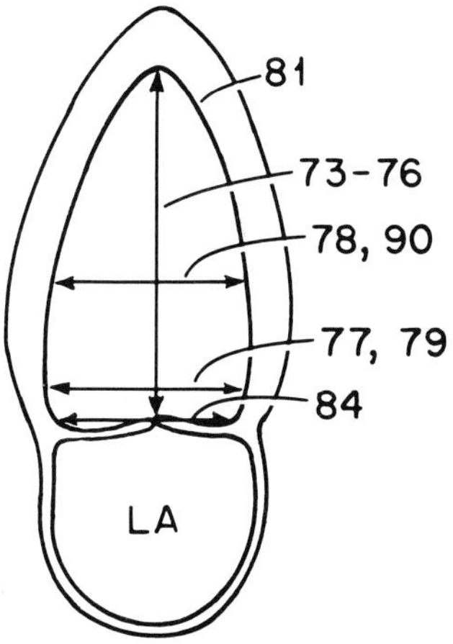

Left Ventricular Length

		N	RANGE		MEAN ± SD
Diastole					
73.	Largest	20	6.8	9.4	8 ± 0.8
74.	Mid	20	6.8	9.4	8 ± 0.8
Systole					
75.	Largest	20	4.4	7.1	5.6 ± 0.9
76.	Mid	20	4.4	7.1	5.6 ± 0.9
Medial-lateral					
77.	Largest	20	3.8	6.1	4.8 ± 0.6
78.	Mid	20	3.8	5.7	4.6 ± 0.6
Systole					
79.	Largest	20	2.6	5.1	3.5 ± 0.6
80.	Mid	20	2.1	4.6	3.2 ± 0.7
Area					
81.	Diastole	20	19.4	48	35.6 ± 6.6
82.	Systole	20	8.9	27	14.3 ± 4.4
83.	Fractional area contraction	20	43.8	69	55.4 ± 7.7
84.	Mitral annulus	18	2	2.7	2.3 ± 0.3

Subcostal View

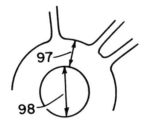

Measurement	N	RANGE		MEAN ± SD
Right Atrium (End-Systole)				
Antero-posterior				
85. Largest	NS‡	NS	NS	NS
86. Mid	NS	NS	NS	NS
Medial-lateral				
87. Largest	14	3.3	4.7	4 ± 0.5
88. Mid	14	3.3	4.7	4 ± 0.4
Pulmonary Artery (End-Diastole)§				
89. RV outflow tract	10	1.4	2.4	1.9 ± 0.4
90. Valvular	10	1.1	1.6	1.3 ± 0.1
91. Supravalvular	11	1.2	2.3	1.5 ± 0.3
92. Right PA	5	0.9	1.5	1.2 ± 0.2
93. Left PA	3	0.8	0.9	0.8 ± 0.1
Inferior Vena Cava				
94. Proximal	16	1.2	2.3	1.7 ± 0.3
95. Distal	13	1.1	2.5	1.6 ± 0.5
96. Hepatic vein	7	0.6	1.1	0.8 ± 0.2

Suprasternal Notch

Measurement	N	RANGE		MEAN ± SD
Aortic Dimension (End-Systole)				
97. Arch	5	2.2	2.7	2.5 ± 0.2
98. Right PA	5	1.8	2.4	2 ± 0.3

§These values are consistently smaller than those obtained from the parasternal transducer location. This is because the pulmonary artery lies in the far field of the scan plane when viewed from the subcostal window and there is significant point-spreading of targets along the vessel walls due to the poor lateral resolution at this level. Therefore, these measurements are more appropriately made from images recorded from the parasternal location, and the subcostal values are included only as a reference for patients in whom the parasternal window is unavailable.

‡NS represents a dimension that is not sufficiently reproducible to be considered a standard.

APICAL TWO-CHAMBER VIEW

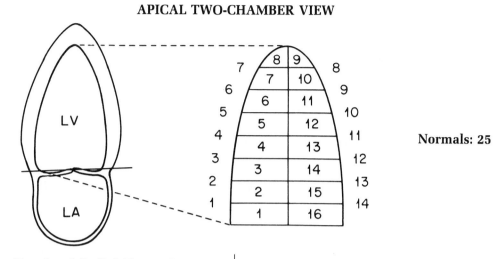

Normals: 25

Fractional Radial Shortening				Fractional Area Contraction			
SEGMENT	MEAN	± SD	RANGE	AREA	MEAN	± SD	RANGE
1	36	9	23–54	1	54	9	39–73
2	39	8	26–54	2	56	9	42–71
3	40	9	26–54	3	59	9	42–72
4	40	10	22–58	4	57	9	41–72
5	40	10	20–59	5	57	9	38–70
6	39	12	12–62	6	58	9	40–74
7	37	11	21–61	7	56	9	40–74
8	33	11	17–55	8	55	14	29–78
9	36	8	18–48	9	51	10	24–67
10	35	10	16–58	10	54	7	43–63
11	33	9	15–53	11	55	7	44–72
12	34	8	19–53	12	53	7	40–71
13	33	9	16–59	13	53	8	42–70
14	31	8	19–51	14	53	9	36–71
15				15	52	9	40–71
16				16	52	16	19–78

APICAL FOUR-CHAMBER VIEW OF THE LEFT VENTRICLE

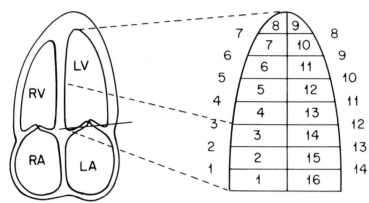

Normals: 25

	Fractional Radial Shortening				Fractional Area Contraction		
SEGMENT	MEAN	±SD	RANGE	AREA	MEAN	±SD	RANGE
1	33	10	16–50	1	51	11	28–67
2	34	11	14–52	2	54	10	38–69
3	35	12	17–58	3	54	11	33–72
4	36	13	12–62	4	55	11	36–74
5	37	12	9–63	5	57	10	37–77
6	37	13	17–60	6	56	9	38–76
7	34	19	10–61	7	57	10	37–77
8*	31	15	−.09–55	8*	56	13	21–78
9*	33	13	−.07–53	9*	51	17	1–72
10	33	10	8–57	10	54	11	25–68
11	35	9	16–58	11	53	9	29–76
12	35	9	16–58	12	56	8	39–69
13	33	8	20–56	13	55	8	37–67
14	31	8	18–49	14	54	8	34–66
15				15	52	8	38–66
16				16	50	16	6–77

*Using this system of segmental analysis, the long-axis length of the ventricle is calculated independently for systole and diastole. This approach fails to account for motion of the apex toward the center of mass of the ventricle; since the end-diastolic radii at the apex are small, it may yield an apparent systolic increase in radial length if there is any slight change in apical shape.

PARASTERNAL SHORT AXIS AT THE LEVEL OF THE MITRAL VALVE

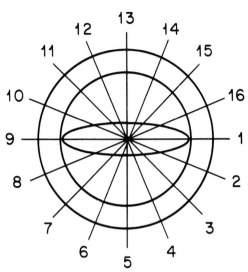

Normals: 25

Fractional Radial Shortening				Fractional Area Contraction			
SEGMENT	MEAN	± SD	RANGE	AREA	MEAN	± SD	RANGE
1	34	8	19–48	1	55	11	36–78
2	33	8	21–49	2	55	9	44–69
3	32	8	14–51	3	51	10	24–69
4	29	8	12–44	4	47	12	23–69
5	28	7	16–40	5	46	10	26–61
6	29	7	17–41	6	42	10	36–67
7	31	7	18–48	7	55	8	39–67
8	34	6	19–45	8	56	10	26–71
9	35	8	17–49	9	54	12	28–73
10	33	10	16–50	10	54	10	35–71
11	29	6	18–44	11	49	8	37–68
12	27	6	18–39	12	44	9	27–81
13	27	8	14–40	13	45	13	26–66
14	28	8	16–44	14	52	11	26–74
15	32	8	13–48	15	56	10	31–70
16	34	8	17–48	16	56	10	32–73

PARASTERNAL SHORT AXIS AT THE LEVEL OF THE PAPILLARY MUSCLES

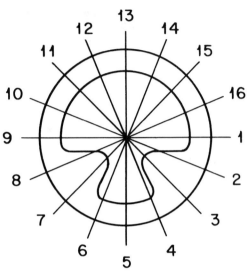

Normals: 25

Fractional Radial Shortening				Fractional Area Contraction			
SEGMENT	MEAN	± SD	RANGE	AREA	MEAN	± SD	RANGE
1	42	9	17–55	1	63	14	24–79
2	41	9	16–55	2	63	13	29–80
3	39	9	23–54	3	60	12	30–78
4	36	8	16–52	4	57	11	30–76
5	36	8	16–52	5	55	13	23–78
6	37	10	10–58	6	59	12	29–79
7	39	11	25–71	7	60	12	34–79
8	39	12	16–67	8	60	13	37–81
9	39	9	24–63	9	59	11	39–76
10	37	9	16–50	10	60	11	40–78
11	37	9	26–58	11	58	10	28–74
12	36	9	23–69	12	56	9	38–71
13	36	10	22–71	13	55	10	31–72
14	37	10	16–51	14	61	11	31–81
15	40	8	20–61	15	63	10	36–83
16	41	8	26–54	16	65	13	31–80

Index

Numerals in *italics* indicate figures; "t" following a page number indicates tabular material.